Mucosal Health in Aquaculture

Mucosal Health in Aquaculture

Edited by

Benjamin H. Beck

Stuttgart National Aquaculture Research Center, Stuttgart, Arkansas, USA

Eric Peatman

School of Fisheries, Aquaculture, and Aquatic Sciences, Auburn University, Alabama, USA

ELSEVIER

AMSTERDAM • BOSTON • HEIDELBERG • LONDON • NEW YORK
OXFORD • PARIS • SAN DIEGO • SAN FRANCISCO • SINGAPORE
SYDNEY • TOKYO

Academic Press is an Imprint of Elsevier

Academic Press is an imprint of Elsevier
125, London Wall, EC2Y 5AS, UK
525 B Street, Suite 1800, San Diego, CA 92101-4495, USA
225 Wyman Street, Waltham, MA 02451, USA
The Boulevard, Langford Lane, Kidlington, Oxford OX5 1GB, UK

British Library Cataloguing-in-Publication Data
A catalogue record for this book is available from the British Library

Library of Congress Cataloging-in-Publication Data
A catalog record for this book is available from the Library of Congress

ISBN: 978-0-12-417186-2

For information on all Academic Press publications visit our website at http://store.elsevier.com/

Typeset by Thomson Digital

Dedication

We dedicate this text to fish that have captivated us since youth.
Slimy and colorful. Resilient and enduring.
Fried, broiled, and blackened.

Contents

List of contributors

Bassem Allam School of Marine and Atmospheric Sciences, Stony Brook University, Stony Brook, New York, USA

María Ángeles Esteban Fish Innate Immune System Group, Department of Cell Biology and Histology, Faculty of Biology, Campus of International Excellence, Campus Mare Nostrum, University of Murcia, Murcia, Spain

Benjamin H. Beck Stuttgart National Aquaculture Research Center, Stuttgart, Arkansas, USA

Christopher Marlowe A. Caipang School of Applied Science, Temasek Polytechnic, Singapore

Rosario Castro Centro de Investigación en Sanidad Animal (CISA-INIA), Valdeolmos, Madrid, Spain

Rebeca Cerezuela Fish Innate Immune System Group, Department of Cell Biology and Histology, Faculty of Biology, Campus of International Excellence, Campus Mare Nostrum, University of Murcia, Murcia, Spain

Emmanuelle Pales Espinosa School of Marine and Atmospheric Sciences, Stony Brook University, Stony Brook, New York, USA

Uwe Fischer Federal Research Institute for Animal Health, Friedrich-Loeffler Institut, Greifswald-Insel Riems, Germany

Matt J. Griffin Thad Cochran National Warmwater Aquaculture Center, Aquatic Research and Diagnostic Laboratory, College of Veterinary Medicine, Mississippi State University, Stoneville, Mississippi, USA

Erling Olaf Koppang Section of Anatomy and Pathology, Faculty of Veterinary Medicine and Biosciences, Norwegian University of Life Sciences, Oslo, Norway

Agnar Kvellestad Section of Anatomy and Pathology, Faculty of Veterinary Medicine and Biosciences, Norwegian University of Life Sciences, Oslo, Norway

Carlo C. Lazado Aquaculture Genomics Research Unit, Faculty of Biosciences and Aquaculture, University of Nordland, Bodø, Norway

Daniel L. Merrifield School of Biological Sciences, Plymouth University, Plymouth, United Kingdom

David Parra Department of Cell Biology, Physiology and Immunology. Universitat Autonoma de Barcelona, Cerdanyola del Valles, Spain

Eric Peatman School of Fisheries, Aquaculture, and Aquatic Sciences, Auburn University, Alabama, USA

Tracy S. Peterson Department of Regulatory Science, University of Arkansas at Pine Bluff, Pine Bluff, Arkansas, USA

Ana Rodiles School of Biological Sciences, Plymouth University, Plymouth, United Kingdom

Irene Salinas Center for Evolutionary and Theoretical Immunology, Department of Biology, University of New Mexico, Albuquerque, New Mexico, USA

Esteban Soto Department of Biomedical Sciences, Ross University School of Veterinary Medicine, West Farms, St. Kitts, West Indies

Kristina S. Sundell Fish Endocrinology Laboratory, Department of Biological and Environmental Sciences, University of Gothenburg, Gothenburg, Sweden

Henrik Sundh Fish Endocrinology Laboratory, Department of Biological and Environmental Sciences, University of Gothenburg, Gothenburg, Sweden

Carolina Tafalla Centro de Investigación en Sanidad Animal (CISA-INIA), Valdeolmos, Madrid, Spain

Jaime A. Tobar Investigación y Desarrollo Biológicos, Laboratorio Centrovet, Santiago, Chile

Jesse Trushenski Center for Fisheries, Aquaculture, and Aquatic Sciences, Southern Illinois University Carbondale, Illinois, USA

Acknowledgments

We would like to thank all the authors for their contributions and their tremendous efforts in shaping this textbook. We also extend our gratitude to Allison Sites, Steve Rawles, and Cindy Ledbetter for reviewing content and providing valuable suggestions.

Why mucosal health?

1

Eric Peatman; Benjamin H. Beck*[†]

[*]School of Fisheries, Aquaculture, and Aquatic Sciences, Auburn University, Alabama, USA

[†]Stuttgart National Aquaculture Research Center, Stuttgart, Arkansas, USA

Chapter Outline

1.1 Why mucosal health?

Aquaculture is the fastest growing sector of agriculture and is expected to maintain its rapid growth in coming decades in the face of rising world populations and declining wildcatch fisheries. Roughly half of all seafood for public consumption is now farmed. An ever-growing number of fish and shellfish species is either being grown commercially or being evaluated for aquaculture potential. The domestication of key species for aquaculture is still in its infancy, however, when compared with more established livestock industries such as poultry or cattle. Market demands for higher volumes of cultured product at lower prices have often come into conflict with the ability of near-wild species to cope with intensive aquaculture environments. Resulting disease outbreaks (whether virus, parasite, or bacteria) inflict significant economic, public perception, and marketing damage to the growing industry. Prioritizing the broad-based health of cultured species is critical in avoiding these boom/bust cycles and establishing the sustainable growth of the aquaculture industry worldwide.

Rather than recapitulating the more familiar textbook and cataloging fish pathogens and their treatments, here we choose to focus on the health and immunity of the cultured organism. *Ultimately, the goal of the aquaculture industry is to optimize environmental parameters, dietary regimens, and host genetics such that disease events are rare. These factors intersect in the mucosal surfaces of cultured aquatic organisms.* The mucosal surfaces (skin, gill, and intestine) constitute the first line of defense against pathogen invasion while simultaneously carrying out a diverse array of other critical physiological processes, including nutrient absorption, osmoregulation, and waste excretion. Aquaculture species depend more heavily on mucosal barriers than their terrestrial agricultural counterparts as they are continuously interacting with the aquatic microbiota. Unlike classical immune centers, such as the spleen and kidney, the accessibility of mucosal surfaces through immersion/dip treatments or dietary changes allows tailored chemical and nutritional strategies to maximize mucosal and, therefore, organismal health. Indeed, many areas of intense research in aquaculture over the last decade have hinged upon a better understanding of mucosal health. Nutritionists are hard at work studying the impacts of antinutritional factors in plant-based fish diets on gut mucosa and how to circumvent them. Feed companies are competing to produce superior immunostimulants, prebiotics, and probiotics that maximize mucosal health and decrease disease prevalence. Microbiologists and immunologists are studying mechanisms of pathogen adherence and entry through mucosal surfaces and designing attenuated mucosal vaccines to stimulate robust mucosal protection. This text cuts across all of these areas in order to capture and bring together our latest understandings of mucosal barriers in aquaculture species and their impacts on nutrition and immunity. Beginning with an in-depth overview of mucosal immunity in fish (Chapter 2, Castro and Tafalla), the book synthesizes our current understanding of the fish structure and function (Chapter 3, Peterson), fish skin (Chapter 4, Esteban and Cerezuela), gill (Chapter 5, Koppang, Kvellestad, and Fischer), and gut/intestinal (Chapter 6, Salinas and Parra) barriers, before looking at the impacts of the environment (Chapter 7, Sundh and Sundell), nutrition (Chapter 8, Trushenski), prebiotics and probiotics (Chapter 9, Caipang and Lazado), and the microbial community (Chapter 10, Merrifield and Rodiles) on these same surfaces. Chapter 11 (Soto, Griffin, and Tobar) considers the progress and potential of new vaccines seeking to protect aquacultured organisms at these barriers. Chapter 12 (Allam and Espinosa) provides a detailed investigation into mucosal health in shellfish.

Studies on immunity in aquacultured species, as a whole, have either been comparative in nature, seeking to catalog the presence or absence of components of immunity expected based on knowledge of mammalian immunology, or oriented around artificial disease challenges, with little or no examination of underlying mechanisms. However, an array of new cellular and molecular tools that has become available over the last several years is rapidly changing this. To close out the book, Chapter 13 (Beck and Peatman) focuses on new, promising approaches to understanding the mucosal interactome, a term used to describe the intricate co-regulation of host immunity, environmental signaling, pathogen dynamics, and the broader microbial community at mucosal surfaces.

The future looks bright for global aquaculture, with a growing middle class and an array of new, more sustainable production models and diets that promise to lower costs and reduce waste output. The key to continued success, however, rests in maintaining the health of cultured organisms season after season. Understanding how culture practices, system specifications, and nutrition can impact mucosal health and enhance or decrease disease prevalence puts control in the hands of producers and brings a needed predictability to a growing industry. It is our hope that this book serves as an important step in that direction.

Overview of fish immunity

2

Rosario Castro; Carolina Tafalla
Centro de Investigación en Sanidad Animal (CISA-INIA), Valdeolmos, Madrid, Spain

Chapter Outline

2.1 Introduction

Fish are a wide and heterogeneous group of vertebrates that comprise about 40,000 species, divided into three classes: Agnatha (jawless fish represented by hagfish and lampreys), Chondrichthyes (cartilaginous fish comprising sharks, rays, and skates), and Osteichthyes (bony fish). Fish heterogeneity is based on many aspects of their biology and habitats. There are fish species adapted to the most diverse aquatic environments with significant differences in morphology, size, physiology, and behavior. These differences evolved in parallel with the fact that fish have undergone a second whole-genome duplication event (2R), following the ancient genome duplication that occurred in early vertebrates (1R), and a further duplication in the teleostean lineage (3R), all of these leading to the subsequent duplication or deletion of various genome parts (Figure 2.1) (Danzmann et al., 2008; Meyer and Van de Peer, 2005; Ravi and Venkatesh, 2008). One of the first consequences of these genomic rearrangements during the evolution of the fish families is that some immune molecular families have expanded tremendously in some fish species, providing important differences with mammals and opening an exciting field to understand the functional effects of this molecular diversification.

In vertebrates, immunity was classically divided into two components: the innate immune response and the adaptive or acquired immune response. Innate immunity is the first line of defense against infection and includes both physical barriers as well as humoral and cellular responses. The adaptive immune response also has humoral and cellular players and is characterized by a specific antigen recognition that drives a stronger and faster secondary pathogen-specific immune response. In light of the discoveries from the past 20 years, an inseparable interrelationship among innate and adaptive components of the immune response has proven more complicated than previously thought, and many of the cells/molecules assigned to either the innate or acquired systems have specific roles in both of them. This is why, in this chapter, we will not make this distinction, but describe each immune cell type or factor indicating their role in either innate or acquired responses.

In a general view, the encounter with a pathogenic organism via mucosal tissues, such as gills, skin, or gut, is primary blocked or limited by physical barriers such as the mucus, the scales, and the epithelium. The mucosal layer interferes with the pathogen not only by trapping it, but also through the action of a variety of antimicrobial factors present in the mucus like lectins, lysozymes, pentraxins, complement proteins, antibacterial peptides, and immunoglobulins, which are destined to directly eliminate the

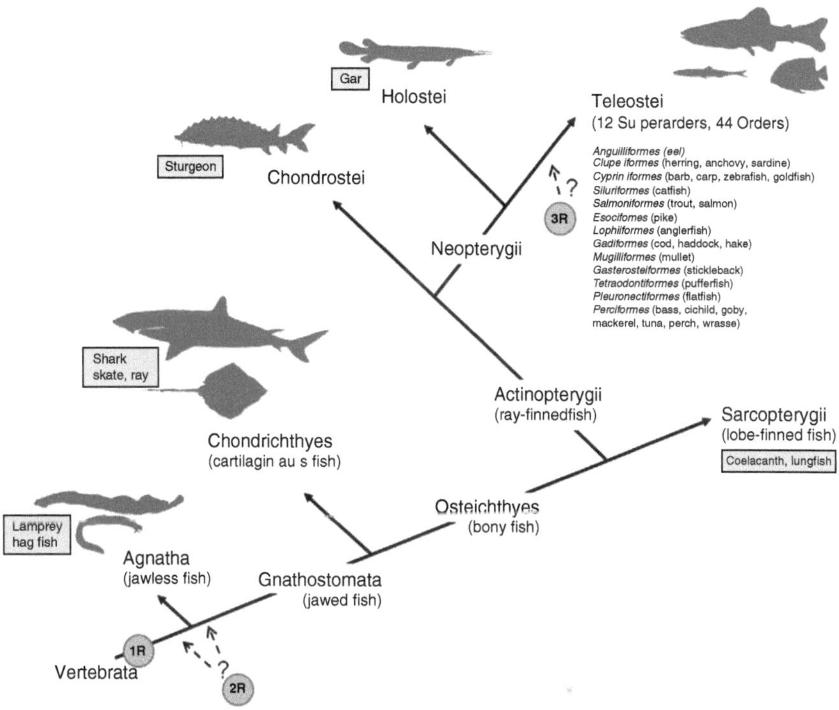

Figure 2.1 Schematic representation of the living-fish phylogeny (Near et al., 2012). Two rounds of whole-genome duplication (WGD) occurred early in the history of vertebrate evolution. WGD event in the ancestral vertebrate lineage duplicated the ancestral possibly cephalochordata-like genome to two (1R), and then to four genomes after a second WGD (2R) before the divergence of fish and tetrapods. Recent findings on lamprey genome sequentiation suggest that this second WGD occurred before the divergence of Agnatha and Gnathostomata (Smith et al., 2013). In the last 10 years evidence has accumulated for a ray-finned- (actinopterygii) specific genome duplication (3R) about 350 million years ago, leading initially to eight copies of the ancestral deuterostome genome. Most duplicated genes were secondarily lost or evolved new functions (Danzmann et al., 2008; Meyer and Van de Peer, 2005; Ravi and Venkatesh, 2008). Whether this third WGD occurred in the whole actinopterygian group or in part of the divergent lineages, in example salmonids and cyprinids, needs further investigation.

infectious agent (Alexander and Ingram, 1992b; Ellis, 2001). If the pathogen succeeds in penetrating the epithelium, it then encounters the complete cellular and humoral machinery of the immune system, triggered first by cell types bearing invariable receptors called pattern recognition receptors, which are able to recognize common conserved molecular characteristics of many microbial agents. Simultaneously, the primary responses of antigen-specific lymphocytes bearing variable receptors that are able to specifically recognize molecules distinctive of a pathogen will also be activated, setting the basis for further secondary responses (Figure 2.2).

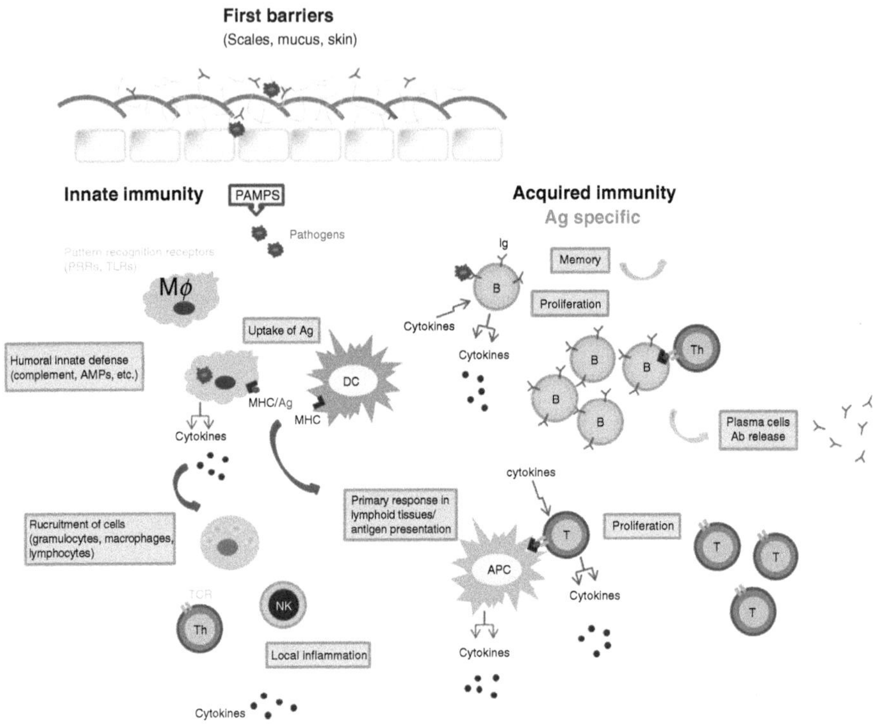

Figure 2.2 General mechanisms of the fish immune response. The encounter with a pathogenic organism via mucosal tissues, such as gills, skin, or gut, is primarily blocked or limited by physical barriers such as the mucus, the scales, and the epithelium. The mucus contains different humoral components with antimicrobial activity such as complement factors, lysozyme or Igs. In case the pathogen succeeds to penetrate the epithelium, it encounters the innate cellular machinery, triggered in a first step by those cell types bearing invariable receptors called pattern recognition receptors (PRRs), able to recognize common conserved molecules (PAMPs) characteristic of many microbial agents. The uptake of the antigen leads, on one hand, to the release of cytokine mediators and attractants for different cell types to unleash the inflammatory process and, on the other hand, to the antigenic presentation through the MHC in the lymphoid tissues for the activation of the primary responses of antigen-specific lymphocytes bearing variable receptors able to specifically recognize molecules distinctive of the pathogen, setting the bases for further secondary responses and memory.

2.2 Organs, tissues, and general structures

In higher vertebrates, the immune system consists of primary (lymphocyte-generating) and secondary (immune response-generating) lymphoid organs. The fetal liver, thymus and bone marrow constitute the primary lymphoid organs, while the spleen, lymph nodes, and mucosal-associated lymphoid tissue (MALT) comprise the secondary lymphoid organs. Fish organization of immune organs is slightly different from higher vertebrates. The main difference is that fish lack bone marrow and lymph nodes and the

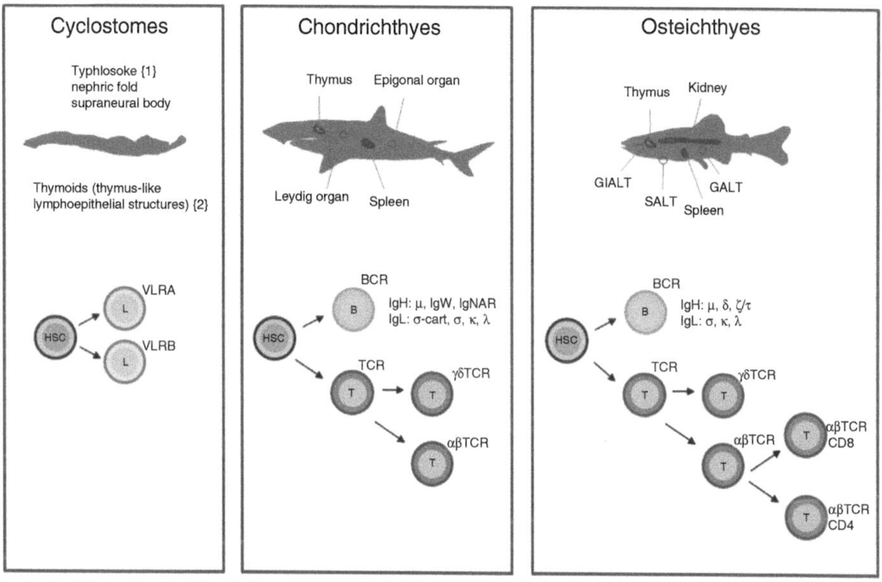

Figure 2.3 Schematic representation of the hematopoietic tissues of the three main fish groups and types of lymphoid cells described for each group. Whether jawless fish have dedicated primary lymphohematopoietic organs is unknown, but several discrete structures have been found in different phases of their development, including the typhlosole (an invagination of the intestinal epithelium), the nephric fold, the supraneural body, and a thymus-like lymphoepithelial structure, termed thymoids, located in the tips of the gill filaments and secondary lamellae of lamprey larvae (Amemiya et al., 2007; Bajoghli et al., 2011). Jawless fish lymphocytes (L), differentiated from hematopoietic stem cells (HSC), bear the variable lymphocyte receptors, in which the basic rearranging element is a leucine-rich repeat cassette, either VLRA or VLRB. Chondrichthyes and Osteichthyes lymphocyte receptor system is based in the presence of variable receptors of the Ig superfamily, either BCR or TCR. The BCR isotypes found in Chondrichthyes are three heavy chains (IgH) and four light chains (IgL), while Osteichthyes have three IgH and three IgL chains. T cells in Chondrichthyes can be $\alpha\beta$ or $\gamma\delta$, and no CD4 or the cytokine system associated to T helper cells has been found to date (Venkatesh et al., 2014). In bony fish, $\alpha\beta$ T cells can differentiate into $CD8^+$ T cytotoxic cells and $CD4^+$ T helper cells.

primary lymphoid organs are the thymus, the head kidney, or pronephros for teleosts, and the Leydig and epigonal organs for chondrichthyes, while secondary lymphoid organs are the spleen, the kidney, and MALT present in peripheral immune tissues (Figure 2.3).

2.2.1 Primary lymphoid organs

2.2.1.1 The thymus

The thymus is the primary organ for functional T lymphocyte development and is present in all jawed vertebrates, but not completely defined in the jawless fish. Cartilaginous fish are the first in evolution to possess a thymus originating from pharyngeal pouches. The structure of the organ is similar to its mammalian counterparts, with a differentiated cortex and medulla and expression of Rag1 (recombination activating gene) and TdT (recombination of terminal deoxyribonucleotidyl transferase) molecules, which are involved in the rearrangement and recombination of B and T cell receptors (Criscitiello et al., 2010; Wyffels et al., 2005; Zapata, 1981). The teleost thymus gland can be uni-, bi-, or trilobed, depending on the species and is situated on the dorsolateral region of the gill chamber. The structure varies from one species to another, but a cortex/medulla architecture is always apparent (Chilmonczyk, 1992; Zapata and Amemiya, 2000). The thymus is comprised of two main populations of cells: the thymic epithelial cells and the lymphoid thymocytes (mainly T cells). Additional cells include the surrounding mesenchymal cells that together with the thymic epithelial cells form an epithelial environmental niche for the support of T cell differentiation. Comparative studies on thymus development performed in mice (*Mus musculus*) and zebrafish (*Danio rerio*) indicate that this process is highly conserved throughout vertebrate evolution and many of the mechanisms and transcription factors involved in this development are common among species (Ma et al., 2013b). The age-related involution process, which characterizes this organ in higher vertebrates, is not as accused in most fish species; however, thymic growth and function may be modulated by crucial factors like aging, sexual maturity, or stress.

2.2.1.2 The kidney

The equivalent to mammalian bone marrow in elasmobranchs is the Leydig organ (nested between the muscular tissue and the mucosa of the esophagus) and the epigonal organ (associated with the gonads). In teleosts, the kidney is the main hematopoietic organ, and, in some species like zebrafish, it is associated with the dorsal aorta to form the "whole-kidney marrow" (Traver et al., 2003). The fish kidney is a complex organ composed of four structurally and functionally distinct systems, including the hematopoietic, reticulo-endothelial, endocrine, and secretory systems. It is commonly located ventrally across the backbone, extending from the base of the cranium along the body axis. The anterior portion of the kidney (defined as anterior kidney, pronephros, or head kidney) is usually bifurcated into two lobes, lacks nephrons, and has no renal function. It houses the main hematopoietic site, and is interdigitated with some adrenal-like endocrine tissue. On the other hand, the posterior kidney possesses a combination of both renal and immune tissue (Grassi Milano et al., 1997; Zapata et al., 1995). B cell development in hematopoietic organs is believed to occur in specialized domains or niches that are spatially separated from environments supporting development of other hematopoietic cell types such as erythroid and myeloid cells. Structurally, the pronephros is supported by a connective tissue capsule and a network of reticular fibers that holds the parenchyma, and is dispersed through an extensive system of sinusoids. Melanomacrophage centers that are formed by totally or partially encapsulated accumulations of pigment-containing macrophages are distributed randomly throughout the lymphohematopoietic tissue. A special organization of B cell maturation within the kidney has been reported in rainbow trout (*Oncorhynchus mykiss*). In this species, the anterior kidney is thought to mostly contain proliferating

B cell precursors and plasma cells, whereas the posterior kidney houses B cells in different states of activation and plasmablast/plasma cells (both antigen-secreting cells, but in different maturation stages). A model for B cell development, differentiation, and distribution was consequently proposed for teleosts. Early B cell development is harbored in the anterior kidney, from where the mature naïve B cells can be distributed via the blood to the spleen and posterior kidney. The activation by an antigen can lead to the plasmablast stage and even further to the more mature plasma cell that can be relocated in a niche of the anterior kidney to become long-lived (Ye et al., 2011a; Zwollo et al., 2008).

2.2.2 Secondary lymphoid organs

2.2.2.1 The spleen

The spleen is a compact, dark red organ located in the peritoneal cavity. Elasmobranchii are compartmentalized into discrete vascularized T cell and B cell zones, although no detectable marginal zone separates red pulp from white pulp (Rumfelt et al., 2002). Teleost spleen structure is similar to the mammalian structure, with blood vessels and differentiated red pulp and white pulp; however, the white pulp is poorly developed. It is surrounded by a fibrous capsule from where small trabeculae extend into the parenchyma. The red pulp occupies the majority of the organ and consists of a reticular cell network that supports blood sinusoids and leukocytes, mainly macrophages and lymphocytes. The white pulp is mainly composed of ellipsoids (terminal capillaries) that have a thin endothelial layer, surrounded by fibrous reticulum and accumulations of macrophages. This part is also rich in melanomacrophage centers. The functions of the spleen are numerous, including blood filtration, erythrocytic destruction, antigen presentation, and antibody production (Zapata, 1982; Zapata et al., 1995).

2.2.2.2 Mucosal-associated lymphoid tissues (MALT)

Fish leukocytes are not only present in immune organs, but have been described in practically all fish tissues, including liver, digestive tract, gills, skin, and gonads (Abos et al., 2013; Ballesteros et al., 2013a; Chaves-Pozo et al., 2003). While in some tissues like liver or gonad there is a spare distribution of leukocytes, more organized structures are found in mucosal tissues such as gut, gills, and skin. Consequently, these structures are usually designated as gut-associated lymphoid tissue (GALT), gill-associated lymphoid tissue (GIALT), and skin-associated lymphoid tissue (SALT). Because the specific composition and functionality of these tissues will be extensively reviewed in successive chapters, we will only name their most important characteristics.

The GALT in fish comprises B and T lymphocytes both in the lamina propria (LP) and as intraepithelial lymphocytes (IEL); however, a singular characteristic of the fish GALT is the absence of organized structures like Peyer's patches and mesenteric lymph nodes present in mammals (Rombout et al., 2011). Although many studies have characterized different aspects of the immune response of the teleost gut in response to diverse pathogens or stimuli (reviewed in Rombout et al., 2011), most studies have focused on the posterior segments exclusively. Recently, it has been revealed that other segments of the digestive tract have numerous leukocyte populations that effectively respond to infection or oral vaccination. For example, in rainbow trout, both B and T lymphocytes are recruited to the pyloric caeca region in response to local viral stimuli (Ballesteros et al., 2013a, 2013b).

Regarding GIALT, fish have been long known to possess all types of leukocytes dispersed within the gill lamellae. In addition, a novel immune structure was recently described in salmonids in association to gills. This structure, designated as interbranchial lymphoid tissue (ILT), is mainly composed of T cells embedded in a meshwork of epithelial cells (Haugarvoll et al., 2008; Koppang et al., 2010). The morphological differences between the thymus and the ILT suggest different roles in the salmonid immune system. Furthermore, the absence of Rag transcription in gills appears to indicate that this tissue would function as a secondary immune organ, even though its specific role in defense has not been elucidated (Koppang et al., 2010).

Due to its lack of keratinization, teleost skin has living epithelial cells in direct contact with the water. Consequently, mucous secretions are produced by different types of epithelial cells, those located in the superficial layer in particular. Furthermore, specific unicellular glands in the skin of gnathostome fish are the goblet cells, the sacciform cells, and the club cells (Zaccone et al., 2001). Additionally, the skin epidermis contains multiple B and T cells that have shown to respond to pathogens in different species (Findly et al., 2013; Jorgensen et al., 2009; Xu et al., 2013).

2.3 Cellular components

The different leukocyte types derived from the lymphoid and myeloid lineages known from mammals have also been recognized in fish, including cells morphologically and functionally equivalent to mammalian B and T lymphocytes, natural killer (NK) cells, monocytes, macrophages, neutrophils, eosinophils, mast cells, and thrombocytes (Secombes, 1996; Whyte, 2007), as well as the recent description of dendritic-like cells in some species (Bassity and Clark, 2012; Lugo-Villarino et al., 2010).

2.3.1 Lymphocytes

The term "lymphocyte" refers to the three types of white blood cells present in mammalian blood, namely B and T lymphocytes and natural killer (NK) cells. The term was prompted because they are the main cellular components of mammalian lymph. In mammals, B and T lymphocytes mediate the specific responses of the adaptive immunity in jawed vertebrates. Both types of lymphocytes share the unique characteristic process of somatic DNA rearrangement of their antigen-specific receptors (members of the Ig superfamily) by the random combination of the variable gene segments present in the receptor locus. B cells express their antigen receptors on their cell surface as B cell receptors (BCR) and secrete them as immunoglobulin (Ig) or antibody, whereas T cell receptors (TCR) are always cell-surface bound. In both cases, one of each multiple variable (V), diversity (D), and joining (J) gene segments are randomly combined together with the constant gene segments (C) that define the type of receptor to form a mature functional VDJC antigen receptor (see Section 2.5.5). This process produces a vast repertoire of B or T cells bearing structurally diverse antigen receptors for specific pathogen recognition. Thus, each lymphocyte carries a unique Ig domain-containing receptor and can originate a clone of cells upon induction that will react specifically with only one antigen. Jawless fish have a lymphoid cellular adaptive immune system based on the rearrangement of a variable lymphocyte receptor (VLR) encoded by genes of a leucine-rich repeat family of proteins not related with the Ig superfamily (Pancer et al., 2004) that does not distinguish between B-like and T-like cells. On the other hand, in Chondrichthyes and Osteichthyes, the lymphocyte receptor system is based on the presence of variable receptors of the Ig superfamily, either BCR or TCR, and, therefore, B-like and T-like cells are present in these species, even though functional differences to their mammalian equivalents have begun to be elucidated. The classical B cell function is the production of antibodies (or Igs) to specifically neutralize pathogens and label them to be removed by the immune system. T cells act mainly as coordinators of the responses of other immune cells and as effector cells to directly kill infected or tagged cells. Hematopoietic stem cells give rise to lymphocyte progenitors that diverge to develop into the T, B, or NK cell subsets.

2.3.1.1 B cells

In cartilaginous fish, three different Ig isotypes have been found, namely IgM, IgW, and IgNAR (Dooley and Flajnik, 2006). Chondrichthyan IgM is homologous to the IgM found in all vertebrates, while IgW has been suggested to be closely related to IgD based on phylogenetic analyses. IgNAR is a shark-specific Ig composed of heavy chains only, with no light chain association. Two different subsets of B cells have been described in sharks, expressing either IgM only or IgNAR only. There is no information available at present on IgW-expressing B cells (Flajnik, 2002; Flajnik and Kasahara, 2010; Ohta and Flajnik, 2006).

In teleosts, three different Igs have been reported, namely IgM, IgD, and IgT, the last designated as IgZ in zebrafish (Warr et al., 1979; Wilson et al., 1997; Hansen et al., 2005; Danilova et al., 2005). While IgM and IgD seem to be essential Igs present in all teleost species, IgZ/T are only present in some of them (Fillatreau et al., 2013). Based on the expression of membrane Igs, three B cell subsets were identified in rainbow trout to date: $IgM^{+}/IgD^{+}/IgT^{-}$ (IgM^{+} cells), $IgM^{-}/IgD^{-}/IgT^{+}$ (IgT^{+} cells), and the recently discovered $IgM^{-}/IgD^{+}/IgT^{-}$ (IgD^{+} cells) (Castro et al., 2014a; Hansen et al., 2005; Zhang et al., 2010). In catfish (*Ictalurus punctatus*), which lack IgT, three subpopulations have been described: IgM^{+}/IgD^{+}, IgM^{+}/IgD^{-}, and IgM^{-}/IgD^{+} (Edholm et al., 2010). In mammals, IgM^{+}/IgD^{+}, which make up the majority of peripheral B cells, down-regulate their IgD expression upon antigen binding; whether this occurs in fish and if IgM^{+}/IgD^{-} cells are present in all fish species is still unknown. Concerning the $IgM^{-}/IgD^{+}/IgT^{-}$ population recently identified in trout, these cells are mainly present in the gills, and, although they still have an unknown function, they are regulated upon viral infection (Castro et al., 2014a). Also in catfish, the role in defense of the IgD^{+}/IgM^{-} described in peripheral blood leukocytes (PBLs) is still unknown (Edholm et al., 2010). In mammals, two types of IgD^{+}/IgM^{-} cells have been described. An IgD^+/IgM^- population present mainly in the upper aerodigestive mucosa arises in humans after active IgM-to-IgD class switch. These plasmablast-like cells that retain IgD in the membrane secrete highly mutated mono- and polyreactive IgD, providing a layer of mucosal protection by interacting with pathogens and are either retained locally or are circulated in the blood, where they can account for up to 0.5–1% of circulating B cells (Chen and Cerutti, 2010; Chen et al., 2009). The second type of IgD^+/IgM^- cells comprise up to 2.5% of circulating B cells in humans. These naïve B cells have antibody variable region genes in an unmutated configuration and are fully mature cells that are autoreactive and functionally attenuated and, therefore, have been cataloged as a new type of anergic (low reactive, tolerance-mediating) B cells (Duty et al., 2009).

In any case, four different subsets of B cells seem to be present in teleosts; three subsets with single surface expression of IgM, IgD, or IgT; and a subset co-expressing surface IgM and IgD. Teleost B cells bearing different membrane Igs correspond to different cell linages because, in fish, there is no Ig isotype switching as in mammals (from IgM to more specific Igs). Concerning fish B cell ontogeny to date, most studies have been directed to studying the presence of IgM-bearing and IgM-secreting cells, and very little is known about the ontogeny or the tissue distribution and population dynamics of IgD and IgT/IgZ populations. Through the study of IgM kinetics, three models of early hematopoiesis have been described in fish: in angelfish, hematopoiesis starts in the yolk sac blood islands; in zebrafish, early hematopoiesis is observed in the intraembryonic intermediate cell mass (ICM); while in trout, hematopoiesis is thought to initiate in the yolk sac for a short time before continuing in the ICM. Hematopoietic activity appears as early as 4 days post-fertilization, giving rise to erythroblasts and myeloid cells (Fillatreau et al., 2013; Salinas et al., 2011; Zapata et al., 2006). After fertilization, B cell lymphopoiesis occurs mainly in the kidney, and detectable membrane IgM-expressing cells appear around three weeks post-fertilization (Razquin et al., 1990). Evidence for B cell development, homing, and maturation in teleost kidney is supported by the expression of conserved molecular markers and transcription factors such as Rag1 and Rag2 genes, TdT, Ikaros, EBF1, Pax5, Blimp1, or $HC\mu$, among others (Hansen, 1997; Hansen et al., 1997; Zwollo et al., 2010). In adult fish, B cells can be found in the anterior and posterior kidney, spleen, liver, MALT tissues, and blood (Abos et al., 2013; Salinas et al., 2011).

The major functions of B cells are antibody production and antigen presentation and, in the case of teleosts, also include active phagocytic and microbicidal capacities (see Section 2.5.2) (Salinas et al., 2011). Once a B cell is activated by an antigen, part of its progeny becomes antibody-secreted cells (ASC), whereas some other cells become mid- or long-term memory cells. The presence and characteristics of these B cell stages have been studied in a few teleost species such as rainbow trout. Different ASC populations have been defined in this species at the cellular and molecular level, including plasmablasts (replicating, low antibody secretors, bearing minimal BCR) and plasma cells (nonreplicating, terminally differentiated, high antibody secretors, bearing no BCR), further divided in short-lived plasma cells and long-lived plasma cells (Bromage et al., 2004; Zwollo et al., 2008, 2010). The B cell development and maturation model proposed for teleost species resembles the one observed in mammalian bone marrow (see Section 2.2.1.2). On the other hand, even though affinity maturation takes place in teleosts, it is modest compared to that of mammals (Kaattari et al., 2002; Malecek et al., 2008; Yang et al., 2006; Ye et al., 2011b). Affinity maturation is the process that allows B cells to produce antibodies with increased affinity for a specific antigen during the course of an immune response. It takes place through a double action: somatic hypermutation in the Ig genes that leads to antibodies with different binding specificities and binding affinities and the consequent clonal selection by which only the B cell progeny with the highest affinities for antigens will be selected to survive.

In those species that express IgT, such as rainbow trout, both IgM^+ and IgT^+ B cells are present in mucosal tissues; however, some infection models have revealed that IgT plays an important role at the mucosal level. Despite these results, IgM also seems to react to some pathogens/antigens at a mucosal level, and recent studies have observed non-mucosal IgT responses to viral infections (Castro et al., 2013) or DNA vaccination (Castro et al., 2014b). Therefore, the exact contribution of IgT to pathogen clearance in both mucosal and systemic infections remains to be further clarified. In any case, IgT^+ cells constitute 16–28% of all trout B cells in the blood, spleen, head kidney, and peritoneal cavity, while they represent the main B cell population (54.3% of all B cells) in the gut (Zhang et al., 2010). Moreover, upon infection with an intestinal parasite, IgT responses were predominant in the gut, while IgM responses were confined to the serum (Zhang et al., 2010). On the other hand, IgM is also modulated in different segments of the digestive tract in response to antigens (Ballesteros et al., 2013a, 2013b). Concerning the skin, again, IgT seems to be the predominant Ig isotype involved in its responsiveness to waterborne pathogens (Xu et al., 2013). However, in the gills, both IgT and IgM were discovered bound to surface structures of *Ichthyophthirius multifiliis* in the gills of infected rainbow trout shortly after invasion (von Gersdorff Jorgensen et al., 2011).

2.3.1.2 T cells

T cells are characterized by the presence of a T cell receptor (TCR) by which they recognize antigens. Unlike B lymphocytes, T lymphocytes fail to recognize antigens in the absence of antigen presentation, with the exception of superantigens (antigens that produce a nonspecific polyclonal T cell activation with a massive cytokine release) because the T cell receptor is restricted to recognizing antigens only when exposed in the context of an isogenic major histocompatibility complex (MHC), either class I or II, present on the cell surface (see Section 2.5.3). A first classification of T cells can be based on the TCR chains they express, either αβ or γδ. αβ-T cells can be cataloged as conventional T cells, whereas γδ-T cells recognize unprocessed antigens in a manner similar to that of pattern recognition receptors. Consequently, in mammals, γδ-T cells are more innate-like immune cells with less dependence on MHC presentation and are mostly present in epithelial and mucosal tissues, representing around 2% of the total T cell population (Bonneville et al., 2010). On the other hand, conventional αβ-T cells can be divided into T cytotoxic (Tc) or T helper (Th) cells, distinguished by the expression of the membrane-bound glycoproteins,

CD8 or CD4, respectively. These molecules act as co-receptors for the TCR, stabilizing the interaction with the MHC and enhancing TCR activation through the CD3 tyrosine phosphorylation pathway. Tc cells, expressing CD8 on the cell surface, are able to kill infected or cancerous cells after recognizing non-self or cancer-associated antigens in the context of MHC class I (Strasser et al., 2009). Th cells, on the other hand, express CD4 and produce cytokines to regulate the action of other immune cells, mainly B cells. They can be further classified in mammals according to the expression of specific transcription factors and the secretion of representative combinations of cytokines. Although there is still some controversy as to whether these Th subsets constitute differential cell lines or cells in a different stage of activation with a certain degree of plasticity (Kleinewietfeld and Hafler, 2013), well-defined subsets in mammals include Th1, Th2, Th17, and T reg. Upon stimulation, Th1 cells secrete effector cytokines, such as interferon γ (IFN-γ) and tumor necrosis factor α (TNF-α), to control intracellular infections and interleukin 2 (IL-2) to induce lymphocyte proliferation. Th2 cells produce IL-4, IL-5, and IL-13 that stimulate B cells and control extracellular infections through the secretion of antibodies. Th17 cells produce IL-17 together with IL-21 and IL-22. These cells appear to be implicated in the control of extracellular bacterial infections, although their precise role is still debated. Finally, the Th22 subset was recently discovered and secretes IL-22, but not IL-17. In mammals, Th22 cells are involved in epidermal repair.

Concerning fish, genomic studies performed in different species have identified most of the components associated with T cell function, making it possible to speculate that fish have all the different T cell subsets (Laing and Hansen, 2011); however, whether the functionalities are maintained is something that needs to be further investigated. All four TCR chains have been identified in different species of teleosts and elasmobranchs (Criscitiello et al., 2006; Flajnik and Kasahara, 2010; Nam et al., 2003), but it is still not known if $\gamma\delta$-T cells exert roles similar to the equivalent mammalian subsets. Mature Tc cells express a heterodimer of CD8 formed by α and β chains (Laing and Hansen, 2011). Different CD8 (both α and β chains) have been sequenced in multiple teleost species (Buonocore et al., 2006; Hansen and Strassburger, 2000; Moore et al., 2005; Patel et al., 2008; Pinto et al., 2006; Somamoto et al., 2006; Suetake et al., 2007; Sun et al., 2007). Furthermore, the combination of specific anti-CD8α antibodies, clonal fish, and MHC class I matching cell lines has permitted the verification that CD8$^+$ Tc cells in fish also kill virus-infected cells when the TCR matches the MHC in which the antigenic peptide is exposed (Fischer et al., 2006). CD4 orthologs have also been identified in different teleost species (Buonocore et al., 2008; Edholm et al., 2007; Laing et al., 2006; Moore et al., 2009; Patel et al., 2009; Sun et al., 2007; Wen et al., 2011); however, there is no data available to date on the functionality of CD4 cells in fish due to the lack of specific antibodies against this molecule. In some species, the presence of an additional CD4 gene has been reported (CD4L or CD 4REL) that could correspond to an ancient CD4 molecule with a different role still not elucidated (Dijkstra et al., 2006; Laing et al., 2006). Finally, most of the cytokine representatives of the various Th populations described in mammals have been identified in teleosts (reviewed in Laing and Hansen, 2011), but again, whether they are being produced by specific Th subsets remains unknown.

T cells in fish have been reported in the thymus, spleen, head kidney, and mucosal tissues such as gills, skin, and gut (reviewed in Laing and Hansen, 2011). They have been detected either through the use of specific CD8 antibodies or in some cases through the use of pan-T antibodies. However, most of these pan-T antibodies were developed against non-IgM expressing lymphocytes and the specific targets they are recognizing are not known (Rombout et al., 1998; Scapigliati et al., 2000). Given the fact that we now know that B cell populations with no IgM on the cell surface are also present in fish, the specific target for these antibodies should be further characterized, despite the fact that some studies performed with some of these antibodies have rendered interesting data on T cell functionality (Abelli et al., 1999; Romano et al., 2011; Scapigliati et al., 2000). On the other hand, some approaches focused on specific molecules have been more successful such as the development of antibodies against CD3, which is present in all T cell subpopulations. Through the use of a polyclonal antibody against the intracellular region of salmonid CD3 epsilon, high numbers of $CD3^+$ cells were identified in the thymus, gills, and intestine, whereas lower numbers were detected in the head kidney, spleen, and peripheral blood leukocytes (Koppang et al., 2010). Surprisingly, the use of another anti-rainbow trout CD3 antibody, in this case a monoclonal, revealed high rations of $CD3^+$ cells in thymus, skin, and posterior kidney and lower rations in head kidney, spleen, gills, and peripheral blood leukocytes (Boardman et al., 2012).

2.3.1.3 Natural killer cells (and natural cytotoxic cells)

Cell-mediated cytotoxicity is a process by which the immune system senses and kills altered, tumor, virus-infected, or foreign cells to maintain homeostasis. Natural killer (NK) cells constitute the first line of defense to carry out such processes as part of the innate immune system. NK cells are effector cells of lymphoid origin characterized by unique surface markers ($CD3^-CD56^+CD16^+$) and the absence of recombined TCR or Ig genes (Vivier et al., 2008). These cells possess cytotoxic granules and their killing activity is similar to the cytotoxic T lymphocytes, except that they utilize innate nonspecific receptors to recognize antigens (Lieberman, 2003). NK cells recognize MHC class I in the surface of the target cells through the action of three different types of receptors: killer cell immunoglobulin-like receptors (KIRs), leukocyte immunoglobulin-like receptors (LIRs), and receptors of the C-lectin-like family. Depending on the receptors involved, receptor binding can lead to activation or inhibitory signals on the cell. Stimulation of the activating receptors, which associate with proteins having an intracellular ITAM motif (CD3ζ, DAP12, or DAP10), results in killing of target cells. Inhibitory signaling receptors all possess cytoplasmic ITIMs (Yoder and Litman, 2011). For example, interaction of NK cells with normal levels of self MHC-I on a cell produces an inhibitory signal, whereas a decrease in MHC-I levels on a cell as a consequence of a tumoral process or viral infection triggers an activation signal that results in killing of the cell by the NK. This mechanism is often called the "missing self." On the other hand, cells infected with an intracellular pathogen display not only a unique repertoire of pathogen-derived peptides in the context of MHC-I (recognized by the TCR on Tc cells), but also peptides that can disrupt the normal assembly of MHC-I, which are then detected by NK cells.

Two types of NK cell homologs have been described in fish, mainly based on channel catfish studies: nonspecific cytotoxic cells (NCCs) and NK-like cells. NCCs have been observed in several species, such as catfish, tilapia and damselfish, and are characterized by their ability to spontaneously kill allogeneic targets and protozoan parasites, but not autologous targets. These cells are small, agranular, and positive for the 5C6 antibody (developed against catfish NCCs). They bear a vimentin-like surface molecule and express a type III membrane protein designated as NCC receptor protein 1 (NCCRP-1) (Evans et al., 1990; Jaso-Friedmann et al., 2001; McKinney and Schmale, 1997; Yoder, 2004). NK-like cells where inferred by the observations made on catfish from long-term alloantigen-stimulated mixed leukocyte cultures initiated with naïve PBLs. The predominant cytotoxic cells in such a culture are large, granular cells that do not express TCR messengers, are negative for both neutrophil and macrophage markers and for reactivity with the 5C6 antibody, and are capable of killing virus-infected autologous cells (Nakanishi et al., 2011; Shen et al., 2003, 2004). Other molecules involved in mammalian NK functions have been described in these and other fish species at the gene level, including the NK cell-enhancing factor (NKEF), immunoglobulin-like receptors, novel immune-type receptors (NITR), novel immunoglobulin-like transcripts (NILT), leukocyte immune-type receptors (LITRs), adaptor molecules like DNAX-activating proteins (DAP), perforins, NK-lysins, granulysin, granzymes, and FasL (reviewed in Fischer et al., 2013; Nakanishi et al., 2011; Yoder and Litman, 2011). Apart from these functional studies in these specific fish species, the contribution of NK cells in the context of an *in vivo* infection has never been evaluated.

2.3.2 Cells of the monocyte–macrophage lineage

2.3.2.1 Monocytes and macrophages

Macrophages (and their precursors, monocytes) are the main phagocytic cells of the immune system. Tissue macrophages are present throughout the body and contribute to tissue homeostasis and immune surveillance. Upon tissue damage or infection, monocytes are rapidly recruited to the tissue where they differentiate into tissue macrophages that can take up antigens and produce cytokines that modulate the action of other recruited cell types. Macrophages are remarkably plastic and can change their functional phenotype depending on the environmental cues they receive. Based on these signals, activated macrophages were traditionally divided into classically activated macrophages induced in a Th1 cytokine environment and alternatively activated macrophages induced in a Th2 cytokine environment; however, recent classifications have introduced novel subtypes. Forlenza et al. (2011) based on the current knowledge on macrophage activation mechanisms in fish, adopted a model with four different phenotypes for activated macrophages.

Innate activated macrophages are induced by pathogens (or a microbial stimulus such as pathogen-associated molecular patterns) alone. The pathogens are recognized through toll-like receptors (TLRs) in macrophages and are phagocytosed. In fish, most of our knowledge regarding innate activation of macrophages comes from stimulating these cells with antigenic molecules like bacterial lipopolysaccharide (LPS), although some studies have also been reported using peptidoglycan, Poly I:C (double stranded RNA), flagellin, or lipoteichoic acid (reviewed in Forlenza et al., 2011). The effects that these molecules provoke in fish macrophages vary between fish species, but generally lead to the production of oxygen and nitrogen radicals, increased phagocytosis, and production of pro-inflammatory cytokines. It is surprising, however, that fish are much less susceptible to LPS stimulation and septic shock than mammals, and this suggests important differences in the way that LPS is sensed in this group of animals that have to survive aquatic environments with a much higher microbial load. For example, toll-like receptor 4 (TLR4), responsible for LPS recognition in mammals (see Section 2.5.1), is thought to be absent in salmonids (Rebl et al., 2010), whereas it has been demonstrated that TLR4 does not recognize LPS in some other species such as zebrafish (Sepulcre et al., 2009).

Classically activated macrophages are induced by a combination of IFN-γ and a microbial stimulus. IFN-γ has been identified in many different teleost species, whereas, in some species, such as zebrafish, catfish, common carp (*Cyprinus carpio*), and goldfish, two types of IFN-γ containing all the conserved IFN-γ signature motifs have been identified (see Section 2.4.1.2). In trout macrophages, recombinant IFN-γ has been shown to induce the transcription of IFN-γ-inducible protein 10 (γIP-10), MHC class IIα chain, and antiviral genes as well as enhanced respiratory burst activity (Zou et al., 2005). In goldfish, recombinant IFN-γ increased the expression of several pro-inflammatory genes and the phagocytic and nitric oxide response of macrophages (Grayfer and Belosevic, 2009). In carp, however, IFN-γ alone produced no effect, whereas in combination with LPS induced a strong synergistic effect on nitric oxide (NO) production, respiratory burst activity, and expression of pro-inflammatory cytokines. In those species that contain a second IFN-γ, important differences on their effects on macrophages have been detected between the two proteins, demonstrating that although both genes produce functionally active molecules with effects on macrophages, their role in immunity is not exactly the same (Forlenza et al., 2011).

Alternatively activated macrophages are differentiated in the presence of the Th2 cytokines IL-4 and/or IL-13 (Forlenza et al., 2011). In mammals, alternatively activated macrophages metabolize L-arginine differently from innate/classically activated macrophages (Modolell et al., 1995). Innate/classically activated macrophages convert L-arginine into L-citrulline and NO, whereas alternatively activated macrophages convert L-arginine into L-ornithine and urea through the activation of arginase, rendering L-arginine unavailable for conversion by iNOS (inducible NO synthase) into NO and, therefore, attenuating the production of NO and acting as an "anti-inflammatory" macrophage (Modolell et al., 1995). Although genes with homology to both IL-4 and IL-13 have been reported in some species (Li et al., 2007; Ohtani et al., 2008), no functional studies have yet been performed with these molecules. Thus, there is no evidence that this activation path is conserved in teleost fish.

Finally, regulatory macrophages are associated with the presence of the regulatory cytokine IL-10 and are, therefore, involved in the down-regulation of inflammation. They can be generated in response to a combination of TLR ligands and second signals such as immune complexes, prostaglandins, apoptotic cells, glucocorticoids, or G-protein-coupled receptor ligands (Mantovani et al., 2004). Again, even though IL-10 is present in different teleost species (Inoue et al., 2005; Lutfalla et al., 2003; Pinto et al., 2007; Savan et al., 2003; Seppola et al., 2008; Zhang et al., 2005; Zou et al., 2003a), there is no evidence that this macrophage activation pathway functions in a similar fashion to that of mammalian macrophages.

2.3.2.2 Melanomacrophages

The functions described for melanomacrophage centers present in immune organs, such as the kidney or the spleen, are numerous, including the possibility of being active phagocytic centers for heterogeneous materials such as cell debris, melanin pigments, hemosiderin granules, and lipofuscin residues as well as diverse lipids, protein aggregates, and mucopolysaccharides, acting as metabolic scavengers. They are also responsible for iron storage, deposition of resistant phases of pathogens, such as bacterial and parasitic spores, and seem to play an active role in antigen processing and presentation. Consequently, they have been proposed as a primitive analog of the germinal centers of mammalian lymph nodes (Agius and Roberts, 2003; Zapata and Amemiya, 2000). Additionally, the fact that melanin is produced *de novo* through enzymes belonging to the tyrosinase gene family at the sites of injury or infection in a wide range of species has led authors to speculate that melanin, and/or its quinone precursors, could have antimicrobial properties, as in mammals (Mackintosh, 2001). Although this has to be further explored in fish, the expression of the tyrosinase gene family that occurs in melanomacrophages during chronic inflammation of Atlantic salmon (*Salmo salar*) (Larsen et al., 2012) and the fact that melanin synthesis is induced in viral disease in this same species (Fagerland et al., 2013) suggests a similar role.

2.3.3 Polymorphonuclear leukocytes

Polymorphonuclear leukocytes (PMNs) are cells of myeloid origin with a distinctive structure based on the polymorphic shape of their nucleus and on the numerous granules present in the cytoplasm. The nomenclature used in mammals for the classification of granulocytes, according to their affinities for acidic or basic dyes, does not always correlate with the characteristics and functions of fish granulocytes; furthermore, the different morphological types of granulocytes are not always present in each fish species. Neutrophils are the predominant type of granulocytes found in most fish species, but some teleost have been reported to have both acidophilic and/or basophilic granulocytes, in addition to neutrophils (Rowley, 1996).

2.3.3.1 Neutrophils

Neutrophils are one of the first recruited cells at inflammation sites and are known to possess a pivotal antimicrobial activity through their strong phagocytic capacity and, at an extracellular level, by the degranulation of their cytoplasmic granules containing a vast array of soluble mediators, including enzymes, antimicrobial peptides, and potent redox molecules, or by the release of the recently discovered neutrophil extracellular traps (NETs) (Henry et al., 2013; Pijanowski et al., 2013). Besides, they provide signals for the activation and maturation of other immune cells. Neutrophils (also called heterophils in some species) are present in almost all fish species studied and are critical components of the innate immune defenses. In fish, these cells possess typical neutrophil capacities such as phagocytosis or degranulation. Their antimicrobial mechanisms also include a strong intracellular (inside the phagosome) and extracellular production of reactive oxygen intermediates (a mechanism called respiratory burst) and nitric oxide metabolites that directly interfere with pathogen survival as well as NET release. Histochemically, neutrophils show strong myeloperoxidase activity, both in elasmobranchs and teleosts (Lieschke et al., 2001). Recently, thanks to the generation of transgenic zebrafish with neutrophils specifically labeled with fluorescent proteins, many advances have been made to understand neutrophil functionality in fish, including the identification of a tissue gradient of hydrogen peroxide for neutrophil recruitment following tissue injury and direct evidence for reverse migration as a mechanism of inflammation resolution (Henry et al., 2013).

2.3.3.2 Eosinophils and basophils

Eosinophils are PMN leukocytes that retain acid dyes such as eosin. In mammals, these cells are primarily involved in the destruction of internal parasites and in the modulation of allergic inflammatory reactions. Eosinophils have been described in several fish species, including cyprinids. Zebrafish eosinophils have been isolated using a transgene of Gata-2, a transcription factor required for differentiation and maintenance of murine eosinophils, in combination with their light/scatter characteristics (Balla et al., 2010). These zebrafish eosinophils degranulate *in vitro* in response to an extract of *Heligmosomoides polygyrus* or *in vivo* in response to either the same extracts or a live infection with *Pseudocapillaria tomentosa*; the latter suggests a common response to helminthic infections in all vertebrate eosinophils. In gilthead sea bream (*Sparus aurata*), cells with the tinctorial properties of eosinophils designated as acidophilic granulocytes show high MHC class II gene expression and phagocytic capacities, suggesting a role for these cells in antigen presentation (Cuesta et al., 2006).

The basophils of vertebrates are uncommon granular leukocytes, containing characteristic large basophilic metachromatic granules. Basophils are rarely described in fish, and most of the characterizations are based on their morphology and ultrastructural characteristics (Ellis, 1977).

2.3.3.3 Mast cells/eosinophilic granule cells

Cells with structural and functional properties resembling those of mammalian mast cells (MCs) have been described in the digestive tract, gills, and other tissues of most teleosts. These cells present a characteristic basic staining of the cytoplasmic granules with alcoholic thionin and toluidine blue, or Alcian blue. After water fixation, the granules present eosinophilic characteristics and, for this reason, these cells have been denominated "eosinophilic granule cells" (EGCs) in some studies (Reite and Evensen, 2006). The granules contain phospholipids and acidic mucopolysaccharides and present acid and alkaline phosphatase, arylsulfatase, and 5N-nucleotidase activities. Several studies made in teleosts suggest that, as in mammals, mast cell precursors leave the hematopoietic system and enter the tissues via blood circulation in order to undergo the maturation process (Bergeron and Woodward, 1983). The acute responses of MCs/EGCs observed in fish after intraperitoneal or intestinal administration of bacteria or after natural infection consists of a typical degranulation, followed by an inflammatory reaction and vasodilatation (Dezfuli and Giari, 2008; Reite and Evensen, 2006). The recruitment and accumulation of MCs/EGCs observed in different species after parasitic infections or dermal lesions indicates that this recruitment is a general response in persistent inflammatory reactions in teleosts.

2.3.3.4 Rodlet cells

In teleost, the rodlet cells are secretory cells located in the endothelium of the cardiovascular system, the intestinal epithelia, and other epithelia of many fish species that release their products at epithelial, mesothelial, or endothelial surfaces. These cells have a characteristic structure with cytoplasmic inclusions that possess a crystalline inner core. The recruitment and accumulation of rodlet cells in tissues has been correlated with the presence of different parasites, including cestodes, trematodes, encysted larvae of helminths, myxosporodian, or copepods, usually parallel to the accumulation of MCs/EGCs (Bielek, 2002; Reite and Evensen, 2006; Yokoya and Ebina, 1981). Additionally, rodlet cells seem to respond to the presence of parasites on epithelial surfaces by degranulation, secreting substances that dampen the infections and contribute to the elimination of parasites (Leino, 1996; Manera and Dezfulli, 2004).

2.3.4 Dendritic cells

Dendritic cells (DCs) in mammals constitute the most important antigen-presenting cell with the broadest range of antigen presentation capacities. Although the presence of a well-defined DC population has not been reported in fish, some recent studies point to subpopulations of leukocytes with characteristics or functions similar to those of DCs. Fish cells positive to human antibodies characteristic of DCs or with DC-like morphology have been reported in salmonids (Haugland et al., 2012; Lovy et al., 2006, 2009). In zebrafish, a cell population with high affinity for the lectin peanut agglutinin (PNA) and the classical morphological features of mammalian DCs has been described and is capable of phagocytizing bacteria and activating T lymphocytes in an antigen-dependent manner (Lugo-Villarino et al., 2010). In rainbow trout, a protocol for the enrichment of head kidney and spleen cultures for DCs was adapted from mammals (Bassity and Clark, 2012). These cells were phagocytic, exhibited a DC-like morphology and were activated by TLR ligands. However, due to the fact that B lymphocytes and phagocytes can also be considered professional antigen-presenting cells capable of phagocytizing antigens and displaying them in the context of MHC class II and having evidence that, in fish, some of these mammalian DC-signature markers do not seem exclusive of DCs (Johansson et al., 2012), the real nature of these cell populations remains unclear until specific fish markers are developed for their in-depth study.

2.3.5 Thrombocytes

Thrombocytes are the equivalent of mammalian platelets and are involved in blood clotting. On the contrary to mammalian platelets, teleost thrombocytes have a nucleus and thus some additional functions have been described for them. Thrombocytes from carp (Stosik et al., 2002), rainbow trout (Hill and Rowley, 1998), and sea bass (*Dicentrarchus labrax)* (Meseguer et al., 1992) showed phagocytic capacity and thus a possible role in antigen presentation has been speculated for them (Kollner et al., 2004). Furthermore, trout thrombocytes express components of the MHC class I pathway, IL-1β, TNF-α, transforming growth factor β (TGF-β), the IL receptor common γ chain, as well as CXC and CC chemokines; however, their exact role in immunity has still not been clearly elucidated (Kollner et al., 2004).

2.4 Soluble mediators of immunity

An important array of regulatory mediators, highly toxic soluble molecules, degradative enzymes, and antimicrobial peptides provide strong immune humoral protection against a wide range of pathogens, orchestrate the majority of the immune mechanisms, and contribute to maintain the host homeostasis. These mediators, constitutively expressed or secreted upon induction by different immune cell types, can be found in all the extracellular body fluids, mainly serum and mucus, and at interstitial spaces.

2.4.1 Cytokines

Within these soluble factors, cytokines include a broad category of small proteins (~5–20 kDa) that mediate cell signaling within the immune system. Cytokines are released by cells (mainly leukocytes) and regulate immune functions through the interaction with a specific receptor on the surface of other cells (paracrine) or the same cell that produced it (autocrine). In some cases, systemic effects can also be produced through their release (endocrine). Each cytokine can be produced by different cell types, but in the same way; its receptor can be expressed on the surface of many different leukocyte types. Finally, several cytokines may exert very similar roles and thus there is a high degree of duplication.

2.4.1.1 Chemokines

Chemokines are a family of cytokines that regulate immune cell migration, maturation, and functionality of the recruited cells in response to inflammation. Constitutively expressed chemokines also play a role in physiological leukocyte transit and microenvironmental segregation within lymphoid organs (Cyster et al., 1999; Warnock et al., 2000). They are produced by different cell types and act on leukocytes through interaction with G-protein-linked chemokine receptors on the cell surface. Additionally, many chemokines also have a role outside the immune system in processes such as angiogenesis (Arenberg et al., 1997; Keane et al., 1998), neurological development and function (Belmadani et al., 2006; Gordon et al., 2009), or organogenesis and germ cell migration (DeVries et al., 2006; Doitsidou et al., 2002; Knaut et al., 2003). They are defined by the presence of four conserved cysteine residues and are divided into four subfamilies depending on the arrangement of the first two conserved cysteines in their sequence, into CXC, CC, C, and CX_3C classes.

The CXC and the CC families constitute the two largest chemokine families, both in mammals and fish. CXC chemokines can contain an ELR (Glu-Leu-Arg) motif at the N-terminus of their sequence responsible for receptor binding and activation of neutrophils, whereas CXC chemokines that lack this motif do not attract neutrophils and act on monocytes and lymphocytes (Clark-Lewis et al., 1991, 1993). There are seven human ELR^+ CXC chemokine genes (CXCL1–5, 5–8) located on the same chromosome and known to act through receptors CXCR1 and CXCR2 and nine ELR^- CXC chemokines that interact with receptors CXCR3–6 (Mackay, 1997; Zlotnik et al., 1999). In fish, this ELR motif is usually replaced by a defective DLR motif (Asp-Leu-Arg) thought, at first, to be active due to the fact that mammalian ELR motifs mutated to DLR retained the capacity to attract neutrophils (Hebert et al., 1991). However, it has been recently demonstrated that this DLR motif is not essential for the attraction of neutrophils by fish CXC chemokines, and, therefore, DLR^+ fish chemokines attract neutrophils even when this motif is eliminated (Cai et al., 2009). Phylogenetic analyses of teleost CXC chemokine sequences have identified six different teleost CXC chemokine clades: CXCa, CXCb, CXCc, CXCd, CXCL12, and CXCL14 (reviewed in Huising et al., 2003). However, chemokines from each clade have not been identified in every species. A wide review of the CXC chemokines identified in fish to date was published in 2011 (Alejo and Tafalla, 2011), and, recently, a unified nomenclature for CXC chemokines in fish, amphibians, and reptiles has been proposed based on an extensive phylogenetic study (Chen et al., 2013).

The CC chemokine family, distinguished by adjacent cysteine residues in a conserved position, has suffered a large increase in some fish species, evidencing extensive, species-specific intrachromosomal duplications. So far, 18 different genes have been identified in rainbow trout (Dixon et al., 1998; Laing and Secombes, 2004b; Liu et al., 2002), 30 in Atlantic salmon (Peatman and Liu, 2007), 26 in channel catfish (*Ictalurus punctatus*) (Bao et al., 2006; Peatman and Liu, 2007), and 81 in zebrafish (Nomiyama et al., 2008). CC chemokines were first divided into "inflammatory" (or "inducible") CC chemokines, which are expressed only after immune stimulation, and "homeostatic" (or "constitutive") CC chemokines, which are produced under normal physiological conditions (Laing and Secombes, 2004a; Zlotnik, 2006). However, as more information becomes available, many chemokines appear to have a dual role. Therefore, seven large groups of fish CC chemokines were established after an extensive phylogenetic analysis: the CCL19/21/25 group, the CCL20 group, the CCL27/28 group, the CCL17/22 group, the macrophage inflammatory protein (MIP) group, the monocyte chemotactic protein (MCP) group, and a fish-specific group (Peatman and Liu, 2007). It was suggested that this "fish CC chemokine group" may represent a subset of ancestral chemokines that carry on important functional roles common to all teleost fish, not yet identified.

Concerning the other two mammalian chemokine families, C and CX_3C, so far in teleost fish, C chemokines have only been identified in zebrafish (Nomiyama et al., 2008), whereas CX_3C chemokines have never been reported. Moreover, a novel family of chemokines named CX, which includes five different members, has been established in zebrafish (Nomiyama et al., 2008). These chemokines differ from the C family in that they lack one of the two N-terminus conserved cysteine residues but retain the third and fourth one, while the C family only retains the second and fourth signature cysteine residues. There is no information available yet on the bioactivity of these chemokines.

Despite the great number of chemokine genes identified in diverse fish species, only very few studies have demonstrated the chemotactic capacity of these molecules (Alejo and Tafalla, 2011). Furthermore, although in some species, such as zebrafish, pufferfish, or rainbow trout (Daniels et al., 1999; DeVries et al., 2006; Dixon et al., 2013; Nomiyama et al., 2008; Zhang et al., 2002), the number of chemokine receptor genes identified also begins to grow, there are only a few of receptor:chemokine pairs revealed so far (Knaut et al., 2003; Perlin and Talbot, 2007). Until this information is available, it will be very difficult to understand the functionality of these molecules.

2.4.1.2 IFNs

Interferons (IFN) are virus-inducible cytokines with antiviral activity that, in mammals, can be classified into three subfamilies (I, II, and III), depending on their genomic structure, the cell types that produce them, and the receptors through which they signal (Zou and Secombes, 2011). In mammals, different type I and III IFNs exist, whilst there is only one single type II IFN gene. In fish, type I and II IFNs have been reported and at least two type II IFN genes are known to be present in some species.

Type I IFNs can be produced by any cell type in response to a viral infection and constitute the main antiviral mechanism in vertebrates. Although type I IFN-like activities were reported many years ago in fish, it was only until 2003 that it was cloned and reported in three independent studies in zebrafish (Altmann et al., 2003), Atlantic salmon (Robertsen et al., 2003), and pufferfish (*Takifugu rubripes*) (Lutfalla et al., 2003). After those reports, type I IFN genes have been identified in multiple fish species (reviewed in Zou and Secombes, 2011). The number of IFN present in one species varies from one to another, but, in general, salmonids and cyprinids appear to have more copies than species of the Acanthopterygian superorder such as pufferfish (Zou and Secombes, 2011). Furthermore, fish IFNs can be divided according to the number of cysteines in their sequence. These two groups are referred to as group I type I IFN (2C) and group II type I IFN (4C), but, so far, group II IFNs have been found only in salmonids and cyprinids where their expression seems to be restricted to specific cell types such as leukocytes (Zou and Secombes, 2011; Zou et al., 2007). Bioactivity studies have mostly focused on group I type I fish IFNs for which antiviral activity, as well as capacity to induce downstream molecules, has been demonstrated (reviewed in Zou and Secombes, 2011). Although the bioactivity of group II type I IFNs has not been studied as extensively, recent evidence suggests they have complementary antiviral effects (Aggad et al., 2009; Levraud et al., 2007; Lopez-Munoz et al., 2009; Zou et al., 2007). The direct antiviral effects of type I IFN in infected and surrounding cells are mediated by the induction of a set of IFN-stimulated genes such as Mx, oligo-2',5'-adenylate synthetase, or protein kinase R (PKR). The direct antiviral effects of these different proteins are not completely clear even in mammals, and, moreover, different viruses exert different sensibilities to their actions (Staeheli, 1990). Mx is the IFN-induced protein most widely studied in teleost fish, and up to three isoforms of Mx proteins have been reported in multiple species (Abollo et al., 2005; Altmann et al., 2004; Chen et al., 2006; Jensen and Robertsen, 2000; Lee et al., 2000; Plant and Thune, 2004; Robertsen et al., 1997; Tafalla et al., 2004; Trobridge et al., 1997; Trobridge and Leong, 1995; Zhang et al., 2004). However, its antiviral activity has been demonstrated only in a few cases (Caipang et al., 2003; Fernandez-Trujillo et al., 2011, 2013; Larsen et al., 2004). Other IFN-induced antiviral proteins reported in fish include the viperin, protein kinases, ISG15, galectins, and finTRIM proteins (reviewed in Verrier et al., 2011).

In mammals, type II IFN (IFN-γ) is produced by Th1 cells and NK cells to promote Th1 responses mainly directed against intracellular pathogens, such as viruses and intracellular bacteria, through the activation of Tc lymphocytes and macrophages (Boehm et al., 1997). Orthologs to IFN-γ have been identified in many teleost species (reviewed in Zou and Secombes, 2011), and, in some species, an additional IFN-γ gene cataloged as IFN-γrel has also been reported (Chen et al., 2010b; Grayfer and Belosevic, 2009; Igawa et al., 2006; Milev-Milovanovic et al., 2006; Stolte et al., 2008; Zou and Secombes, 2011). It is generally accepted that this gene is a second member of the type II IFN family that appeared in teleost after duplication of the IFN-γ gene (Zou and Secombes, 2011). Several IFN-γ have been recombinantly produced and their bioactivity tested, mainly on macrophages. In these cells, fish IFN-γ has been shown to increase the expression of MHC-I and MHC-II (Martin et al., 2007; Zou et al., 2005), the production of nitric oxide (Arts et al., 2010; Grayfer and Belosevic, 2009), the respiratory burst (Grayfer and Belosevic, 2009; Zou et al., 2005), and the phagocytic capacity (Grayfer and Belosevic, 2009). Furthermore, some of the antiviral genes usually induced by type I IFN, such as Mx, can also be induced by type II IFN (Jorgensen et al., 2007), even though the antiviral capacity of this IFN is much weaker than that of type I IFN (Xu et al., 2010).

2.4.1.3 Interleukins

The term "interleukin" (IL) was first coined in 1979 to refer to molecules that signal between different leukocyte types, and, although nowadays it is known that these ILs are not only synthesized nor have effects exclusively on leukocytes, the term has been maintained (Secombes et al., 2011). In mammals, 35 ILs have been identified so far; however, some of these numbers refer to subfamilies of molecules rather than to single molecules. Secombes et al. (2011) excellently reviewed the ILs described to that current date in fish, classifying them into different families; therefore, in this chapter, we will mention only the main roles and members of these IL groups.

The IL-1 family groups 11 members in mammals, namely, IL-1α (IL-1F1), IL-1β (IL-1F2), IL-1 receptor antagonist (IL-1ra/IL-1F3), IL-18 (IL-1F4), IL-1F5-10, and IL-33 (IL-1F11). All these molecules are either pro-inflammatory or agonists of other pro-inflammatory family members. IL-1β was first discovered in fish (rainbow trout) in 1999 (Zou et al., 1999), and it has been reported in many different teleost species since then (reviewed in Secombes et al., 2011). IL-18 has been identified in pufferfish and trout, and, although no functional studies have yet been performed, its transcription is modulated in response to different immune stimuli (Huising et al., 2004; Zou et al., 2004). Although no clear homologs of other family members are present in the locus of IL-1β as occurs in mammals, other family members with high relatedness to IL-1β exist in some fish species in different locus, for example, the molecule named novel IL-1F (nIL-1F), thought to be an IL-1β agonist (Wang et al., 2009a).

There are other pro-inflammatory cytokines outside the IL-1 family such as IL-6. The IL-6 family includes IL-6, IL-11, IL-31, and other mammalian cytokines such as CNTF, LIF, OSM, CT-1, and CT-2 (Secombes et al., 2011). Although not clear in relation to other family members, there seem to be clear homologs of IL-6 and IL-11 in several fish species, which can be modulated in response to diverse stimulation (reviewed in Secombes et al., 2011).

The IL-2 subfamily of cytokines include those that signal via the common gamma chain (γC or CD132), a member of the type I cytokine receptor family expressed on most leukocytes. In mammals, the IL-2 subfamily is formed by IL-2, IL-4, IL-7, IL-9, IL-15, and IL-21. All these molecules are implicated in T cell memory or correspond to molecules released by different Th subsets upon stimulation. All of them, except IL-9, have been found in fish (Secombes et al., 2011).

The IL-10 subfamily groups IL-10, an anti-inflammatory cytokine, and other class II cytokine family members such as IL-19, IL-20, IL-22, IL-24, IL-26, and the IFNs (Lutfalla et al., 2003). The induced transcription of IL-10 in response to LPS or bacterial infection has been demonstrated in several fish species (Inoue et al., 2005; Lutfalla et al., 2003; Pinto et al., 2007; Savan et al., 2003; Seppola et al., 2008; Zhang et al., 2005; Zou et al., 2003a); however, its regulatory or anti-inflammatory effects have not been characterized yet in fish.

The IL-17 cytokine subfamily in mammals is composed of 6 members, IL-17A to IL-17F, with IL-17E also known as IL-25. This gene family is considered very ancient and is the only IL family to have been found in invertebrates as well as in agnatha (Secombes et al., 2011). Several of these family members have been found in fish, even though their homology to mammalian counterparts has been difficult to establish.

Several ILs with very diverse functions, such as IL-12, IL-23, IL-27, and IL-35, can be grouped because they are formed as heterodimers and share some of the peptide chains that form them. These chains include p19, p28 (also called IL-30), p35, p40, and Epstein-Barr virus induced gene 3 (EBI3); consequently, IL-12 is formed by p35 and p40, IL-23 by p19 and p40, IL-27 by p28 and EBI3, and IL-35 by p35 and EBI3 (Secombes et al., 2011). Additionally, the p40 homodimer can function as an inhibitor of IL-12 (Jana and Pahan, 2009). To date no functional studies have been performed with any of these cytokines; however, the p19, p35, p40, and EBI3 chains have been identified in several fish species (reviewed in Secombes et al., 2011).

2.4.1.4 Other cytokines

Other important cytokine families include TNFs, TGFs, and colony-stimulating factors (CSFs).

In mammals, the TNF superfamily groups 19 members with a wide range of functions, including key roles in inflammation, host defense, autoimmunity, organogenesis, cellular apoptosis, and differentiation (Ware, 2003). TNF-α, the best-known family member, has been identified in several fish species, often finding two molecules per species (Kinoshita et al., 2014; Zou et al., 2003b). Zebrafish TNF-α has been shown to mediate virus-induced apoptosis in fish cells, suggesting that the function of this molecule is conserved (Wang et al., 2011). Using two different fish models, it has been shown that TNF-α mediates pro-inflammatory responses through the promotion of E-selectin and chemokine expression in endothelial cells and a subsequent recruitment and activation of phagocytes (Roca et al., 2008). Recently, the inclusion of TNF-α in an oral *Vibrio* vaccine in sea bass produced an extended protective response and higher local IgT transcription levels (Galindo-Villegas et al., 2013).

TGF-β is the best-known cytokine belonging to a family of multifunctional cytokines involved in cell growth, migration, differentiation, and apoptosis (ten Dijke and Hill, 2004). TGF-β also acts as an important regulator in the proliferation of T and B cells, having effects on macrophages, DCs, and NK cells (Kee et al., 2001; Li and Flavell, 2006; Strobl and Knapp, 1999). Although dose-dependent, often these effects on immune cells are anti-inflammatory, restoring lymphocyte homeostasis. Three isoforms of the TGF-β family (e.g., TGF-β1, TGF-β2, and TGF-β3) have been identified in mammals. These isoforms are similar in structure and biological function, with TGF-β1 as the predominant form in the immune system. All isoforms of the TGF-β family have been identified in teleosts, including zebrafish (Kohli et al., 2003), rainbow trout (Hardie et al., 1998), sea bream (Tafalla et al., 2003), grass carp (*Ctenopharyngodon idella*) (Yang and Zhou, 2008), and striped bass (*Morone saxatilis*) (Harms et al., 2000). However, information on biological functions of these molecules in the fish immune system remains limited. In grass carp, it has been demonstrated that TGF-β1 inhibits *in vitro* peripheral blood leukocyte proliferation induced by LPS and PHA, but could up-regulate MHC class I expression and proliferation in nonstimulated peripheral blood leukocytes (Yang and Zhou, 2008).

CSFs are cytokines with a central role in hematopoiesis, activating intracellular signaling pathways that can cause the cells to proliferate and differentiate into a specific kind of blood cell. Additionally, they can influence specific mature cells to modulate immune functions and maintain homeostasis and immune competence (Barreda et al., 2004). Belonging to this group, macrophage-CSF (M-CSF) and granulocyte-CSF (G-CSF) are relatively lineage-specific, having a role in the proliferation, differentiation, and survival of macrophages, neutrophils, and their precursors. On the other hand, granulocyte/macrophage-CSF (GM-CSF) and multi-CSF (IL-3) function at earlier stages of lineage commitment regulating the expansion and maturation of primitive hematopoietic progenitors.

2.4.2 Complement

The complement system is an ancient innate immune mechanism present in both vertebrate and invertebrate species. The mammalian complement system appears more developed and is composed of ~30 different proteins, either plasma- or membrane-associated. The proteins and glycoproteins that constitute the complement system are synthesized by hepatocytes, but significant amounts are also produced by tissue macrophages, blood monocytes, and epithelial cells of the genitourinary tract and gastrointestinal tract. Complement proteins have a wide range of functions, including the elimination of invading pathogens, promotion of inflammatory responses, clearance of cell debris, and modulation of adaptive immune responses (Walport, 2001a, 2001b). They are normally present as inactive precursors until the system is activated by one of the three biochemical activation pathways: the classical pathway, the alternative pathway, and the lectin pathway. The three cascades of activation lead to the formation of a protease complex, the protease C3 convertase, that activates a further cascade of cleavage and activation events, mainly the release of opsonic and chemotactic components and the activation of the C5 component, part of the membrane-attack complex (MAC), which damages the membrane of the target (pathogens or cells). The classical pathway is part of the specific immune response and requires immune complexes (antigen-antibody complexes) for the activation of the C1 complex that, together with C2 and C4 components, lead to the formation of the protease C3 convertase. The alternative and lectin pathways can be activated by C3 hydrolysis or antigens without the presence of antibodies as part of the innate response. In the alternative pathway, the spontaneous activation of C3 and its binding to microbial surfaces leads to the interaction with plasmatic factors B and D and, finally, to the formation of the protease C3 convertase. The lectin pathway is based on the interaction of lectins, such as mannose-binding lectin and ficolins, with sugar moieties found on the surface of microbes, activating in this manner a system of proteases (MBL-associated serine proteases, MASPs) that cleave the C2 and C4 complement components in a similar way as the classical pathway.

Complement components participating in the alternative and lectin pathways have been described in jawless fish, whereas molecules involved in all three pathways have been reported in both Chondrichthyes (Smith, 1998) and Osteichthyes (Nakao et al., 2011). In teleosts, mRNAs encoding complement components show not only a wide tissue distribution in the liver, but also substantial extrahepatic expression in the kidney, intestine, gill, skin, brain, and gonads. Functional assays performed with some of these molecules revealed conserved effector activities recognized in the mammalian system such as opsonization, killing of target cells, and anaphylotoxin leukocyte stimulation (reviewed in Boshra et al., 2006; Nakao et al., 2011). Based on the data obtained in zebrafish, carp, and trout, it is evident that almost all the homologs of the mammalian complement components are present in teleost with the particularity that some of the key components show multiple isoforms in fish species. For example, the components C3, C4, C5, C7, MBL, factor B, and factor I are present in several isoforms being the product of different genes (Nakao et al., 2006; Nakao et al., 2000; Sunyer et al., 1997). Teleost complement is active at very low temperatures, and their alternative pathway titers are several orders of magnitude higher than that of the mammalian order. Different expression studies performed with immunostimulants or microbial infections suggest that fish complement is a powerful defense mechanism against viral, bacterial, or parasitic infections (reviewed in Boshra et al., 2006; Nakao et al., 2011). Furthermore, complement proteins are among the immune factors delivered to eggs from a maternal source. During early egg development and before the transcription and functionality of their own immune factors is established, embryo survival relies on the maternal transfer of several immune molecules, including various complement components (Lovoll et al., 2006; Swain and Nayak, 2009; Wang et al., 2009b).

2.4.3 Antimicrobial peptides

Antimicrobial peptides (AMPs) are small peptides (less than 100 amino acids) with low molecular weight and direct microbicidal activities. They are mostly cationic and amphipathic, although some anionic peptides are included among them. AMPs are synthesized as pre-pro-peptides, and, once the active peptides are released by cleavage, they interact directly with pathogens, leading to rapid destruction of the microorganism, either bacteria, virus, protozoa, fungi or tumor cells (Cuesta et al., 2008; Chia et al., 2010; Mihajlovic and Lazaridis, 2010). Although the main function of AMPs is the direct lytic activity on pathogens, other relevant functions have been described for them such as endotoxin neutralization, chemotactic activity, and immunomodulation. A large number of AMPs have been isolated from fish, including cationic peptides, linear amphipathic α-helical peptides (piscidins, moronecidins, gaduscidins, epinecidin, pleurocidin, chrysophsins, cathelicidins), cationic peptides derived from larger proteins (histone-derived, hemoglobin-derived, hemocyanin-derived peptides) or cationic peptides with cysteines that form intramolecular bonding (defensins, hepcidins) (reviewed in Rajanbabu and Chen, 2011; Valero et al., 2013). Anionic peptides have also been reported in the case of *Setipinna taty* (Song et al., 2012). AMPs are mainly expressed in the skin and mucosal epithelia, but constitutive and inducible expression of different AMPs have been described in many tissues, including liver, kidney, blood, spleen, gills, eyes, gonads, or pituitary gland (Nam et al., 2010; Rajanbabu and Chen, 2011; Valero et al., 2013). The activity of many of these fish AMPs have been demonstrated against a wide number of bacterial, viral, and fungal pathogens (Casadei et al., 2009; Chang et al., 2005; Chia et al., 2010; Cuesta et al., 2008; Jin et al., 2010; Rajanbabu and Chen, 2011; Zhao et al., 2009).

2.4.4 Lectins

Lectins are oligomeric carbohydrate-binding proteins characterized by the presence of a carbohydrate recognition domain that is highly specific for sugar moieties. They are ubiquitous and have been found in animals, plants, and microorganisms. This diversified group of proteins has different roles in animal biology, including the mediation of cell-to-cell interactions, homeostatic regulation, and immune recognition of foreign carbohydrates. Animal lectins are classified in several families, depending on their amino acid sequences and biochemical properties (Zelensky and Gready, 2005). Fish present a greatly diversified lectin repertoire with representatives from most lectin families described so far (C-type lectins, galectins, pentraxins, X-type lectins/intelectins, calnexin, and calreticulin) and also with members of lectin families described for the first time in fish (F-type lectins, rhamnose-binding lectins, and pufflectins) (reviewed in Vasta et al., 2011). The tissue-specific expression of the diverse lectin repertoires in fish suggests distinct biological roles in innate and adaptive immunity. Some lectins bind endogenous ligands, whilst others bind sugars on the surface of potential pathogens; therefore, in addition to pathogen recognition and opsonization, some lectins display additional effector roles such as complement activation and regulation of immune functions. Furthermore, some fish lectins mediate nonimmune processes through the recognition of exogenous ligands, acting, for example, as antifreeze proteins or preventing polyspermy during fertilization (reviewed in Vasta et al., 2011).

2.4.5 Other humoral factors

Lysozyme is a mucolytic enzyme that acts on the peptidoglycan of bacterial walls, catalyzing the hydrolysis of the linkages between the N-acetylmuramic acid and the N-acetyl-D-glucosamine. It is produced mainly by monocyte–macrophages and neutrophils and, consequently, is abundant in lymphoid tissues, serum, mucus, and eggs. Serum lysozyme has been identified in practically all aquacultured species and its modulation, in response to infection and physiological stress, has been demonstrated (Fast et al., 2002; Grinde, 1989; Lie et al., 1989; Saurabh and Sahoo, 2008).

Transferrins are iron-binding proteins that control the level of free iron in biological fluids. They are associated with innate immunity by chelating free iron and thus blocking the survival of many classes of bacteria. Ferritin is another protein related with iron storage that can also have a role in immunity. Both proteins have been identified in several fish species and, surprisingly, are mainly expressed in the liver and brain (Bayne and Gerwick, 2001; Neves et al., 2009). During bacterial infections, these proteins can act as negative or positive acute phase proteins, and, consequently, their protein expression can be either up- or down-regulated. Additionally, fish transferrin exerts a novel role as macrophage activator, which may represent a primitive and evolutionary conserved mechanism for the induction of NO response in macrophages (Stafford and Belosevic, 2003).

There are other mucosal factors, such as α2-macroglobulin, a protease inhibitor that can act against pathogen proteases (Armstrong and Quigley, 1999), or lytic enzymes like the hydrolases chitinase and cathepsin, which have been also described in fish, but their role in the immune system remains essentially unexplored (Magnadottir, 2006).

2.4.6 The mucus

Mucus represents the biochemical interface between fish and the aqueous external environment and is continuously exposed to microbes and stressors. All fish surfaces in contact with the external environment are covered by a mucosal layer, including the skin, the gills, the gut, and the eggs. Mucus composition, structure, and thickness of the mucosal layer can vary depending on the mucosal territory and the physiological, immunological, or environmental conditions. The functions of this mucosal barrier include mechanical, physiological, and immunological aspects. Mucus is produced by secretory cells and is composed of a matrix of glycoproteins (mucins) that confer a gel structure and contain diverse humoral immune factors with biostatic or biocidal activities against pathogen infiltration, including Igs, complement factors, C-reactive protein, lectins, lysozyme, proteolytic enzymes, antimicrobial peptides, phosphatases, and esterases (Alexander and Ingram, 1992a; Jones, 2001; Palaksha et al., 2008).

2.5 Immune mechanisms

2.5.1 Pathogen recognition

Once a pathogen succeeds in breaching the innate physical barriers, it is recognized by pattern recognition receptors on immune cells, this step being the first key factor in the triggering of all subsequent immune responses. These receptors are mainly present in DCs and macrophages, but also in other cell types, such as B lymphocytes or endothelial cells, and are activated in response to conserved motifs in pathogens, designated as pathogen-associated molecular patterns (PAMPs), or in response to damage-associated molecular patterns (DAMPs), cell components released during cell damage. Once these receptors are activated, several intracellular activation routes are triggered. All of them essentially lead to the activation of pro-inflammatory or antimicrobial genes. TLRs are the best-known receptors in this group that also includes C-type lectin receptors, NOD-like receptors, RIG-I-like receptors, and peptidoglycan recognition proteins (PGRPs). All five types of receptors have been reported in teleost fish (Boltana et al., 2011). C-type lectin receptors exist as both soluble and transmembrane proteins. In fish, only seven transmembrane C-type lectin receptors have been described to date, and, although they are expressed in immune tissues and modulated upon infection, their immune role has yet to be elucidated (Chen et al., 2010a; Goetz et al., 2004; Soanes et al., 2004). NOD-like receptors are cytosolic proteins involved in autoimmunity, bacterial and viral responses, as well as apoptosis (Martinon and Tschopp, 2005). In fish, these receptors form a large family with up to 70 members in species such as zebrafish (Laing et al., 2008). RIG-I-like receptors are a type of intracellular pattern recognition receptors involved in the recognition of viruses that activate host IFN upon recognition of viral RNA. The RLH family contains three members, RIG-I, melanoma differentiation-associated gene 5 (MDA5), and laboratory of genetics and physiology 2 (LGP2). Fish also possess RIG-I-like receptors, among which RIG-I has been shown to activate the IFN response via a mitochondrion-associated signaling pathway (Biacchesi et al., 2009; Lauksund et al., 2009). Finally, recent studies performed in trout revealed that MDA5 and LGP2 act as independent positive regulators of the IFN response, while an LGP2 variant identified in this species antagonizes with LGP2 function (Chang et al., 2011). The PGRPs recognize peptidoglycans from both gram-positive and gram-negative bacteria and have a well-conserved structure between invertebrates and vertebrates. In fish, 10 different PGRPs have been identified to date (Boltana et al., 2011). Finally, the TLR group is a well-characterized family that comprises membrane receptors and endolysosomal receptors. In fish, they have been reported in large numbers in more than a dozen different fish species that include modern fish, such as the sea bream, or ancient species such as the lamprey (Boltana et al., 2011; Pietretti and Wiegertjes, 2014; Rebl et al., 2010). Several reviews provide detailed descriptions of the down stream activating routes triggered by TLRs in fish (Collet and Secombes, 2002; Rebl et al., 2010). Most of the studies dealing with TLRs in fish report only transcriptional changes, but of course consistent changes in TLR transcription in the same species or across different fish species should be considered as an indirect indication of functional relevance of this TLR in a defined situation. Thus, it has been mainly through these types of studies that we have seen a high degree of conservation in TLR recognition and functionality in fish compared to their mammalian counterparts. In mammals, TLR3, 7, 8, and 9 are mainly involved in viral detection, whereas TLR1, 2, 4, 5, 6, 7, 8, and 9 recognize highly conserved structures of bacterial origin. Nevertheless, remarkable distinct features of teleostean TLR cascades have been discovered and have been reviewed elsewhere (Pietretti and Wiegertjes, 2014; Rebl et al., 2010). For example, it has been shown that TLR3 in fish can detect bacterial molecular patterns, in addition to viral patterns in contrast to mammalian TLR3. Regarding TLR4, responsible for sensing LPS in mammals, it seems that this receptor is missing from the genome of several fish species (Pietretti and Wiegertjes, 2014), whereas it does not recognize LPS in some others (Sepulcre et al., 2009). Finally, while the orthologs of some human TLRs are missing in teleosts (TLR6 and TLR10), some piscine TLRs are encoded by duplicated genes, such as salmonid TLR22, found in several fish species, but only as a nonfunctional pseudogene in humans (Rebl et al., 2010).

2.5.2 Phagocytosis

The cells that primarily sense the pathogens through receptors, such as DCs and macrophages, are also characterized by a strong phagocytic capacity. This phagocytosis contributes, on one hand, to pathogen clearance, while, at the same time, phagocytosis constitutes a necessary step for antigen presentation by these cells. Since the latter will be addressed in the next section, in this section we will focus on the capacity that cells of the immune system have to clear pathogens through phagocytosis. This mechanism mainly relies on the activities of the two so-called "professional phagocytes," macrophages and neutrophils. Even though the differential features of these two cell types have been extensively studied in mammals, it has been through the use of transgenic zebrafish larvae that it has been revealed that macrophages efficiently engulf bacteria from blood or fluid-filled body cavities; neutrophils barely do so. By contrast, neutrophils are very efficient at sweeping up surface-associated, but not fluid-borne, bacteria (Colucci-Guyon et al., 2011). Furthermore, it is especially the phagocytic ability of neutrophils that is essential for the removal of microbes and damaged tissue needed for the resolution of inflammation. For this, subsequent reduction in neutrophil numbers at a site of tissue injury occurs by several different processes: by neutrophil apoptosis, by removal in inflammatory exudates, or by reverse migration, all of them demonstrated in the zebrafish model (Henry et al., 2013).

Once the pathogen is inside a phagocyte, intracellular killing mechanisms are triggered. It is interesting to note that these intracellular killing mechanisms are triggered, not only when the pathogen has been internalized in a phagosome as a consequence of active phagocytosis, but also when the pathogen itself penetrates the cells (Rieger and Barreda, 2011). In case the pathogen has been phagocytized, lysosome granules migrate towards and fuse with the phagosome, forming a phagolysosome structure, resulting in the release of acidic and enzymatic lysosomal contents into the phagosomal lumen and subsequent degradation of phagolysosome contents. Phagolysosome fusion has been shown to occur in goldfish monocytes and mature macrophages (Rieger et al., 2010). Upon pathogen internalization, phagocytes also trigger the production of oxygen and nitrogen radicals as one of the main intracellular killing mechanisms. The production of oxygen radicals or respiratory burst is a process catalyzed by NADPH-oxidase, a multicomponent enzyme assembled on the inner surface of the plasma membrane following appropriate activation. This activation leads to the production of superoxide anion. NADPH-oxidase has been identified in diverse teleost fish (reviewed in Rieger and Barreda, 2011) and the stimulation of respiratory burst, especially in macrophages, has been widely studied in diverse species, (reviewed in Rieger and Barreda (2011) and Forlenza et al. (2011)). Furthermore, it is known that several fish cytokines can augment this respiratory burst. These include TNF-α (Grayfer et al., 2008), IFN-γ (Arts et al., 2010; Grayfer and Belosevic, 2009; Grayfer et al., 2010; Zou et al., 2005), CSF-1 (Grayfer et al., 2009), and IL-8 (Harun et al., 2008). Interestingly, in some species, TNF-α has no direct effect on phagocytes, but instead it activates endothelial cells, that then lead to an indirect activation of phagocytes (Forlenza et al., 2009; Roca et al., 2008).

It is worth noting that in 2006, the active phagocytic capacity of teleost B cells was revealed as a breakthrough discovery in immunology (Li et al., 2006), posteriorly reported for some subsets of mammalian B cells (Nakashima et al., 2012; Parra et al., 2012). Both IgM^+ (Li et al., 2006) and IgT^+ (Zhang et al., 2010) cells were shown to actively internalize beads or bacteria, leading to phagolysosome fusion. Although the actual contribution of teleost B cell to pathogen clearance in comparison to other professional phagocytes may be low, the phagocytic activity suggests a higher capacity of B cells in fish to present antigens, a hypothesis also supported by the reported high levels of expression of DC-like markers in teleost B cells (Johansson et al., 2012; Zhang et al., 2009).

2.5.3 Antigen presentation

MHC class I molecules are found on nearly every nucleated cell of the body. They bind peptides mainly generated from degradation of cytosolic proteins by the proteasome. The MHC I:peptide complex is then exposed on the cell surface. Thus, the function of the class I MHC is to display intracellular proteins produced during an intracellular infection or through a cell cycle alteration (tumor cells) to Tc lymphocytes. Recognition of antigenic peptides through MHC class I by Tc lymphocytes leads to the killing of the target cell, which is either infected by virus or by intracellular bacteria, or is otherwise damaged or dysfunctional.

MHC class II molecules on the other hand are found only on specific cell types, which in the case of fish could include macrophages, DCs, B cells, thrombocytes, and acidophilic granulocytes (in gilthead sea bream), all of them assumed to have antigen-presenting properties (Cuesta et al., 2006; Forlenza et al., 2011; Kollner et al., 2004; Li et al., 2006; Lugo-Villarino et al., 2010). The antigens presented by class II peptides are derived from extracellular proteins that have been taken up through phagocytosis by these cells. The protein is then processed into the phagolysosome that breaks into smaller peptides, which are then exposed on the cell surface in the context of class II MHC molecules. This MHC:antigen complex is then recognized by T cells, usually $CD4^+$ Th cells that become activated and secrete cytokines to modulate the adaptive immune response. In mammals, this presentation takes place in the spleen or in the lymph nodes. In fish, since there are no lymph nodes, antigen presentation seems to take place locally where the antigen is present (Castro et al., 2014b). Despite the fact that fish DCs have not been clearly characterized, the antigen presenting capacity of the DC-like cells described in fish has been established (Bassity and Clark, 2012; Lugo-Villarino et al., 2010).

The up-regulation of MHC-I and MHC-II levels in response to different pathogens or immunostimulants has been reported in various fish species (Cuesta and Tafalla, 2009; Dixon et al., 1995; Goetz et al., 2004; Ingerslev et al., 2009; Miller et al., 2004; Olsen et al., 2011; Rakus et al., 2009; Stet and Egberts, 1991); however, many details of its regulation remain unsolved. One of the limiting factors in understanding teleost major histocompatibility receptor function is the lack of knowledge about antigen presentation accessory molecules. Some of these molecules have been identified in some fish species and seem to have an expression regulation different from that of tetrapods (Fujiki et al., 2003).

2.5.4 Cytotoxic responses

In the process of recognition of self from non-self, immune cells can detect nonspecifically most pathogens and altered cells via cell surface receptors that recognize expressed pathogen-associated molecular patterns, non-self cells (with heterologous MHC class I molecules in their surface) and foreign molecules presented in the context of MHC class I (intracellular antigens) or MHC class II (extracellular antigens). In this sense, both NK-like cells and Tc lymphocytes are responsible for identifying and killing these cells. NK cells sense the down-regulation or altered expression of MHC-I to identify altered cells, whereas Tc cells identify a certain antigenic peptide exposed in a self MHC-I complex through an interaction with the TCR complex. Furthermore, in comparison to NK cells, Tc cells require priming and clonal expansion for an adequate response. However, their mode of killing is very similar and is based on two different types of mechanisms. On the one hand, granule-exocytosis releases pore-forming molecules, such as perforin, granulysin, and NK-lysin, that disrupt the membrane of the target cells that allow entry of granzymes that provoke cell apoptosis. Perforin and granzyme has been identified in $CD8^+$ Tc lymphocytes and NK cells in various fish species (reviewed in Fischer et al., 2013) and their expression is up-regulated in response to virus infection (Aquilino et al., 2013), suggesting an equivalent role as to that of mammals. On the other hand, the second killing mechanism is mediated through FasL/Fas interaction. FasL proteins produced by cytotoxic cells provoke apoptotic cell death through its interaction with Fas receptor (FasR) on the surface of the target cell. In mammals, FasL can be expressed in a membrane-bound form and as a cytosolic soluble form, whereas in fish only cytosolic forms have been identified (Fischer et al., 2013). This killing mechanism has been demonstrated in catfish and zebrafish.

2.5.5 Antibody production

B cells express Ig either on the cell surface as antigen receptors (BCR) or secrete them as soluble Igs or antibodies. Igs are composed of two identical heavy (H) chains and two identical light (L) chains that are encoded by the IgH locus and IgL locus, respectively. Both the H and L chains are composed of a variable (V) and a constant (C) domain. The V domain is composed of one of each V, D, and J gene segments and is responsible for antigen-binding, whereas the C domain is responsible for binding to effector molecules, triggering complex signaling pathways that lead to the elimination of the antibody-coated foreign material. Two different types of genomic arrangement of the Ig loci have evolved. Mammalian V, D (only in the H chain), J, and C gene segments encoding Ig H or L chains are organized in one type of locus containing multiple consecutive V segments, D segments, and J segments upstream in the constant region in an organization known as translocon arrangement. In cartilaginous fish, successive individual clusters of V-(D)-J-C gene segments are repeated 100–200 times in what has been termed as multicluster arrangement $(VDJ\text{-}C)_n$. IgH genes in teleost are organized in a translocon configuration as in mammals, whereas the Ig L-chain gene organization is of multicluster type (Hsu et al., 2006; Malecek et al., 2008; Warr, 1995). Cartilaginous fish possess three Ig heavy chain isotypes, namely, μ (IgM), δ (IgW), and IgNAR, and four light chain isotypes, namely, σ-cart, σ, κ, and λ. For teleost, three heavy chain isotypes – μ (IgM), δ (IgD), and τ (IgT) – and three light chain isotypes – σ, κ, and λ – have been described (Das et al., 2012). Igs are expressed in the membrane of B cells, defining the different B cell subtypes (see Section 2.3.1.1). Upon the interaction of a pathogen with the variable region of these Igs, the B cell becomes activated and part of its progeny initiates Ig secretion as part of the process that will lead the cell to become an antigen-secreting cell (ASC). The production of specific IgMs in response to antigens has been reported against several types of pathogens, including virus, bacteria, and parasites and in some occasions this antibody production seems to be directly related to protection (Raida et al., 2011; Romstad et al., 2013; Ye et al., 2013). In those cases when protection is mediated by antibodies, they can protect fish against a reinfection with the same pathogen and can last for a long time (Ma et al., 2013a; Ye et al., 2013). In most teleosts, serum IgM is expressed as a tetramer in different redox states, variability suggested as important for their function, although not clearly elucidated yet (Kaattari et al., 1998). IgM can be present in serum and secretions, including mucus, and the antibody response intensity varies among fish species, from salmonids that produce a large amount of specific antibodies to a variety of antigens, to cod that has very low antibody responses, being mainly natural, nonspecific antibodies (Solem and Stenvik, 2006). The secreted antigen bind to the pathogen and in some cases directly interferes with their replication capacity (neutralizing antibodies). Furthermore, antibody-pathogen complexes attract phagocytes through receptors (Fc receptors) that recognize the Fab portion of the antibody bound to the antigen, facilitating phagocytosis. The Fc receptor-antibody complex can also create by-products, such as C3b and C4b, that activate the complement system (Stafford et al., 2006).

Recently, the production of specific IgDs and IgTs have also been described, suggesting that all three Igs cooperate in pathogen clearance even though their specific function is not clear yet (Bromage et al., 2004; Xu et al., 2013; Zhang et al., 2010). Before the identification of an IgD homolog in catfish, IgD was believed to represent a recently evolved Ig described only in primates and rodents (Wilson et al., 1997). Since then, IgD was identified in all vertebrates except birds, indicating that this Ig represents an ancient Ig class. A secreted IgD was identified in serum of catfish as a monomer, although this protein may not contain a functional V-region (Bengten et al., 2002). On the other hand, rainbow trout possess a secretory IgD product that is associated with a Cμ1 exon and a V-region, and its secretory arrangement has been inferred in other teleost species analyzing the IGH locus expressed sequence transcripts (ESTs) (Ramirez-Gomez et al., 2012). This analysis includes Atlantic salmon, Atlantic cod (*Gadus macrocephalus*), and grass carp (*Ctenopharyngodon idella*). A single positive IgD population was recently described in trout. This B cell population, mainly present in the gills, has still an unknown function, although it is regulated upon viral infection. In mammals, a $_{mem}IgD^{+}{}_{mem}IgM^{-}$ population present mainly in the upper aerodigestive mucosa arises in humans after active IgM-to-IgD class switch. These plasmablast-like cells that retain IgD in the membrane secrete highly mutated mono- and polyreactive IgD, providing a layer of mucosal protection by interacting with pathogens, and are either retained locally or are circulated in the blood, where they can account for up to 0.5–1% of circulating B cells (Chen and Cerutti, 2010; Chen et al., 2009). IgT is expressed as a monomer in rainbow trout serum and as a tetramer in gut mucus (Zhang et al., 2010). This Ig has been described as a specialized Ig in mucosal immunity in rainbow trout. So far, IgT positive populations have been described as the prevalent B cell subset in the gut and skin. Although fish do not produce IgA, IgM produced at mucosal sites can be secreted and so does IgT/Z (Rombout et al., 2011). In trout, a strong gut local IgT response was elicited by a gut protozoan parasite, while the IgT levels in serum remained at low levels. In contrast a strong IgM response was restricted to serum (Xu et al., 2013; Zhang et al., 2010). In the case of the skin, IgT responses against a skin parasite were mainly limited to the skin, whereas IgM responses were almost exclusively detected in the serum (Xu et al., 2013). These results suggested that IgT could be an equivalent of IgA; however, systemic IgT responses to either virus (Castro et al., 2013) or DNA vaccination (Castro et al., 2014b) suggest that IgT also plays an important role outside mucosal tissues.

The repertoire of the BCR was inferred in zebrafish and rainbow trout using spectratyping and high-throughput sequencing methods. The expressed variable domain (VDJ region) of the IgHμ, IgHδ, and IgHτ was studied in naïve fish and these repertoires are polyclonal and highly diversified (Castro et al., 2013; Weinstein et al., 2009). The B cell response against a rhabdovirus, viral hemorrhagic septicemia virus (VHSV), was also studied, vaccinating fish with an attenuated strain and challenging them 3 weeks later with the same strain. The study of the BCR repertoire in the spleen of these fish showed a strong IgM response with clonal expansion of several VDJ sequences, a more moderate IgT response, and an IgD repertoire that remained essentially unaltered (Castro et al., 2013).

It is worth noting that what have been designated as natural antibodies are present in the serum of vertebrates at any time without apparent antigenic stimulation. In mammalian species they are mostly of the IgM type, secreted by the long-lived, self-renewing B1 subset of B cells, which are generated during fetal or neonatal development. These antibodies are polyreactive and have low-binding affinity, binding various autoantigens like thyroglobulin, single stranded DNA and heat shock proteins, or haptens like 2,4,6-trinitrophenyl (TNP) or 2,4-dinitrophenyl (DNP) (Boes, 2000; Casali and Schettino, 1996). Their role is mainly to provide local confinement of infection, to enhance IgG response, to take part in homeostasis and clearing of cell debris, and to link innate and adaptive immunity (Boes, 2000; Lutz, 2007; Ochsenbein et al., 1999). Natural antibodies have been described in several species of chondrichthyes and teleosts (Gonzalez et al., 1988; Sinyakov et al., 2002; Vilain et al., 1984). In a comparative study of the natural antibody repertoire of different fish species, it has been shown that teleost natural antibodies have specificity primarily for haptenated protein (TNP-BSA), while those of elasmobranchs and sturgeon show specificity for various self and non-self-antigens but a lower anti-TNP-BSA titre (Gonzalez et al., 1988). The contribution of these natural antibodies in the immune defense against both bacterial and viral diseases has been studied in cod, goldfish, and rainbow trout (Gonzalez et al., 1989; Magnadottir et al., 2009; Sinyakov et al., 2002). In cod, special attention has been paid to natural antibodies because of the peculiarities of the antibody response in this species. When fighting an infection, cod relies more on the quantity than the specificity of the antibody repertoire. Thus, immunization and challenge experiments have resulted in poor acquired antibody response, even if the IgM concentration in serum is relatively high compared with other fish species. In contrast, the activity of natural antibodies against TNP-BSA is commonly high, and these natural antibodies have a broad specificity and relatively strong affinity (Magnadottir et al., 2009).

Acknowledgments

This work was supported by Starting Grant 2011 (Project No. 280469) from the European Research Council and project AGL2011-29676 from the Spanish Ministerio de Economia y Competitividad. Financial support was also from the European Commission under the 7th Framework Programme for Research and Technological Development (FP7) of the European Union (Grant Agreement 311993 TARGETFISH). The authors thank Beatriz Abós for critically reviewing the chapter.

References

Abelli, L., Baldassini, M.R., Mastrolia, L., Scapigliati, G., 1999. Immunodetection of lymphocyte subpopulations involved in allograft rejection in a teleost, *Dicentrarchus labrax* (L.). Cell Immunol. 191, 152–160.

Abollo, E., Ordas, C., Dios, S., Figueras, A., Novoa, B., 2005. Molecular characterisation of a turbot Mx cDNA. Fish Shellfish Immunol. 19, 185–190.

Abos, B., Castro, R., Pignatelli, J., Luque, A., Gonzalez, L., Tafalla, C., 2013. Transcriptional heterogeneity of IgM(+) cells in rainbow trout (*Oncorhynchus mykiss*) tissues. PLoS One 8, e82737.

Aggad, D., Mazel, M., Boudinot, P., Mogensen, K.E., Hamming, O.J., Hartmann, R., Kotenko, S., Herbomel, P., Lutfalla, G., Levraud, J.P., 2009. The two groups of zebrafish virus-induced interferons signal via distinct receptors with specific and shared chains. J. Immunol. 183, 3924–3931.

Agius, C., Roberts, R.J., 2003. Melano-macrophage centres and their role in fish pathology. J. Fish Dis. 26, 499–509.

Alejo, A., Tafalla, C., 2011. Chemokines in teleost fish species. Dev. Comp. Immunol. 35, 1215–1222.

Alexander, J.B., Ingram, G.A., 1992a. Noncellular nonspecific defence mechanisms of fish. Ann. Rev. Fish Dis. 2, 249–279.

Alexander, J.B., Ingram, G.A., 1992b. Noncellular nonspecific defense mechanisms of fish. Ann. Rev. Fish Dis. 2, 249–279.

Altmann, S.M., Mellon, M.T., Distel, D.L., Kim, C.H., 2003. Molecular and functional analysis of an interferon gene from the zebrafish, *Danio rerio*. J. Virol. 77, 1992–2002.

Altmann, S.M., Mellon, M.T., Johnson, M.C., Paw, B.H., Trede, N.S., Zon, L.I., Kim, C.H., 2004. Cloning and characterization of an Mx gene and its corresponding promoter from the zebrafish, *Danio rerio*. Dev. Comp. Immunol. 28, 295–306.

Amemiya, C.T., Saha, N.R., Zapata, A., 2007. Evolution and development of immunological structures in the lamprey. Curr. Opin. Immunol. 19, 535–541.

Aquilino, C., Castro, R., Fischer, U., Tafalla, C., 2013. Transcriptomic responses in rainbow trout gills upon infection with viral hemorrhagic septicemia virus (VHSV). Dev. Comp. Immunol. 44, 12–20.

Arenberg, D.A., Polverini, P.J., Kunkel, S.L., Shanafelt, A., Strieter, R.M., 1997. *In vitro* and *in vivo* systems to assess role of C-X-C chemokines in regulation of angiogenesis. Methods Enzymol. 288, 190–220.

Armstrong, P.B., Quigley, J.P., 1999. Alpha2-macroglobulin: an evolutionarily conserved arm of the innate immune system. Dev. Comp. Immunol. 23, 375–390.

Arts, J.A., Tijhaar, E.J., Chadzinska, M., Savelkoul, H.F., Verburg-van Kemenade, B.M., 2010. Functional analysis of carp interferon-gamma: evolutionary conservation of classical phagocyte activation. Fish Shellfish Immunol. 29, 793–802.

Bajoghli, B., Guo, P., Aghaallaei, N., Hirano, M., Strohmeier, C., McCurley, N., Bockman, D.E., Schorpp, M., Cooper, M.D., Boehm, T., 2011. A thymus candidate in lampreys. Nature 470, 90–94.

Balla, K.M., Lugo-Villarino, G., Spitsbergen, J.M., Stachura, D.L., Hu, Y., Banuelos, K., Romo-Fewell, O., Aroian, R.V., Traver, D., 2010. Eosinophils in the zebrafish: prospective isolation, characterization, and eosinophilia induction by helminth determinants. Blood 116, 3944–3954.

Ballesteros, N.A., Castro, R., Abós, B., Rodriguez Saint-Jean, S., Perez-Prieto, S.I., Tafalla, C., 2013a. The pyloric caeca area is a major site for IgM+ and IgT+ B cell recruitment in response to oral vaccination in rainbow trout. PLoS One 8 (6), e66118.

Ballesteros, N.A., Rodriguez Saint-Jean, S., Perez-Prieto, S.I., Aquilino, C., Tafalla, C., 2013b. Modulation of genes related to the recruitment of immune cells in the digestive tract of trout experimentally infected with infectious pancreatic necrosis virus (IPNV) or orally vaccinated. Dev. Comp. Immunol. 44, 195–205.

Bao, B., Peatman, E., Peng, X., Baoprasertkul, P., Wang, G., Liu, Z., 2006. Characterization of 23 CC chemokine genes and analysis of their expression in channel catfish (*Ictalurus punctatus*). Dev. Comp. Immunol. 30, 783–796.

Barreda, D.R., Hanington, P.C., Belosevic, M., 2004. Regulation of myeloid development and function by colony stimulating factors. Dev. Comp. Immunol. 28, 509–554.

Bassity, E., Clark, T.G., 2012. Functional identification of dendritic cells in the teleost model, rainbow trout (*Oncorhynchus mykiss*). PLoS One 7, e33196.

Bayne, C.J., Gerwick, L., 2001. The acute phase response and innate immunity of fish. Dev. Comp. Immunol. 25, 725–743.

Belmadani, A., Tran, P.B., Ren, D., Miller, R.J., 2006. Chemokines regulate the migration of neural progenitors to sites of neuroinflammation. J. Neurosci. 26, 3182–3191.

Bengten, E., Quiniou, S.M., Stuge, T.B., Katagiri, T., Miller, N.W., Clem, L.W., Warr, G.W., Wilson, M., 2002. The IgH locus of the channel catfish, *Ictalurus punctatus*, contains multiple constant region gene sequences: different genes encode heavy chains of membrane and secreted IgD. J. Immunol. 169, 2488–2497.

Bergeron, T., Woodward, B., 1983. The development of the stratum granulosum of the small intestine of rainbow trout (*Salmo gairdneri*). Can. J. Zool. 60, 1513–1516.

Biacchesi, S., LeBerre, M., Lamoureux, A., Louise, Y., Lauret, E., Boudinot, P., Bremont, M., 2009. Mitochondrial antiviral signaling protein plays a major role in induction of the fish innate immune response against RNA and DNA viruses. J. Virol. 83, 7815–7827.

Bielek, E., 2002. Rodlet cells in teleosts: new ultrastructural observations on the distribution of the cores in trout (*Oncorhynchus mykiss*, *Salmo trutta* L.). J. Submicrosc. Cytol. Pathol. 34, 271–278.

Boardman, T., Warner, C., Ramirez-Gomez, F., Matrisciano, J., Bromage, E., 2012. Characterization of an anti-rainbow trout (*Oncorhynchus mykiss*) CD3epsilon monoclonal antibody. Vet. Immunol. Immunopathol. 145, 511–515.

Boehm, U., Klamp, T., Groot, M., Howard, J.C., 1997. Cellular responses to interferon-gamma. Annu. Rev. Immunol. 15, 749–795.

Boes, M., 2000. Role of natural and immune IgM antibodies in immune responses. Mol. Immunol. 37, 1141–1149.

Boltana, S., Roher, N., Goetz, F.W., Mackenzie, S.A., 2011. PAMPs, PRRs and the genomics of gram negative bacterial recognition in fish. Dev. Comp. Immunol. 35, 1195–1203.

Bonneville, M., O'Brien, R.L., Born, W.K., 2010. Gammadelta T cell effector functions: a blend of innate programming and acquired plasticity. Nat. Rev. Immunol. 10, 467–478.

Boshra, H., Li, J., Sunyer, J.O., 2006. Recent advances on the complement system of teleost fish. Fish Shellfish Immunol. 20, 239–262.

Bromage, E.S., Kaattari, I.M., Zwollo, P., Kaattari, S.L., 2004. Plasmablast and plasma cell production and distribution in trout immune tissues. J. Immunol. 173, 7317–7323.

Buonocore, F., Randelli, E., Bird, S., Secombes, C.J., Costantini, S., Facchiano, A., Mazzini, M., Scapigliati, G., 2006. The CD8alpha from sea bass (*Dicentrarchus labrax L.*): Cloning, expression and 3D modelling. Fish Shellfish Immunol. 20, 637–646.

Buonocore, F., Randelli, E., Casani, D., Guerra, L., Picchietti, S., Costantini, S., Facchiano, A.M., Zou, J., Secombes, C.J., Scapigliati, G., 2008. A CD4 homologue in sea bass (*Dicentrarchus labrax*): molecular characterization and structural analysis. Mol. Immunol. 45, 3168–3177.

Cai, Z., Gao, C., Zhang, Y., Xing, K., 2009. Functional characterization of the ELR motif in piscine ELR + CXC-like chemokine. Mar. Biotechnol. (NY) 11, 505–512.

Caipang, C.M.A., Hirono, I., Aoki, T., 2003. *In vitro* inhibition of fish rhabdoviruses by Japanese flounder, *Paralichthys olivaceus* Mx. Virology 317, 373–382.

Casadei, E., Wang, T., Zou, J., Gonzalez Vecino, J.L., Wadsworth, S., Secombes, C.J., 2009. Characterization of three novel beta-defensin antimicrobial peptides in rainbow trout (*Oncorhynchus mykiss*). Mol. Immunol. 46, 3358–3366.

Casali, P., Schettino, E.W., 1996. Structure and function of natural antibodies. Curr. Top. Microbiol. Immunol. 210, 167–179.
Castro, R., Bromage, E., Abos, B., Pignatelli, J., Gonzalez Granja, A., Luque, A., Tafalla, C., 2014a. CCR7 is mainly expressed in teleost gills, where it defines an IgD+IgM- B symphocyte subset. J. Immunol. 192, 1257–1266.
Castro, R., Jouneau, L., Pham, H.P., Bouchez, O., Giudicelli, V., Lefranc, M.P., Quillet, E., Benmansour, A., Cazals, F., Six, A., Fillatreau, S., Sunyer, O., Boudinot, P., 2013. Teleost fish mount complex clonal IgM and IgT responses in spleen upon systemic viral infection. PLoS Pathog. 9, e1003098.
Castro, R., Martinez-Alonso, S., Fischer, U., Haro, N.A., Soto-Lampe, V., Wang, T., Secombes, C.J., Lorenzen, N., Lorenzen, E., Tafalla, C., 2014b. DNA vaccination against a fish rhabdovirus promotes an early chemokine-related recruitment of B cells to the muscle. Vaccine 32, 1160–1168.
Chang, C.I., Pleguezuelos, O., Zhang, Y.A., Zou, J., Secombes, C.J., 2005. Identification of a novel cathelicidin gene in the rainbow trout, *Oncorhynchus mykiss*. Infect. Immunol. 73, 5053–5064.
Chang, M., Collet, B., Nie, P., Lester, K., Campbell, S., Secombes, C.J., Zou, J., 2011. Expression and functional characterization of the RIG-I-like receptors MDA5 and LGP2 in Rainbow trout (*Oncorhynchus mykiss*). J. Virol. 85, 8403–8412.
Chaves-Pozo, E., Pelegrin, P., Mulero, V., Meseguer, J., Garcia Ayala, A., 2003. A role for acidophilic granulocytes in the testis of the gilthead seabream (*Sparus aurata* L., *Teleostei*). J. Endocrinol. 179, 165–174.
Chen, J., Lu, X.J., Yang, H.Y., Shi, Y.H., 2010a. An interaction between a C-type lectin receptor and leukocyte cell-derived chemotaxin 2 of ayu, *Plecoglossus altivelis*. Fish Shellfish Immunol. 28, 245–248.
Chen, J., Xu, Q., Wang, T., Collet, B., Corripio-Miyar, Y., Bird, S., Xie, P., Nie, P., Secombes, C.J., Zou, J., 2013. Phylogenetic analysis of vertebrate CXC chemokines reveals novel lineage specific groups in teleost fish. Dev. Comp. Immunol. 41, 137–152.
Chen, K., Cerutti, A., 2010. New insights into the enigma of immunoglobulin D. Immunol. Rev. 237, 160–179.
Chen, K., Xu, W., Wilson, M., He, B., Miller, N.W., Bengten, E., Edholm, E.S., Santini, P.A., Rath, P., Chiu, A., Cattalini, M., Litzman, J., J, B.B., Huang, B., Meini, A., Riesbeck, K., Cunningham-Rundles, C., Plebani, A., Cerutti, A., 2009. Immunoglobulin D enhances immune surveillance by activating antimicrobial, proinflammatory and B cell-stimulating programs in basophils. Nat. Immunol. 10, 889–898.
Chen, W.Q., Xu, Q.Q., Chang, M.X., Zou, J., Secombes, C.J., Peng, K.M., Nie, P., 2010b. Molecular characterization and expression analysis of the IFN-gamma related gene (IFN-gammarel) in grass carp *Ctenopharyngodon idella*. Vet. Immunol. Immunopathol. 134, 199–207.
Chen, Y.M., Su, Y.L., Lin, J.H., Yang, H.L., Chen, T.Y., 2006. Cloning of an orange-spotted grouper (*Epinephelus coioides*) Mx cDNA and characterisation of its expression in response to nodavirus. Fish Shellfish Immunol. 20, 58–71.
Chia, T.J., Wu, Y.C., Chen, J.Y., Chi, S.C., 2010. Antimicrobial peptides (AMP) with antiviral activity against fish nodavirus. Fish Shellfish Immunol. 28, 434–439.
Chilmonczyk, S., 1992. The thymus in fish: development and possible function in the immune response. Ann. Rev. Fish Dis 181–200.
Clark-Lewis, I., Dewald, B., Geiser, T., Moser, B., Baggiolini, M., 1993. Platelet factor 4 binds to interleukin 8 receptors and activates neutrophils when its N terminus is modified with Glu-Leu-Arg. Proc. Natl. Acad. Sci. U.S.A. 90, 3574–3577.
Clark-Lewis, I., Schumacher, C., Baggiolini, M., Moser, B., 1991. Structure-activity relationships of interleukin-8 determined using chemically synthesized analogs. Critical role of

NH_2-terminal residues and evidence for uncoupling of neutrophil chemotaxis, exocytosis, and receptor binding activities. J. Biol. Chem. 266, 23128–23134.
Colucci-Guyon, E., Tinevez, J.Y., Renshaw, S.A., Herbomel, P., 2011. Strategies of professional phagocytes *in vivo*: unlike macrophages, neutrophils engulf only surface-associated microbes. J. Cell Sci. 124, 3053–3059.
Collet, B., Secombes, C.J., 2002. Type 1-interferon signalling in fish. Fish Shellfish Immunol. 12, 389–397.
Criscitiello, M.F., Ohta, Y., Saltis, M., McKinney, E.C., Flajnik, M.F., 2010. Evolutionarily conserved TCR binding sites, identification of T cells in primary lymphoid tissues, and surprising trans-rearrangements in nurse shark. J. Immunol. 184, 6950–6960.
Criscitiello, M.F., Saltis, M., Flajnik, M.F., 2006. An evolutionarily mobile antigen receptor variable region gene: doubly rearranging NAR-TcR genes in sharks. Proc. Natl. Acad. Sci. U.S.A. 103, 5036–5041.
Cuesta, A., Angeles Esteban, M., Meseguer, J., 2006. Cloning, distribution and up-regulation of the teleost fish MHC class II alpha suggests a role for granulocytes as antigen-presenting cells. Mol. Immunol. 43, 1275–1285.
Cuesta, A., Meseguer, J., Esteban, M.A., 2008. The antimicrobial peptide hepcidin exerts an important role in the innate immunity against bacteria in the bony fish gilthead seabream. Mol. Immunol. 45, 2333–2342.
Cuesta, A., Tafalla, C., 2009. Transcription of immune genes upon challenge with viral hemorrhagic septicemia virus (VHSV) in DNA vaccinated rainbow trout (*Oncorhynchus mykiss*). Vaccine 27, 280–289.
Cyster, J.G., Ngo, V.N., Ekland, E.H., Gunn, M.D., Sedgwick, J.D., Ansel, K.M., 1999. Chemokines and B-cell homing to follicles. Curr. Top. Microbiol. Immunol. 246, 87–92, discussion 93.
Daniels, G.D., Zou, J., Charlemagne, J., Partula, S., Cunningham, C., Secombes, C.J., 1999. Cloning of two chemokine receptor homologs (CXC-R4 and CC-R7) in rainbow trout *Oncorhynchus mykiss*. J. Leukoc. Biol. 65, 684–690.
Danilova, N., Bussmann, J., Jekosch, K., Steiner, L.A., 2005. The immunoglobulin heavy-chain locus in zebrafish: identification and expression of a previously unknown isotype, immunoglobulin Z. Nat. Immunol. 6, 295–302.
Danzmann, R.G., Davidson, E.A., Ferguson, M.M., Gharbi, K., Koop, B.F., Hoyheim, B., Lien, S., Lubieniecki, K.P., Moghadam, H.K., Park, J., Phillips, R.B., Davidson, W.S., 2008. Distribution of ancestral proto-Actinopterygian chromosome arms within the genomes of 4R-derivative salmonid fishes (Rainbow trout and Atlantic salmon). BMC Genom. 9, 557.
Das, S., Hirano, M., Tako, R., McCallister, C., Nikolaidis, N., 2012. Evolutionary genomics of immunoglobulin-encoding Loci in vertebrates. Curr. Genom. 13, 95–102.
DeVries, M.E., Kelvin, A.A., Xu, L., Ran, L., Robinson, J., Kelvin, D.J., 2006. Defining the origins and evolution of the chemokine/chemokine receptor system. J. Immunol. 176, 401–415.
Dezfuli, B.S., Giari, L., 2008. Mast cells in the gills and intestines of naturally infected fish: evidence of migration and degranulation. J. Fish Dis. 31, 845–852.
Dijkstra, J.M., Somamoto, T., Moore, L., Hordvik, I., Ototake, M., Fischer, U., 2006. Identification and characterization of a second CD4-like gene in teleost fish. Mol. Immunol. 43, 410–419.
Dixon, B., Luque, A., Abos, B., Castro, R., Gonzalez-Torres, L., Tafalla, C., 2013. Molecular characterization of three novel chemokine receptors in rainbow trout (*Oncorhynchus mykiss*). Fish Shellfish Immunol. 34, 641–651.
Dixon, B., Shum, B., Adams, E.J., Magor, K.E., Hedrick, R.P., Muir, D.G., Parham, P., 1998. CK-1, a putative chemokine of rainbow trout (*Oncorhynchus mykiss*). Immunol. Rev. 166, 341–348.

Dixon, B., vanHerp, S.H., Rodrigues, P.N., Egberts, E., Stet, R.J., 1995. Fish major histocompatibility complex genes: an expansion. Dev. Comp. Immunol. 19, 109–133.

Doitsidou, M., Reichman-Fried, M., Stebler, J., Koprunner, M., Dorries, J., Meyer, D., Esguerra, C.V., Leung, T., Raz, E., 2002. Guidance of primordial germ cell migration by the chemokine SDF-1. Cell 111, 647–659.

Dooley, H., Flajnik, M.F., 2006. Antibody repertoire development in cartilaginous fish. Dev. Comp. Immunol. 30, 43–56.

Duty, J.A., Szodoray, P., Zheng, N.Y., Koelsch, K.A., Zhang, Q., Swiatkowski, M., Mathias, M., Garman, L., Helms, C., Nakken, B., Smith, K., Farris, A.D., Wilson, P.C., 2009. Functional anergy in a subpopulation of naive B cells from healthy humans that express autoreactive immunoglobulin receptors. J. Exp. Med. 206, 139–151.

Edholm, E.S., Bengten, E., Stafford, J.L., Sahoo, M., Taylor, E.B., Miller, N.W., Wilson, M., 2010. Identification of two IgD+ B cell populations in channel catfish, *Ictalurus punctatus*. J. Immunol. 185, 4082–4094.

Edholm, E.S., Stafford, J.L., Quiniou, S.M., Waldbieser, G., Miller, N.W., Bengten, E., Wilson, M., 2007. Channel catfish, *Ictalurus punctatus*, CD4-like molecules. Dev. Comp. Immunol. 31, 172–187.

Ellis, A.E., 1977. The leucocytes of fish: a review. J. Fish Biol. 11, 453–491.

Ellis, A.E., 2001. Innate host defense mechanisms of fish against viruses and bacteria. Dev. Comp. Immunol. 25, 827–839.

Evans, D.L., Harris, D.T., Staton, D.L., Friedman, L.J., 1990. Pathways of signal transduction in teleost nonspecific cytotoxic cells. Dev. Comp. Immunol. 14, 295–304.

Fagerland, H.A., Austbo, L., Fritsvold, C., Alarcon, M., Rimstad, E., Falk, K., Taksdal, T., Koppang, E.O., 2013. Pathological pigmentation in cardiac tissues of Atlantic salmon (*Salmo salar* L.) with cardiomyopathy syndrome. Vet. Res. 44, 107.

Fast, M.D., Ross, N.W., Mustafa, A., Sims, D.E., Johnson, S.C., Conboy, G.A., Speare, D.J., Johnson, G., Burka, J.F., 2002. Susceptibility of rainbow trout *Oncorhynchus mykiss*, Atlantic salmon *Salmo salar* and coho salmon *Oncorhynchus kisutch* to experimental infection with sea lice *Lepeophtheirus salmonis*. Dis. Aquat. Organ. 52, 57–68.

Fernandez-Trujillo, M.A., Garcia-Rosado, E., Alonso, M.C., Borrego, J.J., Alvarez, M.C., Bejar, J., 2011. Differential antiviral activity of Mx1, Mx2 and Mx3 proteins from gilthead seabream (*Sparus aurata*) against Infectious Pancreatic Necrosis Virus (IPNV). Mol. Immunol. 49, 107–114.

Fernandez-Trujillo, M.A., Garcia-Rosado, E., Alonso, M.C., Castro, D., Alvarez, M.C., Bejar, J., 2013. Mx1, Mx2 and Mx3 proteins from the gilthead seabream (*Sparus aurata*) show *in vitro* antiviral activity against RNA and DNA viruses. Mol. Immunol. 56, 630–636.

Fillatreau, S., Six, A., Magadan, S., Castro, R., Sunyer, J.O., Boudinot, P., 2013. The astonishing diversity of Ig classes and B cell repertoires in teleost fish. Front. Immunol. 4, 28.

Findly, R.C., Zhao, X., Noe, J., Camus, A.C., Dickerson, H.W., 2013. B cell memory following infection and challenge of channel catfish with *Ichthyophthirius multifiliis*. Dev. Comp. Immunol. 39, 302–311.

Fischer, U., Koppang, E.O., Nakanishi, T., 2013. Teleost T and NK cell immunity. Fish Shellfish Immunol. 35, 197–206.

Fischer, U., Utke, K., Somamoto, T., Kollner, B., Ototake, M., Nakanishi, T., 2006. Cytotoxic activities of fish leucocytes. Fish Shellfish Immunol. 20, 209–226.

Flajnik, M.F., 2002. Comparative analyses of immunoglobulin genes: surprises and portents. Nat. Rev. Immunol. 2, 688–698.

Flajnik, M.F., Kasahara, M., 2010. Origin and evolution of the adaptive immune system: genetic events and selective pressures. Nat. Rev. Genet. 11, 47–59.

Forlenza, M., Fink, I.R., Raes, G., Wiegertjes, G.F., 2011. Heterogeneity of macrophage activation in fish. Dev. Comp. Immunol. 35, 1246–1255.

Forlenza, M., Magez, S., Scharsack, J.P., Westphal, A., Savelkoul, H.F., Wiegertjes, G.F., 2009. Receptor-mediated and lectin-like activities of carp (*Cyprinus carpio*) TNF-alpha. J. Immunol. 183, 5319–5332.

Fujiki, K., Smith, C.M., Liu, L., Sundick, R.S., Dixon, B., 2003. Alternate forms of MHC class II-associated invariant chain are not produced by alternative splicing in rainbow trout (*Oncorhynchus mykiss*) but are encoded by separate genes. Dev. Comp. Immunol. 27, 377–391.

Galindo-Villegas, J., Mulero, I., Garcia-Alcazar, A., Munoz, I., Penalver-Mellado, M., Streitenberger, S., Scapigliati, G., Meseguer, J., Mulero, V., 2013. Recombinant TNFalpha as oral vaccine adjuvant protects European sea bass against vibriosis: insights into the role of the CCL25/CCR9 axis. Fish Shellfish Immunol. 35, 1260–1271.

Goetz, F.W., Iliev, D.B., McCauley, L.A., Liarte, C.Q., Tort, L.B., Planas, J.V., Mackenzie, S., 2004. Analysis of genes isolated from lipopolysaccharide-stimulated rainbow trout (*Oncorhynchus mykiss*) macrophages. Mol. Immunol. 41, 1199–1210.

Gonzalez, R., Charlemagne, J., Mahana, W., Avrameas, S., 1988. Specificity of natural serum antibodies present in phylogenetically distinct fish species. Immunology 63, 31–36.

Gonzalez, R., Matsiota, P., Torchy, C., De Kinkelin, P., Avrameas, S., 1989. Natural anti-TNP antibodies from rainbow trout interfere with viral infection *in vitro*. Res. Immunol. 140, 675–684.

Gordon, R.J., McGregor, A.L., Connor, B., 2009. Chemokines direct neural progenitor cell migration following striatal cell loss. Mol. Cell Neurosci. 41, 219–232.

Grassi Milano, E., Basari, F., Chimenti, C., 1997. Adrenocortical and adrenomedullary homologs in eight species of adult and developing teleosts: morphology, histology, and immunohistochemistry. Gen. Comp. Endocrinol. 108, 483–496.

Grayfer, L., Walsh, J.G., Belosevic, M., 2008. Characterization and functional analysis of goldfish *Carassius auratus* tumor necrosis factor-alpha. Dev. Comp. Immunol. 32, 532–543.

Grayfer, L., Belosevic, M., 2009. Molecular characterization, expression and functional analysis of goldfish (*Carassius aurutus* L.) interferon gamma. Dev. Comp. Immunol. 33, 235–246.

Grayfer, L., Garcia, E.G., Belosevic, M., 2010. Comparison of macrophage antimicrobial responses induced by type II interferons of the goldfish (*Carassius auratus* L.). J. Biol. Chem. 285, 23537–23547.

Grayfer, L., Hanington, P.C., Belosevic, M., 2009. Macrophage colony-stimulating factor (CSF-1) induces pro-inflammatory gene expression and enhances antimicrobial responses of goldfish (*Carassius auratus* L.) macrophages. Fish Shellfish Immunol. 26, 406–413.

Grinde, B., 1989. A lysozyme isolated from rainbow trout acts on mastitis pathogens. FEMS Microbiol. Lett. 51, 179–182.

Hansen, J.D., 1997. Characterization of rainbow trout terminal deoxynucleotidyl transferase structure and expression. TdT and RAG1 co-expression define the trout primary lymphoid tissues. Immunogenetics 46, 367–375.

Hansen, J.D., Landis, E.D., Phillips, R.B., 2005. Discovery of a unique Ig heavy-chain isotype (IgT) in rainbow trout: implications for a distinctive B cell developmental pathway in teleost fish. Proc. Natl. Acad. Sci. U.S.A. 102, 6919–6924.

Hansen, J.D., Strassburger, P., 2000. Description of an ectothermic TCR coreceptor, CD8 alpha, in rainbow trout. J. Immunol. 164, 3132–3139.

Hansen, J.D., Strassburger, P., Du Pasquier, L., 1997. Conservation of a master hematopoietic switch gene during vertebrate evolution: isolation and characterization of Ikaros from teleost and amphibian species. Eur. J. Immunol. 27, 3049–3058.

Hardie, L.J., Laing, K.J., Daniels, G.D., Grabowski, P.S., Cunningham, C., Secombes, C.J., 1998. Isolation of the first piscine transforming growth factor beta gene: analysis reveals tissue specific expression and a potential regulatory sequence in rainbow trout (*Oncorhynchus mykiss*). Cytokine 10, 555–563.

Harms, C.A., Kennedy-Stoskopf, S., Horne, W.A., Fuller, F.J., Tompkins, W.A., 2000. Cloning and sequencing hybrid striped bass (*Morone saxatilis x M. chrysops*) transforming growth factor-beta (TGF-beta), and development of a reverse transcription quantitative competitive polymerase chain reaction (RT-qcPCR) assay to measure TGF-beta mRNA of teleost fish. Fish Shellfish Immunol. 10, 61–85.

Harun, N.O., Zou, J., Zhang, Y.A., Nie, P., Secombes, C.J., 2008. The biological effects of rainbow trout (*Oncorhynchus mykiss*) recombinant interleukin-8. Dev. Comp. Immunol. 32, 673–681.

Haugarvoll, E., Bjerkas, I., Nowak, B.F., Hordvik, I., Koppang, E.O., 2008. Identification and characterization of a novel intraepithelial lymphoid tissue in the gills of Atlantic salmon. J. Anat. 213, 202–209.

Haugland, G.T., Jordal, A.E., Wergeland, H.I., 2012. Characterization of small, mononuclear blood cells from salmon having high phagocytic capacity and ability to differentiate into dendritic like cells. PLoS One 7, e49260.

Hebert, C.A., Vitangcol, R.V., Baker, J.B., 1991. Scanning mutagenesis of interleukin-8 identifies a cluster of residues required for receptor binding. J. Biol. Chem. 266, 18989–18994.

Henry, K.M., Loynes, C.A., Whyte, M.K., Renshaw, S.A., 2013. Zebrafish as a model for the study of neutrophil biology. J. Leukoc. Biol. 94, 633–642.

Hill, D.J., Rowley, A.F., 1998. Are integrins involved in the aggregatory and phagocytic behaviour of fish haemostatic cells? J. Exp. Biol. 201, 599–608.

Hsu, E., Pulham, N., Rumfelt, L.L., Flajnik, M.F., 2006. The plasticity of immunoglobulin gene systems in evolution. Immunol. Rev. 210, 8–26.

Huising, M.O., Stet, R.J., Kruiswijk, C.P., Savelkoul, H.F., Lidy Verburg-van Kemenade, B.M., 2003. Molecular evolution of CXC chemokines: extant CXC chemokines originate from the CNS. Trends Immunol. 24, 307–313.

Huising, M.O., Stet, R.J., Savelkoul, H.F., Verburg-van Kemenade, B.M., 2004. The molecular evolution of the interleukin-1 family of cytokines; IL-18 in teleost fish. Dev. Comp. Immunol. 28, 395–413.

Igawa, D., Sakai, M., Savan, R., 2006. An unexpected discovery of two interferon gamma-like genes along with interleukin (IL)-22 and -26 from teleost: IL-22 and -26 genes have been described for the first time outside mammals. Mol. Immunol. 43, 999–1009.

Ingerslev, H.C., Ronneseth, A., Pettersen, E.F., Wergeland, H.I., 2009. Differential expression of immune genes in Atlantic salmon (*Salmo salar L.*) challenged intraperitoneally or by cohabitation with IPNV. Scand. J. Immunol. 69, 90–98.

Inoue, Y., Kamota, S., Ito, K., Yoshiura, Y., Ototake, M., Moritomo, T., Nakanishi, T., 2005. Molecular cloning and expression analysis of rainbow trout (*Oncorhynchus mykiss*) interleukin-10 cDNAs. Fish Shellfish Immunol. 18, 335–344.

Jana, M., Pahan, K., 2009. Induction of lymphotoxin-alpha by interleukin-12 p40 homodimer, the so-called biologically inactive molecule, but not IL-12 p70. Immunology 127, 312–325.

Jaso-Friedmann, L., Leary, 3rd, J.H., Evans, D.L., 2001. The non-specific cytotoxic cell receptor (NCCRP-1): molecular organization and signaling properties. Dev. Comp. Immunol. 25, 701–711.

Jensen, V., Robertsen, B., 2000. Cloning of an Mx cDNA from Atlantic halibut (*Hippoglossus hippoglossus*) and characterization of Mx mRNA expression in response to double-stranded RNA or infectious pancreatic necrosis virus. J. Interferon Cytokine Res. 20, 701–710.

Jin, J.Y., Zhou, L., Wang, Y., Li, Z., Zhao, J.G., Zhang, Q.Y., Gui, J.F., 2010. Antibacterial and antiviral roles of a fish beta-defensin expressed both in pituitary and testis. PLoS One 5, e12883.

Johansson, P., Corripio-Miyar, Y., Wang, T., Collet, B., Secombes, C.J., Zou, J., 2012. Characterisation and expression analysis of the rainbow trout (*Oncorhynchus mykiss*) homologue of the human dendritic cell marker CD208/lysosomal associated membrane protein 3. Dev. Comp. Immunol. 37, 402–413.

Jones, S.R., 2001. The occurrence and mechanisms of innate immunity against parasites in fish. Dev. Comp. Immunol. 25, 841–852.

Jorgensen, J.B., Johansen, A., Hegseth, M.N., Zou, J., Robertsen, B., Collet, B., Secombes, C.J., 2007. A recombinant CHSE-214 cell line expressing an Mx1 promoter-reporter system responds to both interferon type I and type II from salmonids and represents a versatile tool to study the IFN-system in teleost fish. Fish Shellfish Immunol. 23, 1294–1303.

Jorgensen, T.R., Raida, M.K., Kania, P.W., Buchmann, K., 2009. Response of rainbow trout (*Oncorhynchus mykiss*) in skin and fin tissue during infection with a variant of *Gyrodactylus salaris* (Monogenea: Gyrodactylidae). Folia Parasitol. (Praha) 56, 251–258.

Kaattari, S., Evans, D., Klemer, J., 1998. Varied redox forms of teleost IgM: an alternative to isotypic diversity? Immunol. Rev. 166, 133–142.

Kaattari, S.L., Zhang, H.L., Khor, I.W., Kaattari, I.M., Shapiro, D.A., 2002. Affinity maturation in trout: clonal dominance of high affinity antibodies late in the immune response. Dev. Comp. Immunol. 26, 191–200.

Keane, M.P., Arenberg, D.A., Moore, B.B., Addison, C.L., Strieter, R.M., 1998. CXC chemokines and angiogenesis/angiostasis. Proc. Assoc. Am. Physicians 110, 288–296.

Kee, B.L., Rivera, R.R., Murre, C., 2001. Id3 inhibits B lymphocyte progenitor growth and survival in response to TGF-beta. Nat. Immunol. 2, 242–247.

Kinoshita, S., Biswas, G., Kono, T., Hikima, J., Sakai, M., 2014. Presence of two tumor necrosis factor (tnf)-alpha homologs on different chromosomes of zebrafish (*Danio rerio*) and medaka (*Oryzias latipes*). Mar. Genom. 13, 1–9.

Kleinewietfeld, M., Hafler, D.A., 2013. The plasticity of human Treg and Th17 cells and its role in autoimmunity. Semin. Immunol. 25, 305–312.

Knaut, H., Werz, C., Geisler, R., Nusslein-Volhard, C., 2003. A zebrafish homologue of the chemokine receptor Cxcr4 is a germ-cell guidance receptor. Nature 421, 279–282.

Kohli, G., Hu, S., Clelland, E., Di Muccio, T., Rothenstein, J., Peng, C., 2003. Cloning of transforming growth factor-beta 1 (TGF-beta 1) and its type II receptor from zebrafish ovary and role of TGF-beta 1 in oocyte maturation. Endocrinology 144, 1931–1941.

Kollner, B., Fischer, U., Rombout, J.H., Taverne-Thiele, J.J., Hansen, J.D., 2004. Potential involvement of rainbow trout thrombocytes in immune functions: a study using a panel of monoclonal antibodies and RT-PCR. Dev. Comp. Immunol. 28, 1049–1062.

Koppang, E.O., Fischer, U., Moore, L., Tranulis, M.A., Dijkstra, J.M., Kollner, B., Aune, L., Jirillo, E., Hordvik, I., 2010. Salmonid T cells assemble in the thymus, spleen and in novel interbranchial lymphoid tissue. J. Anat. 217, 728–739.

Laing, K.J., Hansen, J.D., 2011. Fish T cells: recent advances through genomics. Dev. Comp. Immunol. 35, 1282–1295.

Laing, K.J., Purcell, M.K., Winton, J.R., Hansen, J.D., 2008. A genomic view of the NOD-like receptor family in teleost fish: identification of a novel NLR subfamily in zebrafish. BMC Evol. Biol. 8, 42.

Laing, K.J., Secombes, C.J., 2004a. Chemokines. Dev. Comp. Immunol. 28, 443–460.

Laing, K.J., Secombes, C.J., 2004b. Trout CC chemokines: comparison of their sequences and expression patterns. Mol. Immunol. 41, 793–808.

Laing, K.J., Zou, J.J., Purcell, M.K., Phillips, R., Secombes, C.J., Hansen, J.D., 2006. Evolution of the CD4 family: teleost fish possess two divergent forms of CD4 in addition to lymphocyte activation gene-3. J. Immunol. 177, 3939–3951.

Larsen, H.A., Austbo, L., Morkore, T., Thorsen, J., Hordvik, I., Fischer, U., Jirillo, E., Rimstad, E., Koppang, E.O., 2012. Pigment-producing granulomatous myopathy in Atlantic salmon: a novel inflammatory response. Fish Shellfish Immunol. 33, 277–285.

Larsen, R., Rokenes, T.P., Robertsen, B., 2004. Inhibition of infectious pancreatic necrosis virus replication by Atlantic salmon Mx1 protein. J. Virol. 78, 7938–7944.

Lauksund, S., Svingerud, T., Bergan, V., Robertsen, B., 2009. Atlantic salmon IPS-1 mediates induction of IFNa1 and activation of NF-kappaB and localizes to mitochondria. Dev. Comp. Immunol. 33, 1196–1204.

Lee, J.Y., Hirono, I., Aoki, T., 2000. Cloning and analysis of expression of Mx cDNA in Japanese flounder, *Paralichthys olivaceus*. Dev. Comp. Immunol. 24, 407–415.

Leino, R.L., 1996. Reaction of rodlet cells to a myxosporean infection in kidney of the bluegill, *Lepomis macrochirus*. Can. J. Zool. 74, 217–225.

Levraud, J.P., Boudinot, P., Colin, I., Benmansour, A., Peyrieras, N., Herbomel, P., Lutfalla, G., 2007. Identification of the zebrafish IFN receptor: implications for the origin of the vertebrate IFN system. J. Immunol. 178, 4385–4394.

Li, J., Barreda, D.R., Zhang, Y.A., Boshra, H., Gelman, A.E., Lapatra, S., Tort, L., Sunyer, J.O., 2006. B lymphocytes from early vertebrates have potent phagocytic and microbicidal abilities. Nat. Immunol. 7, 1116–1124.

Li, J.H., Shao, J.Z., Xiang, L.X., Wen, Y., 2007. Cloning, characterization and expression analysis of pufferfish interleukin-4 cDNA: the first evidence of Th2-type cytokine in fish. Mol. Immunol. 44, 2078–2086.

Li, M.O., Flavell, R.A., 2006. TGF-beta, T-cell tolerance and immunotherapy of autoimmune diseases and cancer. Exp. Rev. Clin. Immunol. 2, 257–265.

Lie, O., Evensen, O., Sorensen, A., Froysadal, E., 1989. Study on lysozyme activity in some fish species. Dis. Aquat. Organ. 6, 1–5.

Lieberman, J., 2003. The ABCs of granule-mediated cytotoxicity: new weapons in the arsenal. Nat. Rev. Immunol. 3, 361–370.

Lieschke, G.J., Oates, A.C., Crowhurst, M.O., Ward, A.C., Layton, J.E., 2001. Morphologic and functional characterization of granulocytes and macrophages in embryonic and adult zebrafish. Blood 98, 3087–3096.

Liu, L., Fujiki, K., Dixon, B., Sundick, R.S., 2002. Cloning of a novel rainbow trout (*Oncorhynchus mykiss*) CC chemokine with a fractalkine-like stalk and a TNF decoy receptor using cDNA fragments containing AU-rich elements. Cytokine 17, 71–81.

Lopez-Munoz, A., Roca, F.J., Meseguer, J., Mulero, V., 2009. New insights into the evolution of IFNs: zebrafish group II IFNs induce a rapid and transient expression of IFN-dependent genes and display powerful antiviral activities. J. Immunol. 182, 3440–3449.

Lovoll, M., Kilvik, T., Boshra, H., Bogwald, J., Sunyer, J.O., Dalmo, R.A., 2006. Maternal transfer of complement components C3-1, C3-3, C3-4, C4, C5, C7, Bf, and Df to offspring in rainbow trout (*Oncorhynchus mykiss*). Immunogenetics 58, 168–179.

Lovy, J., Savidant, G.P., Speare, D.J., Wright, G.M., 2009. Langerin/CD207 positive dendritic-like cells in the haemopoietic tissues of salmonids. Fish Shellfish Immunol. 27, 365–368.

Lovy, J., Wright, G.M., Speare, D.J., 2006. Morphological presentation of a dendritic-like cell within the gills of chinook salmon infected with *Loma salmonae*. Dev. Comp. Immunol. 30, 259–263.

Lugo-Villarino, G., Balla, K.M., Stachura, D.L., Banuelos, K., Werneck, M.B., Traver, D., 2010. Identification of dendritic antigen-presenting cells in the zebrafish. Proc. Natl. Acad. Sci. U.S.A. 107, 15850–15855.

Lutfalla, G., Crollius, H.R., Stange-Thomann, N., Jaillon, O., Mogensen, K., Monneron, D., 2003. Comparative genomic analysis reveals independent expansion of a lineage-specific gene family in vertebrates: the class II cytokine receptors and their ligands in mammals and fish. BMC Genom. 4, 29.

Lutz, H.U., 2007. Homeostatic roles of naturally occurring antibodies: an overview. J. Autoimmun. 29, 287–294.

Ma, C., Ye, J., Kaattari, S.L., 2013a. Differential compartmentalization of memory B cells versus plasma cells in salmonid fish. Eur. J. Immunol. 43, 360–370.

Ma, D., Wei, Y., Liu, F., 2013b. Regulatory mechanisms of thymus and T cell development. Dev. Comp. Immunol. 39, 91–102.

Mackay, C.R., 1997. Chemokines: what chemokine is that? Curr. Biol. 7, R384–R386.

Mackintosh, J.A., 2001. The antimicrobial properties of melanocytes, melanosomes and melanin and the evolution of black skin. J. Theor. Biol. 211, 101–113.

Magnadottir, B., 2006. Innate immunity of fish (overview). Fish Shellfish Immunol. 20, 137–151.

Magnadottir, B., Gudmundsdottir, S., Gudmundsdottir, B.K., Helgason, S., 2009. Natural antibodies of cod (*Gadus morhua L.*): specificity, activity and affinity. Comp. Biochem. Physiol. B Biochem. Mol. Biol. 154, 309–316.

Malecek, K., Lee, V., Feng, W., Huang, J.L., Flajnik, M.F., Ohta, Y., Hsu, E., 2008. Immunoglobulin heavy chain exclusion in the shark. PLoS Biol. 6, e157.

Manera, M., Dezfulli, B.S., 2004. Rodlet cells in teleosts: a new insight into their nature and functions. J. Fish Biol. 65, 597–619.

Mantovani, A., Sica, A., Sozzani, S., Allavena, P., Vecchi, A., Locati, M., 2004. The chemokine system in diverse forms of macrophage activation and polarization. Trends Immunol. 25, 677–686.

Martin, S.A., Mohanty, B.P., Cash, P., Houlihan, D.F., Secombes, C.J., 2007. Proteome analysis of the Atlantic salmon (*Salmo salar*) cell line SHK-1 following recombinant IFN-gamma stimulation. Proteomics 7, 2275–2286.

Martinon, F., Tschopp, J., 2005. NLRs join TLRs as innate sensors of pathogens. Trends Immunol. 26, 447–454.

McKinney, E.C., Schmale, M.C., 1997. Damselfish with neurofibromatosis exhibit cytotoxicity towards retrovirus infected cells. Dev. Comp. Immunol. 21, 287–298.

Meseguer, J., Esteban, M.A., Garcia-Ayala, A., Lopez-Ruiz, A., 1992. Ultrastructural study of the phagocytotic mechanism in blood thrombocytes of sea bass (*Dicentrarus labrax* L.). Electron Microsc. 3, 589–590.

Meyer, A., Van de Peer, Y., 2005. From 2R to 3R: evidence for a fish-specific genome duplication (FSGD). Bioessays 27, 937–945.

Mihajlovic, M., Lazaridis, T., 2010. Antimicrobial peptides in toroidal and cylindrical pores. Biochim. Biophys. Acta 1798, 1485–1493.

Milev-Milovanovic, I., Long, S., Wilson, M., Bengten, E., Miller, N.W., Chinchar, V.G., 2006. Identification and expression analysis of interferon gamma genes in channel catfish. Immunogenetics 58, 70–80.

Miller, K.M., Winton, J.R., Schulze, A.D., Purcell, M.K., Ming, T.J., 2004. Major histocompatibility complex loci are associated with susceptibility of Atlantic salmon to infectious hematopoietic necrosis virus. Environ. Biol. Fish. 69, 307–316.

Modolell, M., Corraliza, I.M., Link, F., Soler, G., Eichmann, K., 1995. Reciprocal regulation of the nitric oxide synthase/arginase balance in mouse bone marrow-derived macrophages by TH1 and TH2 cytokines. Eur. J. Immunol. 25, 1101–1104.

Moore, L.J., Dijkstra, J.M., Koppang, E.O., Hordvik, I., 2009. CD4 homologues in Atlantic salmon. Fish Shellfish Immunol. 26, 10–18.

Moore, L.J., Somamoto, T., Lie, K.K., Dijkstra, J.M., Hordvik, I., 2005. Characterisation of salmon and trout CD8alpha and CD8beta. Mol. Immunol. 42, 1225–1234.

Nakanishi, T., Toda, H., Shibasaki, Y., Somamoto, T., 2011. Cytotoxic T cells in teleost fish. Dev. Comp. Immunol. 35, 1317–1323.

Nakao, M., Kato-Unoki, Y., Nakahara, M., Mutsuro, J., Somamoto, T., 2006. Diversified components of the bony fish complement system: more genes for robuster innate defense? Adv. Exp. Med. Biol. 586, 121–138.

Nakao, M., Mutsuro, J., Obo, R., Fujiki, K., Nonaka, M., Yano, T., 2000. Molecular cloning and protein analysis of divergent forms of the complement component C3 from a bony fish, the common carp (*Cyprinus carpio*): presence of variants lacking the catalytic histidine. Eur. J. Immunol. 30, 858–866.

Nakao, M., Tsujikura, M., Ichiki, S., Vo, T.K., Somamoto, T., 2011. The complement system in teleost fish: progress of post-homolog-hunting researches. Dev. Comp. Immunol. 35, 1296–1308.

Nakashima, M., Kinoshita, M., Nakashima, H., Habu, Y., Miyazaki, H., Shono, S., Hiroi, S., Shinomiya, N., Nakanishi, K., Seki, S., 2012. Pivotal advance: characterization of mouse liver phagocytic B cells in innate immunity. J. Leukoc. Biol. 91, 537–546.

Nam, B.H., Hirono, I., Aoki, T., 2003. The four TCR genes of teleost fish: the cDNA and genomic DNA analysis of Japanese flounder (*Paralichthys olivaceus*) TCR alpha-, beta-, gamma-, and delta-chains. J. Immunol. 170, 3081–3090.

Nam, B.H., Moon, J.Y., Kim, Y.O., Kong, H.J., Kim, W.J., Lee, S.J., Kim, K.K., 2010. Multiple beta-defensin isoforms identified in early developmental stages of the teleost *Paralichthys olivaceus*. Fish Shellfish Immunol. 28, 267–274.

Near, T.J., Eytan, R.I., Dornburg, A., Kuhn, K.L., Moore, J.A., Davis, M.P., Wainwright, P.C., Friedman, M., Smith, W.L., 2012. Resolution of ray-finned fish phylogeny and timing of diversification. Proc. Natl. Acad. Sci. U.S.A. 109, 13698–13703.

Neves, J.V., Wilson, J.M., Rodrigues, P.N., 2009. Transferrin and ferritin response to bacterial infection: the role of the liver and brain in fish. Dev. Comp. Immunol. 33, 848–857.

Nomiyama, H., Hieshima, K., Osada, N., Kato-Unoki, Y., Otsuka-Ono, K., Takegawa, S., Izawa, T., Yoshizawa, A., Kikuchi, Y., Tanase, S., Miura, R., Kusuda, J., Nakao, M., Yoshie, O., 2008. Extensive expansion and diversification of the chemokine gene family in zebrafish: identification of a novel chemokine subfamily CX. BMC Genom. 9, 222.

Ochsenbein, A.F., Fehr, T., Lutz, C., Suter, M., Brombacher, F., Hengartner, H., Zinkernagel, R.M., 1999. Control of early viral and bacterial distribution and disease by natural antibodies. Science 286, 2156–2159.

Ohta, Y., Flajnik, M., 2006. IgD, like IgM, is a primordial immunoglobulin class perpetuated in most jawed vertebrates. Proc. Natl. Acad. Sci. U.S.A. 103, 10723–10728.

Ohtani, M., Hayashi, N., Hashimoto, K., Nakanishi, T., Dijkstra, J.M., 2008. Comprehensive clarification of two paralogous interleukin 4/13 loci in teleost fish. Immunogenetics 60, 383–397.

Olsen, M.M., Kania, P.W., Heinecke, R.D., Skjoedt, K., Rasmussen, K.J., Buchmann, K., 2011. Cellular and humoral factors involved in the response of rainbow trout gills to Ichthyophthirius multifiliis infections: molecular and immunohistochemical studies. Fish Shellfish Immunol. 30, 859–869.

Palaksha, K.J., Shin, G.W., Kim, Y.R., Jung, T.S., 2008. Evaluation of non-specific immune components from the skin mucus of olive flounder (*Paralichthys olivaceus*). Fish Shellfish Immunol. 24, 479–488.

Pancer, Z., Amemiya, C.T., Ehrhardt, G.R., Ceitlin, J., Gartland, G.L., Cooper, M.D., 2004. Somatic diversification of variable lymphocyte receptors in the agnathan sea lamprey. Nature 430, 174–180.

Parra, D., Rieger, A.M., Li, J., Zhang, Y.A., Randall, L.M., Hunter, C.A., Barreda, D.R., Sunyer, J.O., 2012. Pivotal advance: peritoneal cavity B-1 B cells have phagocytic and microbicidal capacities and present phagocytosed antigen to CD4+ T cells. J. Leukoc. Biol. 91, 525–536.

Patel, S., Overgard, A.C., Nerland, A.H., 2008. CD8alpha and CD8beta in Atlantic halibut, *Hippoglossus hippoglossus*: cloning, characterization and gene expression during viral and bacterial infection. Fish Shellfish Immunol. 25, 570–580.

Patel, S., Overgard, A.C., Nerland, A.H., 2009. A CD4 homologue in Atlantic halibut (*Hippoglossus hippoglossus*): molecular cloning and characterisation. Fish Shellfish Immunol. 26, 377–384.

Peatman, E., Liu, Z., 2007. Evolution of CC chemokines in teleost fish: a case study in gene duplication and implications for immune diversity. Immunogenetics 59, 613–623.

Perlin, J.R., Talbot, W.S., 2007. Signals on the move: chemokine receptors and organogenesis in zebrafish. Sc. STKE 2007, pe45.

Pietretti, D., Wiegertjes, G.F., 2014. Ligand specificities of Toll-like receptors in fish: Indications from infection studies. Dev. Comp. Immunol. 43, 205–222.

Pijanowski, L., Golbach, L., Kolaczkowska, E., Scheer, M., Verburg-van Kemenade, B.M., Chadzinska, M., 2013. Carp neutrophilic granulocytes form extracellular traps via ROS-dependent and independent pathways. Fish Shellfish Immunol. 34, 1244–1252.

Pinto, R.D., Nascimento, D.S., Reis, M.I., do Vale, A., Dos Santos, N.M., 2007. Molecular characterization, 3D modelling and expression analysis of sea bass (*Dicentrarchus labrax L.*) interleukin-10. Mol. Immunol. 44, 2056–2065.

Pinto, R.D., Nascimento, D.S., Vale, A., Santos, N.M., 2006. Molecular cloning and characterization of sea bass (*Dicentrarchus labrax L.*) CD8alpha. Vet. Immunol. Immunopathol. 110, 169–177.

Plant, K.P., Thune, R.L., 2004. Cloning and characterisation of a channel catfish (*Ictalurus punctatus*) Mx gene. Fish Shellfish Immunol. 16, 391–405.

Raida, M.K., Nylen, J., Holten-Andersen, L., Buchmann, K., 2011. Association between plasma antibody response and protection in rainbow trout *Oncorhynchus mykiss* immersion vaccinated against *Yersinia ruckeri*. PLoS One 6, e18832.

Rajanbabu, V., Chen, J.Y., 2011. Applications of antimicrobial peptides from fish and perspectives for the future. Peptides 32, 415–420.

Rakus, K.L., Wiegertjes, G.F., Adamek, M., Siwicki, A.K., Lepa, A., Irnazarow, I., 2009. Resistance of common carp (*Cyprinus carpio L.*) to Cyprinid herpesvirus-3 is influenced by major histocompatibility (MH) class II B gene polymorphism. Fish Shellfish Immunol. 26, 737–743.

Ramirez-Gomez, F., Greene, W., Rego, K., Hansen, J.D., Costa, G., Kataria, P., Bromage, E.S., 2012. Discovery and characterization of secretory IgD in rainbow trout: secretory IgD is produced through a novel splicing mechanism. J. Immunol. 188, 1341–1349.

Ravi, V., Venkatesh, B., 2008. Rapidly evolving fish genomes and teleost diversity. Curr. Opin. Genet. Dev. 18, 544–550.

Razquin, B.E., Castillo, A., Lopez-Fierro, P., Alvarez, F., Zapata, A., Villena, A.J., 1990. Ontogeny of IgM-producing cells in the lymphoid organs of rainbow trout, Salmo gairdneri Richardson: an immuno- and enzyme-histochemical study. J. Fish Biol. 36, 159–173.

Rebl, A., Goldammer, T., Seyfert, H.M., 2010. Toll-like receptor signaling in bony fish. Vet. Immunol. Immunopathol. 134, 139–150.

Reite, O.B., Evensen, O., 2006. Inflammatory cells of teleostean fish: a review focusing on mast cells/eosinophilic granule cells and rodlet cells. Fish Shellfish Immunol. 20, 192–208.

Rieger, A.M., Barreda, D.R., 2011. Antimicrobial mechanisms of fish leukocytes. Dev. Comp. Immunol. 35, 1238–1245.

Rieger, A.M., Hall, B.E., Barreda, D.R., 2010. Macrophage activation differentially modulates particle binding, phagocytosis and downstream antimicrobial mechanisms. Dev. Comp. Immunol. 34, 1144–1159.

Robertsen, B., Bergan, V., Rokenes, T., Larsen, R., Albuquerque, A., 2003. Atlantic salmon interferon genes: cloning, sequence analysis, expression, and biological activity. J. Interferon Cytokine Res. 23, 601–612.

Robertsen, B., Trobridge, G., Leong, J.A., 1997. Molecular cloning of double-stranded RNA inducible Mx genes from Atlantic salmon (*Salmo salar* L.). Dev. Comp. Immunol. 21, 397–412.

Roca, F.J., Mulero, I., Lopez-Munoz, A., Sepulcre, M.P., Renshaw, S.A., Meseguer, J., Mulero, V., 2008. Evolution of the inflammatory response in vertebrates: fish TNF-alpha is a powerful activator of endothelial cells but hardly activates phagocytes. J. Immunol. 181, 5071–5081.

Romano, N., Caccia, E., Piergentili, R., Rossi, F., Ficca, A.G., Ceccariglia, S., Mastrolia, L., 2011. Antigen-dependent T lymphocytes (TcRbeta+) are primarily differentiated in the thymus rather than in other lymphoid tissues in sea bass (*Dicentrarchus labrax* L.). Fish Shellfish Immunol. 30, 773–782.

Rombout, J.H., Abelli, L., Picchietti, S., Scapigliati, G., Kiron, V., 2011. Teleost intestinal immunology. Fish Shellfish Immunol. 31, 616–626.

Rombout, J.H., Joosten, P.H., Engelsma, M.Y., Vos, A.P., Taverne, N., Taverne-Thiele, J.J., 1998. Indications for a distinct putative T cell population in mucosal tissue of carp (*Cyprinus carpio* L.). Dev. Comp. Immunol. 22, 63–77.

Romstad, A.B., Reitan, L.J., Midtlyng, P., Gravningen, K., Evensen, O., 2013. Antibody responses correlate with antigen dose and *in vivo* protection for oil-adjuvanted, experimental furunculosis (*Aeromonas salmonicida* subsp. *salmonicida*) vaccines in Atlantic salmon (*Salmo salar* L.) and can be used for batch potency testing of vaccines. Vaccine 31, 791–796.

Rowley, A.F., 1996. The evolution of inflammatory mediators. Mediators Inflamm. 5, 3–13.

Rumfelt, L.L., McKinney, E.C., Taylor, E., Flajnik, M.F., 2002. The development of primary and secondary lymphoid tissues in the nurse shark *Ginglymostoma cirratum*: B-cell zones precede dendritic cell immigration and T-cell zone formation during ontogeny of the spleen. Scand. J. Immunol. 56, 130–148.

Salinas, I., Zhang, Y.A., Sunyer, J.O., 2011. Mucosal immunoglobulins and B cells of teleost fish. Dev. Comp. Immunol. 35, 1346–1365.

Saurabh, S., Sahoo, P.K., 2008. Lysozyme: an important defence molecule of fish innate immune system. Aquacult. Res. 39, 223–239.

Savan, R., Igawa, D., Sakai, M., 2003. Cloning, characterization and expression analysis of interleukin-10 from the common carp, *Cyprinus carpio* L. Eur. J. Biochem. 270, 4647–4654.

Scapigliati, G., Romano, N., Abelli, L., Meloni, S., Ficca, A.G., Buonocore, F., Bird, S., Secombes, C.J., 2000. Immunopurification of T-cells from sea bass *Dicentrarchus labrax* (L.). Fish Shellfish Immunol. 10, 329–341.

Secombes, C.J., 1996. The non-specific immune system: cellular defences. In: Iwama, G., Nakanishi, T. (Eds.), The fish immune system: organisms, pathogen & enviroment. Academic Press, San Diego. pp. 63–103.

Secombes, C.J., Wang, T., Bird, S., 2011. The interleukins of fish. Dev. Comp. Immunol. 35, 1336–1345.

Seppola, M., Larsen, A.N., Steiro, K., Robertsen, B., Jensen, I., 2008. Characterisation and expression analysis of the interleukin genes, IL-1beta, IL-8 and IL-10, in Atlantic cod (*Gadus morhua* L.). Mol. Immunol. 45, 887–897.

Sepulcre, M.P., Alcaraz-Perez, F., Lopez-Munoz, A., Roca, F.J., Meseguer, J., Cayuela, M.L., Mulero, V., 2009. Evolution of lipopolysaccharide (LPS) recognition and signaling: fish TLR4 does not recognize LPS and negatively regulates NF-kappaB activation. J. Immunol. 182, 1836–1845.

Shen, L., Stuge, T.B., Bengten, E., Wilson, M., Chinchar, V.G., Naftel, J.P., Bernanke, J.M., Clem, L.W., Miller, N.W., 2004. Identification and characterization of clonal NK-like cells from channel catfish (*Ictalurus punctatus*). Dev. Comp. Immunol. 28, 139–152.

Shen, L., Stuge, T.B., Evenhuis, J.P., Bengten, E., Wilson, M., Chinchar, V.G., Clem, L.W., Miller, N.W., 2003. Channel catfish NK-like cells are armed with IgM via a putative FcmicroR. Dev. Comp. Immunol. 27, 699–714.

Sinyakov, M.S., Dror, M., Zhevelev, H.M., Margel, S., Avtalion, R.R., 2002. Natural antibodies and their significance in active immunization and protection against a defined pathogen in fish. Vaccine 20, 3668–3674.

Smith, J.J., Kuraku, S., Holt, C., Sauka-Spengler, T., Jiang, N., Campbell, M.S., Yandell, M.D., Manousaki, T., Meyer, A., Bloom, O.E., Morgan, J.R., Buxbaum, J.D., Sachidanandam, R., Sims, C., Garruss, A.S., Cook, M., Krumlauf, R., Wiedemann, L.M., Sower, S.A., Decatur, W.A., Hall, J.A., Amemiya, C.T., Saha, N.R., Buckley, K.M., Rast, J.P., Das, S., Hirano, M., McCurley, N., Guo, P., Rohner, N., Tabin, C.J., Piccinelli, P., Elgar, G., Ruffier, M., Aken, B.L., Searle, S.M., Muffato, M., Pignatelli, M., Herrero, J., Jones, M., Brown, C.T., Chung-Davidson, Y.W., Nanlohy, K.G., Libants, S.V., Yeh, C.Y., McCauley, D.W., Langeland, J.A., Pancer, Z., Fritzsch, B., de Jong, P.J., Zhu, B., Fulton, L.L., Theising, B., Flicek, P., Bronner, M.E., Warren, W.C., Clifton, S.W., Wilson, R.K., Li, W., 2013. Sequencing of the sea lamprey (*Petromyzon marinus*) genome provides insights into vertebrate evolution. Nat. Genet. 45, 415–421, 421e411–421e412.

Smith, S.L., 1998. Shark complement: an assessment. Immunol. Rev. 166, 67–78.

Soanes, K.H., Figuereido, K., Richards, R.C., Mattatall, N.R., Ewart, K.V., 2004. Sequence and expression of C-type lectin receptors in Atlantic salmon (*Salmo salar*). Immunogenetics 56, 572–584.

Solem, S.T., Stenvik, J., 2006. Antibody repertoire development in teleosts – a review with emphasis on salmonids and *Gadus morhua* L. Dev. Comp. Immunol. 30, 57–76.

Somamoto, T., Yoshiura, Y., Sato, A., Nakao, M., Nakanishi, T., Okamoto, N., Ototake, M., 2006. Expression profiles of TCRbeta and CD8alpha mRNA correlate with virus-specific cell-mediated cytotoxic activity in ginbuna crucian carp. Virology 348, 370–377.

Song, R., Wei, R.B., Luo, H.Y., Wang, D.F., 2012. Isolation and characterization of an antibacterial peptide fraction from the pepsin hydrolysate of half-fin anchovy (*Setipinna taty*). Molecules 17, 2980–2991.

Staeheli, P., 1990. Interferon-induced proteins and the antiviral state. Adv. Virus Res. 38, 147–200.

Stafford, J.L., Belosevic, M., 2003. Transferrin and the innate immune response of fish: identification of a novel mechanism of macrophage activation. Dev. Comp. Immunol. 27, 539–554.

Stafford, J.L., Wilson, M., Nayak, D., Quiniou, S.M., Clem, L.W., Miller, N.W., Bengten, E., 2006. Identification and characterization of a FcR homolog in an ectothermic vertebrate, the channel catfish (*Ictalurus punctatus*). J. Immunol. 177, 2505–2517.

Stet, R.J.M., Egberts, E., 1991. The histocompatibility system in teleostean fihes: from multiple histocompatibility loci to a major histocompatibility complex. J. Fish Shellfih Immunol. 1, 1–16.

Stolte, E.H., Savelkoul, H.F., Wiegertjes, G., Flik, G., Lidy Verburg-van Kemenade, B.M., 2008. Differential expression of two interferon-gamma genes in common carp (*Cyprinus carpio* L.). Dev. Comp. Immunol. 32, 1467–1481.

Stosik, M., Deptula, W., Travnicek, M., Baldy-Chudzik, K., 2002. Phagocytic and bactericidal activity of blood thrombocytes in carps (*Cyprinus carpio*). Vet. Med. 40, 21–25.

Strasser, A., Jost, P.J., Nagata, S., 2009. The many roles of FAS receptor signaling in the immune system. Immunity 30, 180–192.

Strobl, H., Knapp, W., 1999. TGF-beta1 regulation of dendritic cells. Microbes Infect. 1, 1283–1290.

Suetake, H., Araki, K., Akatsu, K., Somamoto, T., Dijkstra, J.M., Yoshiura, Y., Kikuchi, K., Suzuki, Y., 2007. Genomic organization and expression of CD8alpha and CD8beta genes in fugu *Takifugu rubripes*. Fish Shellfish Immunol. 23, 1107–1118.

Sun, X.F., Shang, N., Hu, W., Wang, Y.P., Guo, Q.L., 2007. Molecular cloning and characterization of carp (*Cyprinus carpio* L.) CD8beta and CD4-like genes. Fish Shellfish Immunol. 23, 1242–1255.

Sunyer, J.O., Tort, L., Lambris, J.D., 1997. Diversity of the third form of complement, C3, in fish: functional characterization of five forms of C3 in the diploid fish *Sparus aurata*. Biochem. J. 326 (Pt. 3), 877–881.

Swain, P., Nayak, S.K., 2009. Role of maternally derived immunity in fish. Fish Shellfish Immunol. 27, 89–99.

Tafalla, C., Aranguren, R., Secombes, C.J., Castrillo, J.L., Novoa, B., Figueras, A., 2003. Molecular characterisation of sea bream (*Sparus aurata*) transforming growth factor beta1. Fish Shellfish Immunol. 14, 405–421.

Tafalla, C., Aranguren, R., Secombes, C.J., Figueras, A., Novoa, B., 2004. Cloning and analysis of expression of a gilthead sea bream (*Sparus aurata*) Mx cDNA. Fish Shellfish Immunol. 16, 11–24.

ten Dijke, P., Hill, C.S., 2004. New insights into TGF-beta-Smad signalling. Trends Biochem. Sci. 29, 265–273.

Traver, D., Paw, B.H., Poss, K.D., Penberthy, W.T., Lin, S., Zon, L.I., 2003. Transplantation and *in vivo* imaging of multilineage engraftment in zebrafish bloodless mutants. Nat. Immunol. 4, 1238–1246.

Trobridge, G.D., Chiou, P.P., Leong, J.C., 1997. Cloning of the rainbow trout (*Oncorhynchus mykiss*) Mx2 and Mx3 cDNAs and characterization of trout Mx protein expression in salmon cells. J. Virol. 71, 5304–5311.

Trobridge, G.D., Leong, J.A.C., 1995. Characterization of a rainbow-trout mx-gene. J. Interferon Cytokine Res. 15, 691–702.

Valero, Y., Chaves-Pozo, E., Meseguer, J., Esteban, M.A., Cuesta, A., 2013. Biological role of fish antimicrobial peptides. In: Seong, M.D., Hak, Y.I. (Eds.), Antimicrobial peptides: properties, functions and role in immune response. Nova Science Publishers, New York. pp. 31–60.

Vasta, G.R., Nita-Lazar, M., Giomarelli, B., Ahmed, H., Du, S., Cammarata, M., Parrinello, N., Bianchet, M.A., Amzel, L.M., 2011. Structural and functional diversity of the lectin repertoire in teleost fish: relevance to innate and adaptive immunity. Dev. Comp. Immunol. 35, 1388–1399.

Venkatesh, B., Lee, A.P., Ravi, V., Maurya, A.K., Lian, M.M., Swann, J.B., Ohta, Y., Flajnik, M.F., Sutoh, Y., Kasahara, M., Hoon, S., Gangu, V., Roy, S.W., Irimia, M., Korzh, V., Kondrychyn, I., Lim, Z.W., Tay, B.H., Tohari, S., Kong, K.W., Ho, S., Lorente-Galdos, B., Quilez, J., Marques-Bonet, T., Raney, B.J., Ingham, P.W., Tay, A., Hillier, L.W., Minx, P., Boehm, T., Wilson, R.K., Brenner, S., Warren, W.C., 2014. Elephant shark genome provides unique insights into gnathostome evolution. Nature 505, 174–179.

Verrier, E.R., Langevin, C., Benmansour, A., Boudinot, P., 2011. Early antiviral response and virus-induced genes in fish. Dev. Comp. Immunol. 35, 1204–1214.

Vilain, C., Wetzel, M.C., Du Pasquier, L., Charlemagne, J., 1984. Structural and functional analysis of spontaneous anti-nitrophenyl antibodies in three cyprinid fish species: carp (*Cyrinus carpio*), goldfish (*Carassius auratus*) and tench (*Tinca tinca*). Dev. Comp. Immunol. 8, 611–622.

Vivier, E., Tomasello, E., Baratin, M., Walzer, T., Ugolini, S., 2008. Functions of natural killer cells. Nat. Immunol. 9, 503–510.

von Gersdorff Jorgensen, L., Heinecke, R.D., Skjodt, K., Rasmussen, K.J., Buchmann, K., 2011. Experimental evidence for direct in situ binding of IgM and IgT to early trophonts of *Ichthyophthirius multifiliis* (Fouquet) in the gills of rainbow trout, *Oncorhynchus mykiss* (Walbaum). J. Fish Dis. 34, 749–755.

Walport, M.J., 2001a. Complement. First of two parts. N. Engl. J. Med. 344, 1058–1066.

Walport, M.J., 2001b. Complement. Second of two parts. N. Engl. J. Med. 344, 1140–1144.

Wang, T., Bird, S., Koussounadis, A., Holland, J.W., Carrington, A., Zou, J., Secombes, C.J., 2009a. Identification of a novel IL-1 cytokine family member in teleost fish. J. Immunol. 183, 962–974.

Wang, W.L., Hong, J.R., Lin, G.H., Liu, W., Gong, H.Y., Lu, M.W., Lin, C.C., Wu, J.L., 2011. Stage-specific expression of TNFalpha regulates bad/bid-mediated apoptosis and RIP1/ROS-mediated secondary necrosis in Birnavirus-infected fish cells. PLoS One 6, e16740.

Wang, Z., Zhang, S., Tong, Z., Li, L., Wang, G., 2009b. Maternal transfer and protective role of the alternative complement components in zebrafish *Danio rerio*. PLoS One 4, e4498.

Ware, C.F., 2003. The TNF superfamily. Cytokine Growth Factor Rev. 14, 181–184.

Warnock, R.A., Campbell, J.J., Dorf, M.E., Matsuzawa, A., McEvoy, L.M., Butcher, E.C., 2000. The role of chemokines in the microenvironmental control of T versus B cell arrest in Peyer's patch high endothelial venules. J. Exp. Med. 191, 77–88.

Warr, G.W., 1995. The immunoglobulin genes of fish. Dev. Comp. Immunol. 19, 1–12.

Warr, G.W., De Luca, D., Griffin, B.R., 1979. Membrane immunoglobulin is present on thymic and splenic lymphocytes of the trout *Salmo gairdneri*. J. Immunol. 123, 910–917.

Weinstein, J.A., Jiang, N., White, 3rd, R.A., Fisher, D.S., Quake, S.R., 2009. High-throughput sequencing of the zebrafish antibody repertoire. Science 324, 807–810.

Wen, Y., Fang, W., Xiang, L.X., Pan, R.L., Shao, J.Z., 2011. Identification of Treg-like cells in Tetraodon: insight into the origin of regulatory T subsets during early vertebrate evolution. Cell Mol. Life Sci. 68, 2615–2626.

Whyte, S.K., 2007. The innate immune response of finfish – a review of current knowledge. Fish Shellfish Immunol. 23, 1127–1151.

Wilson, M., Bengten, E., Miller, N.W., Clem, L.W., Du Pasquier, L., Warr, G.W., 1997. A novel chimeric Ig heavy chain from a teleost fish shares similarities to IgD. Proc. Natl. Acad. Sci. U.S.A. 94, 4593–4597.

Wyffels, J.T., Walsh, C.J., Luer, C.A., Bodine, A.B., 2005. *In vivo* exposure of clearnose skates, *Raja eglanteria*, to ionizing X-radiation: acute effects on the thymus. Dev. Comp. Immunol. 29, 315–331.

Xu, C., Guo, T.C., Mutoloki, S., Haugland, O., Marjara, I.S., Evensen, O., 2010. Alpha interferon and not gamma interferon inhibits salmonid alphavirus subtype 3 replication *in vitro*. J. Virol. 84, 8903–8912.

Xu, Z., Parra, D., Gomez, D., Salinas, I., Zhang, Y.A., von Gersdorff Jorgensen, L., Heinecke, R.D., Buchmann, K., LaPatra, S., Sunyer, J.O., 2013. Teleost skin, an ancient mucosal surface that elicits gut-like immune responses. Proc. Natl. Acad. Sci. U.S.A. 110, 13097–13102.

Yang, F., Waldbieser, G.C., Lobb, C.J., 2006. The nucleotide targets of somatic mutation and the role of selection in immunoglobulin heavy chains of a teleost fish. J. Immunol. 176, 1655–1667.

Yang, M., Zhou, H., 2008. Grass carp transforming growth factor-beta 1 (TGF-beta 1): molecular cloning, tissue distribution and immunobiological activity in teleost peripheral blood lymphocytes. Mol. Immunol. 45, 1792–1798.

Ye, J., Kaattari, I., Kaattari, S., 2011a. Plasmablasts and plasma cells: reconsidering teleost immune system organization. Dev. Comp. Immunol. 35, 1273–1281.

Ye, J., Kaattari, I.M., Kaattari, S.L., 2011b. The differential dynamics of antibody subpopulation expression during affinity maturation in a teleost. Fish Shellfish Immunol. 30, 372–377.

Ye, J., Kaattari, I.M., Ma, C., Kaattari, S., 2013. The teleost humoral immune response. Fish Shellfish Immunol. 35, 1719–1728.

Yoder, J.A., 2004. Investigating the morphology, function and genetics of cytotoxic cells in bony fish. Comp. Biochem. Physiol. C Toxicol. Pharmacol. 138, 271–280.

Yoder, J.A., Litman, G.W., 2011. The phylogenetic origins of natural killer receptors and recognition: relationships, possibilities, and realities. Immunogenetics 63, 123–141.

Yokoya, S., Ebina, Y., 1981. Rodlet cells in the teleosts, *Oryzias latipes* and *Salmo gairdneri*. Fukushima J. Med. Sci. 28, 47–54.

Zaccone, G., Kapoor, B.G., Fasulo, S., Ainis, L., 2001. Structural, histochemical and functional aspects of the epidermis of fishes. Adv. Marine Biol. 40, 253–276.

Zapata, A., 1981. Lymphoid organs of teleost fish. I. Ultrastructure of the thymus of *Rutilus rutilus*. Dev. Comp. Immunol. 5, 427–436.

Zapata, A., Amemiya, C.T., 2000. Phylogeny of lower vertebrates and their immunological structures. Curr. Top. Microbiol. Immunol. 248, 67–107.

Zapata, A., Diez, B., Cejalvo, T., Gutierrez-de Frias, C., Cortes, A., 2006. Ontogeny of the immune system of fish. Fish Shellfish Immunol. 20, 126–136.

Zapata, A.G., 1982. Lymphoid organs of teleost fish. III. Splenic lymphoid tissue of *Rutilus rutilus* and *Gobio gobio*. Dev. Comp. Immunol. 6, 87–94.

Zapata, A.G., Torroba, M., Vicente, A., Varas, A., Sacedon, R., Jimenez, E., 1995. The relevance of cell microenvironments for the appearance of lympho-haemopoietic tissues in primitive vertebrates. Histol. Histopathol. 10, 761–778.

Zelensky, A.N., Gready, J.E., 2005. The C-type lectin-like domain superfamily. FEBS J. 272, 6179–6217.

Zhang, D.C., Shao, Y.Q., Huang, Y.Q., Jiang, S.G., 2005. Cloning, characterization and expression analysis of interleukin-10 from the zebrafish (*Danio rerion*). J. Biochem. Mol. Biol. 38, 571–576.

Zhang, H., Thorgaard, G.H., Ristow, S.S., 2002. Molecular cloning and genomic structure of an interleukin-8 receptor-like gene from homozygous clones of rainbow trout (*Oncorhynchus mykiss*). Fish Shellfish Immunol. 13, 251–258.

Zhang, Y.A., Hikima, J., Li, J., LaPatra, S.E., Luo, Y.P., Sunyer, J.O., 2009. Conservation of structural and functional features in a primordial CD80/86 molecule from rainbow trout (*Oncorhynchus mykiss*), a primitive teleost fish. J. Immunol. 183, 83–96.

Zhang, Y.A., Salinas, I., Li, J., Parra, D., Bjork, S., Xu, Z., LaPatra, S.E., Bartholomew, J., Sunyer, J.O., 2010. IgT, a primitive immunoglobulin class specialized in mucosal immunity. Nat. Immunol. 11, 827–835.

Zhang, Y.B., Li, Q., Gui, J.F., 2004. Differential expression of two *Carassius auratus* Mx genes in cultured CAB cells induced by grass carp hemorrhage virus and interferon. Immunogenetics 56, 68–75.

Zhao, J.G., Zhou, L., Jin, J.Y., Zhao, Z., Lan, J., Zhang, Y.B., Zhang, Q.Y., Gui, J.F., 2009. Antimicrobial activity-specific to gram-negative bacteria and immune modulation-mediated NF-kappaB and Sp1 of a medaka beta-defensin. Dev. Comp. Immunol. 33, 624–637.

Zlotnik, A., 2006. Chemokines and cancer. Int. J. Cancer 119, 2026–2029.

Zlotnik, A., Morales, J., Hedrick, J.A., 1999. Recent advances in chemokines and chemokine receptors. Crit. Rev. Immunol. 19, 1–47.

Zou, J., Bird, S., Truckle, J., Bols, N., Horne, M., Secombes, C., 2004. Identification and expression analysis of an IL-18 homologue and its alternatively spliced form in rainbow trout (*Oncorhynchus mykiss*). Eur. J. Biochem. 271, 1913–1923.

Zou, J., Carrington, A., Collet, B., Dijkstra, J.M., Yoshiura, Y., Bols, N., Secombes, C., 2005. Identification and bioactivities of IFN-gamma in rainbow trout *Oncorhynchus mykiss*: the first Th1-type cytokine characterized functionally in fish. J. Immunol. 175, 2484–2494.

Zou, J., Clark, M.S., Secombes, C.J., 2003a. Characterisation, expression and promoter analysis of an interleukin 10 homologue in the puffer fish, *Fugu rubripes*. Immunogenetics 55, 325–335.

Zou, J., Grabowski, P.S., Cunningham, C., Secombes, C.J., 1999. Molecular cloning of interleukin 1beta from rainbow trout *Oncorhynchus mykiss* reveals no evidence of an ice cut site. Cytokine 11, 552–560.

Zou, J., Peddie, S., Scapigliati, G., Zhang, Y., Bols, N.C., Ellis, A.E., Secombes, C.J., 2003b. Functional characterisation of the recombinant tumor necrosis factors in rainbow trout, *Oncorhynchus mykiss*. Dev. Comp. Immunol. 27, 813–822.

Zou, J., Secombes, C.J., 2011. Teleost fish interferons and their role in immunity. Dev. Comp. Immunol. 35, 1376–1387.

Zou, J., Tafalla, C., Truckle, J., Secombes, C., 2007. Identification of a second group of type I interferons in fish sheds light on interferon evolution in vertebrates. J. Immunol. 179, 3859–3871.

Zwollo, P., Haines, A., Rosato, P., Gumulak-Smith, J., 2008. Molecular and cellular analysis of B-cell populations in the rainbow trout using Pax5 and immunoglobulin markers. Dev. Comp. Immunol. 32, 1482–1496.

Zwollo, P., Mott, K., Barr, M., 2010. Comparative analyses of B cell populations in trout kidney and mouse bone marrow: establishing B cell signatures. Dev. Comp. Immunol. 34, 1291–1299.

Overview of mucosal structure and function in teleost fishes

3

Tracy S. Peterson
Department of Regulatory Science, University of Arkansas at Pine Bluff, Pine Bluff, Arkansas, USA

Chapter Outline

3.1 Introduction

The organs and tissues comprising mucosae and mucosal surfaces of teleost fish are both structurally and functionally similar in many respects to their mammalian counterparts including man, despite roughly 450 million years of evolutionary separation. Teleostean fish were among the first vertebrate animals to display mucosal immune defenses, particularly adaptive immunity within the intestinal tract, as a likely consequence of developing jaws and switching to a predatory lifestyle and the introduction of novel pathogens (Matsunaga, 1998; Matsunaga and Rahman, 1998) as well as to develop the cooperative function between host tissues and immune cells, which first arose within mucosal tissues. This cooperative function became necessary to discriminate between nonpathogens (commensals) from pathogenic organisms (Gomez et al., 2013).The primary organizational differences of these mucosal immune tissues occur between man and fish due mostly to the environmental niches that each occupy, as the aquatic environment presents unique immunologic challenges to the mucosal tissues of fish through continuous and intimate surface contact of potential pathogens. It is at this surface interface between the environment and mucosal tissue where first antigenic contact and the immunologic response and processing most often occurs in fish. Functionally, the response amplitude and efficacy of fish mucosal tissues to immunologic challenges, much like the systemic humoral response, demonstrates a compelling dependency on environmental factors and can be remarkably impacted by local environmental cues such as photoperiod, ambient water temperature, and constituents of water quality such as oxygen saturation, pH, and turbidity (Tort et al., 2004; Niklasson et al., 2011; Uribe et al., 2011). Population density, social hierarchies and cohort interactions also act as effectors and regulators on response to immunologic challenges (Uribe et al., 2011). Irrespective of these unique environmental challenges that directly influence outcomes of the mucosal immune response, the first-order constitutive mucosal tissues in teleost fishes that react to immunologic challenges include the gills, integument, and intestine. Although their physiological roles vary, all of these mucosal tissues share structural similarities at the microanatomic level, notably the presence of an organized epithelial surface with supporting stromal tissues or lamina propria, a vascular supply network, musculature, and resident immune cells. As the intestine is regarded as a conventional or prototypical example of a mucosal tissue, emphasis will be placed on its microanatomic structure and concomitant mucosal immune functions.

3.1.1 Gills

Gills are multifunctional mucosal tissue of fish that are richly vascular and have a massive respiratory surface area much like the alveolar sacs of mammalian lungs; indeed, the basic microanatomic structure of gill filaments and lamellae comparatively resembles pulmonary alveoli turned inside out (Figure 3.1). At a basic functional level gill filaments and in particular the lamellae are responsible for diffusive and active gas exchange (oxygen and carbon dioxide), active ionoregulation to maintain osmotic and

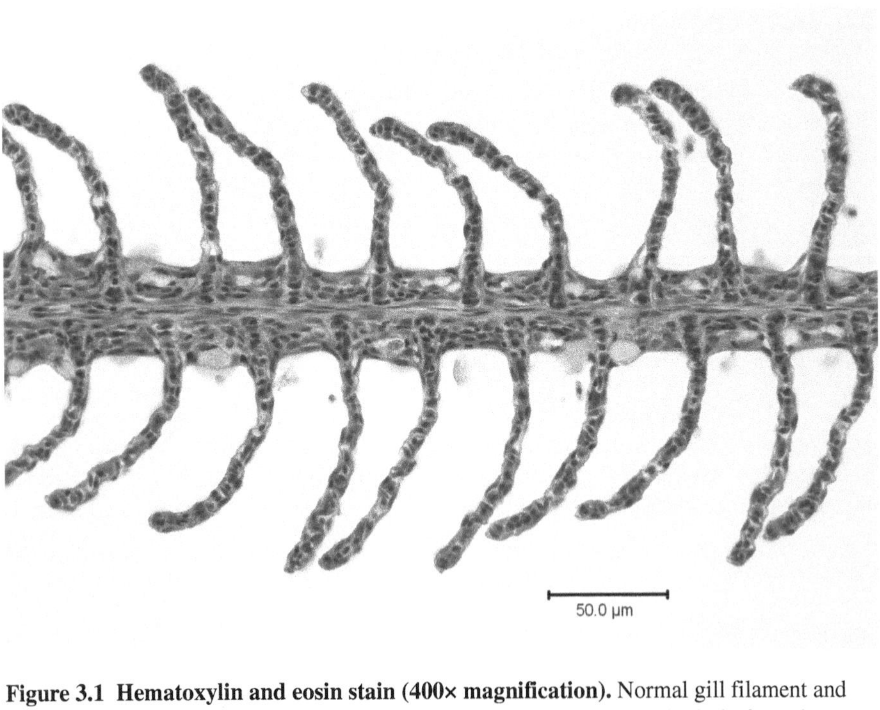

Figure 3.1 Hematoxylin and eosin stain (400× magnification). Normal gill filament and lamellar histoarchitecture. In this view, lamellar leaflets extend perpendicularly from the filament body. The filament and lamellae have a monolayer of simple squamous epithelial cells, with basal reserve populations of epithelial cells. Several goblet cells are basally located between lamellar sulci.

acid–base balance with respect to the environment, localized control of hemodynamics via vasoconstriction and vasorelaxation, and elimination of nitrogenous waste. Structurally, the microarchitecture of the gill filament is a simple design. Each filament proper is supported internally by a cartilaginous core (or "rod") and connective stromal or interstitial tissue, percolated by capillaries comprising the two primary respiratory blood vessels (afferent and efferent) and the interlamellar and nutrient blood vessels. A secondary circulatory system, analogous to mammalian lymphatic vessels, is also present. Arising from the filament body are numerous protruding lamellae or leaflets, which provide the majority of respiratory surface area. These lamellae receive internal support from pillar cells that serve the roles of mechanical support, enable blood circulation, and maintain isolation of the blood plasma from the external environment. A single epithelial layer of simple squamous cells, often referred to as "pavement cells," covers the gill filament and lamellae. Microridges present on the surface of these epithelial cells further increases the surface area and provide a platform that enhances adherence of a stable mucous layer. Interposed among the epithelial cells are a wide variety of specialized cells, including chloride, goblet (mucus-secreting), neuroepithelial, and rodlet cells. Intracellular goblet cells can occasionally be identified in the squamous epithelial cells, depending on the fish species, the unique positioning of which may allow goblet cells to secrete mucus into the environment and avoid compromising the intercellular junctions of epithelium (Lin et al., 1998). Taste buds can also be interspersed among the epithelial cells covering the filament, although they are more commonly found within the gill raker epithelium. The gill rakers, which function to filter particulates and hold prey items, often has abundant lymphocytic aggregates in the subepithelial stromal tissue and may be an anatomic site of primary antigen contact, analogous to the mammalian tonsils.

The surface mucous layer covering the gill filament and lamellar epithelium is an initial physical barrier to pathogen and environmental insults (Dalmo et al., 1997; Magnadottir, 2006) and contains numerous bioactive substances, including enzymes (i.e., lysozyme) and antimicrobial peptides. Preformed antibodies of the IgM isotype, released from systemic circulation, also reside within the mucous layer. Beyond the physical barrier of mucus, there is a full complement of immune cells, including lymphocytes, plasma cells (antibody-secreting cells), macrophages, neutrophils, and eosinophilic granular cells present in both the intraepithelial spaces of the filament and lamellar squamous epithelium and around the perivascular compartments within filaments.

Lymphocytic populations within the gill tissue are particularly numerous and well characterized, with definitive identification of B cells, plasma cells, and antibody-binding macrophages, and the gills have been recognized as a primary organ for the production of antibodies (DosSantos et al., 2001). Intraepithelial resident macrophages with capacity to interact with immunoglobulin IgM serve as a frontline defense against soluble antigens, giving a relatively rapid response when pathogens are encountered. The compact interstitium of lamellae can inhibit progressive mobility and interactions with pathogens. To overcome this, constitutive perivascular plasmacytic cuffs surrounding the interfilament vasculature have an IgM secreting response function to circulating antigens, and antigen trapping occurs within endothelial cells

(Davidson et al., 1997; Grove et al., 2006). The plasma cells and phagocytic endothelial cells likely function in concert to allow an effective, antibody-driven response to pathogens, especially given the constant exposure of the gills to the surrounding aqueous environment. Definable populations of T cells within gill tissue are less certain, although the presence of these cells would be expected, as the expression of interleukins 2, 7, and 15, which drive T cell growth, differentiation, and cytolytic activity, occurs in gill epithelium.

3.2 Integument

The integument of fish is the largest mucosal tissue, respective of surface area, which surrounds the entire animal including fins. Structural organization and dynamic function of the teleost fish integument varies among different species, from having scales to being scaleless (i.e., catfish) as well as the numbers and types of specialized cells, and can be considered to have the most interspecies differences among the mucosal tissues. Despite these inherent species differences, the general organization and microanatomic structures are conserved as are the cell types (Figure 3.2).

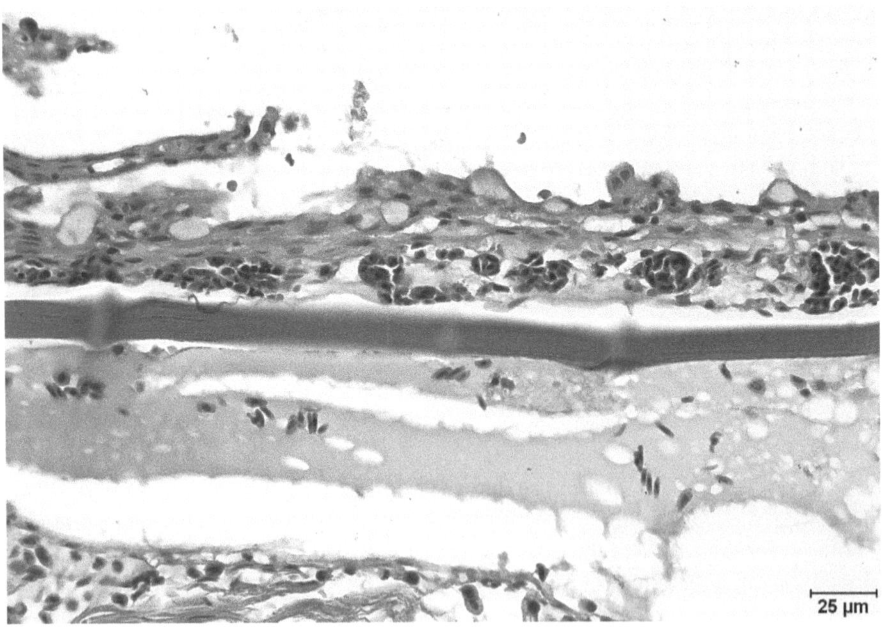

Figure 3.2 Hematoxylin and eosin stain (400× magnification). Normal integument histoarchitecture. In this section, the 5–6 cell thick epidermis is overlying the scale (slightly off-focus in the central photo). Numerous goblet cells punctuate the epidermis and there is multifocal artifactual squamous cell blebbing along the epidermal surface. Wisps of secreted mucus are emanating from some of the goblet cells.

In its simplest organization, fish integument is a comparative precursor to mammalian skin (Rakers et al., 2010) with the notable exceptions of being nonkeratinized (in most species except Asiatic catfish) and containing abundant goblet cells. It is multilayered and has an epidermis with underlying basement membrane, a dermis composed of two discrete tissues, the stratum spongiosum and stratum compactum with an associated subjacent hypodermal space, and a layer of skeletal muscle. The metabolically active, nonkeratinized epidermis is comprised of several cell types; the most abundant are simple stratified squamous epithelial cells, 5–10 cells in average thickness interspersed with goblet (mucus-secreting) cells.

Similar to the simple squamous epithelial cells of the gill filament and lamellae, integumentary squamous epithelial cells have pronounced microridges that function to provide an adherent surface for mucous secretions and is important in maintaining the mucous gel layer that covers the epithelial surface. In addition, the epithelial cells have a phagocytic function that may allow them to eliminate not only pathogens but foreign material from the integument, and as they reach near-capacity of internalized material, the cells are sloughed (Åsbakk, 2001; Esteban, 2012). Goblet cells within the epidermis occur in the outer and intermediate strata of squamous epithelial cells, continuously producing a glycoprotein-rich, viscoelastic mucous secretion. These nonproliferative specialized cells arise from the basal epithelium in early larval life and continuously migrate to their respective epidermal layers, prior to commencing secretory activity (Ottesen and Olafsen, 1997). Both the number of goblet cells and the biochemical composition of their secretory product vary among fish genera and even between species, depending on local environmental conditions (Fast et al., 2002). The dermis contains predominately fibroblasts intermingling with an ordered collagenous matrix that is punctuated by blood vessels, nerves, pigment cells, and intermixed immune cells. Scales emanate from vascularized dermal scale pockets and are retained or "anchored" by collagen filaments within the dermis.

The epidermal mucous layer contributes significantly to the immune defense against pathogens, as a physical barrier and through elaboration of various preformed peptides, enzymes, and agglutinating lectins (Cho et al., 2002; Nakamura et al., 2004). Similar to mammals, the fish epidermis has analogous resident dendritic cells, which phagocytize and process antigens (Davidson et al., 1997). Loose aggregates and individual lymphocytes are present throughout the integument, with B cells and plasma cells being the most populous. Secreted antibodies, consisting of IgM and IgT (trout), localize to the epidermal, epithelial, and mucous layers, conferring more specific and additive protection against pathogens (Hatten et al., 2001; Zhao et al., 2008).

Immunoglobulin IgT remains within the integument, while IgM can participate in systemic immune responses, and IgT is compartmentalized to mucosal pathogen interactions (Xu et al., 2013). Detectable antibodies in the integumentary mucus display a lag phenomenon in contrast to serum antibodies when parenteral systemic vaccinations are given, irrespective of the locally available population of plasma cells in the epidermis, which was thought to result from transport of the antibodies through the epidermis to the mucous layer (Rombout et al., 2010), although this observation is more likely due to timing of antibody production in a given systemic response. Bactericidal activity of immunoglobulin IgM sequestered in the epidermal mucus tends to be more reactive against typical fish pathogens than the corresponding humoral activity (Guardiola et al., 2014).

3.3 Intestine

Organization and structural microanatomic features of the fish intestinal mucosa are similar to that of human embryos (Wallace et al., 2005). The intestinal mucosa of teleost fish is thus comparable to mammals in essential structural elements and cell types, with distinct differences that are unique to fish (Figure 3.3). In basic structural organization, the mucosa is comprised of irregular circumferential and longitudinal folds, which may or may not have periodicity and can occur randomly. Transition to longitudinal folds occurs in the posterior intestinal mucosa and mucosal fold height decreases in prominence from anterior to posterior intestinal segments. On histologic transverse and longitudinal sections, these folds may often resemble the more conventional mammalian villar microarchitecture, and have on occasion been mistaken for villi. Inter-fold sulci create potential spaces between discrete mucosal folds, and may form pseudocrypt structures that can appear similar to mammalian intestinal crypts.

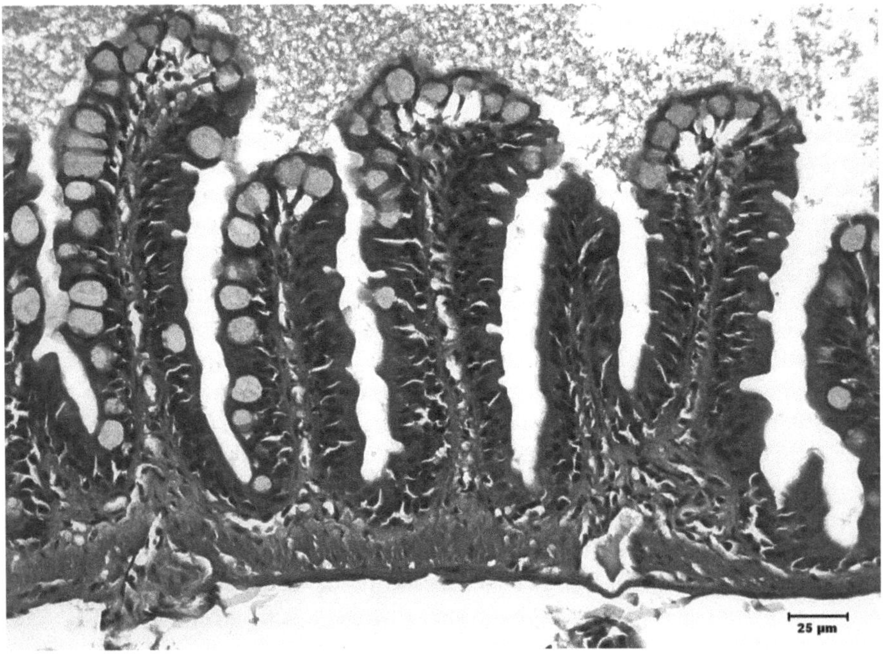

Figure 3.3 Hematoxylin and eosin stain (400× magnification). Normal intestine histoarchitecture. Columnar cells lining the mucosal folds appear pseudostratified in some of the individual folds. Goblet cells are especially prominent at the apices of folds and along lateral aspects. A prominent mucous layer overlies the mucosal folds.

The basal floor of mucosal pseudocrypts contains actively proliferating epithelial cells similar in fashion to mammalian crypts; however, unlike mammals fish do not have characteristic intestinal mucosal crypts.

In salmonids there is a unique circumferential band of homogenously dense and supportive collagenous connective tissue immediately subjacent to the lamina propria, called the stratum compactum, which mirrors the same mammalian microanatomic structure in felids. Variable populations of eosinophilic granule cells intermixed with basophils are frequently located beneath the stratum compactum within the intestinal stromal tissue (Khojasteh et al., 2009; Pirarat et al., 2011), and increases in these inflammatory cells occur during intraluminal parasitic infestation. Additional differences between fish and mammalian intestinal architecture include the lack of a submucosa and muscularis mucosa.

Across most fish species, intestinal mucosal surfaces are covered by a variable surface aqueous boundary layer with an underlying mucous gel layer and lined by a monolayer of simple columnar epithelial cells (enterocytes) that may appear occasionally pseudostratified (Raskovic et al., 2011). Mechanical damage to this mucosal surface layer, from ingestion of hard substances (bone, scales, and gastroliths) and ongoing peristalsis, is thought to enhance local persorption of antigens via the Herbst effect (McLean and Donaldson, 1990). Mucus-secreting goblet cells are interposed between enterocytes throughout the juvenile and adult intestinal mucosa, which differs from the larval life stage, where goblet cells are primarily localized to the intermediate segment. The number of goblet cells tends to decrease from the anterior to posterior intestinal mucosa and total numbers of goblet cells are species dependent (Inami et al., 2009).

In larval and juvenile fish, and during inflammation (enteritis), the mucosal epithelium is more permeable to luminal antigens (Dalmo et al., 1997) and response to acute to subacute injury is often denoted by epithelial hyperplasia. In some cases of more chronic enteritis, there may be focal enterocytic separation from the basement membrane, loss of enterocytes, and goblet cell hyperplasia (Ronza et al., 2011), with subsequent metaplasia in severe enteritis. Mucosal epithelium is bolstered by a supporting simple lamina propria, which contains abundant stromal cells, secretory enteroendocrine cells (i.e., serotonin, somatostatin, and enteroglucagon), collagenous support matrices, blood vessels, nerves, and a primitive lymphatic or secondary circulation system that contains intraluminal leukocytes but not erythrocytes (Wardle, 1971; Vogel and Claviez, 1981). There is some evidence that, at least within trout, intravascular erythrocytes can serve as phagocytic cells for particulate antigens (Jirillo et al., 2007). The existence of a true lymphatic system in fish, comparable to mammals, remains controversial (Press and Evensen, 1999).

Putative M-cell analogs have been observed within the posterior intestinal mucosa of zebrafish, as enterocytes in the posterior segment have supranuclear vacuoles that harbor lumen-derived antigens, and these vacuole-containing enterocytes are thought to act as antigen-presenting cells (Wallace et al., 2005). Resident dendritic cells, another class of antigen-presenting immune cells, are present in relatively low abundance within the intestinal mucosa (Gomez et al., 2013). Gut-associated lymphoid tissue (GALT) is widely assumed to be a constant feature among vertebrates

(Zapata and Cooper, 1990), although its organization in fish differs with respect to GALT found in mammals and other lower vertebrates, mostly by lacking the well-defined Peyer's patches (Lin et al., 2005) or the localized lymphocytic aggregates commonly found in birds and reptiles.

Fish have referential analogs of mammalian GALT, inclusive of frequent intermixed populations of intraepithelial immune cells as well as loosely aggregated and scattered lymphocytes, eosinophilic granule cells, rodlet cells, neutrophils, and macrophages within the intestinal lamina propria (Reite and Evensen, 2006). Intraproprial lymphocytic aggregates are sometimes colloquially referred to as "cryptopatches" (Matsunaga and Rahman, 1998). The intermediate to posterior mucosal epithelium lining the intestine has been postulated as a critical site for the selection and refinement of GALT-analog lymphocyte populations (Fichtelius et al., 1968). Most intraepithelial lymphocytes tend to reside in the apical mucosal folds while aggregated lymphocyte populations are localized to intestinal pseudocrypts. Lymphocytes are often admixed with other immune cells (Matsunaga, 1998). Although transport of serum immunoglobulin IgM to the intestinal mucosa occurs when pathogens are encountered, a subset of lymphocytes, antibody-producing plasma cells, has been positively identified within the intestine of fish.

Locally produced soluble antibodies, such as IgM, are secreted by GALT-analog plasma cells as well as immunoglobulins IgT and IgZ (Flajnik, 2010), which were discovered in trout and zebrafish, respectively. In trout, IgT is preferentially associated with the intestinal mucosa along with compartmentalized IgT-secreting plasma cells (Ye et al., 2013). IgT requires binding to commensal intestinal bacteria in order to interact with potential pathogenic organisms. IgZ is present in the immune organs, including the intestine, of zebrafish and was found on the surface of B cells, indicating that it may have a role as a B cell receptor (Hu et al., 2010). There is a relative paucity of plasma cells secreting immunoglobulin IgD within the intestinal mucosa when compared to other heavy chain isotypes (Ye et al., 2013).

Appearance of mucosa-associated and other lymphomyeloid tissues occurs early in embryonic life prior to hatching and sequential development of mature resident neutrophil populations can be observed within 3 days of initial organogenesis, with lymphocyte populations following by the late larval and juvenile life stages (Uribe et al., 2011), but may decrease in overall number as the fish matures to juvenile and adult life stages. Individual fish genera have been employed for uncovering the interrelationship between intestinal mucosal surface interactions with pathogens. Macromolecule and bacterial antigen uptake, via endocytosis, occurs in the posterior intestinal segment of cyprinids with sequential movement from the intestinal lumen into compartmentalized supranuclear vacuoles, which can vary in size depending on the particle size of the ingested material (Nakamura et al., 2004; Inami, 2011). The contained intravacuolar particles are then subsequently to directed to intraepithelial macrophages for phagocytosis and processing (Joosten et al., 1995). Specific changes can occur to supranuclear vacuoles during inflammatory events, including a decrease in size and gradual disappearance that has been noted in cases of soybean meal enteritis, with a corresponding reduction in endocytosis that resolves once the inciting antigen (soy saponins) has been removed from the diet (Penn, 2005; Uran et al., 2008).

The hindgut, or posterior intestinal segment, was initially discovered as the preferential site of bacterial antigen uptake by Rombout et al. (1989), where they classified the "second gut segment" in carp as playing a key role in antigen uptake and processing as well as the initiation of a systemic immune response (Rombout et al., 1989). This intestinal segment has been demonstrated to be essential in the elicitation of the both systemic and mucosal immune responses to intraintestinal pathogens. In contrast to cyprinids, gilthead seabream (*Sparus aurata*) uptake of bacterial antigens did not occur in supranuclear vacuoles but were diffusely distributed in the cytoplasm of enterocytes (Joosten et al., 1995). Transport of bacterial antigens occurred sequentially from the apical to basal intracytoplasmic locations prior to systemic vascular release (Joosten et al., 1995).

References

Åsbakk, K., 2001. Elimination of foreign material by epidermal malpighian cells during wound healing in fish skin. J. Fish. Biol. 58, 953–966.

Cho, J.H., Park, I.Y., Kim, H.S., Lee, W.T., Kim, M.S., Kim, S.C., 2002. Cathepsin D produces antimicrobial peptide parasin I from histone H2A in the skin mucosa of fish. J. FASEB. 16, 429–431.

Dalmo, R.A., Ingebrigtsen, K., Bogwald, J., 1997. Non-specific defence mechanisms in fish, with particular reference to the reticuloendothelial system (RES). J. Fish. Dis. 20, 241–273.

DosSantos, N.M., Taverne-Thiele, J.J., Barnes, A.C., VanMuiswinkel, W.B., Ellis, A.E., Rombout, J.H.M.W., 2001. The gill is a major organ for antibody secreting cell production following direct immersion of sea bass (*Dicentrarchus labrax,* L.) in a Photobacterium damselae ssp. Piscicida bacterin: an ontogenetic study. Fish Shellfish Immunol. 11, 65–74.

Davidson, G.A., Lin, S.H., Secombes, C.J., Ellis, A.E., 1997. Detection of specific and 'constitutive' antibody secreting cells in the gills, head kidney and peripheral blood leucocytes of dab (*Limanda limanda*). Vet. Immunol. Immunopathol. 58, 363–374.

Esteban, M.A., 2012. An overview of the immunological defenses in fish skin. ISRN Immunol. 2012, 1–29, Published online 2012.

Fast, M.D., Sims, D.E., Burka, J.F., Mustafa, A., Ross, N.W., 2002. Skin morphology and humoral on-specific defence parameters of mucus and plasma in rainbow trout, coho and Atlantic salmon. Comp. Biochem. Physiol. A 132, 645–657.

Fichtelius, K.E., Finstad, J., Good, R.A., 1968. Bursa equivalent of bursaless vertebrates. Lab. Invest. 19, 339–351.

Flajnik, M.F., 2010. All GOD'S creatures got dedicated mucosal immunity. Nat. Immunol. 11, 777–779.

Gomez, D.G., Sunyer, J.O., Salinas, I., 2013. The mucosal immune system of fish: the evolution of tolerating commensals while fighting pathogens. Fish Shellfish Immunol. 35, 1729–1739.

Grove, S., Johansen, R., Reitan, L.J., Press, C.M., 2006. Immune and enzyme histochemical charaterisation of leukocyte populations within lymphoid and mucosal tissues of Atlantic halibut (*Hippoglossus hippoglossus*). Fish Shellfish Immunol. 20, 693–708.

Guardiola, F.A., Cuesta, A., Arizcun, M., Meseguer, J., 2014. Comparative skin mucus and serum humoral defence mechanisms in the teleost gilthead seabream (*Sparus aurata*). Fish Shellfish Immunol. 36, 545–551.

Hatten, F., Fredriksen, A., Hordvir, I., Endresen, C., 2001. Presence of IgM in cutaneous mucus, but not gut mucus of Atlantic salmon, *Salmo salar*, serum IgM is rapidly degraded when added to gut mucus. Fish Shellfish Immunol. 11, 257–268.

Hu, Y.L., Xiang, L.X., Shao, J.Z., 2010. Identification and characterization of a novel immunoglobulin Z isotype in zebrafish: Implications for a distinct B cell receptor in lower vertebrates. Mol. Immunol. 47, 738–746.

Inami, M., 2011. The immune system of Atlantic cod with emphasis in intestinal immunology. Ph.D. Thesis. Norwegian College of Fishery Science. Oslo, Norway.

Inami, M., Taverne-Thiele, A.J., Schroder, M.B., Kiron, V., Rombout, J.H.W.M., 2009. Immunological differences in the intestine and rectum of Atlantic cod (*Gadus morhua* L). Fish Shellfish Immunol. 26, 751–759.

Jirillo, F., Passantino, G., Massaro, M.A., Cianciotta, A., Crasto, A., Perillo, A., Passantino, L., Jirillo, E., 2007. In: vitro elicitation of intestinal immune responses in a teleost fish: evidence for a type I.V hypersensitivity reaction in rainbow trout. Immunopharm. Immunotox. 29, 69–80.

Joosten, P.H.M., Aviles-Trigueros, M., Sorgeloost, P., Rombout, J.H.W.M., 1995. Oral vaccination of juvenile carp (*Cyprinus carpio*) and gilthead seabream (*Sparus aurata*) with bioencapsulated *Vibrio anguillarum* bacterin. Fish Shellfish Immunol. 5, 289–299.

Khojasteh, S.M.B., Sheikhzadeh, F., Mohammadnejad, D., Azami, A., 2009. Histological, histochemical and ultrastructural study of the intestine of rainbow trout (*Oncorhynchus mykiss*). World Appl. Sci. J. 6, 1525–1531.

Lin, S.H., Davidson, G.A., Secombes, C.J., Ellis, A.E., 1998. A morphological study of cells isolated from the perfused gill of dab and Atlantic salmon. J. Fish Biol. 53, 560–568.

Lin, H.T., Lin, H.Y., Yang, H.L., 2005. Histology and histochemical enzyme-staining patterns of major immune organs in *Epinephelus malabaricus*. J. Fish Biol. 66, 729–740.

Magnadottir, B., 2006. Innate immunity of fish (overview). Fish Shellfish Immunol. 20, 137–151.

Matsunaga, T., 1998. Did the first adaptive immunity evolve in the gut of ancient jawed fish? Cytogenet. Cell Genet. 80, 138–141.

Matsunaga, T., Rahman, A., 1998. What brought the adaptive immune system to vertebrates? – the jaw hypothesis and the seahorse. Immunol. Rev. 166, 177–186.

McLean, E., Donaldson, E.M., 1990. Absorption of bioactive proteins by the gastrointestinal tract of fish: a review. J. Aquat. Anim. Health 2, 1–11.

Nakamura, O., Tazumi, Y., Muro, T., Yasuhara, Y., Watanabe, T., 2004. Active uptake and transport of protein by the intestinal epithelial cells in embryo of viviparous fish, Neoditrema ransonneti (Perciformes: Embiotocidae). J. Exp. Zool. 301A, 38–48.

Niklasson, L., Sundh, H., Fridell, F., Taranger, G.L., Sundell, K., 2011. Disturbance of the intestinal mucosal immune system of farmed Atlantic salmon (*Salmo salar*) in response to long-term hypoxic conditions. Fish Shellfish Immunol. 31, 1072–1080.

Ottesen, O.H., Olafsen, J.A., 1997. Ontogenetic development and composition of the mucous cells and the occurrence of saccular cells in the epidermis of Atlantic halibut. J. Fish Biol. 50, 620–633.

Penn, M.H., 2005. The effects of dietary soybean saponins in growth and performance, intestinal histology and immune response of first feeding rainbow trout (*Oncorhynchus mykiss*). Ph.D. Thesis. The Ohio State University.

Pirarat, N., Pinpimai, K., Endo, M., Katagiri, T., Ponpornpisit, A., Chansue, N., Maita, M., 2011. Modulation of intestinal morphology and immunity in the nile tilapia (*Oreochromis niloticus*) by *Lactobacillus rhamnosus* GG. Res. Vet. Sci. 91, 92–97.

Press, C.M., Evensen, O., 1999. The morphology of the immune system in teleost fishes. Fish Shellfish Immunol. 9, 309–318.

Rakers, S., Gebert, M., Uppalapati, S., Meyer, W., Maderson, P., Sell, A.F., Kruse, C., Paus, R., 2010. 'Fish matters': the relevance of fish skin biology to investigative dermatology. Exp. Dermatol. 19, 313–324.

Raskovic, B.S., Stankovic, M.B., Markovic, Z.Z., Poleksic, V.D., 2011. Histological methods in the assessment of different feed effects on liver and intestine of fish. J. Agri. Sci. 56, 87–100.

Reite, O.B., Evensen, O., 2006. Inflammatory cells of teleostean fish: a review focusing on mast cells/eosinophilic granule cells and rodlet cells. Fish Shellfish Immunol. 20, 192–208.

Rombout, J.H.W.M., Abelli, L., Picchietti, S., Scapigliati, G., Kiron, V., 2010. Teleost intestinal immunology. Fish Shellfish Immunol. 31, 616–626.

Rombout, J.H.W.M., Bot, H.E., Taverne-Thiele, J.J., 1989. Immunological importance of the second gut segment of carp. II. Characterization of mucosal leucocytes. J. Fish Biol. 35, 167–178.

Ronza, P., Bermudez, R., Losada, A.P., Robles, A., Quiroga, M.I., 2011. Mucosal CD3+ cell proliferation and gut epithelial apoptosis: implications in rainbow trout gastroenteritis (RTGE). J. Fish Dis. 34, 433–443.

Tort, L., Rotllant, J., Liarte, C., Acerete, L., Hernandez, A., Ceulemans, S., Coutteau, P., Padros, F., 2004. Effects of temperature decrease in feeding rates, immune indicators and histopathological changes of gilthead seabream *Sparus aurata* fed with an experimental diet. Aquaculture 229, 55–65.

Uran, P.A., Goncalves, A.A., Taverne-Thiele, J.J., Schrama, J.W., Verreth, J.A.J., Rombout, J.H.W.M., 2008. Soybean meal induces intestinal inflammation in common carp (*Cyprinus carpio* L). Fish Shellfish Immunol. 25, 751–760.

Uribe, C., Folch, H., Enriquez, R., Moran, G., 2011. Innate and adaptive immunity in teleost fish: a review. Vet. Med. 56, 486–503.

Vogel, W.O., Claviez, M., 1981. Vascular specialization in fish, but no evidence for lymphatics. Z. Naturforsch. Sect. C Bio. 36, 490–492.

Wallace, K.N., Akhter, S., Smith, E.M., Lorent, K., Pack, M., 2005. Intestinal growth and differentiation in zebrafish. Mech. Develop. 122, 157–173.

Wardle, C.S., 1971. New observations on the lymph system of the plaice (*Pleuronactes platessa*) and other teleosts. J. Mar. Biol. Assoc. 51, 977–990.

Xu, Z., Parra, D., Gomez, D., Salinas, I., Zhang, Y.A., vonGersdorff Jergensen, L., Heinecke, R.D., Buchmann, K., LaPatra, S., Sunyer, J.O., 2013. Teleost skin, an ancient mucosal surface that elicits gut-like immune responses. PNAS 110, 13097–13102.

Ye, J., Kaattari, I.M., Ma, C., Kaattari, S., 2013. The teleost humoral immune response. Fish Shellfish Immunol. 35, 1719–1728.

Zapata, A.G., Cooper, E.L., 1990. The immune system: Comparative histophysiology. John Wiley & Sons, Chichester, pp. 232–268.

Zhao, X., Findly, R.C., Dickerson, H.W., 2008. Cutaneous antibody-secreting cells and B cells in a teleost fish. Dev. Comp. Immunol. 32, 500–508.

Fish mucosal immunity: skin

4

María Ángeles Esteban; Rebeca Cerezuela
Fish Innate Immune System Group, Department of Cell Biology and Histology, Faculty of Biology, Campus of International Excellence, Campus Mare Nostrum, University of Murcia, Murcia, Spain

Chapter Outline

4.1 Introduction

Fish are in continuous contact with a wide variety of nonpathogenic and pathogenic microbes present in the aquatic environment, and therefore, have developed mechanisms to guarantee their survival. The normal structure and function of the fish integument reflects the adaptation of the organism to the physical, chemical, and biological properties of the aquatic environment, and the natural history of the organism.

Vertebrate skin with its outermost layer, the epidermis, covers the outer surface of a fish, including the body and fins, separates the individual from its environment, and is one of the organism's crucial interfaces for contact and communication with its external milieu. The skin, sometimes referred to as the integumentary system, is the largest organ of the body. It has a complex structure, being composed of many different tissues. Skin is a multipurpose tissue that encases the body and serves numerous vital functions such as maintaining the body shape, protecting the fish from insults such as physical damage and microorganism invasion, and preservation of hydrodynamics. It also performs many functions that are important in maintaining physiological homeostasis such as osmotic balance. Mucous glands, which offer protection from

Mucosal Health in Aquaculture

microorganisms, are extremely numerous in fish skin, especially in cyclostomes and teleosts. Protection from abrasion and predation is another function of the fish skin, and dermal (skin) bone arose early in fish evolution in response to this need. It is thought that bone first evolved in skin and only later invaded the cartilaginous areas of the body to provide additional support and protection.

Skin is well supplied with blood vessels and nerve endings that receive tactile and thermal stimuli. Some fish breathe, in part through the skin, by the exchange of oxygen and carbon dioxide between the surrounding water and numerous small blood vessels near the skin surface. Skin also serves as protection through the control of coloration. Fish can exhibit an almost limitless range of colors, which allow fish to blend closely with their surroundings, efficiently hiding the animal from predation.

Skin is also a site of mucosal immunity. The fish immune system can be subdivided according to the anatomical location. The mucosal-associated lymphoid tissue (MALT) in teleost fish is subdivided into gut-associated lymphoid tissue (GALT), skin-associated lymphoid tissue (SALT), and gill-associated lymphoid tissue (GIALT).

The innate immune response in fish is considered an essential arm in combating pathogens due to the limitations of the adaptive immune system (e.g., limited repertoire of immunoglobulins, slow proliferation, maturation and memory of lymphocytes, and influence of environmental factors such as temperature). The fish innate immune system can also be divided into three compartments: the mucosal/epithelial barrier (including skin, gills, and gut), the humoral components, and the involved cells (see Chapter 2). Skin and gills act as the first barrier to infection because they are the point of pathogen entry. Since most of pathogens start the process of infection in the mucosal surfaces, the mucosal immune response plays an essential role in the course of the infection, and different studies have begun to examine their cellular and molecular composition. Commensal microflora (normal microflora/indigenous microbiota) present on fish skin will not be discussed in this chapter (see Chapter 10) (Figure 4.1).

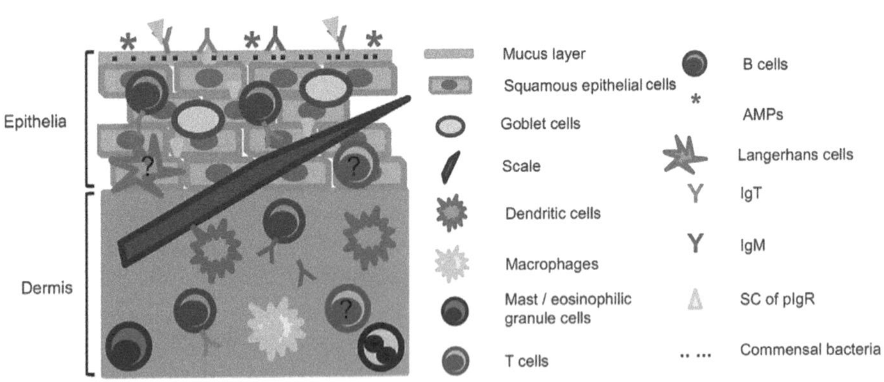

Figure 4.1 Schematic depiction of teleost fish skin highlighting the general structure, components, and cell types present. Elements that are suspected to be present in the skin, but not proven thus far are indicated as (?).
Adapted from (Gomez et al., 2013).

4.2 The mucous layer as a barrier against pathogens

One of the most distinctive features of fish skin is the presence of external mucus. The external mucous gel forms a layer of adherent mucus covering the living epithelial cells. This mucosal layer forms a thin barrier that separates the fish from its aquatic environment. The skin mucus is a semipermeable, physical, chemical, and biological barrier. Mucus is considered the first line of defense against infection through the epidermis (Raj et al., 2011). Skin mucus is impermeable to most bacteria and many pathogens. Mucus captures foreign particles, bacteria, and viruses, which are removed from the skin mucosa by the surrounding water. Due to this effect of mucus, pathogens are immobilized before they can adhere to or make contact with epithelial cells. Moreover, the mucous layer on the surface of the fish is not static, but dynamic both in the quantity and the quality of the substances present. Mucus is continuously secreted and replaced, which prevents colonization by potential infectious agents. Regarding the comprehensive set of innate immune defense mechanisms present at skin mucosal surfaces, the mucus is widely regarded as the most significant (Esteban, 2012).

The mucous layer is secreted by epidermal cells, mainly goblet cells and club cells, which are the unicellular glands present on the epidermis. Mucous composition is very complex and it includes widely varied biologically active substances that function as humoral innate immune factors as well as playing important roles in inhibiting the entry of pathogens. The complete range of immune factors present in the skin mucus is poorly understood. The main molecules present in mucus are high molecular weight and highly glycosylated glycoproteins called mucins. These molecules play a key role in the defense of the mucosa, and confer important adhesive, viscoelastic, and rheological properties to mucosal layers. In fact, mucins act as a mechanical barrier by serving as filters for pathogens (Roussel and Delmotte, 2004).

Knowledge of the immune factors present in the skin mucus and their role in the defense against external insults remains scarce. However, it is known that in teleosts the compartment of innate immune molecules is more diverse than that of mammals. The antimicrobial properties of epidermal mucus against infectious pathogens (bacteria and viruses) have been demonstrated in different fish species (Esteban, 2012). Present among these molecules are lysozymes, complement, lectins, agglutinins, calmodulin, interferons, C-reactive protein, proteolytic enzymes, antimicrobial peptides, vitellogenin, and immunoglobulins (Nigam et al., 2012). Among these substances, lysozyme is one of the most well characterized. Lysozyme is a ubiquitous bactericidal enzyme identified in a wide range of organisms, including fishes. Fish lysozyme exhibits lytic activity against both gram-positive and gram-negative bacteria; it acts as an opsonin (molecules that act as binding enhancers for the process of phagocytosis) and activates the complement system and phagocytic cells, which collectively contribute to the host defense against bacterial infection (Saurabh and Sahoo, 2008; Subramanian et al., 2007). Lysozyme activity has been shown to significantly vary depending on many environmental (such as season, photoperiod, water temperature, pH, toxins) and intrinsic (including sex, age, size, infections, stressors) properties. Furthermore, it has been demonstrated that lysozyme activity showed no significant correlation with other immune substances present in fish mucus, suggesting that lysozyme is constitutively secreted in the skin mucus of fish (Jung et al., 2012).

Fish mucus also contains antimicrobial peptides (AMPs, also called host defense peptides), which are positively charged short-chain amino acid molecules involved in the host defense. Their value in innate immunity lies in their ability to function without either specificity or memory. Teleost skin is a major source of AMPs with approximately 70% of all AMPs expressed in the skin, compared to 52% and 29% expressed in the gills and the gut, respectively (Gomez et al., 2013). They are potent and broad spectrum antimicrobials with little or no toxicity to host cells, and demonstrate potential as novel therapeutic agents. Furthermore, they inhibit DNA, RNA, and protein synthesis. In the skin, AMPs prevent colonization by pathogens, and are produced and stored in granules of phagocytic cells, where they directly kill the phagocytozed pathogens (Bulet et al., 2004). They are also involved in neutralization of endotoxins, leukocyte chemotaxis, immunomodulation, angiogenesis, iron metabolism, and wound repair (Guani-Guerra et al., 2010). In fish skin, several AMPs such as hipposin, piscidin, pleurocidin, parasin, defensin, and hepcidin have been found (Najafian and Babji, 2012; Gomez et al., 2013). Due to their antibiotic properties, fish AMPs could have important applications as antimicrobial and antitumoral agents, vaccine adjuvants, and inactivated vaccines (Rajanbabu and Chen, 2011).

Proteases are proteolytic enzymes that can be found in skin mucus contributing to the natural resistance of fish to infection. These enzymes are able to act directly on bacterial pathogens by cleaving their proteins, leading to death of the bacteria. Proteases also protect against pathogen invasion in an indirect manner by altering mucous consistency, thereby resulting in the increased sloughing of mucus and pathogen removal from bodily surfaces. Proteases can also activate and increase the production of other innate immune components present in fish mucus such as antibacterial peptides, complements, or immunoglobulins.

Trypsin, a serine protease, cleaves peptide chains mainly at the carboxyl side of the amino acids lysine or arginine, except when either is followed by proline. Trypsin comprises more than 25% of the complement system and is reportedly one of the major mucous proteases in several fish species (Nigam et al., 2012). Other proteases, such as cathepsin B and L (cysteine proteases), cathepsin D (aspartic protease), and metalloproteases, have also been identified in fish skin mucus (Esteban, 2012).

Fish mucus is also a rich source of lectins. Lectins are important immune mediators in lower vertebrates and invertebrates, and they may participate in innate or acquired immunity. These proteins are carbohydrate-binding proteins, macromolecules that are highly specific for sugar moieties. They have the ability to bind carbohydrates, which are involved in the attachment to cell walls. Lectins can block the attachment of the potential pathogen to inhibit invasion. Due to these properties lectins are considered potential antimicrobial agents in the skin mucus. Lectins are also involved in cell agglutination and/or precipitation of glycoconjugates. Lectins bind structures on the surface of pathogens, and can opsonize and enhance phagocytic activity, or result in activation of the complement pathway (Matsushita et al., 2004). Different types of lectin have been identified in the skin mucus of fish. Congerin from the conger eel (*Conger myriaster*) and AJL-1 from the Japanese eel (*Anguilla japonica*) were classified as galectins (characterized by its specific binding to b-galactoside). Congerins are produced and secreted into mucus by the club cells in the mucosal epithelium lining the skin (Kamiya et al., 1988).

Other key proteins have been identified in fish mucus, and all of them have major immune functions. For example, lactoferrin is a non-heme iron-binding protein that is part of the transferrin protein family. In addition to inducing systemic immunity, lactoferrin can inhibit allergic responses and promote skin immunity (González-Chávez et al., 2009). Calpain and keratin have also been reported in different tissues of fish (Rajan et al., 2013; Salem et al., 2004). Mucosal-specific calpains present in higher vertebrates are thought to play important roles in mucosal defense, whereas keratin is a cytoskeletal protein whose primary function is to protect cells from mechanical and nonmechanical injuries. Recent reports have also shown that keratin from fish mucus possesses antibacterial activity owing to its pore-forming properties (Molle et al., 2008).

Peroxidase activity has been recently demonstrated in the skin mucus of a marine teleost, and significant differences in peroxidase activity were found between skin mucus and serum samples from the same specimens, which may suggest that this enzyme has an important role in mucosal defense. Other enzymes such as alkaline phosphatase or esterase have also been identified in fish skin mucus (Guardiola et al., 2014).

Immunoglobulins (Ig), the primary humoral component of the acquired immune system, can also be found in skin mucus, and play a pivotal role in the maintenance of mucosal homeostasis (Brandtzaeg, 2009). Moreover, antibodies in cutaneous mucus and the skin of teleosts play a critical role in the protective host defense against surface infections. Up to now, three Ig classes have been identified in teleosts: IgM, IgD, and IgT (also called IgZ in some species) (Salinas et al., 2011; Sunyer, 2013). IgM is the most common Ig in the plasma of teleosts and is the principal Ig involved in systemic immunity. IgM is usually found in high concentrations in fish serum; however, it has been reported to be present at very low levels (from 8 to 90 μg/mL) in the skin mucus of several fish species (Hatten et al., 2001; Zhao et al., 2008). It is thought that the IgM antibodies possess a limited antigen spectrum in fishes. Furthermore, their presence depends on their spatial distribution; Ig levels in channel catfish were found to be highest on lateral skin, lower between pectoral and anal fins, and lowest on the caudal fin and ventral skin (Zilberg and Klesius, 1997). In the earliest studies, no apparent differences between Ig present in skin mucus and serum were reported. More recently, two Igs of different molecular weights were observed in the skin mucus of sheep head. In carp, it was described that the Ig from cutaneous mucus had different protein/carbohydrate composition and antigenicity from that of serum IgM. This tetrameric cutaneous Ig may correspond to one of the two more recently identified carp IgZ (IgZ1 and IgZ2) (Ryo et al., 2010; Savan et al., 2005). A unique redox form consisting of halfmeric constituents (H1L1, ~100 kDa) has been reported in rainbow trout skin mucus (Bromage et al., 2006). IgT, similar to mammalian IgA, is the only teleost Ig isotype with a specialized mucosal function as demonstrated in the gut of rainbow trout (Zhang et al., 2010). In addition, it has been demonstrated that IgT plays the prevailing role in skin mucosal immunity, being the most abundant Ig isotype in the skin mucosa of rainbow trout (Xu et al., 2013). It is expected that additional novel substances present in fish mucus will be described in coming years due to the emerging interest in mucosal fish defense as well as new possibilities of discovering important molecules for human medicine.

4.3 Resident cell types found in the skin

In general, the skin of adult teleosts is divided in three layers: the cuticle or mucous layer, the epidermis, and the dermis. In fish, the outermost layer of cells is alive and it retains the capacity to divide. In that regard, teleost epidermis is a stratified epithelium of variable thickness consisting entirely of live cells, of which the majority is squamous cells and the minority is mucous cells. Squamous cells are characterized by numerous desmosomes and associated cytoplasmic filaments. Teleost epidermis can be subdivided into surface, intermediate, and basal layers. The surface layer is a single-celled layer of squamous cells with only minimal quantities of keratin that develops microridges at the outer surface. These microridges contain mucus and antibacterial substances secreted to the surface from mucous goblet cells located in the intermediate stratum of the epidermis. Cells within this epidermal layer are not periodically renewed, but are replaced individually on cell death. The intermediate layer of epidermis is composed of various types of cells, including but not limited to unicellular glands (such as mucous cells and club cells), sensory cells, ionocytes, immune cells, pigment cells, and undifferentiated cells. The basal part of the epidermis is a single-cell layer (basal layer), which is attached to the basement membrane via hemidesmosomes. The basal layer tightly links the epidermis to dermis (Chang and Hwang, 2011; Esteban, 2012; Salinas et al., 2011).

The dermis is mainly composed of dense connective tissue with a large amount of collagen fibers, although it typically contains relatively little of the connective tissue found in tetrapods. Instead, in most species, it is largely replaced by solid, protective bony scales. In place of true scales, cartilaginous fishes have numerous tooth-like denticles embedded in their skin. The hypodermis consists of both loosely organized collagen fibers and a rich supply of blood vessels and, as the innermost layer, is closest to the striated muscle underneath the skin (Esteban, 2012).

4.3.1 *Leukocytes*

In contrast to mammals, fish lack major lymphoid accumulations in mucosa-associated tissues. Nevertheless, skin-associated lymphoid tissue (SALT) contains a variety of leukocytes, including, but not limited to, lymphocytes (T and B cells), plasma cells, macrophages, and granulocytes. Leukocytes and other amoeboid cells can migrate through normal mucous secretions (Esteban, 2012).

4.3.1.1 *Myeloid cells*

Mast cells, also known as eosinophilic granular cells (EGCs), are tissue-resident cells found throughout the body, particularly in association with structures like blood vessels and nerves that are in proximity to surfaces that interface with the external environment. In fish, mast cells are found in a variety of tissues, including the skin, gut, gills, brain, and in the vicinity of blood vessels. Functionally, teleost EGCs show close similarity to the mast cells of mammals. Mast cells may play an important role in the inflammatory response because they express a variety of functional proteins, including antimicrobial peptides that act against a broad spectrum of pathogens. In fish, mast cells from mucosal tissues have been studied with respect to their AMP content. However, little is known about the biology or function of these innate immune cells in skin mucosa (Esteban, 2012; Gomez et al., 2013).

In mammals, dendritic cells (DCs) act as messengers between the innate and adaptive immune systems. In different tissues, these cells act as sentinels of the immune system. When a pathogen is located and engulfed, antigens are transported to the secondary lymphoid tissues and expressed, which stimulates the production of specific T lymphocytes. Although DCs are of fundamental importance in the mammalian immune response, their presence and function in nonmammalian vertebrates has been poorly studied. Recently, dendritic-like cells have been characterized in zebrafish and rainbow trout, and it has been postulated that zebrafish skin contains DCs that are equivalent to mammalian Langerhans cells (Bassity and Clark, 2012; Lugo-Villarino et al., 2010).

Macrophages and various types of granulocytes, such as neutrophils, are also present in the skin mucosal lymphoid tissue, playing a key role as sentinel cells of the innate immune response. They are phagocytic myeloid cells; therefore, they are involved in different processes such as homeostatic mechanisms, wound healing, and the detection, elimination, and clearance of foreign entities including tumors, virus-infected cells, and invading pathogens. Moreover, macrophages and neutrophils produce hundreds of bioactive molecules that play relevant roles in the processes of pathogen recognition and destruction, cellular communication and activation, initiation of an adaptive immune response, and resolution of the inflammatory response and tissue repair (Katzenback et al., 2012).

4.3.1.2 Lymphoid cells

B and T cells are adaptive immune elements detectable in the skin of both cartilaginous and teleost fish. Among other functions, the main role of B cells in adaptive immunity appears to be the recognition of antigens in their native form and the production of Igs against those antigens. In carp skin, B cells have been detected only in the epithelium. In spotted wolffish, by using *in situ* hybridization, IgM+ cells were found both in the epithelium near the basal membrane and further out in the epidermis (Grontvedt and Espelid, 2003). As B cells are able to produce three types of Igs (IgM, IgD, and IgT/IgZ), there are different B cell subsets based on the Igs that they express. Some teleosts like the channel catfish possess three B cell subsets IgM^+/IgD^+, IgM^+/IgD^-, IgM^-/IgD^+ (Edholm et al., 2011), whereas two populations ($IgD^+/IgM^+/IgT^-$ and $IgD^-/IgM^-/IgT^+$ B cells) have been characterized in rainbow trout (Zhang et al., 2010). Although both IgT^+ and IgM^+ B cells are present at low percentages in the skin of trout, IgT^+ B cells represented the main skin B cell subset in this tissue (Xu et al., 2013).

T cells play an essential role in cell-mediated immunity, and as they interact with the bacteria present on mucosal surfaces, it seems they are very important in creating tolerance or immunity against the commensal microbiota. There are different T cell subsets in mammals (cytotoxic, Th1, Th2, Treg, and Th17) and some of them have also been described in teleost fish. However, teleost skin T cells have not been studied in detail so far (Gomez et al., 2013)

4.3.2 Epithelial cells

The basic cellular element of the fish epidermis is the epithelial cell. Epithelial cells are active orchestrators of homeostasis, commensal colonization, and innate and adaptive immune response through the expression of PRRs, including lectins, NOD-like receptors (NLRs), and toll-like receptors (TLRs). Moreover, they are capable of interacting directly with pathogens and commensal bacteria (Gomez et al., 2013). Contrary to mammals, the epithelial cells in teleost fishes are alive and metabolically active, so they retain the capacity for mitotic division. Cells in any layer of the epidermis can potentially divide, although mitotic activity is most common in the lower layers. In this way, dead cells are regularly sloughed from the epidermal surface and replaced by living cells beneath. The exterior surface of superficial epithelial cells of teleosts is characterized by microridges, which aid in retaining mucous secretions on the skin surface. The epithelial cell is the key element in the unique wound repair mechanism of fish skin. Shortly after damage occurs, epithelial cells migrate from the edges of the wound toward the wound cavity in compact groups. These cells can rapidly cover the wound, providing a protective barrier against infection by opportunistic pathogens during the early stages of wound repair (Elliott, 2011).

4.4 Skin immune responses in diseased fish

Fish are in an intimate contact with their environment and as compared to terrestrial animals, fish "swim" in a sea of pathogens. Thus, any rupture in the normal barrier function of the skin could allow colonization of the skin by infectious agents or invasion by opportunistic microorganisms (microorganisms that normally colonize the skin but are typically of low pathogenicity) (Law, 2001). For this reason, cutaneous disease is relatively more common in fish than in terrestrial vertebrates. Fish skin possesses highly developed antimicrobial features, many of which have been preserved throughout evolution, and immune defense strategies employed by piscine skin are still operative in human skin.

The process of pathogen entry through the skin is being studied by using noninvasive whole-body imaging techniques on living animals. Bioluminescence imaging, typically using luciferase reporter systems/constructs, is now widely used in small-animal models such as rodents and fish. This technique offers the advantage of using the same animal for multiple data collections over the course of the entire experiment. Moreover, luciferin, the substrate of luciferase, has been shown to cross cell membranes allowing this reporter protein to be imaged in different tissues of interest (Costes et al., 2009).

Some observed differences in disease susceptibility between fish species and/or strains have been linked to the differing ability of the fish to prevent pathogen attachment and entry at mucosal epithelial sites. Cutaneous lesions are generally nonspecific and may be indicative of disease that is restricted to the integument or a manifestation of systemic disease. Fish skin is able to react uniquely to different attacks. Changes in the skin are "a priori," the most readily observed clinical features of fish, including traumatic lesions, changes in coloration, and/or changes in one or more parts of the skin (including both humoral factors and different cell types). The perfect combination of mucous composition and the kinetic processes of the epidermis must prevent colonization of the skin surface and, for this reason, prevent infection. In the next subsections, the main changes in the skin mucus as well as those observed in skin epidermis and dermis in response to infection will be described.

4.4.1 Changes in the skin mucus in response to infection

As described above, skin mucus has powerful mechanisms that can immobilize or even kill pathogens before they contact epithelial surfaces. Changes in the amount of mucus (an increase or decrease) are common but the most interesting changes are those affecting the chemical composition of the mucus. These changes, due to the large number of substances that can be involved (many still uncharacterized), are responsible for the varied responses that orchestrate mucosal skin immunity. Furthermore, all of these changes can take place without the pathogen in question making physical contact with the epithelial cells underlying the layer of mucus.

The mechanisms of pathogenicity induced by certain bacteria are still uncertain and frequently those mechanisms are correlated to the ability of bacteria to adhere to mucus (Baffone et al., 2006; Zorilla et al., 2003). *Vibrio alginolyticus* strains show a specific binding capability to gilthead sea bass and gilthead seabream mucus (Snoussi et al., 2008). A strong ability to adhere to the fish skin mucus of different species has been reported for different bacteria pathogenic for fish (e.g., *Flavobacterium columnare*; *Photobacterium damselae*, subsp. *damselae*; *V. vulnificus*; *V. alginolyticus*; *V. anguillarum*; *Aeromonas hydrophila*; *P. damselae*, subsp. *piscicida*; and *Flexibacter maritimus*) (Fouz et al., 2000). However, other studies have demonstrated that the skin mucus of some fish species is able to inhibit the adhesion of certain pathogenic bacteria. For example, seabream skin mucus inhibits the adhesion of *Pasteurella piscicida*, *F. maritimus*, *V. anguillarum*, and *V. damsela*.

Some pathogens have developed strategies to circumvent the mucosal barrier to reach epithelial cells. Specifically, the mucous layer can be amended by the pathogen, allowing the pathogen to move through the mucus and adhere to the epithelial cells (Cone, 2009). In the skin of channel catfish and blue catfish, *A. hydrophila* infection rapidly altered the gene expression of a number of potentially critical lectins, chemokines, interleukins, and other mucosal factors in a coordinated manner predicted to enhance its ability to adhere to and invade catfish hosts (Li et al., 2013a; Li et al., 2013b).

It has also been demonstrated that some bacteria harvested from fish skin are able to degrade the skin mucus of the same fish species (Snoussi et al., 2008). For this reason, their presence in skin mucus can make the fish more vulnerable to colonization by other pathogenic or even opportunistic microorganisms. Furthermore, maintaining homeostasis of the physicochemical factors of mucus is important to avoid the potential invasion and/or adhesion of pathogens to mucosal surfaces. For example, mucous transport requires well-regulated viscoelasticity, which is controlled by hydration. By making the mucus slightly more hydrated, the fluid could have a markedly lower viscoelasticity and be readily penetrable by motile bacteria (Cone, 2009). In fact, in challenge experiments with bacteria, removal of mucus/epidermal cells increased the cumulative mortality in salmonids compared to undamaged fish (Madetoja et al., 2002).

The thickness of the mucous blanket is determined by the balance between the rate of secretion and the rate of degradation and shedding. Toxic and irritating substances can greatly stimulate mucous secretion, increasing the thickness of the mucous blanket. Similarly, many infectious agents can modulate the thickness, or alter mucous layer consistency (apparent when studying fish under polarized light). This effect is particularly evident in protozoal and other parasitic infections.

It is known that a mucous blanket is secreted from goblet cells in the epithelium immediately after the first contact with pathogens. More recently, it was demonstrated (by using histological, histochemical, and biochemical techniques) that carp skin mucosa responds rapidly to high bacterial loads, even if the bacteria involved are considered to be nonpathogenic, with an increased secretion of mucin molecules, especially low-glycosylated variants (Van der Marel et al., 2010). Different studies seem to corroborate that mucin-type molecules excreted by intestinal goblet cells are highly species-specific (e.g., sulphated mucins in shi drum (*Umbrina cirrosa*), or neutral mucins in common dentex (*Dentex dentex*)). To date, no similar studies have been reported in fish skin mucus.

Skin mucus also acts as a medium in which antibacterial effectors may act. The mucosal skin defense system secretes different molecules or components into the mucous layer, although there is still a limited knowledge about these defense mechanisms. There are both intrinsic and constitutive antimicrobial components of the mucus (Ellis, 2001). Furthermore, mucus can also be the vehicle for other innate immune humoral factors secreted in the epidermis or in the dermis. In summary, fish skin mucus features an arsenal of a variety of naturally active substances as well as numerous defense molecules of both the innate and acquired immune system (Palaksha et al., 2008; Subramanian et al., 2007, 2008). These antimicrobial properties of epidermal mucus against infectious pathogens (mainly bacteria and viruses) have been demonstrated in different fish species (Kuppulakshmi et al., 2008) and increased expression of one or more of the above-mentioned antimicrobial components in fish epidermal mucus has been observed following microbial stress (Patrzykat et al., 2001), thus supporting the function of epidermal mucus in defending fish from infectious pathogens.

Among the humoral factors present in fish mucus in the present chapter, we will describe the variations of some enzymes, proteases, antimicrobial peptides, and other molecules more recently studied. Regarding enzymes, the levels of some of them increased in skin mucus as a consequence of injury and/or infection. For example, increased activities of phosphatases (considered to play a protective role) were demonstrated in epidermal cells after and during skin injury and regeneration related to cutaneous wound healing, during stress or parasitic infections. Furthermore, alkaline phosphatase has been demonstrated as a potential stress indicator in skin mucus of Atlantic salmon (Ross et al., 2000). It seems that no significant relationship was observed between the phosphatase activity and other mucosal parameters (Jung et al., 2012).

Secretion of proteases into skin has been described as a consequence of the pathogen recognition. Proteases may act directly on a pathogen (e.g., they can kill bacteria by proteolysis) or may modify mucous consistency or increase the sloughing of the mucus, effectively preventing pathogen invasion and facilitating the removal of pathogens from the bodily surfaces. Proteases also activate and enhance the production of other known innate immune components present in fish mucus (such as complement, antibacterial peptides, or Ig).

Antimicrobial peptides are gradually more recognized as a significant component of the host's defense against infection and they are considered a very important part of the mucus and skin barrier function. AMPs are produced (constitutively or induced upon infection in fish epidermal mucus) to defend against invading pathogens (Sarmas¸ik, 2002).

Lectins interact with pathogenic surface structures (such as those present on bacteria, viruses, or parasites) that result in increased phagocytosis (through opsonisation) or complement activation. Lectins recognize different pathogenic bacteria. For example, congerins recognize marine bacteria such as *V. anguillarum.* Similarly, pufflectin binds to the parasitic trematode (*Heterobothrium okamotoi*). Pufflectin (a mannose-specific lectin isolated from the skin mucus of pufferfish) shows no sequence similarity with any known animal lectins, but unexpectedly shares sequence homology with mannose-binding lectins found in monocotyledonous plants. Recently, a rhamnose-binding lectin expressed in gill/skin was found to play a role in the pathogenesis of columnaris disease in channel catfish *Ictalurus punctatus* (Beck et al., 2012). Intelectin protein is expressed in skin and gill club cells of catfish (*Silurus asotus*). Although the intelectin showed agglutination activity against the pathogenic bacterium *A. salmonicida*, its expression was not induced by *in vivo* bacterial stimulation. Taken together all the available results on lectins present in fish mucus, it seems reasonable to think that mucous lectins in fish have wide molecular diversity (Suzuki et al., 2003). Furthermore, there is evidence that suggest that lectins actively participate in the self-defense system by acting on intra- and extra-body surfaces.

The antimicrobial effect of histones is now well known, but only recently are they being recognized as endogenous antibiotics and, for this property, being linked to the innate immune system of fish (Fernandes et al., 2002, 2003). Histone H2B is present in the skin mucus of Atlantic cod and inhibits important bacterial and fungal pathogens of fish (e.g., *A. hydrophila* and *Saprolegnia spp.*). Curiously, histone fragments can also show antimicrobial properties. For example, levels of N-terminal segments of catfish H2A were increased in the epidermal mucus upon stimulation (Patrzykat et al., 2001) and reduced in the absence of disease (Robinette and Noga, 2001).

The available literature describing the skin mucosal immune response after viral infections is particularly scarce, but it has been demonstrated that AMPs are involved in such responses. It is assumed that viruses bearing capsids can disseminate freely through mucus to effectively enter a fish and cause disease. Thus, capsid viruses appear to have a unique mechanism to enter mucus because they are small enough, neutral in net surface charge, and are coated densely with charged groups that prevent hydrophobic binding to mucins. In addition, they have evolved effective methods for selectively adhering to and entering their target cells (Cone, 2009). However, this is not true for all the viruses. For example, it has been demonstrated that skin mucus of *Cyprinus carpio* inhibits cyprinid herpes virus 3 binding to epidermal cells (Raj et al., 2011).

Three different β-defensins from rainbow trout increase in expression during bacterial and simulated viral challenges (Casadei et al., 2009). It is important to underline that AMPs have a double function in antiviral defense, acting not only directly on the virion, but also on the host cell. However, only a few successful attempts to assess the antiviral activities of fish AMPs have been reported. Fish depend more greatly on their innate immune defenses than mammals, and for this reason, they are seen as a likely rich source of antiviral compounds for fighting not only viral infections in fish, but potentially mammalian viruses (Falco et al., 2009). Future research will add to the understanding of the relationships between viruses and fish skin mucosa, as well as the mucosal immune responses elicited by them.

The literature available on the responses of fish skin against parasites is more abundant than those available for bacteria and viruses. The skin is a very frequent place of parasite invasion despite the barrier functions associated with mucosal epithelia of fish. To minimize the effect of parasitic infection, both innate and adaptive defense mechanisms have to be involved (Jones, 2001). Here, special attention will be paid to ectoparasites, those inhabiting within or on the skin.

Fish can also respond to a parasitic infection by altering the quantity or quality of the mucous secretion and this mucus plays a very important role in limiting the parasite load. Two ectoparasitic taxa have been widely studied and have contributed to the information about host resistance in fish: the gyrodactylid monogeneans and the caligid copepods. For example, infection by the parasite *Trichodina* or the metazoan *Gyrodactylus* can provoke excessive mucous production. Hypersecretion of mucus may be associated with a localized epithelial cell hyperplasia or inflammation (both reactions will be described in the next section of this chapter). Pathogenesis in gyrodactyliasis may be related to skin mucification or to a local reduction of mucous cells, and it is considered that a high mucous turnover may be involved in protecting fish against invasion in a similar way to that described for bacteria.

The ciliate parasite *Ichthyophthirius multifiliis* (which is a common obligate and a highly motile ectoparasite) is one of the most important protozoan pathogens of freshwater fish. Parasitized fish usually die following infection, but animals surviving sublethal parasite exposure become resistant to subsequent challenge. This resistance correlates with the presence of humoral antibodies in the sera and also in the cutaneous mucus of immune fish. In fact, fish vaccinated against *I. multifiliis* by intraperitoneal injection of purified immobilization antigens (i-antigens; the surface proteins targeted by immobilizing antibodies) in Freund's complete adjuvant built up active protective immunity and produced antibodies against i-antigens (Clark et al., 2001) in both the blood and the cutaneous mucus. It has been observed that parasites rapidly leave the skin of *I. multifiliis*-immune fish and the explanation could be an antibody-mediated mechanisms of cutaneous immunity (Dickerson and Clark, 1998).

Although there is experimental evidence supporting the existence of a separate mucosal immune system in fish, it is not known exactly how mucosal antibodies reach the surface epithelia of the skin. Findings suggest that parasite-specific antibodies in the cutaneous mucus of channel catfish do not arise by passive transfer or exudation from the blood. Maki and Dickerson (2003) found that mucosal antibodies were produced following either *I. multifiliis* infection or the injection of purified antigen and that in both cases their occurrence did not exactly coincide with serum antibody production. In addition, when skin explants from channel catfish immunized against *I. multifiliis* are cultured *in vitro*, they release *I. multifiliis*-specific antibodies, implying that antibodies are actively produced by cells in skin rather than diffusing from serum (Xu et al., 2002). However, the appearance of i-antigen-specific antibodies in both skin and serum demonstrate that cutaneous mucosal and systemic immunity are integrated (Zhao et al., 2008). Despite the limited amount of related research to date, it seems that a certain parallelism exists between the response observed in the mucus of a possible bacterial and parasitic infection. Further work will help verify this assumption.

4.4.2 Changes in skin epidermis in response to infection

Most animals have the ability to repair an epidermal lesion (e.g., after an infection or a physical injury). In fish, the keratocyte participation in the epithelialization of the wound gap involves changes in the surface architecture of the epithelial cells. In fact, the epidermal healing response is very rapid in fish. As a quick response to injury, copious mucous secretion and accumulation is observed on the surface of the adjacent epithelial cells, which is also associated with the protective function of mucus against pathogenic microorganisms (Rai et al., 2012). It includes a migration of malpigian cells from the periphery of the wound over the wound surface and this makes possible the repair of the lesion. Besides this, keratocytes can cover fish skin wounds with a new protective layer of cells within hours after wounding by rapid migration from the surrounding wound margins. This capacity of fast epidermal healing of fish is crucial for avoiding subsequent infections, but even more remarkable is the property of regeneration (an exceptional and remarkable cellular event in vertebrates). Teleosts can fully regenerate largely severed appendages (such as fins) with different tissues, as it has been described in several aquatic urodelan amphibians. Fin regeneration is a rapid process in which the wound is first healed by the rapid migration and reorganization of the epithelial cells of the base to cover the surface of the cut, leading to the formation of the wound epidermis (Akimenko et al., 2003).

Regarding the changes that can be observed in skin epidermis in response to infection, it is important to mention that the epidermis of fish is avascular, a characteristic that limits its range of potential responses. Frequently, changes in the epidermis reflect other pathological alterations of other tissues or organs as well as changes in the dermis (which is vascular). Pathological changes in fish epidermis include epidermal degeneration, epidermal erosion, epidermal ulceration, and leukocyte infiltration.

Epidermal degeneration is defined as swollen epidermal cells (intracellular edema) with pyknotic (condensed) nuclei. Epidermal erosion is identified by the sloughing of the epidermal layers, but with an intact basement membrane. Epidermal ulceration involves a complete loss of all epidermal layers including the basement membrane. Lastly, leukocyte infiltration is the presence of a greater number of leucocytes in the epidermal and dermal layers.

At the cellular level, there are two important phenomena that determine the outcome of epithelial cell injury (similar as that which occurs in other cell types): (1) cell membrane damage (with associated fluid and ionic imbalances) and (2) the inability of mitochondria (the source of power of the cell) to restart ATP synthesis. As a tissue, fish skin, similar to most other tissues of the body, responds to injuries and severe tissue damage with an inflammatory response. Inflammation, together with hemorrhages, ulcers, and changes in coloration are the most frequent changes in the skin as a consequence of a bacterial infection.

Inflammation is a protective mechanism that provides fluids to the site of injury to help preserve homeostasis in the damaged cells and tissues. The most common causes of such damage are physical and chemical traumas, microbes and their toxins, death of cells, and immune reactions. The results of acute inflammation can lead to the complete resolution of the problem, or the development of exudative or necrotic lesions and progression to chronic inflammation. When inflammation is countered rapidly, the skin will return to a normal appearance after repair by local proliferation. The earliest sign of an inflammatory response in the teleost epidermis is spongiosis (in other words, intercellular edema, separation of the cells by presence of extracellular liquid).

Exudates are the results of continuous production of inflammatory response and may be of different nature: catarrhal (typical from mucous surfaces as skin), supurative (if predominantly neutrophil cells), fibrinous (if there is high leakage of fibrinogen from capillaries), or serous (abundant watery exudate in peritoneal or pericardial cavities). Necrosis occurs if cellular damage is not immediately lethal. During necrosis, intracellular fluid is accumulated and cells swell. These changes may be reversible but, if they progress, the cells may become vacuolated, and nucleic acid is damaged resulting in cell death. Epithelial cell death can also be caused by toxins produced by gram-negative bacteria (e.g., *Aeromonas* spp., *Pseudomonas* spp., *V. anguillarum*).

Furthermore, different cell types present in fish epidermis can internalize particular matter such as bacteria and other particles. Phagocytosis is a very effective cellular innate immune activity serving to defend against microorganisms or parasites.

Some bacteria (e.g., *F. columnare*) cause lesions in the skin, at the beginning of the infection as small places where they grow and those places appear surrounded by a hyperemic tissue giving rise to hemorrhagic ulcers and necrotic tissue. Many bacteria may also cause hemorrhages in the skin (e.g., *A. hydrophila*), which, when the infection progresses, may ulcerate to form necrotic lesions. Also frequent are the appearance of petechiae, which are small (1–2 mm) red or purple spots on the body, caused by a minor hemorrhages. Other bacteria cause skin ulcers featuring a discontinuity of the skin or a break in the skin, accompanied by the disintegration of tissue. Ulcers can result in a complete loss of the epidermis, portions of the dermis, and even subcutaneous fat. Skin ulcers are often visible as an inflamed tissue with an area of reddened skin. Ulcerative lesions are likely to be initiated by a series of factors that lead to a breach of the normal barrier function of the skin (Law, 2001). Skin ulcers can have many different etiologies, including infectious agents, toxins, physical causes, immunologic causes, and nutritional and metabolic perturbations. For example, the bacteria *Moritella viscosa* is considered to be the agent causing winter ulcer diseases characterized by extensive and chronic ulceration of the skin and septicemia (Ingerslev et al., 2010). Recently, it has been demonstrated that *M. viscosa* (but not *A. wodanis*) affected or inhibited the epidermal regeneration abilities of keratocytes (Karlsen et al., 2012).

Many infectious agents can cause changes in skin pigmentation. The most frequent is skin darkening (e.g., the bacteria *Flavobacterium psychrophilum, P. damselae, Pseudomonas anguilliseptica, V. anguillarum, V. salmonicida, Aeromonas salmonicida, Renibacterium salmoninarum, Mycobacterium marinum*), although some other agents cause depigmentation (e.g., *Edwardsiella tarda, Nocardia kampachi*).

Regarding the most frequent changes in the skin as a consequence of a viral infection are petechial hemorrhages and skin hypertrophy and hyperplasia. Different viruses including redfin perch iridovirus, sheatfish iridovirus, and black catfish herpes virus give rise to the petechial hemorrhages, sometimes with preference to a specific body location (e.g., in the base of the fins, operculum).

One of the most studied and well-known skin responses are the changes provoked by lymphocystis disease virus. This disease is characterized by the appearance of light-colored nodular lesions on the skin. Microscopically, it was demonstrated that each nodule comprises an individual virus-infected cell, which is hypertrophied. The infected cells cease dividing, although continue growing; the cells enlarge and show a hyaline capsule before starting a degeneration phase. In this phase macrophages and other phagocytic cells surround the infected cells. Release of virus occurs when the infected cells break down and this could result in a new infection of adjacent cells. Immunohistochemistry and *in situ* hybridization techniques have been used for the detection of lymphocystis disease virus in different tissues. By using a polyclonal antibody raised against a major capsid protein, the virus was detected in skin dermis and caudal fin (Cano et al., 2009).

White sturgeon iridovirus disease also results in the formation of numerous hypertrophied cells in the epithelium and epidermis, and infected cells are seen by light microscopy separating from the dermis. Turbot herpes virus causes giant cells in the fish malpighian epidermis cells. Furthermore, pike epidermal proliferation herpes virus can cause lesions composed of large hypertrophied cells in the fish epidermis.

Hyperplasia is very common in the fish epidermis and all the cell types may proliferate. Usually, hyperplasia is accompanied by spongiosis. Hyperplasia of epithelial cells minimizes the chances of epidermal disruption. There are many causes such as chemical pollutants, hormonal stimuli, bacteria (e.g., *Flexibacter* sp.), virus (e.g., cod and dab adenoviruses; European catfish herpes virus provokes a thickened epidermis without mucous cells; carp pox disease provokes multiple, focal lesions of benign, noninvasive and nonnecrotizing epidermal hyperplasia; Japanese flounder herpes virus; Pacific cod herpes virus), and even, parasites. For example, *Costia necator* is an ectoparasite, which causes costiasis characterized by hyperplasia of the epithelial cells, exhaustion of goblet cells in the area of the parasite attachment, spongiosis, and sloughing of the epidermis. Sometimes, epidermal hyperplasia results in secondary infection with other bacteria or the abnormal tissue may be infiltrated with numerous foci of melanin. Other factors such as netting damage or skin abrasion by parasites can assist virus transmission.

Most fish alloherpesviruses cause primary pathology to epithelial cells, with cells showing signs of virus replication. Characteristic histological changes in diseased fish with alloherpesvirus infections include epidermal cell necrosis (cell death), syncytia formation (multinucleated epithelial cells), epidermal cell hypertrophy, epidermal hyperplasia, and papillomas (benign tumor cells). Epithelial cells that are infected often display enlarged nuclei with marginated chromatin (Hanson et al., 2011).

Regarding parasites, *I. multifiliis* and *Gyrodactylus salaris* have been used to study the ontogeny of the mucosal immune response. The infection is initiated by invasion of the skin by free swimming, ~40 mm theronts that grow within the epithelium, causing extensive damage to the skin. Besides variations in the physicochemical characteristics of skin mucus, the presence of bioactive molecules (e.g., complement, lysozyme, C-reactive protein, lectins) and epidermal migration of inflammatory cells and their secretions may affect the establishment and propagation of parasites (Dickerson and Clark, 1998; Kania et al., 2010).

There are fish parasitic protozoans that use the fish integument as their environment. While many of them are considered as ectocommensals (may simply use the skin as an anchoring substrate), they can sometimes become very numerous and may interfere with normal skin functions. Flagellated protozoans are usually ectoparasites; they attach to epithelial cells and penetrate them. For example, trophozoites from *I. multifiliis* and *Cryptocaryon irritans* destroy epithelial cells in freshwater and seawater fish, respectively. Some ectoparasites (e.g., monogenean and crustacean) modulate mucous production during attachment by reducing the density of mucous cells in the skin of the host. Pathogenesis in gyrodactyliasis is related to skin mucification or to local reduction of mucous cells. Other parasites cause deposition of melanin pigment around the encysted parasite in the host's skin.

Tumors are among the most frequently reported abnormalities involving the skin. Tumors of the epithelial tissues (including the skin) are characterized by the ability of the cells to grow in clusters or sheets of cells. Furthermore, they are also characterized by their ability to provoke the proliferation of capillaries and a stroma of connective tissue, known as a desmoplastic response. Benign tumors of epithelial cells, such as papillomas, vary in size and shape and project above the skin surface. Papillomas can be single or multiple, soft or firm, and exhibit different colors (depending on whether melanocytes are involved). Papillomas typically consist of a stratified squamous epithelium with a supporting stroma. Immunological findings tend to support histologic observations showing that lesions are ultimately sloughed as a result of a cell-mediated immune response. Papilloma cells were found to be similar to normal epidermis in having interdigitating cell membranes with desmosomes (when observed by transmission electron microscopy). Papillomas are rarely lethal, although major problems correlated to the disfigurement caused in specimens and subsequent economic loss makes the study of these tumors of interest. Clinical signs of papillomas can vary from small raised nodules to large, gray-to-black epithelial growths and can appear on any location of the body. Most epithelial papillomas are a result of viral infection (e.g., smelt papilloma herpesvirus, Atlantic salmon papilloma, Esocid lymphosarcoma, pike epidermal proliferation, or white sucker papilloma) and only in scarce cases have been demonstrated to be oncogenic.

Some tumors affect only the epidermis and consist of a hyperplastic epithelium, while others affect the dermis. For example, walleye dermal sarcoma is a retrovirus causing skin lesions of nodular appearance. Although the initial stage occurs in the epidermis, in the later stages, the tumor cells affect the dermis. Piscine retroviruses comprise both exogenous and endogenous viruses; most of them are associated with proliferative diseases. Because several of these proliferative diseases have a seasonal tendency, they offer an exceptional model for studying tumor development and regression. Numerous proliferative diseases in fish have been associated with one or more retroviruses. Typically, these occur as seasonal epizootics affecting farmed and wild fish and most lesions resolve spontaneously. Natural resolution and lifelong resistance to reinfection are two features of some piscine retrovirus-induced tumors that have motivated research interest in this field. The epidemiological and morphological features of proliferative diseases in fish that have been associated with retroviruses have been recently revised (Coffee et al., 2013).

Other changes visible in skin epidermis as a consequence of an infection are the presence of immune factors and immune cells involved in adaptive immunity. Regarding the adaptive immune response in fish skin, it must be taken into account some peculiarities of their immune system. The lymphatic tissue of teleosts is concentrated around the kidneys. They have neither lymph nodes nor bone marrow. However, in the higher bony fish, an adaptive, predominantly humoral immune response has been found. Skin-associated lymphatic follicles are still lacking, but now ATPase-positive dendritic cells and IgM-positive lymphocytes are seen in the epidermis (Wölfle et al., 2009). Furthermore, although the number of lymphocytes present in the epidermis is usually low, it can be highly variable depending on the severity of the immune reaction. It has also been demonstrated that allogeneic skin grafts are rejected relatively rapidly following a circadian rhythm (Flajnik and du Pasquier, 2004).

Based on several experimental approaches (e.g., intraperitoneal administration of serum antibodies), it has been postulated that IgM molecules are poorly transported to the mucosal secretions. For this reason, it has been proposed that the presence of IgM in skin mucus of fish is a result of some mechanism mediating its secretion into the external fluids, and that cells localized near the skin epithelium are responsible for the production of the cutaneous antibodies. Secreted Ig is locally produced in the skin.

4.4.3 Changes in skin dermis and hypodermis in response to infection

The skin dermis and hypodermis will be considered simultaneously in terms of disease because they usually respond very similarly. In fish, cutaneous lesions are generally nonspecific and may be indicative of disease that is just restricted to the integument or a manifestation of systemic disease (Groff, 2001). In fact, there are different pathogenic microorganisms that are able to produce severe alterations to fish (in occasions, 100% mortality after infection) only by affecting the mucosal surface. For example, infection caused by the bacterium *F. columnare* (columnaris disease agent) causes a chronic, ulcerative, necrotic infection of the body surface. The bacteria are readily detected in skin specimens from infected fish; however, they are infrequently detected in other internal organs (e.g., liver, kidney, or spleen) (Tripathi et al., 2005).

However, other bacterial infections (e.g., *E. tarda*) originate in the epidermis and but can progress to cause ulcers affecting the dermis, even the myonecrosis of the overlying areas characterized by cutaneous lesions that extend down into the musculature and to vital organs like the kidney or the liver. After ulceration of the skin, lesions are often hemorrhagic with fibers of collagen surrounding the infected area of the dermis. Chronic inflammatory lesions of the dermis may cause melanophore damage, lymphocytic infiltration, as well as macrophages in the epidermis that phagocytose melanosomes from damaged cells. Other bacteria can cause hemorrhagic ulcers affecting the epidermis, the dermis and the hypodermis (e.g., *Pseudomonas anguilliseptica*). Furthermore, bacteria like *Vibrio viscosus* originate subdermal focal lesions, which initially are hemorrhagic and progress to more necrotic lesions of the dermis and even of the overlying tissues.

Another change observable in the dermis as a consequence of an infection is the appearance of furuncles; a good example are those caused by *A. salmonicida*. A furuncle results from localization of bacteria in the dermis (although sometimes in the epidermis) where the bacteria cause hyperemia with fibrinous edema and then infiltration of macrophages and granulocytes. The center of the lesions correspond to an area of liquefactive necrosis with characteristic strands of fibrin.

Regarding parasitic infections, hemorrhagic and necrotic dermal lesions are often detected. In *Uronema* infections, appearance of brown patches on the skin coincides with the appearance of a large number of pathogens in skin. Other major clinical/pathological manifestations include severe necrotic lesions in the epidermal and dermal musculature of the posterior half of the affected fish. The parasite reaches the blood stream quickly through the lesions on the skin and the ciliates rapidly invade and proliferate in the skin and gills. Afterward, the parasite consume both host cells and body fluids and can spread to the internal organs in the absence of any additional pathogens such as secondary bacterial invaders (Azad et al., 2007).

Tetrahymena corlissi is the causative agent of scuticociliatosis, parasitizes skin and muscle, and sometimes invades body cavities of freshwater fishes. It has a high potential for systemic invasion, destroying tissues that lead to high mortalities of the host. When the disease manifests, the initial clinical symptoms include dark coloration, excessive mucous production, loss of scales, hemorrhagic lesions and/or bleached spots on the skin, and dermal necrotic lesions that finally destroy tissues leading to high mortalities. This parasite feeds on the epithelium of the skin and grows large enough to be visible to the naked eye. Afterward, some dermal necrotic lesions coalesce to form brownish musky clinical manifestations (Harikrishnan et al., 2010). Similarly, some fungi can give rise to skin lesions when grown on skin cells (e.g., *Saprolegnia*) by invading the epidermis and the dermis.

4.4.4 The embryology of the skin immune system

While the structure, organization, and composition of fish skin have attracted the attention of researchers for a long time, information on skin development remains scarce. During the first half of the last century most studies on fish skin have been limited to morphological descriptions of structural diversity, usually in relation to the environment of the fish. With the introduction of the electron microscope, some authors have investigated the structure of fish skin (mainly epidermis), as well as scale structure and development. However, even at present there are very few studies dealing with fish skin development, and most available descriptions highlight features of adult skin. The origins of these skin layers of teleosts are still unknown and it is also surprising that the teleost dermis has not been well characterized in any species.

One major developmental process of fish is the formation of the neural crest, which is found only in chordates. From this channel-like structure the neural tube is established (which is located between the epidermis and notochord). Cells of the neural crest migrate to different parts of the embryo, where they differentiate into diverse types of cells, like parts of the teeth, cartilage, or sensory cells of the skin. All vertebrates initially have the same type of skin. Only later does the skin develop fish scales, reptilian scales, bird feathers, or the hair, claws, and nails of mammals. The epidermis differentiates from an epidermogenic cell population of the embryonic ectoderm, along with neurogenic cell populations giving rise to the central nervous system and the neural crest. However, the dermis derives from the paraxial mesoderm (dermatome region), except for the head region, where it derives from the (ecto) mesenchyme of neural crest origin. These studies have been done in zebrafish.

In embryos (at 90% epiboly) the epidermis consists of a single layer of more or less polarized cells covered by an external, "enveloping" layer, the periderm. The epidermal cells fuse at the midline approximately at 14-somite stage (Schmitz et al., 1998). The epidermis in embryos and young larvae is very thin (less than 10 μm thick). During week 1 of fish larval development, the epidermis is not differentiated in various layers yet, but by weeks 4–6 the thickness increases and various layers appear, depending upon the region of the body. In consequence, only transmission electron microscopical studies can provide an accurate morphological description of the early development of fish epidermis and dermis (Le Guellec et al., 2004). In very early developmental stages, the osmoregulation relies on the skin integument that is covered by ionocytes, in which the ion pumping activity takes place.

Several types of pigment cells arise from the neural crest, including xanthophores, iridophores and melanocytes. This evolutionary achievement is linked with important features of fish skin: a stratified mucogenic epidermis and an alpha-keratogenic potential. Mucous cells differentiate early in development on the surface of epithelium and contain acid and neutral mucopolysaccharides. Primordial sensory buds are visible within the epithelia of the skin of the head in week 1 larvae, and become numerous during later larval development. Club cells, specialized epidermal cells that have an immune function, appear in the middle layer of the head and trunk epidermis on week 4 (Saadatfar et al., 2010).

The fish immune system is adapted to the fact that fish are free-living organisms from the embryonic stage of life in their aquatic environment. For this main reason, fish rely on their innate immune system for a long period of time, beginning at the early stages of embryogenesis. The barrier defenses and innate immune proteins play critical roles during the early-stage fish embryos prior to the development of functional organ systems. The innate immune proteins present in the yolk of embryos are of maternal origin. Early-stage teleostean embryos are dependent upon the adult female for the formation of the zona pellucida as an essential barrier defense, for their supply of nutrients, and for the innate immune proteins and antibodies that are transferred from the maternal circulation to the oocytes. Maternally derived hormones are also transferred, some of which (e.g., cortisol) are known to exert a suppressive action on some aspects of the immune defenses (Li and Leatherland, 2012).

The adult skin develops from the ectoderm on the surface of the post-gastrulation embryo. Skin is a dynamic structure with proliferation in the basal layer, which is in contact with a basement membrane. The skin stem cells are located in the basal part of the epidermis and in specialized compartments of skin appendages. When cells finish differentiation, they cease proliferation and migrate upward, losing contact with the basement membrane. It is known that epidermis is constantly renewed, with a fine equilibrium between proliferation and differentiation. A key characteristic of this protective outer layer is that it is continually shed by new cells. Skin appendages develop from embryonic skin resulting from sequential epithelial-mesenchymal interactions and help with epidermal repair and regeneration. The teleost dermomyotome has been studied including primary myotome morphogenesis, the relationship between the primary myotome and the dermomyotome, as well as the differentiation of axial and appendicular muscles and dermis from the dermomyotome (comprehensively reviewed in Stellabotte and Devoto, 2007).

In contrast to the considerable knowledge of skin patterning and epithelial appendage development in mammals and birds, little is known about the molecular control of skin patterning and scale morphogenesis in fish. The term "scale" in the fish literature is often used as a widespread term for all the hard, normally flattened, skeletal elements found in the skin of aquatic vertebrates. These include the scales of chondrichthyans (placoid scales), the scales of basal actinopterygians (ganoid scales), the bony scales of some actinopterygian taxa (dermal bony scales and scutes), and the scales of basal sarcopterygian taxa and most actinopterygian species (elasmoid scales). Although all these types of appendages are evolutionary linked as derivatives of a common ancestral type, they have a different structure (Sire and Akimenko, 2004). The establishment of the squamation pattern has been described in several teleost species. In all fish species studied so far, the scales appear very late in ontogeny, that is, several weeks post-fertilization, after metamorphosis, when the juveniles are already miniatures of the adults. In the zebrafish skin, fibroblasts, from which the scale-forming cells will differentiate, invade the primary dermal stroma only 20–26 days post-fertilization (Le Guellec et al., 2004), suggesting that fibroblast invasion (and further skin development) requires a specific state of differentiation of the collagenous stroma, and of the cells of the basal epidermal layer. Alizarin red staining of juvenile zebrafish has revealed that scale appearance is related to a combination of size and age.

4.5 Future directions and conclusions

Numerous laboratory models can be applied to better understand skin immunity but only some of them will be mentioned here. For example, the use of cell lines, which represent valuable biological tools for carrying out multiple experimental comparisons in pathology, carcinogenesis, and transgenics. Teleost fish cell lines have been developed from a broad range of tissues, including skin and most fish cell lines originated from normal tissues (Lakra et al., 2011). It has been shown that freshly harvested rainbow trout scales can be incorporated into fish skin cell cultures and, afterward, both cell types will proliferate and start to build connections with the other cell types. As the authors suggest, this seems to be the initial steps to generate "artificial skin" with two different cell types, potentially leading to the development of a three-dimensional skin (Rakers et al., 2011).

Due to the phylogenetic position of fish in evolution and their atypical properties, fish skin offers a unique opportunity to study the origins of innate immune responses, which will be a very interesting research topic in the near future. Each fish species secretes a different repertoire of mucosal AMPs, which could be used by the pharmaceutical industry to identify novel drugs with antimicrobial functions, or new vaccine adjuvants, as part of inactivated vaccines or as antitumor agents. AMPs could be important when studying bacterial resistance to the drugs (antibiotics) used at present or as a potential source of antiviral compounds (Rajanbabu and Chen, 2011).

Presently, genomic/transcriptomic approaches have propelled studies of different humoral immune components present in fish skin mucus, as well as their regulation after different stimuli, including natural or experimental infections. The available results confirm that complicated local signaling networks are present in the fish skin and these networks are involved in the immune response to different microorganisms. Studies of the skin transcriptome and proteome are scarce in fish, and have only recently begun. Omics-based studies will permit the discovery of new molecules not described by more traditional methods. Similarly, the strategies used by invasive pathogens to penetrate host cells or to evade killing will be studied, as well as molecular signatures related to host responses and host-pathogen interactions during infection.

From a developmental standpoint of the skin, many interesting questions remain. For example, how is the transition achieved, in the early stages of skin development, from two cell layers toward the typical epidermis composed of three strata. Some interesting features of adult stem cells in fishes regarding the regeneration processes (e.g., skin damage) should be further investigated and then compared to the human integument. The study of fish skin reveals an abundance of problems that are also of major relevance to mammalian skin, highlighting potential uses of fish skin models in investigative dermatology. A heightened understanding of the biology of fish skin will enhance basic and clinical skin research, as well as comparative anatomy and physiology.

References

Akimenko, M.A., Mari-Beffa, M., Becerra, J., Geraudie, J., 2003. Old questions, new tools, and some answers to the mystery of fin regeneration. Dev. Dyn. 226, 190–201.

Azad, I.S., Al-Marzouk, A., James, C.M., Almatar, S., Al-Gharabally, H., 2007. Scuticociliatosis-associated mortalities and histopathology of natural infection in cultured silver pomfret (*Pampus argenteus* Euphrasen) in Kuwait. Aquaculture 28, 202–210.

Baffone, W., Tarsi, R., Pane, L., Campana, R., Repetto, B., Mariottini, G.L., Pruzzo, C., 2006. Detection of free-living and plankton-bound vibrios in coastal waters of the Adriatic Sea (Italy) and study of their pathogenicity-associated properties. Environ. Microbiol. 8, 1299–1305.

Bassity, E., Clark, T.G., 2012. Functional identification of dendritic cells in the teleost model, rainbow trout (*Oncorhynchus mykiss*). PLoS One 7, e33196.

Beck, B.H., Farmer, B.D., Straus, D.L., Li, C., Peatman, E., 2012. Putative roles for a rhamnose binding lectin in *Flavobacterium columnare* pathogenesis in channel catfish *Ictalurus punctatus*. Fish Shellfish Immunol. 33, 1008–1015.

Brandtzaeg, P., 2009. Mucosal immunity: induction, dissemination, and effector functions. Scand. J. Immunol. 70, 505–515.

Bromage, E.S., Ye, J., Kaattari, S.L., 2006. Antibody structural variation in rainbow trout fluids. Comp. Biochem. Physiol. B Biochem. Mol. Biol. 143, 61–69.

Bulet, P., Stocklin, R., Menin, L., 2004. Anti-microbial peptides: from invertebrates to vertebrates. Immunol. Rev. 198, 169–184.

Cano, I., Ferro, P., Alonso, M.C., Sarasquete, C., García-Rosado, E., Borrego, J.J., Castro, D., 2009. Application of *in situ* detection techniques to determine the systemic condition of lymphocystis disease virus infection in cultured gilthead seabream, *Sparus aurata* L. J. Fish Dis. 32, 143–150.

Casadei, E., Wang, T.H., Zou, J., Vecino, J.L.G., Wadsworth, S., Secombes, C.J., 2009. Characterization of three novel beta-defensin antimicrobial peptides in rainbow trout (*Oncorhynchus mykiss*). Mol. Immunol. 46, 3358–3366.

Chang, W.J., Hwang, P.P., 2011. Development of zebrafish epidermis. Birth Defects Res. C Embryo Today 93, 205–214.

Clark, T.G., Gao, Y., Gaertig, J., Wang, X., Cheng, G., 2001. The I-antigens of *Ichthyophthirius multifiliis* are GPI-anchored proteins. J. Eukaryot. Microbiol. 48, 332–337.

Coffee, L.L., Casey, J.W., Bowser, P.R., 2013. Pathology of tumors in fish associated with retroviruses: a review. Vet. Pathol. 50, 390–403.

Cone, R.A., 2009. Barrier properties of mucus. Adv. Drug Deliv. Rev. 61, 75–85.

Costes, B., Raj, V.S., Michel, B., Fournier, G., Thirion, M., Gillet, L., Mast, J., Lieffrig, F., Bremont, M., Vanderplasschen, A., 2009. The major portal of entry of koi herpesvirus in *Cyprinus carpio* is the skin. J. Virol. 83, 2819–2830.

Dickerson, H.W., Clark, T.G., 1998. *Ichthyophthirius multifiliis*: a model of cutaneous infection and immunity in fishes. Immunol. Rev. 166, 377–384.

Edholm, E.S., Bengten, E., Wilson, M., 2011. Insights into the function of IgD. Dev. Comp. Immunol. 35, 1309–1316.

Elliott, D.G., 2011. Functional morphology of the integumentary system in fish. Farrel, A.P. (Ed.), Encyclopedia of Fish Physiology: From Genome to Environment, 1, Academic Press, San Diego, pp. 476–488.

Ellis, A.E., 2001. Innate host defense mechanisms of fish against viruses and bacteria. Dev. Comp. Immunol. 25, 827–839.

Esteban, M.A., 2012. An overview of the immunological defenses in fish skin. ISRN Immunol. 2012, 29, Article ID 853470; doi:10.5402/2012/853470.

Falco, A., Ortega-Villaizan, M., Chico, V., Brocal, I., Pérez, L., Coll, J.M., Estepa, A., 2009. Antimicrobial peptides as model molecules for the development of novel antiviral agents in aquaculture. Mini Rev. Med. Chem. 9, 1159–1164.

Fernandes, J.M., Kemp, G.D., Molle, M.G., Smith, V.J., 2002. Anti-microbial properties of histone H2A from skin secretions of rainbow trout, *Oncorhynchus mykiss*. Biochem. J. 368, 611–620.

Fernandes, J.M., Saint, N., Kemp, G.D., Smith, V.J., 2003. Oncorhyncin III: a potent antimicrobial peptide derived from the non-histone chromosomal protein H6 of rainbow trout, *Oncorhynchus mykiss*. Biochem. J. 373, 621–628.

Flajnik, M., du Pasquier, L., 2004. Evolution of innate and adaptive immunity: can we draw a line? Trends Immunol. 25, 640–644.

Fouz, B., Toranzo, A.E., Milán, M., Amaro, C., 2000. Evidence that water transmits the disease caused by the fish pathogen *Photobacterium damselae subsp. damselae*. J. Appl. Microbiol. 88, 531–535.

Gomez, D., Sunyer, J.O., Salinas, I., 2013. The mucosal immune system of fish: the evolution of tolerating commensals while fighting pathogens. Fish Shellfish Immunol. 35, 1729–1739.

González-Chávez, S.A., Arévalo-Gallegos, S., Rascón-Cruz, Q., 2009. Lactoferrin: structure, function and applications. Int. J. Antimicrob. Agents 33, 301.e1–301.e8.

Groff, J.M., 2001. Cutaneous biology and diseases of fish. Vet. Clin. North Am. Exotic Anim. Pract. 4, 321–411.

Grontvedt, R.N., Espelid, S., 2003. Immunoglobulin producing cells in the spotted wolfish (Anarhichas minor Olafsen): localization in adults and during juvenile development. Dev. Comp. Immunol. 27, 569–578.

Guani-Guerra, E., Santos-Mendoza, T., Lugo-Reyes, S.O., Teran, L.M., 2010. Antimi- crobial peptides: general overview and clinical implications in human health and disease. Clin. Immunol. 135, 1–11.

Guardiola, F.A., Cuesta, A., Arizcun, M., Meseguer, J., Esteban, M.A., 2014. Comparative skin mucus and serum humoral defence mechanisms in the teleost gilthead seabream (*Sparus aurata*). Fish Shellfish Immunol. 36, 545–551.

Hanson, L., Dishon, A., Kotler, M., 2011. Herpesviruses that infect fish. Viruses 3, 2160–2191.

Harikrishnan, R., Balasundaram, C., Heo, M.S., 2010. Scuticociliatosis and its recent prophylactic measures in aquaculture with special reference to South Korea Taxonomy, diversity and diagnosis of scuticociliatosis: Part I. Control strategies of scuticociliatosis: Part II. Fish Shellfish Immunol. 29, 15–31.

Hatten, F., Fredriksen, A., Hordvik, I., Endresen, C., 2001. Presence of IgM in cutaneous mucus, but not in gut mucus of Atlantic salmon, *Salmo salar*. Serum IgM is rapidly degraded when added to gut mucus. Fish Shellfish Immunol. 11, 257–268.

Ingerslev, H.C., Lunder, T., Nielsen, M.E., 2010. Inflammatory and regenerative responses in salmonids following mechanical tissue damage and natural infection. Fish Shellfish Immunol. 29, 440–450.

Jones, S.M.R., 2001. The occurrence and mechanisms of innate immunity against parasites in fish. Dev. Comp. Immunol. 25, 841–852.

Jung, T.S., del Castillo, C.S., Javaregowda, P.K., Dalvi, R.S., Nho, S.W., Park, S.B., Jang, H.B., Cha, I.S., Sung, H.W., Hikima, J.I., Aoki, T., 2012. Seasonal variation and comparative analysis of non-specific humoral immune substances in the skin mucus of olive flounder (*Paralichthys olivaceus*). Dev. Comp. Immunol. 38, 295–301.

Kamiya, H., Muramoto, K., Goto, R., 1988. Purification and properties of agglutinins from conger eel, *Conger myriaster* (Brevoort), skin mucus. Dev. Comp. Immunol. 12, 309–418.

Kania, P.W., Evensen, O., Buchmann, K., 2010. Molecular and immunohistochemical studies on epidermal responses in Atlantic salmon *Salmo salar* L. induced by *Gyrodactylus salaris* Malmberg, 1957. J. Helminthol. 84, 166–172.

Karlsen, C., Sørum, H., Willassen, N.P., Sbakk, K.A., 2012. *Moritella viscosa* bypasses Atlantic salmon epidermal keratocyte clearing activity and might use skin surfaces as a port of infection. Vet. Microbiol. 154, 353–362.

Katzenback, B.A., Katakura, F., Belosevic, M., 2012. Regulation of teleost macrophage and neutrophil cell development by growth factors and transcription factors. In: Turker H. (Ed.), New Advances and Contributions to Fish Biology. ISBN: 978-953-51-0909-9, InTech. doi: 10.5772/53589.

Kuppulakshmi, C., Prakash, M., Gunasekaran, G., Manimegalai, G., Sarojini, S., 2008. Antibacterial properties of fish mucus from *Channa punctatus* and *Cirrhinus mrigala*. Eur. Rev. Med. Pharmacol. Sci. 12, 149–153.

Lakra, W.S., Swaminathan, T.R., Joy, K.P., 2011. Development, characterization, conservation and storage of fish cell lines: a review. Fish Physiol. Biochem. 37, 1–20.

Law, M., 2001. Differential diagnosis of ulcerative lesions in fish. Environ. Health Perspect. 109, 681–686.

Le Guellec, D., Morvan-Dubois, G., Sire, J.Y., 2004. Skin development in bony fish with particular emphasis on collagen deposition in the dermis of the zebrafish (*Danio rerio*). Int. J. Dev. Biol. 48, 217–231.

Li, C., Wang, R., Su, B., Luo, Y., Terhune, J., Beck, B., Peatman, E., 2013a. Evasion of mucosal defenses during *Aeromonas hydrophila* infection of channel catfish (*Ictalurus punctatus*) skin. Dev. Comp. Immun. 39, 447–455.

Li, C., Beck, B., Su, B., Terhune, J., Peatman, E., 2013b. Early mucosal responses in blue catfish (*Ictalurus furcatus*) skin to *Aeromonas hydrophila* infection. Fish Shellfish Immunol. 34, 920–928.

Li, M., Leatherland, J.F., 2012. The interaction between maternal stress and the ontogeny of the innate immune system during teleost embryogenesis: implications for aquaculture practice. J. Fish Biol. 81, 1793–1814.

Lugo-Villarino, G., Balla, K.M., Stachura, D.L., Banuelos, K., Werneck, M.B.F., Traver, D., 2010. Identification of dendritic antigen-presenting cells in the zebrafish. Proc. Natl. Acad. Sci. USA 107, 15850–15855.

Madetoja, J., Dalsgaard, I., Wiklund, T., 2002. Occurrence of *Flavobacterium psychrophilum* in fish-farming environments. Dis. Aquat. Org. 52, 109–118.

Maki, J.L., Dickerson, H.W., 2003. Systemic and cutaneous mucus antibody responses of channel catfish immunized against the protozoan parasite *Ichthyophthirius multifiliis*. Clin. Diagn. Lab. Immunol. 10, 876–881.

Matsushita, M., Matsushita, A., Endo, Y., Nakata, M., Kojima, N., Mizuochi, T., Fujita, T., 2004. Origin of the classical complement pathway: lamprey orthologue of mammalian C1q acts as a lectin. Proc. Natl. Acad. Sci. U.S.A. 101, 10127–10131.

Molle, V., Campagna, S., Bessin, Y., Ebran, N., Saint, N., Molle, G., 2008. First evidence of the pore-forming properties of a keratin from skin mucus of rainbow trout (*Oncorhynchus mykiss*, formerly *Salmo gairdneri*). Biochem. J. 411, 33–40.

Najafian, L., Babji, A.S., 2012. A review of fish-derived antioxidant and antimicrobial peptides: their production, assessment, and applications. Peptides 33, 178–185.

Nigam, A.K., Kumari, U., Mittal, S., Mittal, A.K., 2012. Comparative analysis of innate immune parameters of the skin mucous secretions from certain freshwater teleosts, inhabiting different ecological niches. Fish Physiol. Biochem. 38, 1245–1256.

Palaksha, K.J., Shin, G.W., Kim, Y.R., Jung, T.S., 2008. Evaluation of non-specific immune components from the skin mucus of olive flounder (*Paralichthys olivaceus*). Fish Shellfish Immunol. 24, 479–488.

Patrzykat, A., Zhang, L., Mendoza, V., Iwama, G.K., Hancock, R.E., 2001. Synergy of histone-derived peptides of coho salmon with lysozyme and flounder pleurocidin. Antimicrob. Agents Chemother. 45, 1337–1342.

Rai, A.K., Srivastava, N., Nigam, A.K., Kumari, U., Mittal, S., Mittal, A.K., 2012. Healing of cutaneous wounds in a freshwater teleost, *Labeo rohita*: scanning electron microscopical investigation. Microsc. Res. Tech. 75, 890–897.

Raj, V.S., Fournier, G., Rakus, K., Ronsmans, M., Ouyang, P., Michel, B., Delforges, C., Costes, B., Farnir, F., Leroy, B., Wattiez, R., Melard, C., Mast, J., Lieffrig, F., Vanderplasschen, A., 2011. Skin mucus of *Cyprinus carpio* inhibits cyprinid herpesvirus 3 binding to epidermal cells. Vet. Res. 42, 92–101.

Rajan, B., Lokesh, J., Kiron, V., Brinchmann, M.F., 2013. Differentially expressed proteins in the skin mucus of Atlantic cod (*Gadus morhua*) upon natural infection with *Vibrio anguillarum*. BMC Vet. Res. 9, 103.

Rajanbabu, V., Chen, J.Y., 2011. Applications of antimicrobial peptides from fish and perspectives for the future. Peptides 32, 415–420.

Rakers, S., Klinger, M., Kruse, C., Gebert, M., 2011. Pros and cons of fish skin cells in culture: long-term full skin and short-term scale cell culture from rainbow trout, *Oncorhynchus mykis*. Eur. J. Cell Biol. 90, 1041–1051.

Robinette, D.W., Noga, E.J., 2001. Histone-like protein: a novel method for measuring stress in fish. Dis. Aquat. Org. 44, 97–107.

Ross, N.W., Firth, K.J., Wang, A., Burka, J.F., Johnson, S.C., 2000. Changes in hydrolytic enzyme activities of naive Atlantic salmon *Salmo salar* skin mucus due to infection with the salmon louse *Lepeophtheirus salmonis* and cortisol implantation. Dis. Aquat. Org. 41, 43–51.

Roussel, P., Delmotte, P., 2004. The diversity of epithelial secreted mucins. Curr. Org. Chem. 8, 413–437.

Ryo, S., Wijdeven, R.H., Tyagi, A., Hermsen, T., Kono, T., Karunasagar, I., Rombout, J.H., Sakai, M., Kemenade, B.M., Savan, R., 2010. Common carp have two subclasses of bony-fish specific antibody IgZ showing differential expression in response to infection. Dev. Comp. Immunol. 34, 1183–1190.

Saadatfar, Z., Shahsavani, D., Fatemi, F.S., 2010. Study of epidermis development in sturgeon (*Acipenser persicus*) larvae. Anat. Histol. Embryol. 39, 440–445.

Salem, M., Nath, J., Killefer, J., 2004. Cloning of the calpain regulatory subunit cDNA from fish reveals a divergent domain-V. Anim. Biotechnol. 15, 145–157.

Salinas, I., Zhang, Y.A., Sunyer, J.O., 2011. Mucosal immunoglobulins and B cells of teleost fish. Dev. Comp. Immunol 35, 1346–1365.

Sarmaşik, A., 2002. Antimicrobial peptides: a potential therapeutic alternative for the treatment of fish diseases. Turkish J. Biol. 26, 201–207.

Saurabh, S., Sahoo, P.K., 2008. Lysozyme: an important defencemolecule of fish innateimmune system. Aquacult. Res. 39, 223–239.

Savan, R., Aman, A., Nakao, M., Watanuki, H., Sakai, M., 2005. Discovery of a novel immunoglobulin heavy chain gene chimera from common carp (*Cyprinus carpio* L.). Immunogenetics 57, 458–463.

Sire, J.Y., Akimenko, M.A., 2004. Scale development in fish: a review, with description of sonic hedgehog (shh) expression in the zebrafish (*Danio rerio*). Int. J. Dev. Biol. 48, 233–247.

Schmitz, R.J., 1998. Immunohistochemical identification of the cytoskeletal elements in the notochord cells of bony fishes. J. Morphol. 236, 105–116.

Snoussi, M., Noumi, E., Cheriaa, J., Usai, D., Sechi, L.A., Zanetti, S., Bakhrouf, A., 2008. Adhesive properties of environmental *Vibrio alginolyticus* strains to biotic and abiotic surfaces. New Microbiol. 31, 489–500.

Stellabotte, F., Devoto, S.H., 2007. The teleost dermomyotome. Dev. Dynam. 236, 2432–2443.

Subramanian, S., MacKinnon, S.L., Ross, N.W., 2007. A comparative study on innate immune parameters in the epidermal mucus of various fish species. Comp. Biochem. Physiol. B Biochem. Mol. Biol. 148, 256–263.

Subramanian, S., Ross, N.W., MacKinnon, S.L., 2008. Comparison of the biochemical composition of normal epidermal mucus and extruded slime of hagfish (*Myxine glutinosa* L.). Fish Shellfish Immunol. 25, 25–32.

Sunyer, J.O., 2013. Fishing for mammalian paradigms in the teleost immune system. Nat. Immunol. 14, 320–326.

Suzuki, Y., Tasumi, S., Tsutsui, S., Okamoto, M., Suetake, H., 2003. Molecular diversity of skin mucus lectins in fish. Comp. Biochem. Physiol. B Biochem. Mol. Biol. 136, 723–730.

Tripathi, N.K., Latimer, K.S., Gregory, C.R., Ritchie, B.W., Wooley, R.E., Walker, R.L., 2005. Development and evaluation of an experimental model of cutaneous columnaris disease in koi *Cyprinus carpio*. J. Vet. Diagn. Invest. 17, 45–54.

Van der Marel, M., Caspari, N., Neuhaus, H., Meyer, W., Enss, M.L., Steinhagen, D., 2010. Changes in skin mucus of common carp, *Cyprinus carpio* L., after exposure to water with a high bacterial load. J. Fish Dis. 33, 431–439.

Wölfle, U., Martin, S., Emde, M., Schempp, C., 2009. Dermatology in the Darwin anniversary. Part 2: Evolution of the skin-associated immune system. J. Dtsch. Dermatol. Ges. 7, 862–869.

Xu, D.H., Klesius, P.H., Shelby, R.A., 2002. Cutaneous antibodies in excised skin from channel catfish, *Ictalurus punctatus* (Rafinesque), immune to *Ichthyophthirius multifiliis*. J. Fish Dis. 25, 45–52.

Xu, Z., Parra, D., Gómez, D., Salinas, I., Zhang, Y.A., von Gersdorff Jørgensen, L., Heinecke, R.D., Buchmann, K., LaPatra, S., Sunyer, J.O., 2013. Teleost skin, an ancient mucosal surface that elicits gut-like mucosal immune responses. Proc. Natl. Acad. Sci. U.S.A. 110, 13097–13102.

Zhang, Y.A., Salinas, I., Li, J., Parra, D., Bjork, S., Xu, Z., LaPatra, S.E., Bartholomew, J., Sunyer, J.O., 2010. IgT, a primitive immunoglobulin class specialized in mucosal immunity. Nat. Immunol. 11, 827–835.

Zhao, X., Findly, R.C., Dickerson, H.W., 2008. Cutaneous antibody-secreting cells and B cells in a teleost fish. Dev. Comp. Immunol. 32, 500–508.

Zilberg, D., Klesius, P.H., 1997. Quantification of immunoglobulin in the serum and mucus of channel catfish at different ages and following infection with *Edwardsiella ictaluri*. Vet. Immunol. Immunopathol. 58, 171–180.

Zorilla, I., Moriñigo, M.A., Castro, D., Balebona, M.C., Borrego, J.J., 2003. Intraspecific characterization of *Vibrio alginolyticus* isolates recovered from cultured fish in Spain. J. Appl. Microbiol. 95, 1106–1116.

Fish mucosal immunity: gill

5

Erling Olaf Koppang; Agnar Kvellestad*; Uwe Fischer***
*Section of Anatomy and Pathology, Faculty of Veterinary Medicine and Biosciences, Norwegian University of Life Sciences, Oslo, Norway
**Federal Research Institute for Animal Health, Friedrich-Loeffler Institut, Greifswald-Insel Riems, Germany

Chapter Outline

Mucosal Health in Aquaculture

5.1 Introduction

The fish gills serve several purposes as they are not only involved in respiration, but are also major sites for osmoregulation, nitrogenous waste excretion, pH regulation and hormone production (Evans et al., 2005). Forming a semipermeable barrier between the organism and the external milieu, the gills of fish are faced with challenges similar to the gut mucosa. In contrast to the air, water frequently contains a higher burden of antigens (Bergh et al., 1989). In mammals, a considerable number of pathogens infects their host via the gastrointestinal tract and to a lesser extent via the respiratory system. In fish, however, the gills are a portal of entry for several pathogens. The gill surface is estimated to 0.1–0.4 m^2/kg body weight, representing the largest organ-specific surface interacting with the external milieu. In addition, there is a short distance between the blood and water, comprising two to three cell layers, 6 μm on average in lamellae of rainbow trout (*Oncorhynchus mykiss* Walbaum), which is covered by a thin mucus layer. This large area and short distance promote a high efficiency of gas exchange but also allow leakage of ions and water and also facilitate uptake of foreign substances or invasion of infectious agents. All these processes or events are augmented by a continuous pumping of water through the gill chamber. This sophisticated system brings the fish into a dilemma because both a large surface and the delicate gill structure provide an ideal port of entry for molecules, particles, and all kind of pathogens.

Gill diseases, and diseases associated with gill damage, cause substantial losses in the aquaculture industry not only through an increased mortality rate among fish but also through impaired growth and costs related to sanitary and treatment measures. Adverse conditions are commonly characterized by inflammation and epithelial cell hyperplasia. Clearly, adequately regulated immune responses distinguishing between self and non-self are imperative to maintain tissue homeostasis and integrity, and in this way, the gills are very similar to the gut where a number of diseases may occur if these outer barriers get out of balance. In the gut, the concept of immune tolerance is a prominent feature. The immune response in the unaffected gut is regulated in such a way that inflammatory reactions only emerge when pathogens threaten the integrity of the organ (e.g., the gut does not mount inflammatory responses against its abundant content of commensal bacteria or against most food-borne antigens). The benefit of such unresponsiveness has been proven through evolution and is known as oral tolerance. Mucosal tolerance has been described in fish where repeated anal administration of allogeneic cells leads to loss of allospecific cell-mediated cytotoxicity (Sato et al., 2005). In humans with deregulated intestinal immune responses lack of mucosal tolerance may lead to severe disorders such as food intolerance. In mammals, also pulmonary homeostasis is regulated by adequate and non-excessive mucosal immune reactions in order to limit the inflammatory consequences of pathogen inhalation while maintaining tolerance to harmless substances. A breakdown in tolerance may lead to all kinds of allergy and asthma. It is highly plausible that similar mechanisms ensuring a general status of tolerance to the vast number of water-borne molecules and particles also exist in fish gills. If this were not the case, inflammatory responses in fish gills would reduce, e.g., gas exchange over the delicate structures of the lamellae. In fact, it has been shown in salmonids that gills of naïve fish represent a Th2 skewed immune environment where pro-inflammatory reactions are kept under control (Takizawa et al., 2011b).

In this chapter, we review our current conception of immune responses in the gills. As the function of the immune system is highly dependent on the anatomy and physiological processes at the site on which it functions, we will also provide an introduction to these latter aspects.

A substantial challenge in piscine immunoanatomy is the lack of useful cell markers. Much of our knowledge thus relies on transcription analysis of various immune genes usually isolated from crude extracts of gills, which also contain blood cells. In salmonids, such investigations have shown that the gills, compared to other organs, are very high in MHC class I and II expression (Koppang et al., 1998a, 1998b). MHC class II may be induced in many cells, but in mammals and probably also in fish, the molecule is predominantly present in antigen-presenting cells including dendritic cells and macrophages. Later, a number of studies have shown that transcripts for most tested immune-related genes are expressed in teleost gills. The recent description of a large, lymphoid structure – the interbranchial lymphoid tissue (ILT) – mainly containing T cells that are embedded in an epithelial meshwork underscored that even on the gross anatomy level, discoveries are still to be made (Koppang et al., 2010). Also recently, an investigation showed that the chemokine receptor CCR7 is mainly expressed in gill tissue, defining an IgD+ IgM- B lymphocyte subset (Castro et al., 2014). All in all, an increasing flow of information points towards the gills as a major organ involved in the immune response.

During the recent years gill immune responses were more and more shifted into the focus of vaccinologists since the fish farming industry urgently demands efficient and cost-effective vaccines applied by cost-effective delivery systems. One of the most cost-effective delivery methods is bath immunization where the gill with its enormous surface is one of the promising sites of vaccine uptake. Consequently, understanding gill physiology including uptake and immune response mechanisms is of utmost importance for designing effective vaccines and delivery systems.

5.2 Embryology and anatomy

The pharyngeal region, from which the thymus and gills develop, is thought to be the cradle for the adaptive immune system as defined by the presence of molecules belonging to the immunoglobulin superfamily. The thymus, which is the first phylogenetically recognizable solitary lymphoid organ and serves as a primary lymphoid organ in jawed fishes and mammals, develops from the endodermal epithelium of branchial (pharyngeal) pouches at each side of the primitive gut in the pharyngeal region. External vertical furrows develop at the position of each pouch, and in teleost fishes the tissues between pouches and furrows are resorbed thus resulting in vertical slits allowing passage for water flow between the pharyngeal lumen and external environment. The tissues between the slits, defined as the pharyngeal (embryonic) arches, develop into gills and pseudobranchiae. The gills, developing from the lateral and well-vascularized pharyngeal arches, finally take over respiratory functions. With the development of jawed fishes, it has been proposed that the need for a more sophisticated immune system in this region was warranted due to mucosal trauma caused by ingested feed being much more crude compared to that ingested by members of cyclostomata species (Matsunaga and Rahman, 2001). Jawless vertebrates do not possess a thymus, but in the gills of lampreys, a thymus-like tissue has been identified in the distal portion of filaments (Bajoghli et al., 2011). This finding underscores the close functional relationship between different tissues of the pharyngeal region.

In mammals, the entrance of the gastrointestinal tract, the pharynx, is protected by a number of secondary lymphoid structures, such as the tubal and palatine tonsils, that have developed from the first and second branchial pouches, respectively, contributing to the Waldeyer's ring of lymphoid tissue in the pharynx. A similar structure has not been reported in fish. On the contrary, it has been generally accepted that fish do not possess secondary mucosa-associated macroscopically recognizable immunological structures hallmarked by germinal centers (proliferating and differentiating B cells) like in mammals.

In the following, we will limit our description to teleosts, which on each side have four gill arches and five slits (Evans et al., 2005; Hughes, 1984; Laurent, 1984; Pisam et al., 1988; Wilson and Laurent, 2002). Each arch (Figure 5.1) develops into a gill by outgrowth of a septum and two rows of filaments, often termed "primary lamellae." The first filaments form midway along the arch, which dorsal to the middle has a flexure with anterior concavity, and during the life-long growth of the fish new filaments are added both dorsally and ventrally. Each gill therefore contains two caudolaterally projecting rows of filaments and between the proximal parts of the filaments a more or less developed septum. The arches and filaments have cores of cartilage (which may ossify), connective tissue, blood vessels, nerves and immune cells. The filaments possess an apical branchiogenic zone where they elongate. At the ventral and dorsal

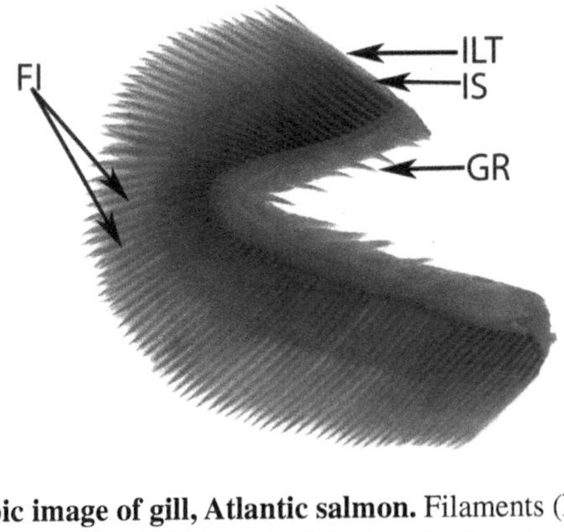

Figure 5.1 Macroscopic image of gill, Atlantic salmon. Filaments (FI) are attached to the gill arch and fused in their proximal third by the interbranchial septum (IS). The location of the interbranchial lymphoid tissue (ILT) is marked and gill rakers (GR) are craniomedially orientated towards the pharynx.
Source: Original image is a courtesy from Professor Trygve T. Poppe.

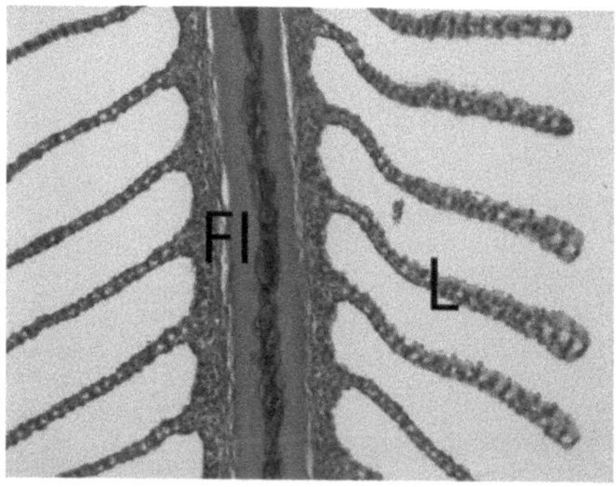

Figure 5.2 Histologic image of gill filament (FI) containing cartilage (cells shown in the center) and adjacent bone tissue. Lamellae are marked (L).

sides numerous lamellae (secondary lamellae, respiratory units) develop as the filaments elongate. They are arranged transversely and in parallel at regular intervals. They are thin plates of a microcirculation enclosed by a fold of basement membrane and commonly a low respiratory epithelium (Figure 5.2). Blood flow in the lamellar microcirculation and water flow in the interlamellar spaces are described as countercurrent.

Intraepithelial aggregations of T cells are located at the terminal (caudolateral) end of the interbranchial septum of salmonids, (Figures 5.3 and 5.4) (Koppang et al., 2010). This structure, termed the interbranchial lymphoid tissue (ILT), does not seem to have any equivalent among lymphoid tissues, and its function is so far unknown although it has has some properties in common with secondary lymphoid sructures (Aas et al. 2014).

5.3 Vascular system

Within the gills, three circulatory systems have been described (Olson, 2002). (A) The arterio-arterial or primary pathway includes afferent and efferent arteries located close to filamental trailing (water outlet) and leading (water inlet) edges, respectively, and the interposed lamellar microcirculation patterned by collagenous columns and pillar cells, a type of endothelial cell. The columns are arranged in many circular clusters

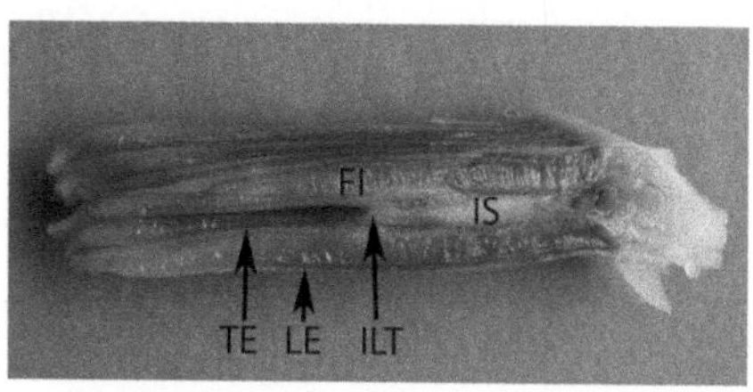

Figure 5.3 Transversal section of a gill arch, Atlantic salmon, 9 kg. The interbranchial septum (IS), terminating in the visible interbranchial lymphoid tissue (ILT) is located between the filaments (FI). The leading (LE) and trailing (TE) edges of the filaments are marked.

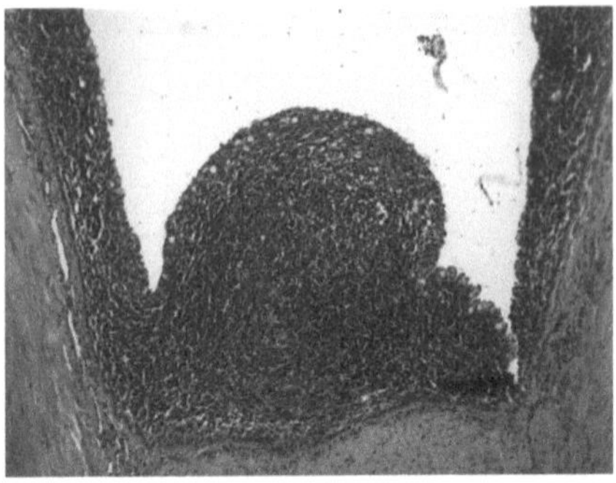

Figure 5.4 Histological image of a transversal section of the interbranchial lymphoid tissue (ILT). As an intraepithelial structure, the ILT is devoid of vessels.

and connect the basement membrane of the opposite sides. These clusters contain pillar cell perikarya, from which cytoplasm extends to envelope the columns and cover the underside of the basement membrane, thus confining the vascular lumen. Argyrophilia indicates reticular fibers, which afford structural maintenance in expansible organs (Mescher, 2010). The tubular structures of pillar cells have also been found to be formed of cytokeratin-like molecules (Köllner et al., 1998). This arrangement in combination with blood pressure probably serves to keep the lamellae inflated but also prevents ballooning (Hughes, 1984). The pillar cells appear to be rather static (Conte and Lin, 1967), but erythrocyte deformation has been observed within the arteriolar luminae (Nilsson et al., 1995). (B) Arterioles selectively filter out blood cells to supply the secondary vessels with plasma (Rasmussen et al., 2013). This secondary vascular system consists of thin-walled but wide vessels (central venous sinus) traversing the filaments underneath the interlamellar epithelium in a ladder-like pattern, and branch around afferent and efferent filamental arteries. It drains into veins. (C) The third system is nutritive and also drains into the branchial veins.

Pillar and other endothelial cells of filamental arteries of rainbow trout gills express high levels of MHC class I protein suggesting that these cells are actively involved in antigen presentation to the adaptive immune system (Dijkstra et al., 2003). On the other hand, distinct MHC class I expression in healthy fish might help to keep NK-like cells in a stage of anergy by triggering NK cell receptors with inhibitory motifs. However, under inflammatory conditions (e.g., when endothelial cells are artificially activated by TNF-α), this may result in an increase of MHC class II and CD83 as shown in gilthead seabream (*Sparus aurata* L.) and zebrafish (*Danio rerio* Hamilton) primary endothelial cell cultures (Roca et al., 2008).

5.4 Epithelium

Common types of differentiated epithelial cells are squamous or cuboidal pavement cells (PEs), mitochondria-rich cells (MRCs) and mucus-producing cells, frequently referred to as goblet cells (Figure 5.5). Their total cell masses and turnover rates

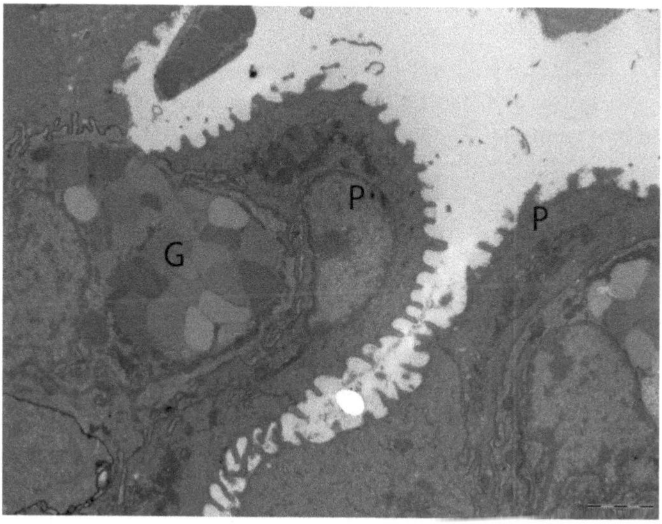

Figure 5.5 Transmission electron microscopy image of gill epithelium, here from the interbranchial lymphoid tissue (ILT). Pavement cells (P) and goblet cells (G) are marked.

depend on proliferation, cell death, growth of the organ and adaptive or preadaptive responses to altered environments (e.g., when freshwater Atlantic salmon *Salmo salar* L. preadapt (smoltify) to a life in seawater before migration to the sea). Cell division is best documented in the interlamellar filamental epithelium (Conte and Lin, 1967) and to a lesser extent in the lamellar epithelium (Wilson and Laurent, 2002). Cell death with morphology resembling apoptosis has been reported as part of the normal cell turnover (Wendelaar Bonga and van der Mej, 1989).

Mucous surfaces in mammals contain specialized epithelial cells (M or microfold cells) facilitating antigen uptake and transport through the upper epithelial layer. M cells contain pockets at their basal portion where T cells, B cells, macrophages, or dendritic cells are situated and where the antigen is delivered to the antigen-presenting cells. Cells with some M cell properties have been identified in fish gut (Fuglem et al., 2010), but so far, no reports have been published with respect to the gills.

All nucleated cells in vertebrates express MHC class I in various degrees. Epithelial cells on filaments and lamellae of rainbow trout express high amounts of this protein (Dijkstra et al., 2003). In Atlantic salmon, fewer but distinctly labeled epithelial cells have been identified (Hetland et al., 2010). Also, MHC class II is detected by IHC in gill epithelial cells of salmon (Koppang et al., 2003). Along with the pro-inflammatory cytokine IL-1β gene another mediator of inflammation gene COX-2 can be highly expressed in gills of Atlantic salmon compared with head kidney and spleen (Ingerslev et al., 2006). Furthermore, the antimicrobial lectins ladderlectin and intelectin have been detected by immunohistochemistry in rainbow trout epithelial cells, especially in their apical parts, where it is possibly secreted to the epithelial surface (Russell et al., 2009).

5.4.1 Glycocalyx

The external gill surface consists of apical plasma membranes of all uppermost cells. A glycocalyx is attached to those membranes. Glycocalyx is defined as a carbohydrate-rich layer that forms the outer coat of cells (Alberts et al., 2008). It is composed of oligosaccharides (including one or more sialic acid residues) present in glycolipids, oligosaccharides present in glycoproteins (N-glycosyl linkage to asparagine, O-glycosyl linkages to serine or threonine), and glycosaminoglycans (repeating disaccharide units of a hexosamine and an uronic acid) and polysaccharides (with carboxylate and sulfate groups) present in proteoglycans.

The oligosaccharide chains are enormously diverse in their arrangement of sugars and have a variety of functions (e.g., they may serve as receptors for pathogenic agents (Alberts et al., 2008)). The glycocalyx has a net negative charge due to carboxylate and sulfate groups and therefore attracts cationic substances. Methods used to visualize sugars (by detecting vicinal diols) and the anionic groups will commonly stain both the glycocalyx and mucus in tissue sections. This, and the mixing of mucus with glycocalyx, makes it a challenge to separately characterize the morphology of either glycocalyx or mucus. By transmission electron microscopy investigations, material consistent with location of the glycocalyx has been shown to contain both vicinal diols, and anionic groups – presumptive being carboxylate and sulfate (Petrik and Bucher, 1969; Pisam et al., 1980; Sardet et al., 1979). The presence of glycoproteins and proteoglycans in the glycocalyx of MRCs has been indicated by the detection of ^{3}H-glucosamine and ^{3}H-fucose in Golgi apparatus and subsequently at the apical surface (Pisam et al., 1980, 1983). In freshwater rainbow trout, Powell et al. (1994) measured the thickness of the glycocalyx at pavement cells to 0.58–0.65 μm and at MRCs to 0.58–0.90 μm, and could not detect a glycocalyx at goblet cells.

5.4.2 Mucus

There are many proposed roles of mucus in fish, including respiration, ionic and osmotic regulation, reproduction, locomotion, and defense against infections (Shephard, 1994). Most examinations on mucous composition have been performed on that from skin, presumptively due to the easy collection. However, mucus has also been analyzed from gills of rainbow trout (Lumsden and Ferguson, 1994). The amino acid profile was similar to that of skin mucus from eel (*Anguilla japonica* Temminck and Schlegel) and charr (*Salvelinus alpinus* L.) but also of mammalian intestinal mucus; serine plus threonine constituted 35% and alanine plus proline constituted 28% of total amino acids. The carbohydrates (except sialic acid) consisted of 26% galactose, 23% galactosamine, 17% glucose, 16% fucose, 12% glucosamine, 5% mannose and 1% uronic acid. Sialic acid amounted 0.06g/g of mucous protein. Most of the mucus at the gill surface consists of gel-forming mucin secreted from mucus cells and mixed with water, it probably also contains substances released from other cell types, and it contains solid material shed from the gill tissue or trapped from surrounding water (Shephard, 1994; Speare and Ferguson, 2006). Possibly it also contains mucus from the oral and pharyngeal mucous membranes along which the inspiratory water moves.

And in cases of high fish densities, mucus shed from other individuals can theoretically be adsorbed. A continuous mucous layer is claimed to exist and to be anchored by the microridges of PEs (Hughes and Wright, 1970), but the thickness that probably offers more protection must be balanced against the advantages of short diffusion distances for gas exchange. The presence of material consistent with a continuous mucous layer over the filaments and lamellae but with random pits was later detected in freshwater rainbow trout (Lumsden et al., 1994; Powell et al., 1992, 1994). The maintenance of the mucus layer distant from the source of production, especially from leading and trailing edges of filaments, requires attraction of the mucus to the surface and to itself. Similarly, the presence of a mucus layer on lamellae that normally have few goblet cells is explained by secreted mucus flowing over distant epithelial areas (Lumsden et al., 1994). Since it is known that the secretion of mucus may increase under certain stressful situations (Speare and Ferguson, 2006), the question arises whether the handling and stunning of fish prior to sampling in the cited studies might have increased the secretion. Thus, it seems to be a challenge to examine for a mucous layer in unstressed and undisturbed fish. Comparatively, a stratified layer of skin mucus with a thickness of 0.8–1.3 μm at the top of the microridges has been detected by transmission electron microscopy in rainbow trout (Sanchez et al., 1997).

Although mucus may contain substances from other epithelial cells, a role of goblet cells in immune defense can be concluded from the presence of antimicrobial peptides in mucin granules of skin MCs detected in a marine fish (Cole et al., 2000). The content of immune molecules in gill mucus has not been examined to the same extent as that of skin mucus. However, a long list of common molecules in both compartments indicates high similarities between skin and gill mucus. In plaice (*Pleuronectes platessa* L.), lysozyme has been demonstrated in skin and gill epithelium as well as in skin mucus (Murray and Fletcher, 1976). Lysozyme has also been detected in gill mucus of juvenile Atlantic salmon (Costa et al., 2011) but the role of MCs in lysozyme secretion remains unknown since components present in the mucus layer are not necessarily secreted by the MCs. Skin mucus has also been reported to contain both main Ig classes in fish, IgM and IgT (Xu and Klesius, 2013).

Given the similarities to other mucous membranes such as that of the skin and intestinal tract it is conceivable that a mucous layer is present all over the filaments, but its distribution and thickness has not been documented in healthy and undisturbed fish. If continuously present in all places, one might think that it is thinnest at the lamellar epithelium where few MCs are present and a short diffusion distance for gases should be an advantage.

5.5 Blood cells and other immune cells

The traditional classification of human blood cells – which is based on morphology, staining patterns by use of Romanowsky-type methods, and the presence of certain enzymes (Mescher, 2010) – can neither be applied to all mammalian species nor to birds, reptiles, amphibians (Claver and Quaglia, 2009; Messick, 2006), or fish, especially when dealing with granulocytes (Burrows et al., 2001; Claver and Quaglia, 2009; Esteban et al., 2000; Tavares-Dias, 2006). However, human and mammalian monocytes, macrophages, neutrophils, T and B lymphocytes, platelets and erythrocytes (Mescher, 2010) are generally accepted to have their approximate counterparts in teleosts (Boehm, 2011; Ellis, 2001; Ferguson, 2006; Koppang et al., 2007; Secombes and Wang, 2012; Whyte, 2007). However, thrombocytes and erythrocytes are nucleated, and thrombocytes are considered to belong to the leukocyte fraction in fish. In addition, dendritic-like cells, nonspecific cytotoxic cells (NCC)/natural killer (NK)-like cells, eosinophilic granule cells (EGCs), rodlet cells, eosinophilic sacciform cells, and melanin-containing cells have been described in teleosts.

Morphological and functional criteria for the more exact classification of circulating leukocytes and the other immune cell types should be established for each fish species in question (Burrows et al., 2001). Until now, it appears that there is no agreement on classification criteria for immune cells in any fish species. Thus cells should be denoted macrophage-like etc. when no other than morphological methods are used. Each cell type comprises populations of varying degrees of differentiation or activity, reflected by different morphologies and functions. Fish leukocytes can also be morphologically divided into polymorphonuclear cells (PMNCs) represented by granulocytes and mononuclear cells (MNCs) comprising lymphocytes, monocytes and macrophages although some fish macrophages may have a somewhat lobulated nucleus.

The cell types to be described, except thrombocytes and erythrocytes, will collectively be designated inflammatory cells when dealing with inflammation. Studies of immune cells in fish have largely been based on cells in or obtained from head kidney, spleen, blood, and peritoneal cavity (i.e., places from which cells are easily harvested). The following review on gill immune cells will therefore also refer to results obtained on cells from these places. Most studies addressing immune reactions in gills have applied tissue extractions, but with no previous perfusion to eliminate peripheral blood content. Therefore, a number of reports may be misleading with respect to the true nature of gill tissue. This must be taken into account when interpreting the literature.

5.5.1 Monocytes and macrophages

Monocytes are commonly the largest leukocyte type in blood of teleosts, being rounded with a large, excentric kidney-shaped nucleus and slightly basophilic cytoplasm (Romanowsky-stain) (Burrows et al., 2001; Esteban et al., 2000; Palić et al., 2011; Tavares-Dias, 2006; Zinkl et al., 1991). Phagocytes belonging to the same cell lineage are referred to as macrophages, or macrophage-like cells, when found outside the circulatory system in tissues. Also, monocytes migrating to the extravasal tissue are referred to as macrophages. These cells are present in teleosts displaying respiratory burst activity (Brattgjerd et al., 1994; Bridle et al., 2005; Jang et al., 1995). Salmon macrophages secrete lysozyme to the blood, and this secretion can be stimulated by lipopolysaccharide and beta-glucan (Paulsen et al., 2001). Ladderlectin and intelectin have been detected within cytoplasmic granules of blood monocytes in rainbow trout (Russell et al., 2009). Cells of the macrophage lineage execute several functions within the immune response ranging from phagocytosis and respiratory burst to antigen processing and presentation (through MHC class I and II) resulting in the expression of several costimulatory receptors (e.g., CD80) and the production of pro-inflammatory (e.g., IL-1, IL-12, IL-18 and TNF-α) and anti-inflammatory (e.g., IL-10) cytokines. Consequently, they represent a central control unit of the immune system thereby linking innate and adaptive elements of the immune system (Huising et al., 2006; Scapigliati et al., 2006). Resident populations of leukocytes have been studied in the peritoneal cavity. Here, macrophages and polymorphonucleated cells (PMNCs) in sea bass (*Dicentrarchus labrax* L.) and rainbow trout are not easily distinguished when stained according to Wright's method (Afonso et al., 1998; do Vale et al., 2002) since few macrophages have polymorphic nuclei similar to granulocytes (Afonso et al., 1997). Some macrophages may also display peroxidase activity due to phagocytosis of PMNCs, and, if small, they may also look similar to lymphocytes (do Vale et al., 2002; Meseguer et al., 1994). MHC class I is detected by immunofluorescence in rainbow trout leukocytes tentatively identified as monocytes, lymphocytes, and neutrophils (Dijkstra et al., 2003). Interestingly, macrophage-like cells in anterior kidney, blood and peritoneal cavity display an increasing capacity for phagocytosis of bacteria in the order that they are listed (Esteban and Meseguer, 1997). This is probably connected with their maturation. However, gills have not been included in such investigations.

Low numbers of putative resident macrophage-like cells have been detected in the gill epithelium of presumptive healthy teleosts including salmonids (Goldes et al., 1986; Wendelaar Bonga and van der Mej, 1989). In gill epithelium of salmonids, high numbers of MHC class II positive cells have been detected (Haugarvoll et al., 2008; Hetland et al., 2010; Koppang et al., 2003; Morrison et al., 2006; Olsen et al., 2011) and may represent resident macrophages. To the best of our knowledge, the presence of MHC class II protein has not been confirmed in cells fulfilling the classical criteria for macrophages. Macrophage-like cells resident in the epithelium appear to be involved in uptake of waterborne macromolecules such as bovine serum albumin conjugated to FITC (Ototake et al., 1996), bovine serum albumin conjugated to 1 μm fluorescent latex microspheres (Moore et al., 1998), 1 μm fluorescent microspheres with or without extract of bacterium *Ewardsiella ictaluri* outer membrane protein (Glenney and Petrie-Hanson, 2006), and to particles such as fluorescent microspheres (Kiryu et al., 2000) and mineral particles (Goldes et al., 1986).

5.5.2 Granulocytes

Granulocyte-like cells reported from the blood of teleost fish include neutrophils, heterophils, eosinophils, and basophils. Cells with staining properties similar to eosinophils and basophils, if detected, are rare. All three cell types are described in Atlantic salmon (Conroy and Conroy, 2006; Tavares-Dias, 2006; Zinkl et al., 1991). Teleost fish blood granulocytes, with rounded to elongated or characteristically multilobulated nuclei and weakly to unstained cytoplasm, are denoted neutrophils or heterophils (Burrows et al., 2001; Esteban et al., 2000; Palić et al., 2011; Tavares-Dias, 2006; Zinkl et al., 1991). However, they lack peroxidase activity (Tavares-Dias, 2006; Zinkl et al., 1991), a characteristic feature of neutrophils in humans and many other mammalian species (Mescher, 2010; Messick, 2006).

The multilobulation apparently occurs in cells undergoing a maturation process as seen in warm-blooded animals (Mescher, 2010). PMNCs are phagocytes (Afonso et al., 1998; do Vale et al., 2002). Among salmonids myeloperoxidase activity has been demonstrated in PMNCs present in the anterior kidney of rainbow trout (Yasutake and Wales, 1983), in peripheral blood of Arctic grayling (*Thymallus arcticus* Pallas) and cutthroat trout (*Oncorhynchus clarkii* Richardson) (Palić et al., 2011) and in the peritoneal cavity of rainbow trout (Afonso et al., 1997). However, in one study peroxidase activity in peripheral blood PMNCs of rainbow trout and coho salmon (*Oncorhynchus kisutch* Walbaum) (Zinkl et al., 1991) could not be demonstrated, possibly explained by immaturity of the cells (Meseguer et al., 1994). Ladderlectin and intelectin have been detected by IHC within cytoplasmic granules of PMNCs present in blood of rainbow trout (Russell et al., 2009). Respiratory burst activity (Hamdani et al., 1998; Palić et al., 2011) and migratory activity (Hamdani et al., 1998) has been demonstrated in blood PMNCs from salmonids. Peroxidase positive PMNCs are present among resident peritoneal leukocytes in rainbow trout (Afonso et al., 1997). Only low numbers of putative resident granulocyte-like cells have been detected in the gill epithelium of presumptive healthy salmonids by transmission electron microscopy (Morgan and Tovell, 1973; Speare and Ferguson, 2006).

Cells denoted basophils are reported as present or absent in non-salmonid teleosts (Claver and Quaglia, 2009). Cells denoted basophils and eosinophils are also reported as rare in Atlantic salmon (Conroy and Conroy, 2006). It should be mentioned that eosinophilic granule cells (EGCs) may erroneously be referred to as eosinophils (Claver and Quaglia, 2009).

5.5.3 Eosinophilic granule cells (EGCs)

Eosinophilic granule cells (EGCs) are large cells with numerous cytoplasmic eosinophilic granules and a dense nucleus (Reite and Evensen, 2006). However, metachromasia characteristic of granules in mammalian and human mast cells (Mescher, 2010) can be demonstrated in tissues treated with alcoholic fixatives (Reite and Evensen, 2006). In granules of salmonid EGCs alkaline and acid phosphatases, arylsulphatase and 5-nucleotidase have been demonstrated and it has been indicated the presence of 5-hydroxytryptamine and lysozyme. Exposure to bacteria, bacterial products or degranulating agents used for mammalian mast cells provokes degranulation and subsequent vasodilation and inflammation. In the filaments of salmonids, such cells have been observed in both the epithelium and further within the perivascular connective tissue of secondary blood vessels and in the endothelium (Powell et al., 1990; Reite, 1997). They may undergo local mitosis (Reite, 1998).

In more advanced teleosts, antimicrobial peptides of the piscidin type have been found within cytoplasmic granules of EGCs (Silphaduang et al., 2006). Histamine has only been detected in gilthead seabream so far (Mulero et al., 2007), while this allergic response substance was absent in salmonids (Reite and Evensen, 2006). The EGCs in the core of gill filament explants from rainbow trout increased in number after treatment with LPS and TNF-α but also after short-term (> 6 h) handling stress (Holland

and Rowley, 1998). EGCs of the posterior intestinal lamina propria of rainbow trout display aryl sulphatase B and peroxidase activity arising from their granule. EGCs were also shown to phagocytose latex beads (Sire and Vernier, 1995). EGCs can be recruited to places with chronic inflammation (Reite and Evensen, 2006).

5.5.4 Lymphocytes

Lymphocytes are small rounded cells with condensed nuclei, high nucleus-to-cytoplasm ratios and sparse amounts of basophilic cytoplasm (Zinkl et al., 1991) while plasma cells are larger, with higher amounts of a more basophilic cytoplasm and an excentrically located nucleus. A portion of the resident peritoneal lymphocytes in rainbow trout is positive for nonspecific esterase and acid phosphatase, and all are negative for peroxidase and alkaline phosphatase (Afonso et al., 1997). Low numbers of putative resident lymphocyte-like cells have been detected in the gill epithelium of presumptive healthy teleosts including salmonids by TEM (Newstead, 1967). The gill resident lymphocyte population consists mainly of T cells (Lin et al., 1999).

5.5.5 B lymphocytes and plasma cells

B lymphocytes and plasma cells in teleosts are associated with three classes of immunoglobulins; IgM, IgD, and IgT (IgZ), all present in plasma membrane receptors and IgM and IgT also secreted to the extracellular environment (Fillatreau et al., 2013). IgM is the predominant isotype found in blood (Secombes and Wang, 2012). B cells in rainbow trout also display phagocytic and microbicidal capabilities (Li et al., 2006; Øverland et al., 2010). Cells termed 'constitutive' IgM secreting plasma-like cells constitute a minor fraction of circulating blood cells in dab (*Limanda limanda* L.) (2700 per million cells). They are also present in the gills, where they apparently correspond to resident cells (Davidson et al., 1997). B lymphocytes or plasmacytes positive for IgM are found around filamental blood vessels in the Mandarin fish (*Siniperca chuatsi* Basilewsky) (Tian et al., 2009), in filamental epithelium of Atlantic halibut (*Hippoglossus hippoglossus* L.) (Grove et al., 2006), in luminae of the lamellar capillary network of parasitized rainbow trout (Olsen et al., 2011) and very few IgM^+ cells can be detected in the salmonid ILT (Koppang et al., 2010). The IgT class has been described in different teleost species including salmonids (Danilova et al., 2005; Flajnik, 2005; Hansen et al., 2005). It is abundantly secreted in gills and other mucosal organs of salmonids (Tadiso et al., 2011a) and thus it has been suggested to act as a mucosal antibody (Zhang et al., 2010). In Atlantic salmon (Tadiso et al., 2011a) IgM and IgT are up to 200 and 20 times, respectively, as abundant as IgD, and the abundance in gills and other organs were ≤ approx. 10% that of kidney and spleen. Consistent with the secretion of immunoglobulins into the mucus of teleosts transcripts for polymeric immunoglobulin receptor (pIgR) mediating the transport of immunoglobulins across epithelia have been detected (Feng et al., 2009a; Rombout et al., 2008; Tadiso et al., 2011b).

5.5.6 T lymphocytes

Teleost T cells are described as two main types, helper T cells and cytotoxic T cells, expressing the plasma membrane-bound glycoproteins with extracellular Ig-like domains, CD4 and CD8, respectively. CD4 and CD8 act as co-receptors for T cell receptors when binding to MHC class II and I, respectively (Castro et al., 2011). Expression of CD4 transcripts has been detected in a number of teleost fish species (Randelli et al., 2008), including Atlantic salmon (Moore et al., 2009). The existence of Th1, Th2, Th17, and Treg cells in fish can be concluded from the presence of respective cytokine and transcription factor genes (Wang and Secombes, 2013). Importantly, high expression of salmonid IL-4/13A and GATA3 transcripts in gills and skin suggests a Th2 skewed environment (Takizawa et al., 2011b) preventing the gill from overwhelming pro-inflammatory reactions toward harmless waterborne antigens. However, high numbers of cytotoxic T cells may diffuse into the epithelium as indicated by the presence of CD8-positive cells, particularly at the leading edges of the filaments in healthy Atlantic salmon (Hetland et al., 2010; 2011). Few CD8-positive cells have been observed in filamental and lamellar epithelium of freshwater rainbow trout (Olsen et al., 2011; Takizawa et al., 2011a). These findings correspond to the observed few scattered CD3-positive T lymphocytes in filamental and lamellar epithelium of Atlantic salmon. However, considerable aggregates of CD3-positive T cells are found in the ILT of salmonid fishes, embedded between epithelial cells forming a meshwork much resembling that of the thymus (Koppang et al., 2010). A high percentage of these T cells is CD8 positive (Takizawa et al., 2011a). However, the function of T cells at this location is still unknown. Future studies have to determine if the ILT represents a primary or secondary lymphoid structure, even though present information suggests it to be the latter (Aas et al., 2014; Austbø et al., 2014) and if similar structures are found in other fish species.

5.5.7 Natural killer (NK)-like cells and nonspecific cytotoxic cells (NCCs)

NK-like cytotoxic lymphocytes belonging to the innate immune system have been shown to kill allogeneic and virus-infected cells in a few fish species (Fischer et al., 2013). They are represented by NK-like cells that are found in the peripheral blood (Yoshida et al., 1995) and by tissue-derived NCCs (Jaso-Friedmann et al., 1993). The latter are agranular small monocyte-like cells in channel catfish (*Ictalurus punctatus* Rafinesque) and of highly variable morphology in gilthead seabream (Whyte, 2007). NCCs bear a vimentin-like surface molecule (Jaso-Friedmann et al., 1993) and express a type III membrane protein termed NCC receptor protein 1 (NCCRP-1) (Jaso-Friedmann et al., 1997). Resident peritoneal lymphocytes in rainbow trout with phosphatase-positive cytoplasmic granules have also been suggested to correspond to NK cells (Afonso et al., 1997). Homologs to the NK cell-enhancing factor (NKEF) have been described in several fish species (Chen et al., 2009). This factor has been shown to be upregulated in the gills and other organs in carp (*Cyprinus carpio* L.) infected with spring viremia of carp virus (SVCV) (Huang et al., 2009). Further NK cell function associated with the gills has not been investigated.

5.5.8 Dendritic-like cells

The presence of dendritic-like cells is indicated in teleosts by the expression of a CD83 homolog in salmonids (Haugarvoll et al., 2006; Ohta et al., 2004) and in turbot (*Psetta maxima* L.), where gill expression correlates with antigen stimulation (Hu et al., 2010). The existence of dendritic-like cells has also been suggested in the intestinal epithelium of Atlantic salmon, in which cells with certain features of mammalian M-cells were detected in their close neighborhood (Fuglem et al., 2010). Cells with a dendritic-like morphology have also been detected in spleen and kidney of salmonids; and in epithelial and connective tissues of rainbow trout gills infected with the microsporidium *Loma salmonae* (Lovy et al., 2008). MHC class II expression is a common feature of mammalian dendritic cells and MHC class II positive cells resembling dendritic-like cells have been detected in filamental and lamellar epithelium of rainbow trout and in uvea of Atlantic salmon (Koppang et al., 2004; Olsen et al., 2011). Some of the MHC class II positive cells seen in hyperplastic epithelia of amoebic gill disease-affected Atlantic salmon also display a dendritic-like morphology (Morrison et al., 2006). Another dendritic cell marker in humans is CD207 (langerin), which is highly conserved among vertebrates. Using an anti-human-CD207 antibody the corresponding intracellular protein was detected in spleen and anterior kidney of two salmonid fish species, but neither in gills nor in any other organ (Lovy et al., 2009).

5.5.9 Rodlet cells

Rodlet cells (Figure 5.6) may already be seen in carp embryos (Mazon et al., 2007). In many adult teleost species they may be observed in the gill epithelium, but there is wide individual variation in their numbers (Manera and Dezfuli, 2004). The origin, nature and function of rodlet cells have been controversially discussed in the past, but their endogenous origin is now broadly accepted. Immature rodlet cells differentiate in the basal part of the gill epithelium and later migrate to their upper part. The mature cells are oval, frequently oriented with their long axis perpendicularly to the epithelial surface. They are attached to adjacent epithelial cells by desmosomes and tight

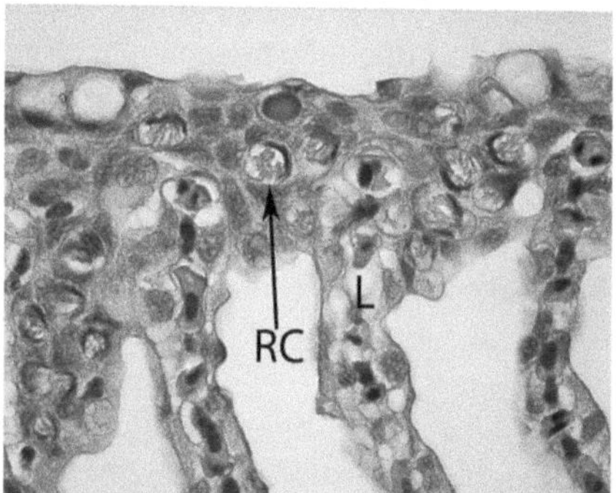

Figure 5.6 Histological image of rodlet cells (RC) in the gills. The lamella is marked (L).

junctions, and have microvilli at their apical surface getting in contact with the water (Bielek, 2008; Karlsson, 1983; Leino, 1974). The characteristic eosinophilic rodlets consist of a club-like sac with a central electron dense core and are ejected to the gill surface when the cell is stimulated (Bielek, 2008; Leino, 1974). Their number seems to depend on the fish species, season, and stress (Leino, 1974). Their nature and function is still a matter of debate. Since rodlet cells have been reported in association with parasitic and viral infections, but also with inflammation they are considered to participate in host defense (Manera and Dezfuli, 2004; Reite, 2005; Reite and Evensen, 2006).

5.5.10 Eosinophilic sacciform cells

Eosinophilic sacciform cells containing a single inclusion of eosinophilic and electron dense material occupying most of the cytoplasm are found in the epithelium of diseased gills of several fish species (Speare and Ferguson, 2006) and in highly varying numbers in the epithelium of wild salmonids (Kvellestad and Larsen, 1999). Although they appear to secrete material onto the gill surface their exact nature and function is still unclear (Speare and Ferguson, 2006).

5.5.11 Melanin-containing cells

Melanin-containing cells present in visceral organs consist of at least two types: melanomacrophages in salmonid and non-salmonid species and melanocyte-like cells as described only in salmonids so far, but probably also present in other species. While melanomacrophages in advanced teleosts contain hemosiderin, lipofuscin and highly varying amounts of melanin (Agius and Agbede, 1984; Agius and Roberts, 2003), it is debatable if melanocyte-like cells only contain high amounts of melanin granules as some authors argue (Agius and Agbede, 1984; Oguri, 1976), or if they also may act as phagocytes as suggested by *in vitro* experiments (Haugarvoll et al., 2006). Melanins bind to metals and are potent antioxidants. Accumulations of melanomacrophages in organs such as the kidney and the spleen are denoted melanomacrophage centers (Agius and Roberts, 2003) or macrophage aggregates (Wolke, 1992). The accumulations are well circumscribed in advanced teleost species while in species of Salmoniformes and Clupeiformes they are irregular and poorly-confined (Agius and Roberts, 2003; Wolke, 1992). In gills, melanin-containing cells are present in septum and filaments of presumptive healthy salmonids and are apparently restricted to connective tissue (Figure 5.7). Upon infection, melanin also appears in the lamellar microcirculation, either in melanin-containing cells present in the vascular lumen or in pillar cells. In fish, melanin synthesis has not only been demonstrated *in vivo* but also *in vitro* using a macrophage-like cell line (Thorsen et al., 2006).

5.5.12 Thrombocytes

Thrombocytes in teleost blood are nucleated cells involved in hemostasis (Meseguer et al., 2002). In salmonids they are oval to elongated cells with sparse cytoplasm that

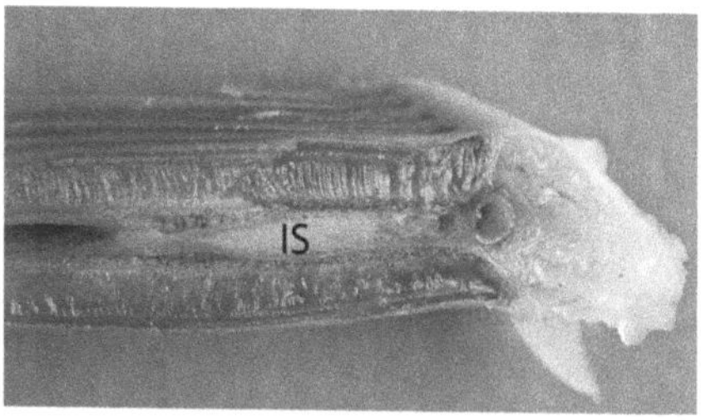

Figure 5.7 Transversal section of a gill arch, Atlantic salmon, 9 kg. On each side of the interbranchial septum, black spots, representing melanized cells, are visible.

stains slightly basophilic or not and they possess acid phosphatase activity (Zinkl et al., 1991). In non-salmonid species cytoplasmic vesicular and microtubular structures have been demonstrated that contain alkaline phosphatase indicating the presence of glycogen (Tavares-Dias et al., 2007). Thrombocytes are able to take up carbon particles (Burrows et al., 2001) and cellular debris (Tavares-Dias et al., 2007) while further fate of the foreign material is unknown (Meseguer et al., 2002). Different thrombocyte surface molecules have been indicated, of which two are involved in collagen-induced aggregation of the cells. Moreover, thrombocytes express MHC class I and IL1β and TNFα and may increase in number after antigenic stimulation (Köllner et al., 2004). However, thrombocyte function has not been investigated in association with the gills.

5.5.13 Erythrocytes

Erythrocytes are present in teleosts with few exceptions (Antarctic ice fishes) and in most teleosts are nucleated. They are generally oval in shape with an oval to rounded nucleus (Claver and Quaglia, 2009). Erythrocytes in rainbow trout appear to display immune responses. Erythrocytes *in vitro* exposed to the fungus *Candida albicans* tend to cluster around macrophage-like cells, thus stimulating their phagocytic activity toward the fungus (Passantino et al., 2002). Erythrocytes exposed to different antigens do subsequently express pathogen recognition receptor (PRR) mRNA transcripts, and stimulation by poly (I:C) may result in secretion of molecules that can modify antiviral responses of macrophages (Morera et al., 2011). Another defense mechanism of erythrocytes is displayed by respiratory proteins that can mediate the production of reactive oxygen species even in invertebrates following activation by microbial proteases and pathogen-associated molecular patterns (PAMPS) (Jiang et al., 2007).

5.5.14 Intravascular occurrence of cell types

The hitherto described cell types are reported from peripheral blood, but the relative numbers of the different cell types vary a lot in decreasing order from erythrocytes, to thrombocytes and other leukocytes. Erythrocyte numbers in fish blood vary between 1×10^9 and 5×10^9 per mL (Claver and Quaglia, 2009) and rainbow trout blood may contain 10^9 erythrocytes and 10^8 leukocytes (thrombocytes included) per mL (Lin et al., 1999). Lymphocytes are the most common circulating leukocyte in fish (Claver and Quaglia, 2009) followed by PMN cells and monocytes in low and approximately equal numbers in this species and coho salmon (Zinkl et al., 1991).

Antibody-labeled PMN cells detected by flow cytometry have been found to amount 28% of the peripheral blood leukocyte population (thrombocytes included) in rainbow trout (Hamdani et al., 1998) and 11–34% in groups of out-of-season salmon post-smolts (Pettersen et al., 2005). B cells detected by an IgM-specific monoclonal antibody averaged 7–47% in the same fish species. In turbot, a total leukocyte concentration of 10^8 cells per mL consists of 52% thrombocytes, 40.8% lymphocytes, 5.6% granulocytes, and 1.6% monocytes (Burrows et al., 2001).

5.6 Mucosal immunity and the gills

Before we go into detail with some selected conditions, we will briefly address the key steps of infection establishment in gills, including mechanisms for attachment and uptake. In this respect, molecules of different kinds, particles and pathogens have been studied. Present knowledge is scarce, especially for the attachment phase. In a number of studies of exposure to waterborne pathogens, the organisms have been re-isolated from peripheral blood but morphological methods allowing the demonstration of organisms in the gills have not always been used. Specialized gill epithelial cells such as M cells involved in antigen uptake have not been identified, but it is highly likely that such cells are present. This question should be a major challenge for the scientific community in the years to come. Further, we should like to emphasize the recent discovery of the teleost IgA-analog IgT, which already and by all rights has attracted considerable attention. IgT has been detected in cells of filamental and lamellar epithelium in parasitized rainbow trout (Olsen et al., 2011), but the positive cells display rather a PE-like rather than a lymphocyte-like morphology, possibly indicating transepithelial transport, a mechanism previously suggested (Hughes and Wright, 1970). We have just started to understand some of the mucosal humoral immune responses in fish, a field that probably is of greatest importance for future vaccine development. Therefore, future research on gill immunity should be put on elucidating mechanisms for waterborne antigen uptake showing that such events may trigger cellular and humoral immune responses.

Concerning uptake of particles from the gill circulatory system after systemic administration, latex (0.81 μm) or colloidal carbon has been demonstrated in the basally located pillar cells, but never in endothelial cells located at the lamellar-free margin of rainbow trout gills (Chilmonczyk and Monge, 1980). Many particles were present in the cytoplasm of the phagocytic cells, of which some also contained cytoplasmic melanin-like granules. In another study where FITC-conjugated bovine serum albumin was injected to rainbow trout, fluorescent particles were detected in endothelial cells of filamental secondary vessels (Ototake et al., 1996).

Uptake and distribution to other organs of waterborne agents or substances over the gills through mucosal surfaces have been observed after exposure to high concentrations of macromolecules, particles or microorganisms. There is limited knowledge about the underlying mechanisms, but receptor-mediated uptake of selected antigens or nonselective phagocytosis of material has been suggested (Anderson et al., 1984). The latter option, however, was considered to make fish survival impossible in waters with high concentrations of suspended solids. Several authors have argued for selective uptake processes. McIntosh and colleagues noted that gill epithelium apparently is impermeable for *Renibacterium salmoninarum* (McIntosh et al., 2000), while *Aeromonas salmonicida* seems to infect Atlantic salmon over the gills (Hodgkinson et al., 1987). In addition to *Yersinia ruckeri*, which is described in a separate paragraph, a number of bacterins and bacteria attach to the gills. *Pasteurella piscicida* antigens have been observed in gill tissues of yellowtail (*Seriola quinqueradiata* Temminck and Schlegel) (Kawahara and Kusuda, 1988) after immersion vaccination. These results suggest that the fish gills represent a main site of pathogen entry into the host. Uptake across the gills and subsequent systemic distribution of radiolabeled *Listonella anguillarum* bacterin has been indicated in marine fish (Tatner and Horne, 1983). These findings were supported by immunostaining of sections demonstrating a transient presence of antigen in mucus at the gill surface and occurrence in the kidney after 3 hours (Nelson et al., 1985). Also, *Vibrio anguillarum* bacterin is taken up via the gills of Japanese flounder (*Paralichthys olivaceus* Temminck and Schlegel) resulting in subsequent immune responses (Kato et al., 2013). Similarly, *Edwardsiella tarda* apparently uses the gills as a site of entry into the fish. However, only virulent but not avirulent *Edwardsiella tarda* adhered to the gills and other mucosal surfaces and could subsequently be re-isolated from internal organs (Ling et al., 2001).

The transport into the organism seems to appear rapidly as bacteria have been isolated in peripheral blood as early as 1-minute post-infection. Interestingly, *Yersinia ruckeri* has been demonstrated to bind more efficiently to gill mucus than to skin mucus (Tobback et al., 2010). In the corresponding study, the ability to adhere or invade the gill tissue was not different between virulent and avirulent strains of *Y. ruckeri* as described in *E. tarda* (Ling et al., 2001). Nevertheless, Hodgkinson and colleagues observed that uptake of *Aeromonas salmonicida* was enhanced by culturing the bacterium in low levels of nutrient (Hodgkinson et al., 1987). The uptake was further enhanced by mixing the bacterium with latex beads while the explanation of this effect remains an enigma. Differences between bacteria species, between different activation stages and between live and inactivated bacteria regarding uptake across the gills suggests selective mechanisms. Such selectivity has been demonstrated in the mammalian gut where for instance *Salmonella* species and *Yersinia enterocolitica* entered the submucosa through specialized epithelial cells termed M cells. Recently, cells with some M cell properties have been identified in the salmonid gut (Fuglem et al., 2010).

Besides bacteria, uptake of many other particulate and soluble substances by the gills has been reported in a series of studies. After bath exposure if fish to radiolabeled proteins ranging from 66 bovine serum albumin to 900 (glycoproteins) kDa these macromolecules appear in the epithelium and subsequently in the kidney and the spleen of freshwater fish. Uptake was shown to be enhanced when the molecules were bound to 0.8 μm latex particles or when fish were pre-exposed to a salinity of 8% (Smith, 1982). The uptake of lipopolysaccharides (LPS) by gills and subsequent distribution to internal organs has been demonstrated in marine fish (Al-Harbi and Austin, 1992; Kawahara and Kusuda, 1988), using anti-LPS antibodies. In the first investigation, LPS from *Pasteurella piscicida* was demonstrated in the gill lamellae. In the latter, LPS from *Cytophaga*-like bacteria was detected in gill and to lesser extent in skin. While FITC-conjugated BSA is vigorously taken up by macrophage-like cells in the skin of freshwater rainbow trout such cells were also shown to contribute to bovine serum albumin uptake in the filamental gill epithelium of rainbow trout (Ototake et al., 1996). Bovine serum albumin conjugated to 1 μm fluorescent latex microspheres was ingested by epithelial cells and by intra-epithelial macrophage-like cells in rainbow trout (Moore et al., 1998). Also, 1 μm fluorescent microspheres (uncoated or coated with an extract from *Ewardsiella ictaluri* outer membrane protein) were detected within macrophage-like cells of filamental and lamellar gill epithelia (Glenney and Petrie-Hanson, 2006). All these proteins or particles were identified in internal organs later on. However, portals of entry might have been extrabranchial too.

Both local gill and systemic immune responses have been reported following bacterial gill disease and immunizations with bacterins. Increased levels of antibodies in gill mucus and to lesser extent in serum have been detected following experimental bacterial gill disease caused by *Flavobacterium branchiophilium*, and a poor correlation between levels in mucus and serum in the same individuals was interpreted as the existence of a specific, inducible gill antibody response, which is independent of systemic antibody production (Lumsden et al., 1993). The latter assumption has been supported by results from experiments with both bath exposure and intraperitoneal immunization with bacterins of *F. branchiophilium* (Lumsden et al., 1995) and *Vibrio harvey* (Xu et al., 2009), with strongest gill and systemic responses obtained from bath and injection, respectively. The responses were measured by detecting immunoglobulins in gill mucus and serum (Lumsden et al., 1995) and by counting immunoglobulin-containing cells in the gills, head kidney, and peripheral blood (Xu et al., 2009). From these results transportation in either direction between gills and anterior kidney of antigens and/or migration of immune cells was interpreted, and that local immune responses in gills are more or less independent from the systemic responses. Feng and colleagues (Feng et al., 2009b) obtained similar results (Xu et al., 2009) after exposure to *Edwardsiella tarda* bacterin as a bath immunization gave a significant increase in immunoglobulin-containing cells in the gills only and intraperitoneal injection resulted in a significant increase in the head kidney and blood only. And dos Santos and colleagues (dos Santos et al., 2001) detected significantly higher numbers of immunoglobulin-containing cells in gills compared to the kidney and spleen after bath immunization with *Photobacterium damselae* ssp. *piscicida* bacterin. Immunization by both immersion and intraperitoneal injection of bacterin provided protective immunity in subsequent challenge by bath exposure to live bacteria of the above-mentioned species (Lumsden et al., 1995; Xu et al., 2009). In the immunoassays in these investigations anti-immunoglobulin polyclonal antibodies presumably directed against all Ig isotypes (Lumsden et al., 1993; 1995; Xu et al., 2009) or anti-IgM monoclonal antibodies (dos Santos et al., 2001; Feng et al., 2009b) were used. Local and systemic responses would possibly be better distinguished by use of separate antibodies against IgM and IgT.

In the following part of the chapter, the initial responses of the gills to waterborne infectious organisms will be described and discussed. Such pathogens may remain on the gills, either causing unnoticeable or minor responses, or provoking local and generalized responses even if they do not infect other sites, such as during amoebic gill disease (AGD). Alternatively, the pathogens may enter the host through the gills. Some bacteria and viruses may enter the fish body through the huge mucosal surface of the gill, but may still leave the gill undisturbed. However, when serving as a port of entry, gills may also be heavily affected as in some bacterial diseases. Viruses with mucosal tropism such as koi herpes virus may cause serious pathological changes in the gill. Otherwise, parasites with a common mucosal tropism like *Ichthyophthirius multifiliis* do not only parasitize in the gills but also in the skin.

Thus, immune responses or pathological changes in the gills will never be strictly local but will frequently affect the whole organism by triggering systemic immune responses. Agents, replicating or not, and cell and tissue injury will display their PAMPs and DAMPs, respectively. This in concert with local cytokine responses will activate local and systemic immune reactions where immune cells are recruited from central lymphoid organs (thymus, spleen, head kidney). It is also a question if the ILT may be heavily involved in the recruitment of immune cells. We will discuss this possibility further when dealing with infectious salmon anemia virus (ISAV).

As the gills contain a variety of different immune cells, local responses to antigen challenge may be highly diversified and fine-tuned according to the different challenges they are exposed to. A vast number of works have in particular addressed transcriptional responses to different pathogens, but the distribution of these transcripts to different cell types and tissues is frequently unknown and may well belong to blood cells as they are transported through the gills. Common features include induction of innate and adaptive immune responses. However, the general lack of useful antibodies in the characterization of immune responses has impaired morphological studies in connection with disease. Likewise, limited information clearly linking immune cells to pathological changes exists. To illustrate such events, we have selected examples from four different pathogens in the following where gene expression has been studied at the transcript and/or protein (effector molecule) level and in association with description of pathological changes.

Considering that the above mentioned is a dilemma when writing a chapter on gills we will still concentrate on local gill reactions as a response to pathogens and describe systemic responses only when we feel the necessity to do so.

5.7 Infectious salmon anemia

Infectious salmon anemia (ISA) is a disease mainly affecting Atlantic salmon. After ISA virus (ISAV) has entered the fish using different mucosal surfaces including gill epithelia (Aamelfot et al., 2014), a non-cytolytic virus replication in endothelial cells occurs throughout the body, including gill pillar cells (Aamelfot et al., 2012).

To a lesser extent, ISAV also replicates in leukocytes (Aamelfot et al., 2012; Moneke et al., 2005) and gill epithelial cells (Aamelfot et al., 2012; Weli et al., 2013). ISAV attaches to its target cells using glycoprotein-bound 4-O-acetylated sialic acids (Hellebø et al., 2004). This receptor is also found in gill endothelial and epithelial cells (Aamelfot et al., 2012).

Several studies on ISA pathogenesis have been performed in Atlantic salmon where gill responses were studied following exposure to waterborne virus. A transient replication in few epithelial cells followed by increasing replication in endothelial cells of the gills has been observed by immunohistochemistry (Aamelfot et al., 2012; Weli et al., 2013). In a study by Austbø et al. (2014), replicating ISAV was detected by PCR in gills immediately after bath infection and at high levels after 2, 8, and 24 days, but never in laser-dissected intraepithelial lymphoid tissue (ILT). Mortality only occurred from day 20 on. These authors demonstrated that innate immune responses were characterized by an up-regulation of IFN-α, IFN–γ, viperin, and RIG-1 genes in filaments and laser-dissected ILT 8 days after infection. Components of the adaptive immune response such as MHC class I were found to be slightly up-regulated in whole filaments and in ILT. In agreement with this study, Hetland et al. (2010) recorded increasing numbers of MHC class I-positive cells in filamental and lamellar epithelia using immunohistochemistry. At the same time, there was a decrease in the number of MHC class I expressing cells in the filamental trailing edge epithelium and in the ILT. It has been speculated that ISAV proteins with type I interferon antagonizing activity may delay this innate immune response (Austbø et al., 2014; García-Rosado et al., 2008; McBeath et al., 2006). In another study viperin, but not IFN-α, IFN–γ, and RIG-1 transcripts were up-regulated (Lauscher et al., 2011), while Jørgensen et al. (2007) reported an up-regulation of IFN-α but not of IFN–γ, and of the IFN-associated Mx protein in moribund fish. These differences may reflect different experimental procedures or times of sampling, as the fish of the first study were sampled 3 days after mortality emerged, while the fish of the second study were sampled 6 days before mortality started.

Unaltered expression of CD8 mRNA (Lauscher et al., 2011) or even depletion of CD8-positive cells in the ILT and in filamental epithelia (Aamelfot et al., 2012; Hetland et al., 2010) has been attributed to reduced numbers of circulating lymphocytes in salmon infected by i.p. injection (Aamelfot et al., 2012).

Controversial results were reported in studies on MHC class II expression in the gills after ISAV infection. While no changes in mRNA expression were seen in the filaments (Austbø et al., 2014; Jørgensen et al., 2007; Lauscher et al., 2011), increased levels were recorded for the ILT (Austbø et al., 2014). In contrast, (Hetland et al., 2010) found deceasing numbers of MHC class II-positive cells by immunohistochemistry both in the ILT and in filamental and lamellar epithelia. ISAV infection has not been found to alter the protein expression of IgT and IgM (Austbø et al., 2014), and the mRNA expression of CD4, IgM, IgT, and IgD (Lauscher et al., 2011).

Taken together, these results indicate that ISAV does neither induce a strong adaptive cell-mediated nor a humoral immune response in gills during the early phase of infection. However, survival of fish can be attributed to increased Ig-related transcripts in gills and other organs during the late phase of infection (Jørgensen et al., 2008) and to protective immune responses recorded in extrabranchial organs (Falk and Dannevig, 1995; LeBlanc et al., 2012). This also explains why intraperitoneal vaccination of salmon offers protection against ISA (Lauscher et al., 2011).

5.8 Red mouth disease (yersiniosis)

Yersiniosis or red mouth disease (RMD) is a septicemia affecting salmonids cultured in freshwater and is caused by the bacterium *Yersinia ruckeri* (Tobback et al., 2007). Fish of different ages are susceptible to natural infection (bath). Although some authors do not regard the gills as the primary sites of *Y. ruckeri* uptake (Khimmakthong et al., 2013), others have shown that both *in vivo* and *in vitro* bath exposure to live *Y. ruckeri* results in an immediate presence of pathogens in gill mucus, subsequent invasion of gill epithelium and further the lamellar vascular system (Ohtani et al., 2014; Tobback et al., 2009; 2010).

Following bath exposure to live *Y. ruckeri*, the corresponding bacterial antigen can be detected by IHC in a moderate number of scattered lamellar epithelial cells already 1 minute after exposure (Ohtani et al., 2014). The antigen-containing cells were described as pavement cells (PEs) but it remained unclear if these were of the columnar or squamous type. At the same early time point bacteria could be re-isolated from peripheral blood. Fernandez et al. (2003) suggested that the bacterial protease Yrp1 is important for this rapid tissue invasion and spread into the vascular system.

Also bacterins are taken up by the gill epithelium (Khimmakthong et al., 2013; Torroba et al., 1993; Zapata et al., 1987). The corresponding cell types were identified as PE-like cells and epithelial macrophage-like cells (Torroba et al., 1993; Zapata et al., 1987). Interestingly, *Y. ruckeri* is a facultative intracellular bacterium, which may reside in macrophages (Ryckaert et al., 2010). Thus, uptake into gill macrophages may be yet an additional component in the pathogenesis of this pathogen or in the immunization with its bacterin.

According to a number of authors (Bridle et al., 2011; 2012; Chettri et al., 2012; Wiens et al., 2006), local gill immune responses upon bacterial infection occur before the onset of a severe septicemia. In a study on the expression of immune relevant molecules upon *Y. ruckeri* infection in rainbow trout (Deshmukh et al., 2013), a general Th2-driven immune response has been observed in internal organs. Although gills were not investigated in this study, a Th2 environment can also be suggested for this organ because gills of healthy salmonids have been shown to constitutively express genes that are typical for a Th2-skewed environment (Takizawa et al., 2011b). Bath vaccination with *Y. ruckeri* bacterin or challenge with live bacteria did not increase expression of CXCd in gills (Wiens et al., 2006), which additionally may explain the rather weak attraction of inflammatory cells to the gills upon infection.

The antimicrobial peptides cathelicidin 1 and 2, of which the second is constitutively expressed in gills, undergo up-regulation during the early phase following bath exposure to *Y. ruckeri* (Bridle et al., 2011). Since direct antimicrobial activity of cathelicidins against *Y. ruckeri* could not be demonstrated, it was hypothesized that these molecules have an immunomodulatory role by stimulating the expression of IL-8.

Other antimicrobial immune responses during the early phase of infection include the up-regulation of C-type lectin and collagenase 3 precursor (Bridle et al., (2012).

A sequential study of rainbow trout fry infected with *Y. ruckeri* over 25 days has been provided by Chettri et al. (2012). However, while gene expression studies referred to whole larvae, tissue sections revealed no differences in IgT and CD8 expression between gills of infected and uninfected fry. Nevertheless, a constitutively high expression of IgT molecules was suggested to be of high importance in mucosal antibacterial immune defenses.

5.9 Amoebic gill disease

Amoebic gill disease (AGD) occurs in salmonids and some non-salmonid species and is caused by the ectoparasite *Neoparamoeba perurans* (Nowak, 2012). The pathogen causes significant losses in salmon aquaculture, especially in Tasmania. It vegetates at the gill epithelial surface, and up to a few million trophozoites have been recorded in one fish. The degrees of pathological changes, clinical signs and mortality display a wide range of variation in infected salmon depending on factors such as age and salinity (Nowak, 2012; Palmer et al., 1997; Rodger and McArdle, 1996).

Pathological changes start in multiple focal infected sites of the gills and may first be observed as hyperplasia of apparently poorly differentiated epithelial cells, but also inflammation, adhesions between lamellae, excessive mucous production, and death of cells in contact with amoebae (Adams and Nowak, 2001, 2003, 2004; Kent et al., 1988; Lovy et al., 2007; Morrison et al., 2006; Munday et al., 1990; Rodger and McArdle, 1996; Roubal et al., 1989). Focal changes expand along portions of filaments, developing to become confluent, with highest parasite numbers and epithelial edema and inflammatory (macrophage-, granulocyte-, lymphocyte- and eosinophil-like) cell infiltrations at advancing ends.

These adhesions frequently occur between the apical parts of lamellae, resulting in partly enclosed interlamellar spaces. Such spaces are lined by squamous pavement cells and may contain remnants of amoebae and desquamated cells. These extensive pathological changes are accompanied with inflammatory immune responses, which have been documented in a number of studies. In gills of healthy salmon, pro-inflammatory cytokines such as TNF-α (Morrison et al., 2007) and IL-1β (Bridle et al., 2006) are constitutively expressed. IL-1β mRNA has been localized by *in situ* hybridization to pavement cells of filamental and lamellar epithelia (Bridle et al., 2006) and was found to be highly up-regulated in filamental segments with extensive changes of AGD, especially in cells that are located at the top of the hyperplastic epithelium. Following experimental infection of salmon, not only pro-inflammatory cytokine genes (IL-1β and TNF-α), but also genes indicating adaptive cell-mediated (MHC class I, MHC class II, TCR-α, CD8-α, CD4) and humoral (IgM, IgT) immune responses were up-regulated. Expectedly, Mx gene expression which is rather up-regulated during viral infections was not significantly different from control groups (Pennacchi et al., 2014).

While IL-1β and TNF-α were up-regulated in gill segments with light, medium, or severe pathological changes, all other investigated genes were expressed at highest levels at sites with negligible to moderate changes. Thus, decreased levels of MHC class I and II pathway genes in the most severe lesions (Pennacchi et al., 2014) may be a result of immune attrition agreeing with a secondary down-regulation of immune genes reported from chronic AGD in an earlier study (Young et al., 2008). Some degree of immunity or other types of host resistance has been indicated from survivor fish after natural outbreaks or experimental challenge (Bridle et al., 2005; Munday et al., 1990). It has also been observed that Atlantic salmon transferred to seawater netpens in spring are more vulnerable to AGD infection during the following 6 months compared to fish transferred to seawater the previous year (Palmer et al., 1997; Steinum et al., 2008). This may indicate adaptive immunity (given fish have been exposed to the amoebae during their first year in seawater) or some kind of age-dependent resistance.

In Tasmania repeated freshwater exposure is used therapeutically in order to reduce the number of amoebae during the seawater grow out phase of salmon (Nowak, 2012). However, numbers of amoebae and the pathological changes increase again after each freshwater exposure and return to seawater. This suggests that fish can neither mount an efficient innate nor an adaptive immune response against the parasite or that immune responses are strongly affected by salinity (Nowak, 2012).

5.10 Ichthyophthiriasis ("white spot disease")

The ciliated protozoan *Ichthyophthirius multifiliis* Fouquet infects several species of freshwater fish worldwide (Dickerson and Findly, 2014). It causes high mortality associated with ichthyophthiriasis ("white spot disease") in farmed fish, while low-level infections occur in wild fish. The parasite has a direct life cycle including different morphological forms, all being motile. These include the waterborne theronts, which infect gill and skin epithelia, the trophonts, which feed extracellularly within these epithelia (for approximately 7 days at 20°C), and the tomonts, which are released to the aquatic environment where they further divide and differentiate into theronts. The severity of pathological changes and mortality correlates with the numbers of parasite invading the fish. The immune reactions and pathological changes have been extensively studied especially in channel catfish, rainbow trout, and carp. Since many studies in ichthyophthiriasis refer to skin mucosa, we include the corresponding findings for comparative reasons.

5.10.1 Innate immunity

Theronts invade the space between epithelial cells of the filaments and cause immediate death of cells at the site of invasion but are surrounded by intact epithelial cells within 5 minutes post-exposure (Ewing et al., 1985; Hines and Spira, 1974a). Large quantities of hyaluronidase within the parasite are believed to be of importance for rapid invasion of the epithelia and parasite expansion (Uspenskaya 1963). However, in the gills of channel catfish an approximately 50% decline in parasite numbers has been observed within 10 minutes following invasion (Ewing et al., 1986). The mechanism behind this decline in the very early phase of infection remains unknown but points towards immune response mechanisms against the parasite. Although NCCs have a potential to kill the parasite *in vitro* (Graves et al., 1985), no significant NCC activities have yet been demonstrated *in vivo*.

Following the initial pathological changes in the gills, hyperplasia of goblet cells and apparently poorly differentiated epithelial cells result in filling of the entire interlamellar spaces, as observed in mirror carp, and this hyperplasia is not restricted to the areas in vicinity of the parasites (Hines and Spira, 1974a). Spaces containing cellular debris from the ongoing host cell damage form between trophonts and the epithelial cells (Ewing and Kocan, 1986, 1987). High numbers of neutrophil-like cells accumulate around filamental vessels of infected gills. They invade the proliferating epithelium after 8–12 days no matter if parasites are present or not. Lymphocyte-like cells may also infiltrate the epithelium but with high interindividual variations. Finally, fish with a high parasite burden show filamental necrosis and inflammation. In mirror carp, infected fish develop blood lymphopenia and neutrophilia with an apparent shift toward immature cells within 2 days post-infection (Hines and Spira, 1973) further underlining the importance of granulocytes. However, there is no evidence that neutrophil-like cells kill the parasite, but instead dead granulocytes and other cellular debris are subsequently engulfed by the trophonts (Dickerson, 2012). This is remarkable since granulocytes possess very efficient mechanisms to neutralize other single cell invaders such as bacteria. The exact role of neutrophil-like cells thus remains to be demonstrated.

The development of innate immune mechanisms and inflammation is further indicated by differentially regulated transcripts of immune relevant molecules in gills and skin of infected fish. In gills of rainbow trout (8.5 g), up-regulation of transcripts for IL-8, C3, SAA, IFN-γ, and iNOS has been detected while IL-22 remained unaltered at 4 days post-infection (Olsen et al., 2011). When whole larvae of rainbow trout were examined 3–72 h post infection, an up-regulation of transcripts for IL-1β from 3 hours and subsequently for IL-8, cathelicidin-2, TNF-α, hepcidin, IL-6, iNOS and SAA was recorded (Heinecke and Buchmann, 2013), suggesting an induction of inflammatory responses. Transcripts for a number of TLRs have been found to be differently regulated in gills and skin of infected channel catfish (Zhao et al., 2013a). Two signaling molecules (TRAF6 and TAK1) involved in TLR, BCR, and TCR signaling pathways and known to initiate the expression of inflammatory genes are up-regulated in gills and skin following infection of grass carp (Zhao et al., 2013b). Along with extravasation of neutrophil-like cells during the acute phase of white spot disease, an up-regulation of chemokines (CXCa and its receptor CXCR1) was detected in the skin of carp 36 h after infection (Gonzalez et al., 2007). Also in the skin, pro-inflammatory cytokines (IL-1β and TNF-α) were up-regulated 36 h p.i. in rainbow trout kept at 12°C (Sigh et al., 2004) and 96 h p.i. in carp kept at 23°C (Gonzalez et al., 2007), respectively, reflecting a difference in host species or other factors. Similarly, IL-1 receptor transcripts, iNOS and C3, were up-regulated in the skin 4 days after infection in rainbow trout (Gonzalez et al., 2007; Sigh et al., 2004), respectively.

5.10.2 Adaptive immunity

Adaptive protective immunity develops within 3–4 weeks after a waterborne infection, and also following intraperitoneal (i.p.) injection of live theronts or immobilization antigen (i-antigen) (Clark and Dickerson, 1997; Dickerson and Findly, 2014). The i-antigen is a single polypeptide chain that – in combination with adjuvant – is a protective immunogen when administered i.p. into channel catfish (Wang and Dickerson, 2002). Despite lymphopenia (Hines and Spira, 1973) both systemic and mucosal antibody production has been shown after infection, and antibodies seem to play a major role in protective immunity (Dickerson and Findly, 2014). Interestingly, Cross and Matthews (1992) and Wahli and Matthews (1999) found that immune responses following exposure to sublethal levels of live theronts do not seem to prevent theronts from penetrating into the epidermis of carp during subsequent challenge with a lethal level but promote exit of most trophonts within 2 h. These exited trophonts were still infective (Wahli and Matthews, 1999).

In mirror carp subjected to a sublethal experimental infection, serum antibodies were found to reach levels sufficient for *in vitro* immobilization of the parasite after 10 to 22 days, a period during which the parasites usually disappear from the skin (Hines and Spira, 1974b).

High titers of serum antibodies have also been detected in channel catfish following immunization with live theronts by i.p. injection or bath exposure (Xu and Klesius, 2013). Following bath exposure the trophonts were allowed to vegetate for a period of time before inactivation by formalin treatment of the fish. Very low parasite prevalence was observed in the skin following a second challenge with live parasites, and serum antibodies titers were found to correlate with survival of fish (Xu and Klesius, 2013). In a sequential study in channel catfish, in which infection was controlled with formalin treatment, serum antibodies (IgM) reached a maximum after 14 weeks and were able to immobilize the parasite *in vitro* (Maki and Dickerson, 2003). After 7 weeks of infection a transient increase in antibody titers in skin mucus coincided with parasite clearance. Since no correlation between IgM levels in serum and skin mucus has been recorded, it was suggested that a mucosal response is independent of the systemic response, and that mucous antibodies are not the result of passive diffusion from the blood. Similar observations have also been made following i.p. injection of i-antigen (Maki and Dickerson, 2003).

Already several years ago binding of IgM antibodies to the cilia has been shown (Clark et al., 1988). More recently, this observation has been confirmed and also IgT has been found to bind to trophonts (especially to their cilia) as early as 2 h after invasion of immune rainbow trout gills (von Gersdorff Jørgensen et al., 2011). In rainbow trout, immunoglobulins might have been released from IgM and IgT positive cells found in small blood vessels and epithelia of the gills (Olsen et al., 2011). In gills of rainbow trout, MHC class II and IgT expressing cells were found to be associated with trophonts following waterborne infection in rainbow trout (Heinecke and Buchmann, 2013). Interestingly, most trophonts exited from the epidermis of channel catfish within 12 hours following i.p. injection of a mouse monoclonal antibody raised against the i-antigen although *in vitro*, this antibody has been shown to bind to cilia and to immobilize the parasite (Clark et al., 1996).

Observations on adaptive immune responses against the parasite described above are supported by a sequential study during 47 days following i.p. immunization with live theronts (Olsen et al., 2011). While transcripts for MHC II, CD4, IgM, and IgT in gills were up-regulated no clear tendency could be recorded for CD8. Similarly in the skin of rainbow trout, MHC II and IgM transcripts were up-regulated (Sigh et al., 2004), while increased plasma IgM protein levels were detected (von Gersdorff Jørgensen et al., 2008). Consequently, observations on adaptive immune responses following infection or treatment with parasite antigens raised hopes in vaccine development.

Immunization of channel catfish followed by formalin treatment, resulted in protective immunity that was retained for years (Findly et al., 2013). Serum IgM antibodies directed against i-antigen were present after 5 weeks, returned to control levels after 1 year and again rose to high levels following a second challenge after 3 years. The numbers of antibody-secreting cells in the head kidney and the skin recognizing i-antigen declined to control levels after 2–3 years. Following the second challenge, they increased in number in the skin but not in the kidney. Transcripts for IgM heavy chain and TCRβ were detected in the basal layer of epidermis containing putative lymphocytes, indicating that B and T cells were present. This suggests that specific memory B cells might have differentiated into Ig-secreting cells after 3 years.

5.11 Concluding remarks

The gills should be obvious prime targets for the development of future immersion vaccines for the aquaculture industry. Still, we do not know key features related to antigen targeting and uptake over the epithelium. Apparently, pavement cells are involved in antigen uptake, but it remains unclear if such cells need a special form of differentiation or if special molecules on their surfaces are involved in this process. To reveal the nature of ILT, upcoming investigations should address functions of this structure. These are highly relevant questions in future research on the pathogenesis of different diseases and for the development of mucosal vaccines. Mucosal vaccines mimic waterborne infections and promote local mucosal immune reactions, which in the case of bacteria result in a stronger response compared to other delivery methods. Mucosal vaccination is also more simple and more cost effective than traditional delivery systems. Particularly intraperitoneal injection, often requiring the use of oil-adjuvants, may cause significant side effects, which are unacceptable from a fish welfare viewpoint.

References

Aamelfot, M., Dale, O.B., Falk, K., 2014. Infectious salmon anaemia – pathogenesis and tropism. J. Fish Dis. 37, 291–307.

Aamelfot, M., Dale, O.B., Weli, S.C., Koppang, E.O., Falk, K., 2012. Expression of the infectious salmon anemia virus receptor on Atlantic salmon endothelial cells correlates with the cell tropism of the virus. J. Virol. 86, 10571–10578.

Aas, I.B., Austbø, L., König, M., Syed, M., Falk, K., Hordvik, I., Koppang, E.O., 2014. Transcriptional characterization of the T cell population within the salmonid interbranchial lymphoid tissue. J. Immunol. 193, 3463–3469.

Adams, M.B., Nowak, B.F., 2001. Distribution and structure of lesions in the gills of Atlantic salmon, *Salmo salar* L., affected with amoebic gill disease. J. Fish Dis. 24, 535–542.

Adams, M.B., Nowak, B.F., 2003. Amoebic gill disease: sequential pathology in cultured Atlantic salmon *Salmo salar* L., J. Fish Dis. 26, 601–614.

Adams, M.B., Nowak, B.F., 2004. Experimental amoebic gill disease of Atlantic salmon, *Salmo salar* L.: further evidence for the primary pathogenic role of *Neoparamoeba* sp. (Page, 1987). J. Fish Dis. 27, 105–113.

Afonso, A., Ellis, A.E., Silva, M.T., 1997. The leucocyte population of the unstimulated peritoneal cavity of rainbow trout (*Oncorhynchus mykiss*). Fish Shellfish Immunol. 7, 335–348.

Afonso, A., Lousada, S., Silva, J., Ellis, A.E., Silva, M.T., 1998. Neutrophil and macrophage responses to inflammation in the peritoneal cavity of rainbow trout *Oncorhynchus mykiss*. A light and electron microscopic cytochemical study. Dis. Aquat. Org. 34, 27–37.

Agius, C., Agbede, S.A., 1984. An electron microscopical study on the genesis of lipofuscin, melanin and hemosiderin in the hematopoietic tissues of fish. J. Fish Biol. 24, 471–488.

Agius, C., Roberts, R.J., 2003. Melano-macrophage centres and their role in fish pathology. J. Fish Dis. 26, 499–561.

Al-Harbi, A.H., Austin, B., 1992. Distribution of formalized cells and lipopolysaccharide (LPS) of a fish pathogenic *Cytophaga* – like bacterium in tissues of turbot (*Scophthalmus maximus* L.) following uptake by inection, immersion and the oral route. Bull. Europ. Ass. Fish Pathol. 12, 100–103.

Alberts, B., Johnson, A., Lewis, J., Raff, M., Roberts, K., Walter, P., 2008. Molecular Biology of the Cell. New York, Garland Science Taylor & Francis Group, 1268 pp.

Anderson, D.P., Van Muiswinkel, W.B., Roberson, B.S., 1984. Effects of chemically induced immune modulation on infectious diseases of fish. Progr. Clin. Biol. Res. 161, 187–211.

Austbø, L., Aas, I.B., König, M., Weli, S.C., Syed, M., Falk, K., Koppang, E.O., 2014. Transcriptional response of immune genes in gills and the interbranchial lymphoid tissue of Atlantic salmon challenged with infectious salmon anaemia virus. Dev. Comp. Immunol. 45, 107–114.

Bajoghli, B., Guo, P., Aghaallaei, N., Hirano, M., Strohmeier, C., McCurley, N., Bockman, D.E., Schorpp, M., Cooper, M.D., Boehm, T., 2011. A thymus candidate in lampreys. Nature 470, 90–94.

Bergh, Ø., Børsheim, K.Y., Bratbak, G., Heldal, M., 1989. High abundance of viruses found in aquatic environments. Nature 340, 467–468.

Bielek, E., 2008. Membrane transformations in degenerating rodlet cells in fishes of two teleostean families (Salmonidae, Cyprinidae). Anat. Rec. Adv. Integrative Anat. Evol. Biol. 291, 1693–1706.

Boehm, T., 2011. Design principles of adaptive immune systems. Nat. Rev. Immunol. 11, 307–317.

Brattgjerd, S., Evensen, O., Lauve, A., 1994. Effect of injected yeast glucan on the activity of macrophages in Atlantic salmon, *Salmo salar* L., as evaluated by *in vitro* hydrogen peroxide production and phagocytic capacity. Immunol. 83, 288–294.

Bridle, A., Nosworthy, E., Polinski, M., Nowak, B., 2011. Evidence of an antimicrobial-immunomodulatory role of Atlantic salmon cathelicidins during infection with *Yersinia ruckeri*. Plos One 6.

Bridle, A.R., Carter, C.G., Morrison, R.N., Nowak, B.F., 2005. The effect of beta-glucan administration on macrophage respiratory burst activity and Atlantic salmon, *Salmo salar* L., challenged with amoebic gill disease – evidence of inherent resistance. J. Fish Dis. 28, 347–356.

Bridle, A.R., Koop, B.F., Nowak, B.F., 2012. Identification of surrogates of protection against yersiniosis in immersion vaccinated Atlantic salmon. Plos One 7.

Bridle, A.R., Morrison, R.N., Cunningham, P.M.C., Nowak, B.F., 2006. Quantitation of immune response gene expression and cellular localisation of interleukin-1β mRNA in

Atlantic salmon, *Salmo salar* L., affected by amoebic gill disease (AGD). Vet. Immunol. Immunopathol. 114, 121–134.

Burrows, A.S., Fletcher, T.C., Manning, M.J., 2001. Haematology of the turbot *Psetta maxima* (L.): ultrastructural, cytochemical and morphological properties of peripheral blood leucocytes. J. Appl. Ichthyol. 17, 77–84.

Castro, R., Bernard, D., Lefranc, M.P., Six, A., Benmansour, A., Boudinot, R., 2011. T cell diversity and TcR repertoires in teleost fish. Fish Shellfish Immunol. 31, 644–654.

Castro, R., Bromage, E., Abós, B., Pignatelli, J., Granja, A.G., Luque, A., Tafalla, C., 2014. CCR7 Is mainly expressed in teleost gills, where it defines an IgD(+)IgM(-) B lymphocyte subset. J. Immunol. 192, 1257–1266.

Chen, J., Wu, H.Q., Niu, H., Shi, Y.H., Li, M.Y., 2009. Increased liver protein and mRNA expression of natural killer cell-enhancing factor B (NKEF-B) in ayu (Plecoglossus altivelis) after Aeromonas hydrophila infection. Fish Shellfish Immunol. 26, 567–571.

Chettri, J.K., Raida, M.K., Kania, P.W., Buchmann, K., 2012. Differential immune response of rainbow trout (*Oncorhynchus mykiss*) at early developmental stages (larvae and fry) against the bacterial pathogen *Yersinia ruckeri*. Dev. Comp. Immunol. 36, 463–474.

Chilmonczyk, S., Monge, D., 1980. Rainbow trout gill pillar cells: demonstration of inert particle phagocytosis and involvement in viral infection. J. Reticuloendothelial Soc. 28, 327–332.

Clark, T.G., Dickerson, H.W., 1997. Antibody-mediated effects on parasite behavior: evidence of a novel mechanism of immunity against a parasitic protist. Parasitol. Today 13, 477–480.

Clark, T.G., Dickerson, H.W., Findly, R.C., 1988. Immune response of channel catfish to ciliary antigens of *Ichthyophthirius multifiliis*. Dev. Comp. Immunol. 12, 581–594.

Clark, T.G., Lin, T.-L., Dickerson, H.W., 1996. Surface antigen cross-linking triggers forced exit of a protozoan parasite from its host. Proc. Natl. Acad. Sci. USA 93, 6825–6829.

Claver, J.A., Quaglia, A.I.E., 2009. Comparative morphology, development, and function of blood cells in nonmammalian vertebrates. J. Exot. Pet Medic. 18, 87–97.

Cole, A.M., Darouiche, R.O., Legarda, D., Connell, N., Diamond, G., 2000. Characterization of a fish antimicrobial peptide: gene expression, subcellular localization, and spectrum of activity. Antimicr. Agents Chemother. 44, 2039–2045.

Conroy, D.A., Conroy, G., 2006. Basic Atlas of Atlantic Salmon (*Salmo salar* L.) Blood Cells. Patterson Peddie Consulting Ltd, Northern Ireland, UK.

Conte, F.P., Lin, D.H.Y., 1967. Kinetics of cellular morphogenesis in gill epithelium during sea water adaptation on Oncorhynchus (Walbaum). Comp. Biochem. Physiol. 23, 945–957.

Costa, A.A., Leef, M.J., Bridle, A.R., Carson, J., Nowak, B.F., 2011. Effect of vaccination against yersiniosis on the relative percent survival, bactericidal and lysozyme response of Atlantic salmon. Salmo salar. Aquacult. 315, 201–206.

Cross, M.L., Matthews, R.A., 1992. Ichthyophthiriasis in carp, *Cyprinus carpio* L.: fate of parasites in immunized fish. J. Fish Dis. 15, 497–505.

Danilova, N., Bussmann, J., Jekosch, K., Steiner, L.A., 2005. The immunoglobulin heavy-chain locus in zebrafish: identification and expression of a previously unknown isotype, immunoglobulin Z. Nat. Immunol. 6, 295–302.

Davidson, G.A., Lin, S.H., Secombes, C.J., Ellis, A.E., 1997. Detection of specific and 'constitutive' antibody secreting cells in the gills, head kidney and peripheral blood leucocytes of dab (*Limanda limanda*). Vet. Immunol. Immunopathol. 58, 363–374.

Deshmukh, S., Kania, P.W., Chettri, J.K., Skov, J., Bojesen, A.M., Dalsgaard, I., Buchmann, K., 2013. Insight from molecular, pathological, and immunohistochemical studies on cellular and humoral mechanisms responsible for vaccine-induced protection of rainbow trout against *Yersinia ruckeri*. Clin. Vacc. Immunol. 20, 1623–1641.

Dickerson, H.W., 2012. Ichthyophthirius multifiliis. In: Woo, P.T.K., Buchmann, K. (Eds.), Fish Parasites: Pathobiology and Protection. CABI Publishing, Cambridge, MA, pp. 55–72.
Dickerson, H.W., Findly, R.C., 2014. Immunity to *Ichthyophthirius* infections in fish: a synopsis. Dev. Comp. Immunol. 43, 290–299.
Dijkstra, J.M., Köllner, B., Aoyagi, K., Sawamoto, Y., Kuroda, A., Ototake, M., Nakanishi, T., Fischer, U., 2003. The rainbow trout classical MHC class I molecule Onmy-UBA*501 is expressed in similar cell types as mammalian classical MHC class I molecules. Fish Shellfish Immunol. 14, 1–23.
do Vale, A., Afonso, A., Silva, M.T., 2002. The professional phagocytes of sea bass (*Dicentrarchus labrax* L.): cytochemical characterisation of neutrophils and macrophages in the normal and inflamed peritoneal cavity. Fish Shellfish Immunol. 13, 183–198.
dos Santos, N.M.S., Taverne-Thiele, J.J., Barnes, A.C., Van Muiswinkel, W.B., Ellis, A.E., Rombout, J.H.W.M., 2001. The gill is a major organ for antibody secreting cell production following direct immersion of sea bass (*Dicentrarchus labrax.* L.) in a *Photobacterium damselae* ssp *piscicida* bacterin: an ontogenetic study. Fish Shellfish Immunol. 11, 65–74.
Ellis, A.E., 2001. Innate host defense mechanisms of fish against viruses and bacteria. Dev. Comp. Immunol. 25, 827–839.
Esteban, M.A., Meseguer, J., 1997. Factors influencing phagocytic response of macrophages from the sea bass (*Dicentrarchus labrax* L.): An ultrastructural and quantitative study. Anat. Rec. 248, 533–541.
Esteban, M.A., Munoz, J., Meseguer, J., 2000. Blood cells of sea bass (*Dicentrarchus labrax* L.). Flow cytometric and microscopic studies. Anat. Rec. 258, 80–89.
Evans, D.H., Piermarini, P.M., Choe, C.P., 2005. The multifunctional fish gill: dominant site of gas exchange, osmoregulation, acid–base regulation, and excretion of nitrogenous waste. Physiol. Rev. 85, 97–177.
Ewing, M.S., Kocan, K.M., 1986. *Ichthyophthirius multifiliis* (Ciliophora) development in gill epithelium. J. Protozool. 33, 369–374.
Ewing, M.S., Kocan, K.M., 1987. *Ichthyophthirius multifiliis* (Ciliophora) exit from gill epithelium. J. Protozool. 34, 309–312.
Ewing, M.S., Kocan, K.M., Ewing, S.A., 1985. *Ichthyophthirius multifiliis* (Ciliophora) invasion of gill epithelium. J. Protozool. 32, 305–310.
Ewing, M.S., Lynn, M.E., Ewing, S.A., 1986. Critical periods in development of *Ichthyophthirius multifiliis* (Ciliophora) populations. J. Protozool. 33, 388–391.
Falk, K., Dannevig, B.H., 1995. Demonstration of a protective immune response in infectious salmon anaemia (ISA)-infected Atlantic salmon *Salmo salar*. Dis. Aquat. Org. 21, 1–5.
Feng, L.-N., Lu, D.-Q., Bei, J.-X., Chen, J.-L., Liu, Y., Zhang, Y., Liu, X.-C., Meng, Z.-N., Wang, L., Lin, H.-R., 2009a. Molecular cloning and functional analysis of polymeric immunoglobulin receptor gene in orange-spotted grouper (*Epinephelus coioides*). Comp. Biochem. Physiol. B-Biochem. Mol. Biol. 154, 282–289.
Feng, S.-M., Zhan, W.-B., Sheng, X.-Z., Yang, K., Han, J.-G., Wei, J.-L., Li, J., Qiao, X.-T., 2009b. Response of mucosal and systemic sIgM-positive cells in turbot (*Scophthalmus maximus* L.) immunization with *Edwardsiella tarda*. Vet. Immunol. Immunopathol. 129, 108–114.
Ferguson, H.W., 2006. Introduction. In: Ferguson, H. W (Ed.), Systemic pathology of fish: a text and atlas of normal tissues in teleosts and their responses in disease. London, Scotian Press, pp. 11–22.
Fernandez, L., Lopez, J.R., Secades, P., Menendez, A., Marquez, I., Guijarro, J.A., 2003. *In vitro* and *in vivo* studies of the Yrp1 protease from *Yersinia ruckeri* and its role in protective immunity against enteric red mouth disease of salmonids. Appl. Environ. Microbiol. 69, 7328–7335.

Fillatreau, S., Six, A., Magadan, S., Castro, R., Sunyer, J.O., Boudinot, P., 2013. The astonishing diversity of Ig classes and B cell repertoires in teleost fish. Front. Immunol. 4, 28.

Findly, R.C., Zhao, X., Noe, J., Camus, A.C., Dickerson, H.W., 2013. B cell memory following infection and challenge of channel catfish with *Ichthyophthirius multifiliis*. Dev. Comp. Immunol. 39, 302–311.

Fischer, U., Koppang, E.O., Nakanishi, T., 2013. Teleost T and NK cell immunity. Fish Shellfish Immunol. 35, 197–206.

Flajnik, M.F., 2005. The last flag unfurled? A new immunoglobulin isotype in fish expressed in early development. Nat. Immunol. 6, 229–230.

Fuglem, B., Jirillo, E., Bjerkås, I., Kiyono, H., Nochi, T., Yuki, Y., Raida, M., Fischer, U., Koppang, E.O., 2010. Antigen-sampling cells in the salmonid intestinal epithelium. Dev. Comp. Immunol. 34, 768–774.

García-Rosado, E., Markussen, T., Kileng, O., Baekkevold, E.S., Robertsen, B., Mjaaland, S., Rimstad, E., 2008. Molecular and functional characterization of two infectious salmon anaemia virus (ISAV) proteins with type I interferon antagonizing activity. Vir. Res. 133, 228–238.

Glenney, G.W., Petrie-Hanson, L., 2006. Fate of fluorescent microspheres in developing *Ictalurus punctatus* following prolonged immersion. Fish Shellfish Immunol. 20, 758–768.

Goldes, S.A., Ferguson, H.W., Daoust, P.-Y., Moccia, R.D., 1986. Phagocytosis of the inert suspended clay kaolin by the gills of rainbow trout, *Salmo gairdneri* Richardson. J. Fish Dis. 9, 147–151.

Gonzalez, S.F., Buchmann, K., Nielsen, M.E., 2007. Real-time gene expression analysis in carp (*Cyprinus carpio* L.) skin: inflammatory responses caused by the ectoparasite *Ichthyophthirius multifiliis*. Fish Shellfish Immunol. 22, 641–650.

Graves, S.S., Evans, D.L., Dawe, D.L., 1985. Antiprotozoan activity of nonspecific cytotoxic cells (NCC) from the channel catfish (*Ictalurus punctatus*). J. Immunol. 134, 78–85.

Grove, S., Johansen, R., Reitan, L.J., Press, C.M., 2006. Immune- and enzyme histochemical characterisation of leukocyte populations within lymphoid and mucosal tissues of Atlantic halibut (*Hippoglossus hippoglossus*). Fish Shellfish Immunol. 20, 693–708.

Hamdani, S.H., McMillan, D.N., Pettersen, E.F., Wergeland, H., Endresen, C., Ellis, A.E., Secombes, C.J., 1998. Isolation of rainbow trout neutrophils with an anti-granulocyte monoclonal antibody. Vet. Immunol. Immunopathol. 63, 369–380.

Hansen, J.D., Landis, E.D., Phillips, R.B., 2005. Discovery of a unique Ig heavy-chain isotype (IgT) in rainbow trout: Implications for a distinctive B cell developmental pathway in teleost fish. Proc. Natl. Acad. Sci. USA 102, 6919–6924.

Haugarvoll, E., Bjerkås, I., Nowak, B.F., Hordvik, I., Koppang, E.O., 2008. Identification and characterization of a novel intraepithelial lymphoid tissue in the gills of Atlantic salmon. J. Anat. 213, 202–209.

Haugarvoll, E., Thorsen, J., Laane, M., Huang, Q., Koppang, E.O., 2006. Melanogenesis and evidence for melanosome transport to the plasma membrane in a CD83+ teleost leukocyte cell line. Pigm. Cell Res. 19, 214–225.

Heinecke, R.D., Buchmann, K., 2013. Inflammatory response of rainbow trout *Oncorhynchus mykiss* (Walbaum, 1792) larvae against Ichthyophthirius multifiliis. Fish Shellfish Immunol. 34, 521–528.

Hellebø, A., Vilas, U., Falk, K., Vlasak, R., 2004. Infectious salmon anemia virus specifically binds to and hydrolyzes 4-O-acetylated sialic acids. J. Virol. 78, 3055–3062.

Hetland, D.L., Dale, O.B., Skjodt, K., Press, C.M., Falk, K., 2011. Depletion of CD8 alpha cells from tissues of Atlantic salmon during the early stages of infection with high or low virulent strains of infectious salmon anaemia virus (ISAV). Dev. Comp. Immunol. 35, 817–826.

Hetland, D.L., Jørgensen, S.M., Skjødt, K., Dale, O.B., Falk, K., Xu, C., Mikalsen, A.B., Grimholt, U., Gjøen, T., Press, C.M., 2010. *In situ* localisation of major histocompatibility complex class I and class II and CD8 positive cells in infectious salmon anaemia virus (ISAV)-infected Atlantic salmon. Fish Shellfish Immunol. 28, 30–39.

Hines, R., Spira, D., 1973. Ichthyophthiriasis in the mirror carp. II. Leukocyte response. J. Fish Biol. 5, 527–534.

Hines, R.S., Spira, D.T., 1974a. Ichthyophthiriasis in mirror carp *Cyprinus carpio* (L). III. Pathology. J. Fish Biol. 6, 189–196.

Hines, R.S., Spira, D.T., 1974b. Ichthyophthiriasis in mirror carp *Cyprinus carpio* (L). 5. Acquired immunity. J. Fish Biol. 6, 373–378.

Hodgkinson, J.L., Bucke, D., Austin, B., 1987. Uptake of the fish pathogen, *Aeromonas salmonicida*, by rainbow trout (*Salmo gairdneri* L.). FEMS Microbiol. Lett. 40, 207–210.

Holland, J.W., Rowley, A.F., 1998. Studies on the eosinophilic granule cells in the gills of the rainbow trout, *Oncorhynchus mykiss*. Comp. Biochem. Physiol. C-Pharmacol. Toxicol. Endocrinol. 120, 321–328.

Hu, Y.H., Zhang, M., Sun, L., 2010. Expression of *Scophthalmus maximus* CD83 correlates with bacterial infection and antigen stimulation. Fish Shellfish Immunol. 29, 608–614.

Huang, R., Gao, L.Y., Wang, Y.P., Hu, W., Guo, Q.L., 2009. Structure, organization and expression of common carp (*Cyprinus carpio* L.) NKEF-B gene. Fish Shellfish Immunol. 26, 220–229.

Hughes, G.M., 1984. General anatomy of the gills. In: Hoar, W.S., Randall, D.J. (Eds.), Fish Physiology. Volume X. Gills. Part A. Anatomy, Gas Transfer, and Acid–Base Regulation. Orlando, Florida, D.J. Academic Press, pp. 1–72.

Hughes, G.M., Wright, D.E., 1970. A comparative study of the ultrastructure of the water-blood pathway in the secondary lamellae of teleost and elasmobranch fishes – benthic forms. Z. Zellforsch. 104, 478–493.

Huising, M.O., van Schijndel, J.E., Kruiswijk, C.P., Nabuurs, S.B., Savelkoul, H.F.J., Flik, G., Verburg-van Kemenade, B.M.L., 2006. The presence of multiple and differentially regulated interleukin-12p40 genes in bony fishes signifies an expansion of the vertebrate heterodimeric cytokine family. Mol. Immunol. 43, 1519–1533.

Ingerslev, H.C., Cunningham, C., Wergeland, H.I., 2006. Cloning and expression of TNF-alpha, IL-1 beta and COX-2 in an anadromous and landlocked strain of Atlantic salmon (*Salmo salar* L.) during the smolting period. Fish Shellfish Immunol. 20, 450–461.

Jang, S.I., Hardie, L.J., Secombes, C.J., 1995. Elevation of rainbow trout *Oncorhynchus mykiss* macrophage respiratory burst activity with macrophage-derived supernatants. J. Leukoc. Biol. 57, 943–947.

Jaso-Friedmann, L., Leary, J.H., III, Evans, D.L., 1993. Nonspecific cytotoxic cells in fish: antigenic cross-reactivity of a function associated molecule with the intermediate filament vimentin. Cell. Immunol. 148, 208–217.

Jaso-Friedmann, L., Leary, J.H., Evans, D.L., 1997. NCCRP-1: A novel receptor protein sequenced from teleost nonspecific cytotoxic cells. Mol. Immunol. 34, 955–965.

Jiang, N., Tan, N.S., Ho, B., Ding, J.L., 2007. Respiratory protein-generated reactive oxygen species as an antimicrobial strategy. Nat. Immunol. 8, 1114–1122.

Jørgensen, S.M., Afanasyev, S., Krasnov, A., 2008. Gene expression analyses in Atlantic salmon challenged with infectious salmon anemia virus reveal differences between individuals with early, intermediate and late mortality. BMC Genomics 9.

Jørgensen, S.M., Hetland, D.L., Press, C.M., Grimholt, U., Gjøen, T., 2007. Effect of early infectious salmon anaemia virus (ISAV) infection on expression of MHC pathway genes and type I and II interferon in Atlantic salmon (*Salmo salar* L.) tissues. Fish Shellfish Immunol. 23, 576–588.

Karlsson, L., 1983. Gill morphology in the zebrafish, *Brachydanio rerio* (Hamilton-Buchanan). J. Fish Biol. 23, 511–524.

Kato, G., Takano, T., Sakai, T., Matsuyama, T., Nakayasu, C., 2013. *Vibrio anguillarum* bacterin uptake via the gills of Japanese flounder and subsequent immune responses. Fish Shellfish Immunol. 35, 1591–1597.

Kawahara, E., Kusuda, R., 1988. Location of *Pasteurella piscicida* antigens in tissues of yellowtail *Seriola quinqueradiata* vaccinated by immersion. Nippon Suisan Gakkaishi 54, 1101–1105.

Kent, M.L., Sawyer, T.K., Hedrick, R.P., 1988. *Paramoeba pemaquidensis* (Sarcomastigophora, Paramoebidae) infestation of the gills of coho salmon *Oncorhynchus kisutch* reared in sea water. Dis. Aquat. Org. 5, 163–169.

Khimmakthong, U., Deshmukh, S., Chettri, J.K., Bojesen, A.M., Kania, P.W., Dalsgaard, I., Buchmann, K., 2013. Tissue specific uptake of inactivated and live *Yersinia ruckeri* in rainbow trout (*Oncorhynchus mykiss*): visualization by immunohistochemistry and *in situ* hybridization. Microb. Pathogen. 59–60, 33–41.

Kiryu, I., Ototake, M., Nakanishi, T., Wakabayashi, H., 2000. The uptake of fluorescent microspheres into the skin, fins and gills of rainbow trout during immersion. Fish Pathol. 35, 41–48.

Köllner, B., Fischer, U., Rombout, J.H.W.M., Taverne-Thiele, J.J., Hansen, J.D., 2004. Potential involvement of rainbow trout thrombocytes in immune functions: a study using a panel of monoclonal antibodies and RT-PCR. Dev. Comp. Immunol. 28, 1049–1062.

Köllner, B., Mundt, E., Fischer, U., 1998. A monoclonal antibody recognizing a complex tubular structure in rainbow trout pillar cells. J. Fish Biol. 53, 853–865.

Koppang, E.O., Fischer, U., Moore, L., Tranulis, M.A., Dijkstra, J.M., Köllner, B., Aune, L., Jirillo, E., Hordvik, I., 2010. Salmonid T cells assemble in the thymus, spleen and in novel interbranchial lymphoid tissue. J. Anat. 217, 728–739.

Koppang, E.O., Fischer, U., Satoh, M., Jirillo, E., 2007. Inflammation in fish as seen from a morphological point of view with special reference to the vascular compartment. Curr. Pharmac. Design 13, 3649–3655.

Koppang, E.O., Haugarvoll, E., Hordvik, I., Poppe, T.T., Bjerkås, I., 2004. Granulomatous uveitis associated with vaccination in the Atlantic salmon. Vet. Pathol. 41, 122–130.

Koppang, E.O., Hordvik, I., Bjerkås, I., Torvund, J., Aune, L., Thevarajan, J., Endresen, C., 2003. Production of rabbit antisera against recombinant MHC class II [beta] chain and identification of immunoreactive cells in Atlantic salmon (*Salmo salar*). Fish Shellfish Immunol. 14, 115–132.

Koppang, E.O., Lundin, M., Press, C.M., Rønningen, K., Lie, Ø., 1998a. Differing levels of Mhc class II beta chain expression in a range of tissues from vaccinated and non-vaccinated Atlantic salmon (*Salmo salar* L.). Fish Shellfish Immunol. 8, 183–196.

Koppang, E.O., Press, C.M., Rønningen, K., Lie, Ø., 1998b. Expression of Mhc class I mRNA in tissues from vaccinated and non-vaccinated Atlantic salmon (*Salmo salar* L.). Fish Shellfish Immunol. 8, 577–587.

Kvellestad, A., Larsen, B.M., 1999. Histologisk undersøking av gjeller frå fisk som del av overvaking av ungfiskbestandar i lakseførande vassdrag (Histologic examination of fish gills as part of monitoring of juvenile fish populations in salmon-rearing stretch of Norwegian rivers). Report 036. Norwegian Institute for Nature Research, Trondheim.

Laurent, P., 1984. Gill internal morphology. In: Hoar, W.S., Randall, D.J. (Eds.), Fish physiology. Volume X. Gills. Part A. Anatomy, gas transfer, and acid-base regulation. Orlando, Florida, D.J. Academic Press, pp. 73–183.

Lauscher, A., Krossøy, B., Frost, P., Grove, S., König, M., Bohlin, J., Falk, K., Austbø, L., Rimstad, E., 2011. Immune responses in Atlantic salmon (*Salmo salar*) following protective vaccination against infectious salmon anemia (ISA) and subsequent ISA virus infection. Vaccine 29, 6392–6401.

LeBlanc, F., Arseneau, J.R., Leadbeater, S., Glebe, B., Laflamme, M., Gagné, N., 2012. Transcriptional response of Atlantic salmon (*Salmo salar*) after primary versus secondary exposure to infectious salmon anemia virus (ISAV). Mol. Immunol. 51, 197–209.

Leino, R.L., 1974. Ultrastructure of immature, developing, and secretory rodlet cells in fish. Cell Tiss. Res. 155, 367–381.

Li, J., Barreda, D.R., Zhang, Y.-A., Boshra, H., Gelman, A.E., LaPatra, S., Tort, L., Sunyer, J.O., 2006. B lymphocytes from early vertebrates have potent phagocytic and microbicidal abilities. Nat. Immunol. 7, 1116–1124.

Lin, S.-H., Ellis, A.E., Davidson, G.A., Secombes, C.J., 1999. Migratory, respiratory burst and mitogenic responses of leucocytes isolated from the gills of rainbow trout (*Oncorhynchus mykiss*). Fish Shellfish Immunol. 9, 211–226.

Ling, S.H.M., Wang, X.H., Lim, T.M., Leung, K.Y., 2001. Green fluorescent protein-tagged *Edwardsiella tarda* reveals portal of entry in fish. FEMS Microbiol. Lett. 194, 239–243.

Lovy, J., Becker, J.A., Speare, D.J., Wadowska, D.W., Wright, G.M., Powell, M.D., 2007. Ultrastructural examination of the host cellular response in the gills of Atlantic salmon, *Salmo salar*, with amoebic gill disease. Vet. Pathol. 44, 663–671.

Lovy, J., Savidant, G.P., Speare, D.J., Wright, G.M., 2009. Langerin/CD207 positive dendritic-like cells in the haemopoietic tissues of salmonids. Fish Shellfish Immunol. 27, 365–368.

Lovy, J., Wright, G.M., Speare, D.J., 2008. Comparative cellular morphology suggesting the existence of resident dendritic cells within immune organs of salmonids. Anat. Rec. -Adv. Integr. Anat. Evol. Biol. 291, 456–462.

Lumsden, J.S., Ferguson, H.W., 1994. Isolation and partial characterization of rainbow trout (*Oncorhynchus mykiss*) gill mucin. Fish Physiol. Biochem. 12, 387–398.

Lumsden, J.S., Ferguson, H.W., Ostland, V.E., Byrne, P.J., 1994. The mucous coat on gill lamellae of rainbow trout (*Oncorhynchus mykiss*). Cell Tiss. Res. 275, 187–193.

Lumsden, J.S., Ostland, V.E., Byrne, P.J., Ferguson, H.W., 1993. Detection of a distinct gill-surface antibody response following horizontal infection and bath challenge of brook trout *Salvelinus fontinalis* with *Flavobacterium branchiophilum*, the causative agent of bacterial gill disease. Dis. Aquat. Org. 16, 21–27.

Lumsden, J.S., Ostland, V.E., Macphee, D.D., Ferguson, H.W., 1995. Production of gill-associated and serum antibody by rainbow trout (*Oncorhynchus mykiss*) following immersion immunization with acetone-killed *Flavobacterium branchiophilum* and the relationship to protection from experimental challenge. Fish Shellfish Immunol. 5, 151–165.

Maki, J.L., Dickerson, H.W., 2003. Systemic and cutaneous mucus antibody responses of channel catfish immunized against the protozoan parasite *Ichthyophthirius multifiliis*. Clin. Diagn. Lab. Immunol. 10, 876–881.

Manera, M., Dezfuli, B.S., 2004. Rodlet cells in teleosts: a new insight into their nature and functions. J. Fish Biol. 65, 597–619.

Matsunaga, T., Rahman, A., 2001. In search of the origin of the thymus: the thymus and GALT may be evolutionarily related. Scandinavian. J. Immunol. 53, 1–6.

Mazon, A.F., Huising, M.O., Taverne-Thiele, A.J., Bastiaans, J., Verburg-van Kemenade, B.M.L., 2007. The first appearance of rodlet cells in carp (*Cyprinus carpio* L.) ontogeny and their possible roles during stress and parasite infection. Fish Shellfish Immunol. 22, 27–37.

McBeath, A.J.A., Collet, B., Paley, R., Duraffour, S., Aspehaug, V., Biering, E., Secombes, C.J., Snow, M., 2006. Identification of an interferon antagonist protein encoded by segment 7 of infectious salmon anaemia virus. Virus Res. 115, 176–184.

McIntosh, D., Austin, B., Flaño, E., Villena, A., Martínez-Pereda, J.A., Tarazona, J.V., 2000. Lack of uptake of *Renibacterium salmoninarum* by gill epithelia of rainbow trout. J. Fish Biol. 56, 1053–1061.

Mescher, A.L., 2010. Junqueira's Basic Histology: Text and Atlas. New York, McGraw-Hill Company, Inc, 467 pp.

Meseguer, J., Esteban, M.A., Rodríguez, A., 2002. Are thrombocytes and platelets true phagocytes? Microsc Res. Techn. 57, 491–497.

Meseguer, J., López-Ruiz, A., Esteban, M.A., 1994. Cytochemical characterization of leucocytes from the seawater teleost, gilthead seabream (*Sparus aurata* L.). Histochem. Cell Biol. 102, 37–44.

Messick, J., 2006. Blood and bone marrow. In: Eurell, J.A., Frappier, B.L. (Eds.), Dellmann's textbook of veterinary histology. Ames, Iowa, Blackwell Publishing, pp. 61–78.

Moneke, E., Ikede, B.O., Kibenge, F.S.B., 2005. Viremia during infectious salmon anemia virus infection of Atlantic salmon is associated with replicating virus in leucocytes. Dis. Aquat. Org. 66, 153–157.

Moore, J.D., Ototake, M., Nakanishi, T., 1998. Particulate antigen uptake during immersion immunisation of fish: The effectiveness of prolonged exposure and the roles of skin and gill. Fish Shellfish Immunol. 8, 393–407.

Moore, L.J., Dijkstra, J.M., Koppang, E.O., Hordvik, I., 2009. CD4 homologues in Atlantic salmon. Fish Shellfish Immunol. 26, 10–18.

Morera, D., Roher, N., Ribas, L., Balasch, J.C., Doñate, C., Callol, A., Boltaña, S., Roberts, S., Goetz, G., Goetz, F.W., MacKenzie, S.A., 2011. RNA-Seq reveals an integrated immune response in nucleated erythrocytes. Plos One 6.

Morgan, M., Tovell, P.W.A., 1973. The structure of the gill of the trout *Salmo gairdneri* (Richardson). Zeitschr. Zellforsch. 142, 147–162.

Morrison, R.N., Koppang, E.O., Hordvik, I., Nowak, B.F., 2006. MHC class II+ cells in the gills of Atlantic salmon (*Salmo salar* L.) affected by amoebic gill disease. Vet. Immunol. Immunopathol. 109, 297–303.

Morrison, R.N., Zou, J., Secombes, C.J., Scapigliati, G., Adams, M.B., Nowak, B.F., 2007. Molecular cloning and expression analysis of tumour necrosis factor-α in amoebic gill disease (AGD)-affected Atlantic salmon (*Salmo salar* L.). Fish Shellfish Immunol. 23, 1015–1031.

Mulero, I., Sepulcre, M.P., Meseguer, J., García-Ayala, A., Mulero, V., 2007. Histamine is stored in mast cells of most evolutionarily advanced fish and regulates the fish inflammatory response. Proc. Natl. Acad. Sci. USA 104, 19434–19439.

Munday, B.L., Foster, C.K., Roubal, F.R., Lester, R.J.G., 1990. Paramoebic gill infection and associated pathology of Atlantic salmon, *Salmo salar*, and rainbow trout *Salmo gairdneri* Tasmania. In: Perkins, F.O., Cheng, T.C. (Eds.), Pathology in Marine Science. San Diego, Academic Press, Inc, pp. 215–222.

Murray, C.K., Fletcher, T.C., 1976. Immunohistochemical localization of lysozyme in plaice (*Pleuronectes platessa* L.) tissues. J. Fish Biol. 9, 329.

Nelson, J.S., Rohovec, J.S., Fryer, J.L., 1985. Tissue location of vibrio bacterin delivered by intraperitoneal injection, immersion and oral routes to *Salmo gairdneri*. Fish Pathol. 19, 263–269.

Newstead, J.D., 1967. Fine structure of the respiratory lamellae of teleostean gills. Zeitschr. Zellforsch. 79, 396–428.

Nilsson, G.E., Lofman, C.O., Block, M., 1995. Extensive erythrocyte deformation in fish gills observed by *in vivo* microscopy: apparent adaptations for enhancing oxygen uptake. J. Exp. Biol. 198, 1151–1156.

Nowak, B.F., 2012. Neoparamoeba perurans. In: Woo, P.T.K., Buchmann, K. (Eds.), Fish parasites: pathobiology and protection CABI. Cambridge MA, Wallingford, pp. 1–18.

Oguri, M., 1976. Histochemical observations on dark brown pigment granules found in kidney tissue of rainbow trout. Bull. Jap. Soc. Sci. Fish. 42, 1223–1227.

Ohta, Y., Landis, E., Boulay, T., Phillips, R.B., Collet, B., Secombes, C.J., Flajnik, M.F., Hansen, J.D., 2004. Homologs of CD83 from elasmobranch and teleost fish. J. Immunol. 173, 4553–4560.

Ohtani, M., Villumsen, K.R., Strøm, H.K., Raida, M.K., 2014. 3D Visualization of the initial *Yersinia ruckeri* infection route in rainbow trout (*Oncorhynchus mykiss*) by optical projection tomography. Plos One 9.

Olsen, M.M., Kania, P.W., Heinecke, R.D., Skjoedt, K., Rasmussen, K.J., Buchmann, K., 2011. Cellular and humoral factors involved in the response of rainbow trout gills to *Ichthyophthirius multifiliis* infections: Molecular and immunohistochemical studies. Fish Shellfish Immunol. 30, 859–869.

Olson, K.R., 2002. Vascular anatomy of the fish gill. J. Exp. Zool. 293, 214–231.

Ototake, M., Iwama, G.K., Nakanishi, T., 1996. The uptake of bovine serum albumin by the skin of bath-immunised rainbow trout *Oncorhynchus mykiss*. Fish Shellfish Immunol. 6, 321–333.

Øverland, H.S., Pettersen, E.F., Ronneseth, A., Wergeland, H.I., 2010. Phagocytosis by B-cells and neutrophils in Atlantic salmon (*Salmo salar* L.) and Atlantic cod (*Gadus morhua* L.). Fish Shellfish Immunol. 28, 193–204.

Palić, D., Beck, L.S., Palić, J., Andreasen, C.B., 2011. Use of rapid cytochemical staining to characterize fish blood granulocytes in species of special concern and determine potential for function testing. Fish Shellfish Immunol. 30, 646–652.

Palmer, R., Carson, J., Ruttledge, M., Drinan, E., Wagner, T., 1997. Gill disease associated with *Paramoeba*, in sea reared Atlantic salmon in Ireland. Bull. Eur. Ass. Fish Pathol. 17, 112–114.

Passantino, L., Altamura, M., Cianciotta, A., Patruno, R., Tafaro, A., Jirillo, E., Passantino, G.F., 2002. Fish immunology. I. Binding and engulfment of Candida albicans by erythrocytes of rainbow trout (*Salmo gairdneri* Richardson). Immunopharmacol. Immunotoxicol. 24, 665–678.

Paulsen, S.M., Sveinbjørnsson, B., Robertsen, B., 2001. Selective staining and disintegration of intestinal eosinophilic granule cells in Atlantic salmon after intraperitoneal injection of the zinc chelator dithizone. J. Fish Biol. 58, 768–775.

Pennacchi, Y., Leef, M.J., Crosbie, P.B.B., Nowak, B.F., Bridle, A.R., 2014. Evidence of immune and inflammatory processes in the gills of AGD-affected Atlantic salmon *Salmo salar* L. Fish Shellfish Immunol. 36, 563–570.

Petrik, P., Bucher, O., 1969. A propos des "chloride cells" dans l'epithelium des lamelles branchiales du poisson rouge. Zeitschr. Zellforsch. 96, 66–74.

Pettersen, E.F., Bjørløw, I., Hagland, T.J., Wergeland, H.I., 2005. Effect of seawater temperature on leucocyte populations in Atlantic salmon post-smolts. Vet. Immunol. Immunopathol. 106, 65–76.

Pisam, M., Chretien, M., Rambourg, A., Clermont, Y., 1983. Two anatomical pathways for the renewal of surface glycoproteins in chloride cells of fish gills. Anat. Rec. 207, 385–397.

Pisam, M., Prunet, P., Boeuf, G., Rambourg, A., 1988. Ultrastructural features of chloride cells in the gill epithelium of the Atlantic salmon, *Salmo salar*, and their modifications during smoltification. Am. J. Anat. 183, 235–244.

Pisam, M., Sardet, C., Maetz, J., 1980. Polysaccharidic material in chloride cell of teleostean gill: modifications according to salinity. Am. J. Physiol. 238, R213–R218.

Powell, M.D., Speare, D.J., Burka, J.F., 1992. Fixation of mucus on rainbow trout (*Oncorhynchus mykiss* Walbaum) gills for light and electron microscopy. J. Fish Biol. 41, 813–824.

Powell, M.D., Speare, D.J., Wright, G.M., 1994. Comparative ultrastructural morphology of lamellar epithelial, chloride and mucous cell glycocalyx of the rainbow trout (*Oncorhynchus mykiss*) gill. J. Fish Biol. 44, 725–730.

Powell, M.D., Wright, G.M., Burka, J.F., 1990. Eosinophilic granule cells in the gills of rainbow trout, *Oncorhynchus mykiss*: evidence of migration? J. Fish Biol. 37, 495–497.

Randelli, E., Buonocore, F., Scapigliati, G., 2008. Cell markers and determinants in fish immunology. Fish Shellfish Immunol. 25, 326–340.

Rasmussen, K.J., Steffensen, J.F., Buchmann, K., 2013. Differential occurrence of immune cells in the primary and secondary vascular systems in rainbow trout, *Oncorhynchus mykiss* (Walbaum). J. Fish Dis. 36, 675–679.

Reite, O.B., 1997. Mast cells/eosinophilic granule cells of salmonids: staining properties and responses to noxious agents. Fish Shellfish Immunol. 7, 567–584.

Reite, O.B., 1998. Mast cells/eosinophilic granule cells of teleostean fish: a review focusing on staining properties and functional responses. Fish Shellfish Immunol. 8, 489–513.

Reite, O.B., 2005. The rodlet cells of teleostean fish: their potential role in host defence in relation to the role of mast cells/eosinophilic granule cells. Fish Shellfish Immunol. 19, 253–267.

Reite, O.B., Evensen, Ø., 2006. Inflammatory cells of teleostean fish: A review focusing on mast cells/eosinophilic granule cells and rodlet cells. Fish Shellfish Immunol. 20, 192–208.

Roca, F.J., Mulero, I., López-Muñoz, A., Sepulcre, M.P., Renshaw, S.A., Meseguer, J., Mulero, V., 2008. Evolution of the inflammatory response in vertebrates: fish TNF-α is a powerful activator of endothelial cells but hardly activates phagocytes. J. Immunol. 181, 5071–5081.

Rodger, H.D., McArdle, J.F., 1996. An outbreak of amoebic gill disease in Ireland. Vet. Rec. 139, 348–349.

Rombout, J.H.W.M., van der Tuin, S.J.L., Yang, G., Schopman, M., Mroczek, A., Hermsen, T., Taverne-Thiele, J.J., 2008. Expression of the polymeric immunoglobulin receptor (pIgR) in mucosal tissues of common carp (*Cyprinus carpio* L.). Fish Shellfish Immunol. 24, 620–628.

Roubal, F.R., Lester, R.J.G., Foster, C.K., 1989. Studies on cultured and gill-attached *Paramoeba* sp. (Gymnamoebae: Paramoebidae) and the cytopathology of paramebic gill disease in Atlantic salmon, *Salmo salar* L., from Tasmania. J. Fish Dis. 12, 481–492.

Russell, S., Hayes, M.A., Lumsden, J.S., 2009. Immunohistochemical localization of rainbow trout ladderlectin and intelectin in healthy and infected rainbow trout (*Oncorhynchus mykiss*). Fish Shellfish Immunol. 26, 154–163.

Ryckaert, J., Bossier, P., D'Herde, K., Diez-Fraile, A., Sorgeloos, P., Haesebrouck, F., Pasmans, F., 2010. Persistence of *Yersinia ruckeri* in trout macrophages. Fish Shellfish Immunol. 29, 648–655.

Sanchez, J.G., Speare, D.J., Sims, D.E., Johnson, G.J., 1997. Adaptation of a fluorocarbon-based non-aqueous fixation regime for the ultrastructural study of the teleost epithelial mucous coat. J. Comp. Pathol. 117, 165–170.

Sardet, C., Pisam, M., Maetz, J., 1979. The surface epithelium of teleostean fish gills. Cellular and junctional adaptations of the chloride cell in relation to salt adaptation. J. Cell Biol. 80, 96–117.

Sato, A., Somamoto, T., Yokooka, H., Okamoto, N., 2005. Systemic priming of alloreactive cytotoxic cells in carp, following anal administration of allogeneic cell antigens. Fish Shellfish Immunol. 19, 43–52.

Scapigliati, G., Buonocore, F., Mazzini, M., 2006. Biological activity of cytokines: an evolutionary perspective. Curr. Pharm. Design 12, 3071–3081.

Secombes, C.J., Wang, T., 2012. The innate and adaptive immune system of fish. In: Austin, B. (Ed.), Infectious disease in aquaculture. Prevention and control. Woodhead Publishing, Oxford, Cambridge, Philadelphia, New Delhi, pp. 3–68.

Shephard, K.L., 1994. Functions for fish mucus. Rev. Fish Biol. Fish. 4, 401–429.

Sigh, J., Lindenstrom, T., Buchmann, K., 2004. The parasitic ciliate *Ichthyophthirius multifiliis* induces expression of immune relevant genes in rainbow trout, *Oncorhynchus mykiss* (Walbaum). J. Fish Dis. 27, 409–417.

Silphaduang, U., Colorni, A., Noga, E.J., 2006. Evidence for widespread distribution of piscidin antimicrobial peptides in teleost fish. Dis. Aquat. Org. 72, 241–252.

Sire, M.-F., Vernier, J.-M., 1995. Partial characterization of eosinophilic granule cells (EGCs) and identification of mast cells of the intestinal lamina propria in rainbow trout (*Oncorhynchus mykiss*). Biochemical and cytochemical study. Biol. Cell 85, 35–41.

Smith, P.D., 1982. Analysis of the hyperosmotic and bath methods for fish vaccination - comparison of uptake of particulate and non-particulate antigens. In: Van Muiswinkel, W.B., Cooper, E.L., (Eds.), Immunology and Immunization of Fish; Dev. Comp. Immunol. (suppl. 2), 181–186.

Speare, D.J., Ferguson, H.W., 2006. Gills and pseudobranchs. In: Ferguson, H.W. (Ed.), Systemic pathology of fish: a text and atlas of normal tissues in teleosts and their responses in disease. London, UK, Scotian Press, pp. 25–62.

Steinum, T., Kvellestad, A., Rønneberg, L.B., Nilsen, H., Asheim, A., Fjell, K., Nygård, S.M.R., Olsen, A.B., Dale, O.B., 2008. First cases of amoebic gill disease (AGD) in Norwegian seawater farmed Atlantic salmon, *Salmo salar* L., and phylogeny of the causative amoeba using 18S cDNA sequences. J. Fish. Dis. 31, 205–214.

Tadiso, T.M., Lie, K.K., Hordvik, I., 2011a. Molecular cloning of IgT from Atlantic salmon, and analysis of the relative expression of τ, μ, and δ in different tissues. Vet. Immunol. Immunopathol. 139, 17–26.

Tadiso, T.M., Sharma, A., Hordvik, I., 2011b. Analysis of polymeric immunoglobulin receptor- and CD300-like molecules from Atlantic salmon. Mol. Immunol. 49, 462–473.

Takizawa, F., Dijkstra, J.M., Kotterba, P., Korytár, T., Kock, H., Köllner, B., Jaureguiberry, B., Nakanishi, T., Fischer, U., 2011a. The expression of CD8 α discriminates distinct T cell subsets in teleost fish. Dev. Comp. Immunol. 35, 752–763.

Takizawa, F., Koppang, E.O., Ohtani, M., Nakanishi, T., Hashimoto, K., Fischer, U., Dijkstra, J.M., 2011b. Constitutive high expression of *interleukin-4/13A* and *GATA-3* in gill and skin of salmonid fishes suggests that these tissues form Th2-skewed immune environments. Mol. Immunol. 48, 1360–1368.

Tatner, M.F., Horne, M.T., 1983. Factors influencing the uptake of ^{14}C-labelled *Vibrio anguillarum* vaccine in direct immersion experiments with rainbow trout, *Salmo gairdneri* Richardson. J. Fish Biol. 22, 585–591.

Tavares-Dias, M., 2006. A morphological and cytochemical study of erythrocytes, thrombocytes and leukocytes in four freshwater teleosts. J. Fish Biol. 68, 1822–1833.

Tavares-Dias, M., Ono, E.A., Pilarski, F., Moraes, F.R., 2007. Can thrombocytes participate in the removal of cellular debris in the blood circulation of teleost fish? A cytochemical study and ultrastructural analysis. J. Appl. Ichthyol. 23, 709–712.

Thorsen, J., Høyheim, B., Koppang, E.O., 2006. Isolation of the Atlantic salmon tyrosinase gene family reveals heterogenous transcripts in a leukocyte cell line. Pigm. Cell Res. 19, 327–336.

Tian, J.Y., Xie, H.X., Zhang, Y.A., Xu, Z., Yao, W.J., Nie, P., 2009. Ontogeny of IgM-producing cells in the mandarin fish *Siniperca chuatsi* identified by *in situ* hybridisation. Vet. Immunol. Immunopathol. 132, 146–152.

Tobback, E., Decostere, A., Hermans, K., Haesebrouck, F., Chiers, K., 2007. *Yersinia ruckeri* infections in salmonid fish. J. Fish Dis. 30, 257–268.

Tobback, E., Decostere, A., Hermans, K., Ryckaert, J., Duchateau, L., Haesebrouck, F., Chiers, K., 2009. Route of entry and tissue distribution of *Yersinia ruckeri* in experimentally infected rainbow trout *Oncorhynchus mykiss*. Dis. Aquat. Org. 84, 219–228.

Tobback, E., Hermans, K., Decostere, A., Van den Broeck, W., Haesebrouck, F., Chiers, K., 2010. Interactions of virulent and avirulent *Yersinia ruckeri* strains with isolated gill arches and intestinal explants of rainbow trout *Oncorhynchus mykiss*. Dis. Aquat. Org. 90, 175–179.

Torroba, M., Anderson, D.P., Dixon, O.W., Casares, F., Varas, A., Alonso, L., del Moral, M.G., Zapata, A.G., 1993. *In vitro* antigen trapping by gill cells of the rainbow trout: an immunohistochemical study. Histol. Histopathol. 8, 363–367.

Uspenskaya, A.V., 1963. Hyaluronidase in different stages of the life cycle of *Ichthyophthirius multifiliis*. Dokl. Akad. Nauk SSSR 151, 1476–1478.

von Gersdorff Jørgensen, L., Heinecke, R.D., Skjødt, K., Rasmussen, K.J., Buchmann, K., 2011. Experimental evidence for direct *in situ* binding of IgM and IgT to early trophonts of *Ichthyophthirius multifiliis* (Fouquet) in the gills of rainbow trout, *Oncorhynchus mykiss* (Walbaum). J. Fish Dis. 34, 749–755.

von Gersdorff Jørgensen, L., Nemli, E., Heinecke, R.D., Raida, M.K., Buchmann, K., 2008. Immune-relevant genes expressed in rainbow trout following immunisation with a live vaccine against *Ichthyophthirius multifiliis*. Dis. Aquat. Org. 80, 189–197.

Wahli, T., Matthews, R.A., 1999. Ichthyophthiriasis in carp *Cyprinus carpio*: infectivity of trophonts prematurely exiting both the immune and non-immune host. Dis. Aquat. Org. 36, 201–207.

Wang, T., Secombes, C.J., 2013. The cytokine networks of adaptive immunity in fish. Fish Shellfish Immunol. 35, 1703–1718.

Wang, X.T., Dickerson, H.W., 2002. Surface immobilization antigen of the parasitic ciliate *Ichthyophthirius multifiliis* elicits protective immunity in channel catfish (*Ictalurus punctatus*). Clin. Diagn. Lab. Immunol. 9, 176–181.

Weli, S.C., Aamelfot, M., Dale, O.B., Koppang, E.O., Falk, K., 2013. Infectious salmon anaemia virus infection of Atlantic salmon gill epithelial cells. Virol. J. 10, 1–5.

Wendelaar Bonga, S.E., van der Mej, C.J.M., 1989. Degeneration and death, by apoptosis and necrosis, of the pavement and chloride cells in the gills of the teleost *Oreochromis mossambicus*. Cell Tiss. Res. 255, 235–243.

Whyte, S.K., 2007. The innate immune response of finfish – a review of current knowledge. Fish Shellfish Immunol. 23, 1127–1151.

Wiens, G.D., Glenney, G.W., LaPatra, S.E., Welch, T.J., 2006. Identification of novel rainbow trout (*Onchorynchus mykiss*) chemokines, CXCd1 and CXCd2: mRNA expression after *Yersinia ruckeri* vaccination and challenge. Immunogen. 58, 308–323.

Wilson, J.M., Laurent, P., 2002. Fish gill morphology: inside out. J. Exp. Zool. 293, 192–213.

Wolke, R.E., 1992. Piscine macrophage aggregates: a review. Ann. Rev. Fish Dis. 2, 91–108.

Xu, D.-H., Klesius, P.H., 2013. Comparison of serum antibody responses and host protection against parasite *Ichthyophthirius multifiliis* between channel catfish and channel x blue hybrid catfish. Fish Shellfish Immunol. 34, 1356–1359.

Xu, Z., Chen, C.-F., Mao, Z.-J., Zhu, W.-Y., 2009. Detection of serum and mucosal antibody production and antibody secreting cells (ASCs) in large yellow croaker (*Pseudosciaena crocea*) following vaccination with *Vibrio harveyi* via different routes. Aquaculture 287, 243–247.

Yasutake, W.T., Wales, J.H., 1983. Microscopic Anatomy of Salmonids: An Atlas. Washington DC, United States Department of the Interior, Fish and Wildlife Service.

Yoshida, S.H., Stuge, T.B., Miller, N.W., Clem, L.W., 1995. Phylogeny of lymphocyte heterogeneity – cytotoxic activity of channel catfish peripheral blood leukocytes directed against allogeneic targets. Dev. Comp. Immunol. 19, 71–77.

Young, N.D., Cooper, G.A., Nowak, B.F., Koop, B.F., Morrison, R.N., 2008. Coordinated down-regulation of the antigen processing machinery in the gills of amoebic gill disease-affected Atlantic salmon (*Salmo salar* L). Mol. Immunol. 45, 2581–2597.

Zapata, A.G., Torroba, M., Alvarez, F., Anderson, D.P., Dixon, O.W., Wisniewski, M., 1987. Electron microscopic examination of antigen uptake by salmonid gill cells after bath immunization with a bacterin. J. Fish Biol. 31, 209–217.

Zhang, Y.-A., Salinas, I., Li, J., Parra, D., Bjork, S., Xu, Z., LaPatra, S.E., Bartholomew, J., Sunyer, J.O., 2010. IgT, a primitive immunoglobulin class specialized in mucosal immunity. Nat. Immunol. 11, 827–882.

Zhao, F., Li, Y.-W., Pan, H.-J., Shi, C.-B., Luo, X.-C., Li, A.-X., Wu, S.-Q., 2013a. Expression profiles of toll-like receptors in channel catfish (*Ictalurus punctatus*) after infection with *Ichthyophthirius multifiliis*. Fish Shellfish Immunol. 35, 993–997.

Zhao, F., Li, Y.-W., Pan, H.-J., Wu, S.-Q., Shi, C.-B., Luo, X.-C., Li, A.-X., 2013b. Grass carp (*Ctenopharyngodon idella*) TRAF6 and TAK1: molecular cloning and expression analysis after *Ichthyophthirius multifiliis* infection. Fish Shellfish Immunol. 34, 1514–1523.

Zinkl, J.G., Cox, W.T., Kono, C.S., 1991. Morphology and cytochemistry of leucocytes and thrombocytes of six species of fish. Comp. Haematol. Internat. 1, 187–195.

Fish mucosal immunity: intestine

6

*Irene Salinas**; David Parra***
*Center for Evolutionary and Theoretical Immunology, Department of Biology, University of New Mexico, Albuquerque, New Mexico, USA
**Department of Cell Biology, Physiology and Immunology, Universitat Autonoma de Barcelona, Cerdanyola del Valles, Spain

Chapter Outline

Mucosal Health in Aquaculture

6.1 Introduction

The gastrointestinal tract of vertebrates is a multifunctional organ, which carries many important and diverse physiological functions (Grosell et al., 2010). Among these functions, defense is arguably one of the most important, since the gut is a physical barrier to pathogen entry that also contains a gut-associated lymphoid tissue (GALT). GALT is one of the three mucosa-associated lymphoid tissues (MALT) of teleosts and its study is critical for the fish farming industry for a number of reasons. First, the gut is one of the main portals of entry of pathogens. Second, farmed fish are generally fed commercial pellets, which gives farmers the ability to manipulate fish health by incorporating drugs and vaccines into the feed. Third, the gut immune system of teleosts allows microbial colonization by symbionts, and this microbial community can be regarded as a mechanism to modulate fish pathogens. Moreover, the fish gut-associated microbial communities can be manipulated via the food and the water. Altogether, these features make the intestinal immune system intricate while, at the same time, very attractive and prone to manipulation in aquaculture. The rules that govern mucosal immunity, however, are very different from those that govern systemic immunity. Thus, implementing effective mucosal immunotherapies for finfish aquaculture requires a thorough understanding of the mucosal immune system of fish.

Historically, the presence of immune cells in the gut of fish was first reported in elasmobranchs in the early 1900s (Drzewina, 1905; Jacobshagen, 1915). It was not until the 1970s that the first reports on diffuse lymphoid accumulations in the gut of teleost species, such as the Australian catfish (*Tachysurus australis*) (Diconza and Halliday, 1971), channel catfish (*Ictalarus punctatus*) (Krementz and Chapman, 1975), and roach (*Rutilus rutilus*) (Zapata, 1979), were published. During the same years, the first studies on immune molecules present in gut mucus were performed. An immunoglobulin (Ig) was detected in the intestinal mucus of the Australian catfish (Diconza and Halliday, 1971), and Harris (Harris, 1972) demonstrated the presence of specific antibodies in the gut mucus of chub (*Leuciscus cephalus*) against the acanthocephalan *Pomphoryhnchus*.

As it has been the case in the history of human immunology, immunologists enjoyed successful stories (i.e., the discovery of very effective vaccines that eradicated small pox) prior to understanding how and why they actually worked. Similarly, at a time when fish immunologists knew very little about the gut immunity of fish, the first vaccination experiments began. The very first fish vaccine was surprisingly an oral vaccine performed by Duff (1942) in a teleost, the cutthroat trout. Orally vaccinated trout were challenged by adding *Bacterium salmonicida* (*Aeromonas salmonicida*) to the tank water. This first attempt at oral vaccination resulted in 75% protection in vaccinated fish, compared to 25% in the unvaccinated control group. Moreover, vaccination induced specific agglutinins in serum. Duff's original success has not been reliably reproduced despite many trials with furunculosis vaccines (Ellis, 1988). Seventy years later, fish oral vaccines continue to show poor potency compared to other vaccination methods.

Other than furunculosis, vibriosis has been one of the biggest bacterial disease problems for aquaculture fish around the world. Thus, development of vaccines against vibriosis has attracted the attention of many researchers throughout the years. Early trials delivered *Vibrio* antigens to the plaice (*Pleuronectens platessa*) orally and showed specific antibody production in both serum and gut mucus (Fletcher and White, 1973).

During the 1980s, several studies were performed to evaluate the efficacy of oral vaccines (Amend and Jhonson, 1981; Davina et al., 1982; Georgopoulou and Vernier, 1986; Rombout et al., 1986) and to identify the mechanisms of antigen absorption by the gut (Hart et al., 1988; Watanabe, 1982) that were continued during the 1990s until the present. The lower efficacy of the oral vaccine formulations compared to the already established delivery methods (injection and immersion vaccination) was likely the trigger for subsequent studies that aimed to further understand how the gut immune system of teleosts functions.

As we will explain later in this chapter, our knowledge on the mucosal immune system of fish has increased tremendously since the 1980s, and the field of fish gut immunology is currently blooming. The combination of genomic and immunological tools is quickly advancing our basic knowledge on teleost mucosal immunity. We are starting to identify the molecules and cells that rule mucosal immunity, and this knowledge should soon be translated into new health management practices for the aquaculture industry.

6.2 The mucus layer as a barrier against mucosal pathogens

The gastrointestinal tract of animals is continuously challenged with food antigens as well as bacteria, viruses, parasites, and toxins. Gut epithelial cells are protected by a mucus layer, which creates a physical and chemical barrier to any offense from the environment (Ellis, 2001). Furthermore, this layer acts as an important mechanism of innate defense that maintains tissue homeostasis (Gomez et al., 2013).

Therefore, teleost intestinal mucus has some functions similar to the gut, gills, and skin, including physical and chemical barriers, osmoregulation, and lubrication. However, there are additional processes in which gut mucus is specifically implicated such as nutrient uptake and digestion (Bakke et al., 2010) or, in air-breathing fish, uptake of oxygen from the air (Nelson and Dehn, 2010). Thus, intestinal mucus is permeable to macromolecules that are required for digestion and absorption, but, at the same time, acts as an effective barrier to particulate matter, including microorganisms.

The chemical composition of teleost mucosal secretions differs slightly from that of humans (Allen, 1983). Mucus is composed of water (around 95%) and glycoproteins (mainly mucins, up to 5%), which confer mucus its viscosity. Other substances are present in smaller quantities, including innate and adaptive immune factors, such as antimicrobial molecules or secretory immunoglobulins (sIgs), (Gomez et al., 2013; Salinas et al., 2011).

Mucins are high molecular weight proteins composed of a long peptide chain with tandem repeats, known as the mucin domain. This domain is significantly *O*-glycosylated and differs in length and sequence from one mucin to another.

Glycosylation of mucins' carbohydrate chains is necessary for the role of mucus as a mechanical barrier as well as for its interactions with the environment (Roussel and Delmotte, 2004). Thus, changes in glycosylation levels of mucins due to, for example, parasite infection modulate bacteria attachment to the mucus layer (Estensoro et al., 2013; Schroers et al., 2008). Based on their structural and functional features, mucins are grouped in two different families: secreted mucin glycoproteins, which are large, highly *O*-glycosylated glycoproteins assembled in oligomers that give mucus its viscosity (Thornton et al., 2008), and membrane-bound forms, which are cell-surface mucins and contain an extracellular *O*-glycosylated domain. These are likely to form long filaments carrying oligosaccharides that may be ligands for microbial adhesions (McGuckin et al., 2011). It is interesting to point out that secreted forms appear earlier in evolution, and membrane-bound mucins provide an additional layer of defense to protect epithelial cells (Lang et al., 2007). The secretion of mucins by goblet cells in the intestine lumen seems to be continuous and constitutes a loose layer, which leads to physical removal of attached pathogens or toxins (Jutfelt, 2011).

Chemical properties of fish mucins have been widely described in the literature and are very similar to those found in mammals (Neuhaus et al., 2007). However, mucin genes have only been identified in a few teleost species, including carp (*Cyprinus carpio L.*), seabream (*Sparus aurata*), and zebrafish (*Danio rerio*). Unfortunately, the gene expression of mucins in mucosal sites has been scarcely studied in fish. In the intestine, two secreted mucins, Muc2 and Muc2-like, are expressed in gilthead seabream (Perez-Sanchez et al., 2013), while only one, Muc2, has been described in common carp (Marel et al., 2012). As far as membrane-bound mucins are concerned, two different molecules have been discovered in gilthead seabream, Muc13 and Muc18 (Perez-Sanchez et al., 2013). The structure and location of these mucins are very similar to their homologous counterparts in humans. In this vein, Muc2 in humans has the capacity of delivering tolerogenic signals to antigen-sampling dendritic cells, constraining the immunogenicity of gut antigens (Shan et al., 2013). Importantly, some pathogens have developed factors capable of degrading mucins to facilitate their entry into the epithelium (Ashida et al., 2012).

Although the intestinal mucus of fish contains a number of immune molecules, for the purposes of this chapter, we are going to focus on two: antimicrobial molecules and sIgs.

6.2.1 Antimicrobial molecules present in teleost gut mucus

Several molecules implicated in innate immunity are found in the intestine of some fish species, such as lysozymes in Asian sea bass (*Lates calcarifer*) (Fu et al., 2013) and Atlantic salmon (*Salmo salar* L.) (Sveinbjornsson et al., 1996); complement components in grass carp (*Ctenopharyngodon idella*)(Shen et al., 2012), rainbow trout (*Oncorhynchus mykiss*) (Kania et al., 2010; Lovoll et al., 2006), and Asian sea bass (Xia et al., 2013); cytokines in Atlantic cod (*Gadus morhua*) (Lokesh et al., 2012) and rainbow trout (Mulder et al., 2007); lectins in several species (reviewed in Vasta et al., 2011); or antimicrobial peptides (AMPs) in rainbow trout (Casadei et al., 2013) and grouper (*Epinephelus coioides*) (Pan et al., 2007). However, due to the numerous proteases from luminal bacteria and their capacity to cleave and degrade all of these immune factors, the presence and levels of these molecules in teleost gut mucus has been scarcely demonstrated. AMPs play a critical role in mucosal immunity, and the presence of teleost AMPs can be observed inside intestinal goblet cells in common carp (van der Marel et al., 2013), grouper (Pan et al., 2007), and winter flounder (*Pleuronectes americanus*) (Cole et al., 2000), indicating that they are likely secreted into the mucus.

6.2.2 Immunoglobulins present in teleost gut mucus

Fish have three immunoglobulin isotypes: IgM, IgD, and IgT/Z (reviewed in Parra et al., 2013). Out of these three isotypes, two are present in rainbow trout gut mucus as secreted forms, IgM and IgT. IgM is the main immunoglobulin in serum and the key player in systemic immune responses. IgM is also present in mucosal secretions (reviewed in Salinas et al., 2011), although, as we mentioned before for other proteins, its detection has been challenging due to the fact that proteases in gut mucus are capable of degrading IgM in a very short period of time (Hatten et al., 2001). Thus, the technique for mucus isolation is crucial to obtaining accurate quantification and functional analysis of proteins in gut mucus, and different collection methods may account for variable results among different laboratories. Even though total IgM levels are higher than those of IgT in rainbow trout mucus, only specific IgT titers are found in rainbow trout gut mucus after an enteric parasite infection (Zhang et al., 2010), as it will be discussed later.

Interestingly, both teleost sIgs are present in intestinal secretions as polymers. In the case of IgT, this is in sharp contrast to the monomers found in plasma. Teleost sIgs are likely to play a number of biological roles other than specific immunity. The best role characterized is perhaps their ability to interact with the microbiota and to perform immune exclusion of luminal bacteria (Zhang et al., 2010), a process by which immunoglobulins attach to bacteria, preventing them from entering the epithelium. As the chief mucosal immunoglobulin, IgT covers the majority of bacteria, while IgM accounts only for a small percentage of them (Zhang et al., 2010). IgT seems to be strategically designed to help teleosts maintain homoeostasis with the microbiota.

Transportation of both Igs to the lumen takes place through a receptor present in the surface of intestinal epithelial cells, named the polymeric immunoglobulin receptor (pIgR), by a process called transcytosis (Johansen and Kaetzel, 2011). Intestinal pIgR is described in rainbow trout (Zhang et al., 2010), common carp (Rombout et al., 2008), and grouper (Feng et al., 2009). This receptor binds IgT and IgM in the lamina propria (LP), and the complex pIgR-Ig is carried across the cell to the apical surface where it is proteolytically cleaved and secreted to the intestine lumen as sIgT or sIgM, constituted by the Ig and the secretory component of the pIgR (Zhang et al., 2010). Interestingly, while transport of Igs to the lumen in higher vertebrates requires the joining (J)-chain, which is linked by disulfide bridges to the Fc region of these Ig molecules, teleost and amphibian mucosal Igs do not present this peptide on their Igs, and it is not required for their interaction with pIgR and posterior secretion (Flajnik, 2010).

6.3 Resident cell types found in the gastrointestinal tract of teleosts

Teleost GALT consists of diffuse elements and lacks organized ones such as Peyer's patches and mesenteric lymph nodes present in endotherms. Similar to mammals, the teleost gut harbors two main populations of immune cells: lamina propia leukocytes (LPLs), which include a variety of immune cells, such as macrophages, granulocytes, lymphocytes, and plasma cells; and the intraepithelial lymphocytes (IEL), composed mostly by T cells and a few B cells located among epithelial cells. Together with these immune cells, epithelial cells, mucus-producing cells, and neuroendocrine cells also take an active part in teleost gut immune responses.

6.3.1 *Leukocytes*

6.3.1.1 *Myeloid cells*

Macrophages: The lack of specific markers for the study of teleost macrophages continues to limit our knowledge of their localization and their specific role in gut immune responses. Based on their morphological features, resident macrophages are described in the gut LP of several fish species such as Atlantic cod (Inami et al., 2009), rainbow trout (Georgopoulou and Vernier, 1986), and common carp (Rombout et al., 1986). In cyprinids, a particular type of macrophage, called "large macrophage," has been described (Rombout et al., 1993), but its presence in other fish species is not clear.

In mammals, gut macrophages are in a quiescent phase in the intestine and cannot induce inflammation unless exposed to a stimulus (Mowat and Bain, 2011). Although this peculiar characteristic has not yet been described in fish macrophages, when comparing mucosal and systemic responses to yeast in rainbow trout, the mucosal compartment leukocytes show lower innate immune activities than the systemic ones (Martin et al., 2012), indicating a possible analogy with mammalian macrophages. Moreover, a second population of gut macrophages exists under inflammatory conditions when monocytes get recruited to the gut mucosa to aid resident macrophages. These two populations will be further discussed in Section 6.4.2.1.

Granulocytes: The existence of neutrophils, eosinophils, basophils, and mast cells has been reported in the intestine LP of several fish species, including, but not limited to, rainbow trout (Sire and Vernier, 1995), brown trout (*Salmo trutta trutta* L.) (Dezfuli and Giari, 2008), and zebrafish (Hedrera et al., 2013). Similarly to mammalian granulocytes, the staining pattern of fish granulocytes differs between major groups (Crowhurst et al., 2002). Importantly, eosinophils are named basophils in common carp because they do not stain with eosin after standard fixation techniques (Rombout et al., 1989). In general, fish gut contains less resident neutrophils than eosinophils/basophils, although neutrophils penetrate the epithelium more easily (Rombout et al., 1989).

Despite the fact that teleosts lack IgE, histamine is present in the granules of immune cells of a few fish species, such as rainbow trout (Vallejo and Ellis, 1989) or gilthead seabream (Mulero et al., 2007), which has led to the consensus that mast cells (also called eosinophilic granule/granular cells) exist in fish. Little is known about the function of these cells in mucosal immunity, although their implication in the immune response against gut parasites will be explained later in Section 6.4.2.1. Fish mast cells can release important innate immune molecules, such as tryptase (Dobson et al., 2008), lysozymes (Uran et al., 2009), AMPs (i.e., piscidin (Silphaduang and Noga, 2001)), and pleurocidin (Murray et al., 2003), and they react strongly upon inflammation via migration and granule release.

Rodlet cells: These cells are unique to teleost fish. Although there are differences in rodlet cell morphology in different species of fish, the general pattern is the same in all species in which they have been described (Reite, 2005). They are ovoid cells with a basally located nucleus and several conspicuous "rodlets" enclosed in a fibrous capsule. For a long time, rodlet cells were described as a parasite in fish intestinal tissue (Bannister, 1966) until the 1970s when they were classified as host cells (Leino, 1974). Rodlet cells are associated to epithelial tissues (although they have also been seen in the blood) and appear to be present in the intestinal epithelium of a number of teleost species, including generous salmonids, cyprinids, gadids, and labrids (reviewed in Reite, 2005). The specific function of these cells is not clear, but most authors point to a role against parasites (reviewed in Reite and Evensen, 2006).

Dendritic cells: Intestinal dendritic cells are a key player in mammalian mucosal response due to their capability of acquiring antigens and regulating immune responses (Coombes and Powrie, 2008). While dendritic cells have been described in trout and zebrafish (Bassity and Clark, 2012; Lugo-Villarino et al., 2010), their presence and role in the intestine of fish is still unknown.

6.3.1.2 Lymphoid cells

B cells: As aforementioned, teleosts express three different Ig heavy chains able to generate three immunoglobulin isotypes, IgM, IgT/Z, and IgD. The structure of the trout and zebrafish IgH locus predicts that the expression of IgM isotypes blocks the generation of IgT/IgZ transcripts, and vice versa (Danilova et al., 2005; Hansen et al., 2005). This has been confirmed in rainbow trout (Xu et al., 2013; Zhang et al., 2010) and zebrafish (Schorpp et al., 2006), which have a lineage of B cells uniquely expressing IgT/Z. Teleosts have two populations of IgD B cells: IgD^+/IgM^- B cells, present only in channel catfish (*I. punctatus*) (Edholm et al., 2010) and rainbow trout (Castro et al., 2014), and IgD^+/IgM^+ B cells, which are present in all teleost species analyzed thus far.

In the intestine of rainbow trout, two populations of B cells exist, IgT^+ and IgM^+ (Zhang et al., 2010). They are primarily located in the LP (Figure 6.1) and can infiltrate the epithelium after parasite infection (Zhang et al., 2010). As resident cells, IgT^+ are the dominant population of B cells (54% of the total gut B cells) and are the main responders against enteric pathogens (Zhang et al., 2010). These two populations of B cells secrete IgT and IgM into the lumen through the pIgR pathway (see Section 6.2.2). No IgD^+/IgM^- B cells or secreted IgD are present in intestine or gut secretions.

Plasma cells: Plasma cells secreting IgM have been identified in the intestine of a number of fish species after vaccination, including rainbow trout (Davidson et al., 1993) or carp (Joosten et al., 1997), as well as the naïve intestine of carp (Rombout et al., 1993). Although specific IgT titers are present in trout gut mucus (Zhang et al., 2010), the presence of resident IgT plasma cells in teleost intestines has not been demonstrated so far. It is important to point out that plasma cells are scarce in the intestine, and, in some studies, these cells were not detected in naïve fish (Davidson et al., 1993). Interestingly, in the Emerald rockcod (*Trematomus bernacchii*), an accumulation of plasma cells in the liver and Ig in bile conduct are present, indicating the possible implication of the liver in intestine antibody responses (Abelli et al., 2005).

T cells: Presence of T cells in fish intestine is corroborated by the expression of T cell-specific markers in sea bass (*Dicentrarchus labrax*) whole intestine tissue, including CD4,

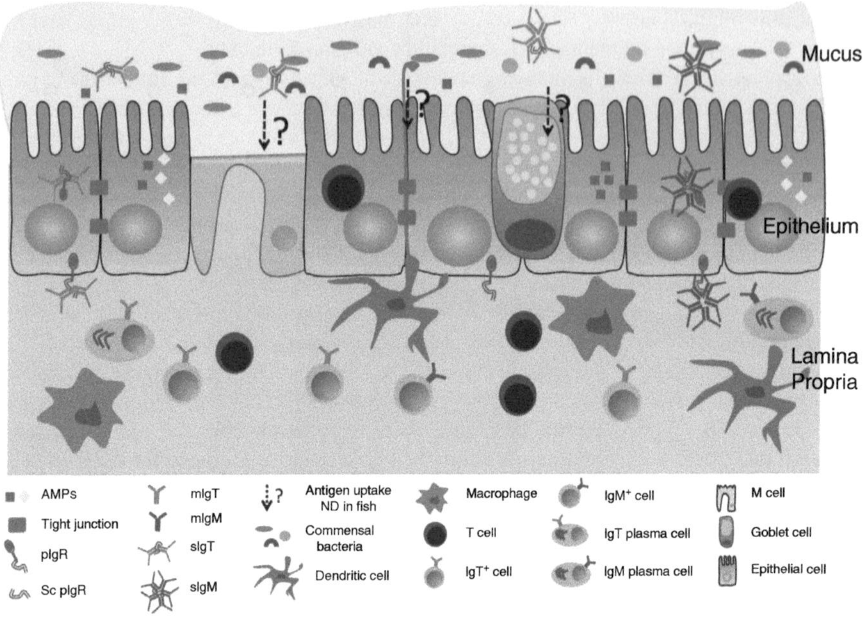

Figure 6.1 Schematic representation of GALT in teleost fish. Intestine epithelium structure and main resident cells implicated in mucosal immune responses in fish are represented (epithelial cells macrophages, goblet cells, B cells, T cells, and plasma cells) as well as the mucus layer and gut-associated microbiota. M cells and dendritic cells, crucial cell subsets in mammalian GALT, are shown, although their presence in fish intestine is not demonstrated yet. Some humoral components of immune response are represented as well (Igs and AMPs). Possible routes of antigen uptake are suggested (?). AMPs, antimicrobial peptides; pIgR, polymeric Ig receptor; mIgT/M, membrane-bound immunoglobulin; sIgT/M, secreted immunoglobulin; ND, not determined.

CD8-α, rag-1, TCR-β, and TCR-γ (Boschi et al., 2011). Additionally, rainbow trout IELs have been isolated and express T cell transcripts, including CD3-e, CD4, CD8, CD28, TCR-β, TCR-γ, and TCR-ζ (Takizawa et al., 2011). In teleost gut mucosa, resident T cells are present in several teleost species such as sea bass (Picchietti et al., 2011), common carp (Rombout et al., 1998), Atlantic salmon (Bakke-McKellep et al., 2007), and rainbow trout (Takizawa et al., 2011). T cells, as mentioned before, comprise the main subset of the total IELs, although they are also present in the LP. For instance, T cells constitute the main lymphocyte subset in the gut of sea bass, accounting for more than 50% of gut IELs (Romano et al., 2011), whereas cytotoxic $CD8^+$ T cells account for ~55% of gut lymphocytes in trout (Takizawa et al., 2011).

The two main lineages of T cells, αβ- and γδ-T cells, are present in teleost intestines as confirmed by the expression of their T cell receptor chains. More recent studies have investigated sea bass intestinal T cell subsets (Buonocore et al., 2012), and this model continues to produce valuable and pioneer information on the intestinal T cell biology of teleosts. However, the roles that these two lineages play in intestinal immune responses of fish are still not well known.

Based on their cytokine profile, main $CD4^+$ T cells subset in mammals are Th1, Th2, Th17, and Tregs. *In vitro* studies of $CD4^+$ T cells in Japanese pufferfish (*Takifugu rubripes*) show the same production of Th1, Th2, Th17, and Treg cytokines after stimulation (Kono and Korenaga, 2013). The first *in vivo* evidence for these subsets and their differential role in gut immunity was recently published on zebrafish and turbot (*Scophtalmus maximus*) following bath or injection vaccination (Zhang et al., 2014). Thus, it appears that the aquaculture industry could benefit from further advances in the field of intestinal Th17 responses, since this knowledge is likely to help design and implement new mucosal immunotherapies. **Natural killer (NK) cells:** Two types of NK cells homologous to mammalian ones have been observed in fish: nonspecific cytotoxic cells (NCC) that spontaneously kill a variety of xenogeneic targets, and NK-like cells (reviewed in Fischer et al., 2013). NCC activity has been described in several fish species, including rainbow trout, carp, channel catfish, and tilapia (*Oreochromis niloticus*) (reviewed in Shen et al., 2002). Expression of nonspecific cytotoxic cell receptors, such as (NCCRP)-1, in tilapia intestine (Ishimoto et al., 2004) indicates the presence of NK cells in this tissue. The cytotoxic activity observed in isolated intestinal leukocyte suspensions is even higher than that observed in head kidney leukocytes, suggesting the substantial presence of NK cells in fish intestine (Martin et al., 2012). The existence of resident NK cells in the intestine is further supported by the expression of an important factor for NK activation, NK cell-enhancing factor (NKEF), in several fish species (Chen et al., 2009) and its constitute expression in the intestine of fish (Esteban et al., 2013).

6.3.2 Other cell types

6.3.2.1 Epithelial cells

The intestinal epithelium of fish consists of a single layer of columnar epithelial cells, called enterocytes, with a prominent brush border (Figure 6.1). These cells are tall and narrow with stretched nuclei located near the LP in the basal region and lamellar structures running parallel to the lateral plasma membrane. Cytoplasm, especially the apical part, possesses numerous aggregations of lipid droplets important for lipid digestion (Olsen et al., 1999). Enterocytes show a high basolateral expression of Na/K-ATPase, which is necessary for transport processes implicated in nutrient uptake and ion regulation (Feng et al., 2013). The enterocyte apical membrane is characterized by the presence of microvilli, which form a brush border that contributes to nearly 90% of total intestinal surface area, although it can vary depending on the area of the intestine and the fish species (German et al., 2010). Enzymatic activity has been localized at the brush border membrane, including alkaline phosphatase, disaccharidase, leucine aminopeptidase, and tri- and dipeptidase, which is produced by the epithelial cells (Kuz'mina and Gelman, 1997).

In the distal intestine of fish, some epithelial cells present large vacuoles and participate in macromolecule uptake. These cells are characterized by presenting numerous microvilli, an overdeveloped vesicular network, vacuoles, and lysosomes. Proteins can be taken up via different routes such as transcytosis or pinocytosis. This absorption of macromolecular proteins by enterocytes is important for antigen collecting and initiating immune response (Rombout et al., 1985). Thus, after oral vaccine administration, antigens can be detected inside enterocytes. Depending on the species, this internalization can take 16 h, in the case of common carp, or up to 24 h, in the case of rainbow trout (Joosten et al., 1997).

The interaction of epithelial cells with intestinal bacteria is continuous and triggers different processes in the cells. Therefore, resident bacteria enhance the stability of β-catenin in enterocytes and promote cell proliferation during intestine development (Cheesman et al., 2011). Mammalian epithelial cells can sense luminal bacteria and take part in immune response through their pattern recognition receptors (PRRs) that includes lectins, nod-like receptors (NLRs), and toll-like receptors (TLRs). Only NOD1/NOD2 receptors are described as PRRs in zebrafish enterocytes (Oehlers et al., 2011), and no TLRs have been found. However, zebrafish lacking Myd88, a key molecule implicated in the TLR signal, present a delayed proliferation of intestinal epithelial cells (Cheesman et al., 2011), suggesting the possible existence of TLRs on enterocyte surfaces that could interact with luminal bacteria and induce cell proliferation. On the other hand, some viruses induce apoptosis in fish epithelial cells (Holopainen et al., 2012). Enterocytes can regulate immune responses through expression of intestinal alkaline phosphatase, which has been shown to prevent intestinal inflammation in response to resident microbiota by detoxifying LPS from these bacteria (Bates et al., 2007). Also, as we mentioned before, a very important role of epithelial cells in the control of luminal bacteria is their role in the transport of mucosal Igs to the lumen by expressing pIgR (Zhang et al., 2010).

6.3.2.2 Mucus-producing cells

Goblet cells are the dominant mucus cell type in fish intestine epithelium. Their nucleus is located in the basal portion, and, in the middle area, cells widen and then constrict to form an apical pore through which mucus is discharged. As mentioned before, the main molecules in the mucus are mucins, which play an important role in the maintenance of the epithelial barrier against pathogens. Mucin granules, which are predominate in the cell, can be of variable electron density and aggregate in the characteristic goblet cell thecae. Granules are secreted constitutively and, in response to extracellular stimuli, through a highly regulated process that involves the transport of granules via actin remodeling, granule tethering to the membrane, and granule exocytosis (McGuckin et al., 2011). The amount of goblet cells varies in fish intestine infected with a parasite, increasing in number around the site infection (Dezfuli et al., 2010). In mammals, differences exist in goblet cells from the same tissues in terms of mucin type or glycosylation levels of secreted mucin (McGuckin et al., 2011), a fact not yet demonstrated in fish. In the same vein, goblet cells in mammals are capable of delivering soluble antigens to dendritic cells in the LP (McDole et al., 2012), and it is possible that this function is conserved in fish goblet cells.

6.3.2.3 Neuroendocrine cells

Gut neural and endocrine systems in fish are very similar to those of higher vertebrates. Despite some species-specific differences, the basic histological structure of the neuroendocrine system studied so far appears conserved. Differences observed at the species level may be a consequence of different food regimes, body weight, or body shape. For instance, the family Cyprinidae is probably entirely agastric and, in these animals, the bile duct is found in the gut region immediately distal to the esophagus (Abad et al., 1987). As a consequence of both this extraordinary diversity in morphology, physiology, and biochemistry and the limited number of species that have been examined, the scope of our knowledge on the topic of neuroendocrine systems associated to the gut in fish is still incomplete.

In fish, the vast majority of activities involved in the physiological control of gut function during feeding or fasting periods are mediated by the neuroendocrine system. Thus, they play important roles in the overall regulation of digestive processes such as nutrient absorption, gut motility, and intestinal blood flow. In the gut of vertebrate, epithelial cells belonging to the diffuse endocrine system (DES) interact with components of the enteric nervous system (ENS). Concerning fish, several peptides are produced by structures of the neuroendocrine system and are involved in the communication between DES and ENS. Some of these peptides are associated with the modulation of fish alimentary behavior (Dezfuli et al., 2003). Gastrointestinal hormones are secreted by enteroendocrine cells, which are distributed throughout the intestinal tract. They are located in the epithelium, and they synthesize several hormones and other molecules that regulate physiological functions of the digestive tract. For example, several peptides and hormones have been identified as products of enteroendocrine cells in the intestine of flower fish (*Pseudophoxinus antalyae*) (Cinar et al., 2006), pejerrey (*Odontesthes bonariensis*) (Vigliano et al., 2011), and other fish species (reviewed in Holmgren and Olsson, 2009).

Although it is not well understood yet, it seems that this neuroendocrine system in the gut interacts with the local immune system, and changes in hormone secretion, such as cortisol, might regulate gut immune responses (Kvamme et al., 2013).

6.4 Gut immune responses in diseased fish

Despite the obvious relevance to mucosal health and fish welfare, very little is known about the immune responses that different pathogens elicit in the gut of teleosts. The majority of studies thus far consist of histological observations from wild-caught or farmed fish uninfected or infected with a particular gut pathogen. Due to the growing interest in probiotics for use in aquaculture over the past 10 years, most work has been done with probiotic bacteria, either dead or alive. The gut immune responses of fish following probiotic or immunostimulant oral administration are outlined in a later chapter of this book. Overall, most studies remain highly descriptive, and more mechanistic and functional investigations should be the next step. This is a major problem because it currently hinders our ability to deliver targeted interventions that specifically stimulate the arms of the immune system that are critical to overcome diseases.

6.4.1 Changes in the gut mucus of fish in response to infection

The gut mucus layer acts as a first line of defense against pathogen attachment and invasion. At the same time, gut mucus can be utilized as a nutrient source by bacterial pathogens (Garcia et al., 1997), and, therefore, there is a very dynamic and delicate balance between gut mucosal secretions and gut microorganisms. It is important to bear in mind that marine teleosts, in contrast to their freshwater counterparts, are known to continuously drink water, which directly exposes the gut mucus of these species to waterborne infectious agents. This may imply fundamental differences between marine and freshwater fish species with regards to the gut mucus properties and mucus responses to infection, and these differences deserve investigation.

It has been long known that the amount and properties of fish mucosal secretions change in response to environmental factors (i.e., stress) as well as infectious agents. Perhaps the best examples come from parasitic infections of vertebrate where the parasite benefits from the changes in mucus composition and quantity. Scrutiny of fish literature reveals that enhanced mucus secretion occurs in the intestines of tench infected with the cestode *Monobothrium wageneri* (Dezfuli et al., 2011). Myxozoan parasites also induce changes in the gut mucus of marine species such as seabream and turbot. Particularly, the gut mucus of seabream and turbot infected with *E. leei* and *E. scophthalmi*, respectively, had higher glycosylation levels than uninfected individuals (Redondo and Alvarez-Pellitero, 2010). Changes in glycosylation status of mucus have been associated with a number of diseases in mammals, yet the functional consequences of these changes in the mucus of diseased fish remain unknown.

As mentioned above, fish gut mucus is mostly composed of large glycoproteins, called mucins, secreted by goblet cells or other secretory cells. Thus, any infectious agent capable of altering mucin gene expression and/or mucin secretion has the potential to change the thickness and physicochemical properties of the gut mucus layer in fish. Unfortunately, mucin genes have only recently been found in a number of teleost species (Lang et al., 2007; Perez-Sanchez et al., 2013; van der Marel et al., 2013), and their gene expression regulation and functions are still poorly understood. Surprisingly, down-regulation of mucin gene expression occurs in the gut of seabream as a response to the parasite *E. leei* and diet (Perez-Sanchez et al., 2013). These fluctuations in mucin expression could affect not only the mucosal layer as a physical barrier, but also the immune response downstream as well. This finding led the authors to propose mucins as reliable markers of fish intestinal health. Further studies will have to refine how to use mucins in a diagnosis context for aquaculture.

Bacteriophages can adhere to the mucus of a number of vertebrate species, including teleosts (Barr et al., 2013); however, we know very little about the role of these viruses in controlling fish gut homeostasis and mucus secretion. Similarly, our current knowledge of fish viral pathogens and their interactions with the gut mucus layer is scant.

Teleost gut mucus contains innate and adaptive immune molecules as explained earlier in this chapter. One of the targets of dietary interventions in aquaculture is the modulation of the innate immune molecules of fish gut mucus by immunostimulant or probiotic delivery. For instance, it is possible to modulate the number of goblet cells, the composition of the gut mucus, and its lysozyme content by oral administration of immunostimulants, such as MOS (mannan oligosaccharides) (Torrecillas et al., 2011), or probiotic bacteria (Newaj-Fyzul et al., 2007).

Recent studies have successfully demonstrated the presence of specific antibodies against a gut myxozoan parasite, *C. shasta*, in rainbow trout gut mucus. In particular, gut mucosal antibodies belong to the IgT class, which, as we know, is the predominant Ig in the mucosal lymphoid organs and mucosal secretions of fish.

Finally, it is worth mentioning that, in laboratory zebrafish, as discussed later in this chapter, a few models of chemically induced enterocolitis have been developed. In these models, changes in the number of goblet cells, as well as the type of mucosal secretions they produce, have recently been shown (Oehlers et al., 2012).

6.4.2 Innate immune responses in the gut of fish

6.4.2.1 Innate effector cells in the gut of fish

Regarding lymphoid cells, all cell types necessary for a local innate immune response are present in the gut mucosa of several teleost species, and local innate immune responses can be observed after intestinal immunization or infection (Rombout et al., 2011).

Macrophages: Intestinal macrophages represent the largest pool of tissue macrophages in the body of a mammal (Smith et al., 2011). They play a critical role in maintaining gut homeostasis and have a peculiar phenotype described as "inflammatory anergic" or "tolerogenic" macrophages. Under inflammatory or infection scenarios, however, resident macrophages receive help from monocyte/macrophages that infiltrate the gut mucosa participating in the local immune response. It is assumed that these two populations (resident macrophages and infiltrating monocytes/macrophages) both exist in fish. Whether or not they are phenotypically different from each other (one tolerogenic, one proinflammatory) remains to be investigated.

It is clear, however, that gut macrophages appear to be important antigen uptaking cells in teleosts as demonstrated in a number of fish species using a variety of antigen types (Azad et al., 2000; Georgopoulou and Vernier, 1986; Rombout et al., 2011; Rombout and van den Berg, 1989). These are putative resident macrophages since a number of observations were made at early time points following antigen delivery, and, therefore, the identified cells were likely resident and not infiltrated macrophages.

Accumulations of macrophages can be observed in the wall of *C. carpio* experimentally infected with the tapeworm *B. acheilognathi* (Hoole and Nisan, 1994), and these macrophages appear to be able to migrate to the gut lumen and adhere to the parasite tegument. Similarly, macrophages are involved in the gut immune response of the gibel carp (*Carassius gibelio*) against the metacestode parasite *Neogryporhynchus cheilancristrotus* (Molnar, 2005). In *Goussia carpelli*-infected carp, macrophages and granulocytes infiltrate into infected tissue areas (Jendrysek et al., 1994; Lom and Dykova, 1992). These cells have enhanced phagocytic activity *in vivo* (Jendrysek et al., 1994) and *in vitro* (Stelnhagen and Hespe, 1997; Studnicka and Siwicki, 1990). Increased numbers of macrophages are found in the foregut of Atlantic salmon incubated *ex vivo* with the bacterial pathogen *A. salmonicida* (Salinas et al., 2008).

Overall, the role of intestinal macrophages during the course of an infection has rarely been investigated. Our current knowledge on the matter originates from laboratory vaccination experiments or *ex vivo* studies using model antigens, and, therefore, the basic biology of these cells remains largely obscure.

Granulocytes and rodlet cells: Granulocytes (neutrophils, eosinophils, and basophils) as well as rodlet cells are present in the gut of teleost fish as resident cell populations. These innate cell types change in response to infection. It is presumed that granulocytes, mast cells, and rodlet cells commonly play a role in the inflammatory immune response of most fish species against different gut parasites since increased numbers of granulocytes, mast cells, and rodlet cells can be typically observed in the gut of parasite-infected feral or farmed fish (Reite, 1998; Reite and Evensen, 2006; Salinas et al., 2011). These inflammatory cells can migrate and degranulate in response to intestinal helminthes. For instance, rainbow trout infected with the acanthocephalan *Pomphorhynchus laevis*, brown trout infected with the acanthocephalans *Dentitruncus truttae* and *Echinorhynchus truttae*, respectively (Dezfuli and Giari, 2008; Dezfuli et al., 2008; Wanstall et al., 1986), tench infected with the cestode *Monobothrium wageneri* (Dezfuli et al., 2011) or unidentified digenean trematodes (Dezfuli et al., 2013), and powan (*Coregonus lavaretus*) infected with the acanthocephalan *Dentitruncus truttae* (Dezfuli et al., 2009) are all examples of how gut parasites elicit inflammatory cellular immune responses in the gut tissue of teleosts with enteritis and how eosinophils/basophils seem to play a crucial role in this intestinal inflammation model (Bakke-McKellep et al., 2000; Hedrera et al., 2013; Uran et al., 2008). Finally, chronic inflammation due to hypoxia in the gut of fish results in neutrophil infiltration (Niklasson et al., 2011).

Dendritic cells: There are dendritic cells in teleost lymphoid organs as recently described in zebrafish and salmonids (Bassity and Clark, 2012; Lugo-Villarino et al., 2010). Dendritic cells are one of the most important cell types found in vertebrate mucosal surfaces since they receive signals from the microbiota, pathogens, epithelial cells, and other immune cells, and they orchestrate immune homeostasis. Gut dendritic cells are well characterized in mammals with a number of subsets described in functional studies that support the idea of their pivotal function in both innate and adaptive immunity (Tezuka et al., 2007; Uematsu et al., 2008). Unfortunately, there are no reports concerning the characteristics and roles of mucosal dendritic cells in teleosts. The latter, therefore, remains an open field that should be explored in the near future.

NK cells: NK cells have cytotoxic killing capacities and are part of the mucosal immune system of mammals. In teleosts, as mentioned earlier in this chapter, NK can be identified by the expression of the nonspecific cytotoxic cell receptor protein-1 (NCCRP-1). The expression of NCCRP-1 increases in the distal intestine of Atlantic cod 1 and 3 days after intraperitoneal (IP) injection of killed *V. anguillarum*. This indicates that infiltration of NCC or increased expression of this receptor in resident NCC cells takes place in response to IP injection of killed pathogenic bacteria (Caipang, 2013).

Epithelial cells: The innate immune properties of intestinal epithelial cells are well recognized in mammals. In fact, intestinal epithelial cells contribute to recruitment, maintenance, and regulation of effector functions of various intestinal immune cells, and recently, some researchers have regarded intestinal epithelial cells as innate immune cells themselves. How epithelial cells sense and respond to antigens in the fish gut has barely been studied.

Many pathogens enter the host by adhering and invading epithelial cells (intracellular route) or by breaking the tight junctions located in between them (paracellular route). Infected or damaged epithelial cells must release danger signals for the immune system to control the infection. In response to infection, epithelial cells via pattern recognition receptors (i.e., TLRs and NOD receptors) initiate signaling cascades that lead to the initiation of mucosal inflammation. This involves the expression of transcription factors (i.e., NFκ-B), cytokines (i.e., interleukins and interferons), and chemical mediators (i.e., prostaglandins and nitric oxide). Ultimately, surrounding cytotoxic T cells must specifically eliminate infected epithelial cells in the gut mucosa. These pathways have been well characterized in mammals. Recently, an epithelial cell line (RTgutGC) derived from the intestine of *O. mykiss* was developed, allowing for the study of gut epithelial immune responses *in vitro* (Kawano et al., 2011; Komatsu et al., 2009). Trout epithelial cells express cytokines and respond to bacterial infection with *A. salmonicida* by producing IL-1β and TNFα2 (Komatsu et al., 2009).

To date, very few studies have evaluated the innate immune responses that take place in fish gut epithelial cells in response to viral infection. Carp gut epithelial cells increase the expression of the cytokines IFN-α2 and IL-1β, as well as iNOS, upon cyprinid herpes virus 3 infection (Syakuri et al., 2013).

Some knowledge comes from parasitic infections of feral fish. Teleost gut epithelial cells undergo important changes in response to parasitic infections as evidenced by recent studies in wild brown trout infected with the acanthocephalan *Dentitruncus truttae*. The production of the proliferating cell nuclear antigen (PCNA), a protein involved in protein synthesis, within intestinal epithelia appears to provide an early warning indication of altered gut homeostasis since changes in expression of this protein were found in infected compared to uninfected individuals (Dezfuli et al., 2012). Overall, there is an urgent need to increase our understanding of the cross talk between epithelial cells and leukocytes during gut infections in fish.

B cells: Teleost B cells, like their mammalian counterparts, have innate immune functions such as phagocytic and microbial killing capacities (Li et al., 2006). Although these functions have only been studied *in vitro* or in B cells isolated from systemic lymphoid organs (Li et al., 2006; Zhang et al., 2010), the contribution of B cells to the gut innate immunity of fish remains unexplored.

6.4.2.2 Innate effector molecules

Innate effector molecules are known to play crucial roles in the gut immune responses of mammals. Most of these effector molecules are expressed in teleost fish, although most studies have looked at systemic rather than mucosal sites.

Enzymes: A number of enzymes, such as proteases, oxidases, peroxidases, and phosphatases, are important innate immune mechanisms found on the mucosal surfaces of vertebrates. Many of these enzymes have been studied in laboratory zebrafish and, to a lesser extent, in farmed teleost species. For the purposes of this chapter, two enzymes, the dual oxidase and the alkaline phosphatase, will be discussed.

Dual oxidase (duox) allows non-phagocytic cell types, such as epithelial cells, to produce superoxide anion and, therefore, have oxidative killing responses. In teleosts, duox is present and depletion of the receptors NOD1 or NOD2 decreases duox expression and leads to increased bacterial infection burdens in the intestine, presumably due to lower ROS production (Oehlers et al., 2011).

The intestinal specific enzyme intestinal alkaline phosphatase (IAP) is a marker for enterocyte maturation with important roles in intestinal immune homeostasis. This enzyme is able to dephosphorylate LPS from gut commensal bacteria. Dephosphorylated LPS has a lower TLR4 activation ability than native LPS, and, therefore, it can modulate inflammatory responses in the gut, including neutrophil infiltration (Bates et al., 2007). In mammals, IAP is present in vesicles released by the tips of enterocyte microvilli into the gut lumen (McConnell, et al., 2009).

Cytokines: Cytokines are innate immune molecules with many pleiotropic functions, which determine the type of adaptive immune responses that a pathogen elicits. Due to the specific characteristics of mucosal lymphoid tissues, certain cytokines appear to be even more important at mucosal sites than systemic lymphoid tissues. The balance between proinflammatory and anti-inflammatory cytokines is known to determine the immune status and health of the gut in mammals. In teleosts, studies are limited to gene expression profiles in response to infection or vaccination. For instance, a classic profile of proinflammatory cytokine up-regulation is observed in the proximal intestine of trout when infected by bath challenge with the bacterial pathogen *A. salmonicida* with increased expression levels of IL-1β, IL-8, TNF-α, and IFN-γ (Mulder et al., 2007). Mixed cytokine profiles were detected in the distal intestine of Atlantic cod after IP vaccination with heat-killed *V. anguillarum* (Caipang, 2013). In particular, significantly lower levels of IL-1β and significantly higher levels of IL-8 at 1 and 3 days and at 3 and 7 days, respectively, were detected in the aforementioned study.

In contrast with the observation of proinflammatory responses in response to antigenic stimulation, some studies have reported anti-inflammatory cytokine profiles. For instance, the gut of Atlantic cod IP infected with *Francisella noatunensis* undergoes anti-inflammatory responses characterized by increased IL-10 gene expression and decreased IL-1β and IFN-γ expression (Ellingsen et al., 2011). Similarly, chronic infection with myxozoan parasites, such as *E. leei*, results in down-regulation of intestinal IL-1 β, TNF-α, and GRP-75 (Sitja-Bobadilla, 2008).

IL-22 is a cytokine with specific gut mucosal immune functions in mammals (Sonnenberg et al., 2011). This molecule has recently been characterized in rainbow trout, and a recombinant protein as well as an antibody are now available (Monte et al., 2011). In the near future, the specific contribution of IL-22 to teleost gut immunity should be unraveled.

Chemokines: Chemokines are small molecules that direct the migration of lymphocytes to intestinal tissues and are also inflammation mediators. In mammalian gut, intestinal chemokines and their receptors have been studied in a number of infection models and are known to be secreted by both epithelial cells and immune cells.

Some of the mammalian mucosal chemokine pathways appear conserved in teleosts. For instance, the Cxcl8 signaling pathway is conserved in zebrafish and plays a role in intestinal inflammatory responses (Oehlers, 2010, p. 216). Teleost intestinal epithelial cells, like their mammalian counterparts, express Cxcl8, and its expression is up-regulated during inflammation in a laboratory zebrafish model (Oehlers et al., 2010).

Another example of conserved mucosal chemokines in teleosts and mammals is the CCL25 and CCR9 pair. CCL25/CCR9 is involved in T cell development and in gut-associated immune responses. The intimate relationship between this chemokine and its receptor is conserved in fish gut immunity as shown in recent studies on sea bass. Sea bass recombinant TNFα delivered as an oral vaccine increased IEL homing through CCL25/CCR9 activation (Galindo-Villegas et al., 2013).

CK12 is a rainbow trout chemokine highly expressed in mucosal tissues. In the gastrointestinal tract, the highest levels of expression are found in the foregut (Montero et al., 2011). CK12 is most closely related to the CCL19/21/25 chemokine group of mammalian chemokines, and a family that carries important mucosal immunity functions in mammals. Thus far, no functional studies on fish CK12 in response to infection have been conducted, limiting the use of this molecule for the control of aquatic infectious diseases.

It is clear that our understanding of the functional role of mucosal chemokines in fish is at its infancy. For instance, a vital question for memory responses in response to vaccination is: which chemokines attract plasmablasts and plasma cells to the gut mucosa? CCL28/CCR10 is a critical gut immunity chemokine pair in mammals. This pair directs the migration and maturation of IgA plasmablasts into the intestine (Hu et al., 2011; Lazarus et al., 2003). Although CCL28 has been identified in Atlantic salmon, its role in gut mucosal immunity of fish needs to be investigated.

Finally, chemokines control the overall integration and compartmentalization of mucosal immune responses in vertebrates. Thus far, the possible chemokine pairs that govern the connection between gut, skin, and gill mucosal immune responses of fish have not been found.

6.4.3 Adaptive immune responses in fish gut

6.4.3.1 Adaptive effector molecules

Adaptive humoral immunity relies on the presence of specific antibodies in body fluids that can neutralize, agglutinate, precipitate, or block the entry of a pathogen. As explained earlier in this chapter and in a number of reviews, immunoglobulins consist of two identical heavy chains and two identical light chains. Igs are present as a cell surface protein (part of the B cell receptor) or as secreted proteins. The two cell types responsible for Ig secretion are the plasmablast and the plasma cell (see Section 6.3.1.2).

In endotherms, adaptive immunity matures upon subsequent exposure to the same pathogen. This means that a secondary encounter to the same pathogen elicits a faster, stronger, and more effective immune response than that recorded during primary exposure. The processes of class switching, somatic hypermutation, and gene conversion are responsible for the maturation of the adaptive immune response in birds and mammals. These processes are not present in teleost fish, and, thus, the secondary and tertiary humoral adaptive immune responses of fish are somehow different from those of endotherms.

Secreted or secretory Igs are those Igs secreted by plasmablasts and plasma cells that are then transported across epithelial barriers to the mucosal secretions. Both IgM and IgT are secreted across the gut epithelium and found in the intestinal mucus of fish. Generally speaking, Ig titers from mucosal secretions are significantly lower than those found in serum. IgT, nevertheless, clearly plays a preponderant role in gut adaptive immunity (Zhang et al., 2010). Specific IgT responses appear confined to the gut as shown in rainbow trout that survive *C. shasta* infection. The mechanism by which specific IgT antibodies contribute to the clearance of *C. shasta* is yet unknown.

Specific IgM titers have also been reported in the gut (explants and/or mucosal secretions) in a number of vaccination studies and laboratory immunizations (reviewed by Salinas et al., 2011).

In summary, the recent breakthroughs in teleost mucosal Igs have revealed how critical it is to measure specific IgT levels in gut mucus in order to evaluate the health status of fish. Importantly, rational design of oral vaccines for fish should now be on target towards eliciting potent and long-lasting IgT adaptive immunity to the gut mucosa.

6.4.3.2 Adaptive effector cells

All jawed animals have two major arms of their adaptive immune system: B cells and T cells. Both cell types are present on mucosal surfaces and in systemic lymphoid organs, but mucosal B and T cells have evolved to better defend mucosal epithelia as well as to receive signals from the microbiota.

B cells: As explained earlier, teleosts have three different B cell subsets (Parra et al., 2013). IgM B cell numbers increase both in the anterior and posterior intestine of carp in response to the protozoan parasite *G. carpelli*, peaking at 15 days post-infection (Steinhagen and Rombout, 1994). Numbers of IgM^+ and IgT^+ B cells increase in the gut tissue of trout orally vaccinated with IPNV (Ballesteros et al., 2014). IgM and IgT B cells are recruited to the pyloric caeca of rainbow trout following oral vaccination with an alginate-encapsulated DNA vaccine against infectious pancreatic necrosis virus (Ballesteros et al., 2013). It is unclear how fish whose digestive tracts lack pyloric caeca or a stomach differ from those species that do have these structures.

Plasmablasts and plasma cells: Despite the importance of these two cell types for antibody production and establishing long-lasting humoral immunity, there are no studies on gut plasma cells during the course of an immune response. The current literature is limited to the description of when these cells appear during ontogeny.

T cells: There are two main types of T cells in vertebrates: the αβ and the γδ T cells. Both express CD3 on their surface and both are present in fish as discussed earlier in this chapter. Among the αβ T cells, a number of different subpopulations are well described in mammals. Of particular interest for the gut environment are Th17 T cells with largely innate proinflammatory functions. A second vital subset is the regulatory T cell (Treg), previously known as suppressor T cells. Tregs are responsible for the tolerogenic state of the gut mucosa, remaining highly irresponsive to harmless food and commensal antigens. Tregs are induced in the gut by the secretion of cytokines such as IL-10 and TGFβ. Due to the lack of cell markers and immune tools, the biology of mucosal T cells of fish is yet to be investigated. The numbers of $CD3^+$ cells increase in the gut of trout as a result of oral vaccination with IPNV (Ballesteros et al., 2013). Of relevance to the fish farming industry is the recent finding that, compared to injection vaccination, bath vaccination elicited intense Th17-like immune responses in the gut tissue of zebrafish and turbot, while Th1- and Th2-like responses were not remarkable (Zhang et al., 2014). However, these *in vivo* results are limited to gene expression profiles and should be further supported by studies at the protein level once tools are made available.

Cytotoxic T cells are characterized by the expression of CD8 on their surface, and they recognize antigenic peptides presented by all nucleated cells via MHC class I molecules. In the gut, most IELs are $CD8^+$ T cells responsible for the clearance of infected epithelial cells. The expression levels of CD8 may be indicative of specific cytotoxic T cell responses. The TCRβ repertoire of rainbow trout IELs is highly diverse in naïve individuals, and expanded clones are found in the gut during a response to a systemic infection with VHSV conducted in the laboratory. Modifications of the IEL TCRβ repertoire occur after laboratory infection with VHSV, suggesting that the trout gut epithelium contains responsive αβ T cells, like those found in systemic lymphoid tissues (Bernard et al., 2006). In mammals, γδ T cells represent 1–10% of all T cells in the blood and up to 30% in the intestine. These cells play a major role in mucosal immunity and recognize unconventional antigens without need for MHC presentation. Recent work on sea bass shows that expression levels of the TCR γ chain gene decrease in the gut following *in vivo* infection with betanodavirus (Buonocore et al., 2012). This is the only functional study concerning teleost γδ T cells and, since no specific antibodies are available, this field is not likely to advance in the near future.

6.5 The embryology and ontogeny of the gut immune system

Understanding how teleost gut immunity develops and acquires functional maturity is critical for the development of oral vaccines for use in aquaculture. Because development is directly related to temperature and different fish species have very different dietary requirements and gut anatomy and physiology, extrapolation from one species to another is likely an unsatisfactory approach. Generally speaking, the ontogeny of fish GALT is not well understood. It is generally assumed that mucosal immunity appears later during development compared to systemic immunity. Out of all the fish mucosal surfaces, it seems that the gut gets populated with immune cells earlier than the gills and the skin. However, this rule of thumb may not be universal to all teleost species. The lack of organized structures, such as Peyer's patches or lymph nodes present in mammals, complicates fish ontogeny studies, and very limited literature regarding this topic has been published. Common carp and zebrafish are the most widely used fish species for ontogenic studies. In this section, we will first discuss the embryology of the gastrointestinal system of fish. Next, the appearance of innate immune components in the gut of teleosts will be summarized. Finally, the presence of adaptive immune cells and markers, also in the gut, will be reviewed.

Gut tissue development in teleosts follows, at the molecular level, similar patterns to those described in higher vertebrates (amniotes). Thus, several transcription factors homologous to mammalian ones, such as *sox17*, *sox32*, *gata-4*, *-5*, and *-6*, and *foxA2*, are implicated in mesoderm development and consequent intestine ontogeny in zebrafish (Kikuchi et al., 2001; Reiter et al., 2001) and medaka fish (*Oryzias latipes*) (Kobayashi et al., 2006). However, some differences in morphogenesis exist between fish and amniotes. Thus, in fish, the pharynx and esophagus develop separately from the posterior gut tube, whereas, in amniotes, the pharynx, esophagus, and intestine primordium arise from the foregut. Additionally, intestine tube formation in fish requires the rearrangement of newly polarized cells rather than the folding of an endodermal sheet in amniotes (Wallace and Pack, 2003). Another important difference is that no apoptotic cells or cell debris are detected in the developing intestinal tract (Ng et al., 2005). This observation suggests that tubular morphogenesis in the zebrafish intestinal tract is independent of programmed cell death, in contrast to amniotes where apoptosis is required for the formation of intestinal epithelium (de Santa Barbara et al., 2003).

We can draw a timeline for gut development in zebrafish (Wallace and Pack, 2003; Ng et al., 2005). Zebrafish gut progenitors are identified already at 18 h post-fertilization (hpf). Then, the foregut is formed at 21 hpf, while the hindgut appears at 26 hpf. At 58 hpf, the pharynx, esophagus, and developing intestine with a visible lumen are contiguous. From 52–76 hpf, cells polarize to form the intestinal epithelium, and some enteroendocrine cells can be observed. At 76–126 hpf, the intestinal epithelium is differentiated with columnar epithelial cells and goblet cells, although not throughout the entire length of the intestine. Until 12 days post-fertilization (dpf), in fact, the mid-intestine is the sole site of goblet cell differentiation. However, by 120 hpf, it begins to perform its vital function of nutrient absorption. Goblet cells in these early stages are important not only for digestion, but also for innate immune responses thanks to the secretion of mucins that create an acidic environment.

Mucosal surfaces are colonized by millions of commensal bacteria that help to maintain homeostasis of the epithelium, control GALT development, and modulate the host's immune system (Hill and Artis, 2010). Thus, mice lacking commensal bacteria (germ-free animals) present impaired development of GALT tissue and a reduction in IgA in mucus secretions (Round and Mazmanian, 2009). In the same vein, gnotobiotic zebrafish present more comparable responses to microbiota than those observed in mice (Rawls et al., 2004), indicating that commensals, as well as pathogenic microbes, can up-regulate the activity of immune cells in intestine at these early stages (Kanther and Rawls, 2010).

Mucosal sites are the first line of defense at hatching. However, GALT and other MALT defenses do not start to develop in fish until the main lymphoid organs (i.e., head kidney, thymus, and spleen) have already commenced development. Overall, it is thought that fish GALT adaptive immunity develops after the GALT innate immunity. The first immune cells to populate the intestine of carp are macrophages at 4 dpf, and these macrophages are believed to originate in the head kidney (Huttenhuis et al., 2006b). Another cell from the myeloid lineage, the neutrophil, is present at high proportions in the gut 10 dpf, but, after that, the number of these cells in the intestine decreases (Huttenhuis et al., 2006c). In the early stages of gut development, other myeloid cells, such as eosinophils, basophils, and mast cells, do not appear to be present in this tissue. Together with some macrophages, few innate immune factors, such as complement factor 3 (C3), a_2-macroglobulin, and serum amyloid A (Huttenhuis et al., 2006a), have been detected early during development (4 dpf).

Regarding lymphoid cells in the intestine, rag-1 expression, an enzyme necessary for Ig and TCR formation, can be detected from 4 dpf, and *in situ* hybridization showed rag-1+ cells in the basal membrane from 7 dpf (Huttenhuis et al., 2005). However, in zebrafish, TCR transcripts can only be detected in the intestine at 9 dpf (Danilova et al., 2004). Using a monoclonal antibody (WCL38) against carp mucosal T cells, their presence in the intestine was detected as early as 3 dpf. Surprisingly, this occurs before the thymus gets populated by thymocytes. Zebrafish thymus is completely developed by 60 hpf and, by 68 hpf, is colonized by T lymphocyte progenitors, which begin to transcribe rag1 and rag2 at about 72 hpf (Schorpp et al., 2000; Trede and Zon, 1998). Carp WCL38$^+$ cells are very abundant in mucosal organs even before adaptive immunity is detected. Thus, some authors suggest that WCL38$^+$ carp cells could be homologs of mammalian $\gamma\delta$-T cells (Rombout et al., 1998). In the same vein, trout cells showing rag and TdT expression in the gut may be extrathymically developing $\gamma\delta$-intraepithelial T cell homologs (Hansen, 1997). Interestingly, in sea bass, which present a slower developmental rate than carp, in part due to differences in temperature, the first TCR transcripts in the intestine can be detected at 28 days post-hatching (dph) (Rombout et al., 2005).

Concerning B cells, as we described before, the structure of the trout and zebrafish heavy chain locus predicts the existence of at least two B cell subsets, one expressing IgT/Z and the other IgM. Thus, development of these two subsets could be different, and, in fact, as we will explain later, they do not appear at the same time during development. Some initial studies suggest that B cells originate in the kidney, although more recent studies suggest a lack of progenitors in the kidney due to the lack of rag-1 expression in early stages of development (Hansen and Zapata, 1998; Zapata et al., 2006). However, making use of GFP expression technology in zebrafish, the kidney is the first organ (after the thymus) that expresses rag-2 8 dpf (Trede et al., 2004). Danilova and Steiner (2002) observed rag-1 expression and the first rearrangement of genes encoding IgM at 4 and 10 dpf, respectively, in zebrafish pancreas, although the same authors later suggested that the rearrangement likely corresponds to IgZ instead of IgM (Danilova et al., 2005), indicating that IgT/Z B cells could appear before IgM B cells during development. However, in common carp, IgZ seems to appear later than IgM during ontogeny (Ryo et al., 2010). In zebrafish, the first IgM^+ B cells appear between the dorsal aorta and posterior cardinal vein and also in the kidney around 20 dpf (Page et al., 2013), while, in carp, the first IgM B cells are detected around 15 dpf (Huttenhuis et al., 2005; Romano et al., 1997). In carp, the first B cells appear in the intestine around 35 dpf (Huttenhuis et al., 2006b; Rombout et al., 2011). In sea bass, as occurs with T cells, the first B cells appear later than in carp or zebrafish, then first in the spleen and head kidney by 45 dph, and later in the intestine at 90 dph (Rombout et al., 2005). In trout, sequences of IgM^+ B cells appearances are similar to that of sea bass (Castillo et al., 1993).

6.6 Laboratory models that can contribute to our knowledge of gut immunity in aquaculture fish

The two most used laboratory models for the study of mucosal immunity are the zebrafish and the rainbow trout. Since rainbow trout is a farmed species, the translational value of laboratory experiments is potentially higher than that of zebrafish. Here, both strengths and weaknesses of each model are highlighted.

6.6.1 Zebrafish

Zebrafish is a widely used vertebrate model in biology. For a number of logistical reasons, studies on zebrafish are clearly increasing every year, yet the greatest value of this model so far has been for human medicine rather than aquaculture. Zebrafish can be raised under germ-free conditions, which brings unique opportunities for the study of interactions between host and microbes (pathogens or commensals) (Meijer et al., 2013). Zebrafish have been proposed as a model for a number of human gut disorders, such as Crohn's disease and inflammatory bowel disease, as well as infectious organisms such as *Giardia duodenalis V. cholerae* and herpes simplex virus (Antoine et al., 2014; Fleming et al., 2010; Oehlers et al., 2011; Runft et al., 2014; Tysnes et al., 2012). To date, the model has been mostly used to unravel mechanisms of innate intestinal immunity such as dual oxidase, alkaline phosphatase, mucus production, NOD receptors, and recruitment of inflammatory cells following chemical or microbial insults. Studies on the gut adaptive immune system of zebrafish are so far lacking.

Zebrafish have been adapted under laboratory conditions to be used as a host for important aquaculture-relevant infectious agents. For instance, *A. hydrophila*, *Mycobacterium marinum*, *Vibrio anguillarum*, *Edwardsiella ictaluri*, spring viraemia carp virus, VHSV, and IHNV can infect zebrafish (Chinchilla et al., 2013; Ludwig et al., 2011; O'Toole et al., 2004; Pressley et al., 2005; Sanders et al., 2003). The zebrafish is, therefore, a useful model organism that can help scientists understand the biology of pathogens and fish immunity and help fish farmers control infectious diseases. Currently, the use of this model for the study of teleost gut immunity is still at its infancy.

6.6.2 Rainbow trout

The discovery of IgT in rainbow trout and further development of immune tools, such as antibodies specific against the different B and T cell subsets, have established rainbow trout as the most used model for the study of teleost gut adaptive immunity. The studies concerning the trout gut immune system published in 2010 have translated into similar findings in the skin. Since rainbow trout is phylogenetically close to Atlantic salmon and salmonids are a commercially important farmed species worldwide, this laboratory model has the potential to advance and improve current mucosal health practices in fin-fish aquaculture. Further use of this model will require development of new tool kits, such as antibodies, against key gut mucosal health markers available in mammals.

6.6.3 The immunologist perspective: considering the hygiene hypothesis when translating lab gut immunity research to aquaculture fish

Both zebrafish and rainbow trout laboratory models have their own strengths, but they have one drawback if we consider the microbial environment in which these fish are raised and maintained. Microbial stimuli are known to be critical in developing and maintaining homeostasis of the gut immune system. The hygiene hypothesis, first proposed in the 1980s, is gaining support based on new studies that have compared the immune system of wild versus laboratory animals. This hypothesis postulates that early exposure in life to a "dirty" environment (rich in microorganisms) is critical for the onset of a tolerogenic immune status in the gut (Yazdanbakhsh et al., 2002). This tolerogenic state is achieved by the presence of a robust anti-inflammatory network and the consequent induction of Tregs that suppress Th1 and/or Th2 immune responses (Yazdanbakhsh et al., 2002). Thus, in humans, it has been proposed that the Western lifestyle eliminates exposure to microbes early in life. Laboratory animals, in turn, can be regarded as the Western counterparts of wild or farmed animals.

Wild fish, farmed fish, and laboratory fish encounter very different microbial environments throughout their lives (Figure 6.2). Laboratory fish can be regarded as the most "Westernized" of all three groups, farmed fish being the equivalent to a "developing country" exposed to high microbial burdens. Wild fish, in turn, likely face a broad spectrum of microbial environments during development, ranging from low microbial loads to highly contaminated, microbial-rich waters, depending on the habitat. Thus, wild fish may exhibit different forms of gut immunity that may fall within the spectrum of laboratory and farmed fish.

If the hygiene hypothesis is extended to the aquaculture context, a number of predictions can be made. The following predictions are pertinent to laboratory fish that have been hatched, weaned, and grown in laboratory conditions throughout their

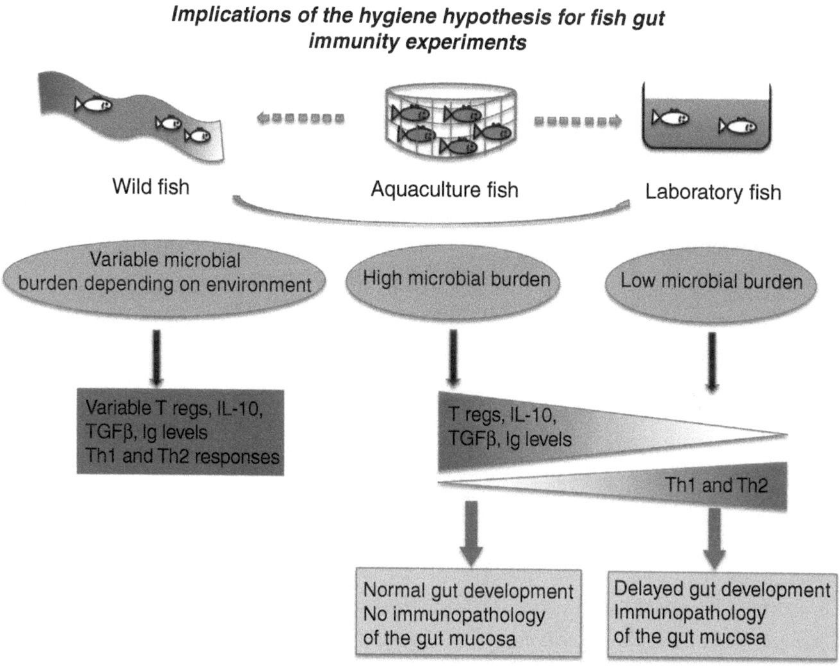

Figure 6.2 Potential implications of the hygiene hypothesis for the study of gut immunity in teleosts. The teleost gut immune system is often studied in research laboratory environments. Laboratory fish are born and maintained in water with a relatively low microbial burden. This is in sharp contrast with the microbial burdens to which farmed fish and wild fish are exposed. According to the hygiene hypothesis, the differences in the microbial burdens to which the gut of laboratory, farmed, and wild fish are exposed imply that the GALT development, as well as GALT function, of these animals is essentially different. Laboratory animals, according to the same hypothesis, are likely to be more prone to intestinal inflammation and unbalanced gut immune responses due to the absence of adequate regulatory T cells. This model is only a hypothetical extrapolation proposed here, and, therefore, its validation will require experimental testing. Intermittent arrows indicate that farmed fish are sometimes transported into laboratory aquaria or used to restock wild aquatic habitats. Full arrows indicates that, in some instances, wild fish can be transported to laboratory facilities to perform certain immune studies.

entire life span. Fish obtained from hatcheries and farms and then transported to laboratory facilities during adulthood are likely to not follow these predictions, at least not entirely. First, under farming conditions, the overall microbial load of the water is higher than in laboratory systems; therefore, the gut immune system of farmed fish is fundamentally different from that of laboratory fish. Second, laboratory fish lack the adequate microbial exposure required for the induction of tolerogenic gut immunity during development. Third, and as a consequence, laboratory fish may be more prone to mucosal inflammation and other gut disorders. Fourth, it is expected that the microbiome of farmed versus laboratory fish is different, and, furthermore, the Th1, Th2, and Treg balance must differ considerably from that of laboratory specimens.

In conclusion, according to the hygiene hypothesis and assuming that farmed fish are generally exposed to higher microbial burdens than laboratory fish, farmed fish should develop a more balanced and tolerogenic gut immune system, whereas laboratory fish are likely to display more gut disorders and be more prone to inflammation. It is obvious that important implications should derive from this hypothesis if knowledge generated in laboratory trials is to be translated into better health management for farmed fish. Comparisons between fish model organisms and farmed species need to be carried out in order to further underpin the limitations and value of laboratory investigations.

6.7 Concluding remarks

In spite of the critical relevance of understanding the gut immune system of fish for aquaculture management and disease prevention, our current knowledge remains patchy and circumstantial. Original oral vaccination success prompted the study of the GALT of wild and farmed teleosts. Today, commercial oral vaccines continue to be a promise. Current efforts to refine oral vaccines for use in aquaculture should be coupled with or pioneered by basic studies of the fish gut immune system.

Whereas significant advances have been made in recent years with respect to fish B cells and antibody responses in the gut mucosa, our current view of teleost gut immunity is far from complete. Important areas of research include: the role of different T cell subsets in the gut of fish, the biology of plasmablasts and plasma cells also in the gut, the role of gut macrophages and dendritic cells in bridging innate and adaptive immunity, and the chemokines and chemokine receptors that govern lymphocyte trafficking to the gut mucosa. In the near future, mucosal intervention on the gut mucosal surface of fish will require development of new research tools, such as monoclonal antibodies, and a deeper understanding of the unique aspects of teleost gut immunity with an emphasis on T cell subsets and long-lasting memory responses against commercially relevant infectious agents.

It is fair to say that the zebrafish model continues to increase our understanding of teleost gut innate immunity. Yet, translation of zebrafish-derived knowledge to the aquaculture industry needs to take place. In this respect, according to the hygiene hypothesis, the different microbial environments present in laboratory compared to fish farm facilities may severely limit the applicability of laboratory models to the aquaculture industry.

References

Abad, M.E., Binkhorst, F.M., Elbal, M.T., Rombout, J.H., 1987. A comparative immunocytochemical study of the gastro-entero-pancreatic (GEP) endocrine system in a stomachless and a stomach-containing teleost. Gen. Comp. Endocr. 66, 123–136.

Abelli, L., Coscia, M.R., De Santis, A., Zeni, C., Oreste, U., 2005. Evidence for hepato-biliary transport of immunoglobulin in the antarctic teleost fish *Trematomus bernacchii*. Dev. Comp. Immunol. 29, 431–442.

Allen, A., 1983. Mucus – a protective secretion of complexity. Trends Biochem. Sci. 8, 169–173.

Amend, D., Jhonson, K., 1981. Current status and future needs of *Vibrio anguillarum* bacterin. Dev. Biol. Stand. 49, 403–417.

Antoine, T.E., Jones, K.S., Dale, R.M., Shukla, D., Tiwari, V., 2014. Zebrafish: modeling for herpes simplex virus infections. Zebrafish 11, 17–25.

Ashida, H., Ogawa, M., Kim, M., Mimuro, H., Sasakawa, C., 2012. Bacteria and host interactions in the gut epithelial barrier. Nat. Chem. Biol. 8, 36–45.

Azad, I.S., Shankar, K.M., Mohan, C.V., Kalita, B., 2000. Uptake and processing of biofilm and free-cell vaccines of *Aeromonas hydrophila* in Indian major carps and common carp following oral vaccination – antigen localization by a monoclonal antibody. Dis. Aquat. Organ. 43, 103–108.

Bakke, A., Glover, C., Krogdahk, A., 2010. Feeding, Digestion and Absorption of Nutrients. Elservier Academic Press, Amsterdam.

Bakke-McKellep, A., McL Press, C., Baeverfjord, G., Krogdahl, Å., Landsverk, T., 2000. Changes in immune and enzyme histochemical phenotypes of cells in the intestinal mucosa of Atlantic salmon, *Salmo salar* L., with soybean meal-induced enteritis. J. Fish. Dis. 23, 115–127.

Bakke-McKellep, A.M., Froystad, M.K., Lilleeng, E., Dapra, F., Refstie, S., Krogdahl, A., Landsverk, T., 2007. Response to soy: T-cell-like reactivity in the intestine of Atlantic salmon, *Salmo salar* L. J. Fish. Dis. 30, 13–25.

Ballesteros, N.A., Castro, R., Abos, B., Saint-Jean, S.S.R., Perez-Prieto, S.I., Tafalla, C., 2013. The pyloric caeca area is a major site for IgM(+) and IgT(+) B cell recruitment in response to oral vaccination in rainbow trout. PloS one 8, e66118.

Ballesteros, N.A., Rodriguez Saint-Jean, S., Perez-Prieto, S.I., Aquilino, C., Tafalla, C., 2014. Modulation of genes related to the recruitment of immune cells in the digestive tract of trout experimentally infected with infectious pancreatic necrosis virus (IPNV) or orally vaccinated. Dev. Comp. Immunol. 44, 195–205.

Bannister, L.H., 1966. Is *Rhabdospora thelohani* (Laguesse) a sporozoan parasite or a tissue cell of lower vertebrates? Parasitology 56, 633–638.

Barr, J.J., Auro, R., Furlan, M., Whiteson, K.L., Erb, M.L., Pogliano, J., Stotland, A., Wolkowicz, R., Cutting, A.S., Doran, K.S., Salamon, P., Youle, M., Rohwer, F., 2013. Bacteriophage adhering to mucus provide a non-host-derived immunity. Proc. Natl. Acad. Sci. U.S.A. A110, 10771–10776.

Bassity, E., Clark, T.G., 2012. Functional identification of dendritic cells in the teleost model, rainbow trout (*Oncorhynchus mykiss*). PloS one 7, e33196.

Bates, J.M., Akerlund, J., Mittge, E., Guillemin, K., 2007. Intestinal alkaline phosphatase detoxifies lipopolysaccharide and prevents inflammation in zebrafish in response to the gut microbiota. Cell Host Microbe 2, 371–382.

Bernard, D., Six, A., Rigottier-Gois, L., Messiaen, S., Chilmonczyk, S., Quillet, E., Boudinot, P., Benmansour, A., 2006. Phenotypic and functional similarity of gut intraepithelial and systemic T cells in a teleost fish. J. Immunol. 176, 3942–3949.

Boschi, I., Randelli, E., Buonocore, F., Casani, D., Bernini, C., Fausto, A.M., Scapigliati, G., 2011. Transcription of T cell-related genes in teleost fish, and the European sea bass (*Dicentrarchus labrax*) as a model. Fish Shellfish Immunol. 31, 655–662.

Buonocore, F., Castro, R., Randelli, E., Lefranc, M.P., Six, A., Kuhl, H., Reinhardt, R., Facchiano, A., Boudinot, P., Scapigliati, G., 2012. Diversity, molecular characterization and

expression of T cell receptor gamma in a teleost fish, the sea bass (*Dicentrarchus labrax* L.). PloS one 7, e47957.
Caipang, C., 2013. Expression of genes involved in the early immune response at the distal segment of the gut in Atlantic cod, *Gadus morhua* L. after vaccination with a bacterial antigen. Aquacul. Int. 21, 591–603.
Casadei, E., Bird, S., Vecino, J.L., Wadsworth, S., Secombes, C.J., 2013. The effect of peptidoglycan enriched diets on antimicrobial peptide gene expression in rainbow trout (*Oncorhynchus mykiss*). Fish Shellfish Immunol. 34, 529–537.
Castillo, A., Sanchez, C., Dominguez, J., Kaattari, S.L., Villena, A.J., 1993. Ontogeny of IgM and IgM-bearing cells in rainbow trout. Dev. Comp. Immunol. 17, 419–424.
Castro, R., Bromage, E., Abos, B., Pignatelli, J., Gonzalez Granja, A., Luque, A., Tafalla, C., 2014. CCR7 is mainly expressed in teleost gills, where it defines an IgD + IgM-B lymphocyte subset. J. Immunol. 192, 1257–1266.
Cheesman, S.E., Neal, J.T., Mittge, E., Seredick, B.M., Guillemin, K., 2011. Epithelial cell proliferation in the developing zebrafish intestine is regulated by the Wnt pathway and microbial signaling via Myd88. Proc. Natl. Acad. Sci. U.S.A. A108 (Suppl 1), 4570–4577.
Chen, J., Wu, H.Q., Niu, H., Shi, Y.H., Li, M.Y., 2009. Increased liver protein and mRNA expression of natural killer cell-enhancing factor B (NKEF-B) in ayu (*Plecoglossus altivelis*) after *Aeromonas hydrophila* infection. Fish Shellfish Immunol. 26, 567–571.
Chinchilla, B., Gomez-Casado, E., Encinas, P., Falco, A., Estepa, A., Coll, J., 2013. *In vitro* neutralization of viral hemorrhagic septicemia virus by plasma from immunized zebrafish. Zebrafish 10, 43–51.
Cinar, K., Senol, N., Ozen, M.R., 2006. Immunohistochemical study on distribution of endocrine cells in gastrointestinal tract of flower fish (*Pseudophoxinus antalyae*). World J. Gastroenterol. 12, 6874–6878.
Cole, A.M., Darouiche, R.O., Legarda, D., Connell, N., Diamond, G., 2000. Characterization of a fish antimicrobial peptide: gene expression, subcellular localization, and spectrum of activity. Antimicrob. Agents Chemother. 44, 2039–2045.
Coombes, J.L., Powrie, F., 2008. Dendritic cells in intestinal immune regulation. Nat. Rev. Immunol. 8, 435–446.
Crowhurst, M.O., Layton, J.E., Lieschke, G.J., 2002. Developmental biology of zebrafish myeloid cells. Int. J. Dev. Biol. 46, 483–492.
Danilova, N., Bussmann, J., Jekosch, K., Steiner, L.A., 2005. The immunoglobulin heavy-chain locus in zebrafish: identification and expression of a previously unknown isotype, immunoglobulin Z. Nat. Immunol. 6, 295–302.
Danilova, N., Hohman, V.S., Sacher, F., Ota, T., Willett, C.E., Steiner, L.A., 2004. T cells and the thymus in developing zebrafish. Dev. Comp. Immunol. 28, 755–767.
Danilova, N., Steiner, L.A., 2002. B cells develop in the zebrafish pancreas. Proc. Natl. Acad. Sci. U.S.A. A99, 13711–13716.
Davidson, G.A., Ellis, A.E., Secombes, C.J., 1993. Route of immunization influences the generation of antibody secreting cells in the gut of rainbow trout (*Oncorhynchus mykiss*). Dev. Comp. Immunol. 17, 373–376.
Davina, J., Parmentier, H., Timmermans, L., 1982. Effect of oral administration of vibrio bacterin on the intestine of cyprinid fish. Dev. Comp. Immunol. 2, 157–166.
de Santa Barbara, P., van den Brink, G.R., Roberts, D.J., 2003. Development and differentiation of the intestinal epithelium. Cell. Mol. Life Sci. 60, 1322–1332.
Dezfuli, B., Pironi, F., Campisi, M., Shinn, A., Giari, L., 2010. The response of intestinal mucous cells to the presence of enteric helminths: their distribution, histochemistry and fine structure. J. Fish. Dis. 33, 481–488.

Dezfuli, B.S., Giari, L., 2008. Mast cells in the gills and intestines of naturally infected fish: evidence of migration and degranulation. J. Fish Dis. 31, 845–852.
Dezfuli, B.S., Giari, L., Arrighi, S., Domeneghini, C., Bosi, G., 2003. Influence of enteric helminths on the distribution of intestinal endocrine cells belonging to the diffuse endocrine system in brown trout *Salmo trutta* L. J. Fish Dis. 26, 155–166.
Dezfuli, B.S., Giari, L., Lui, A., Squerzanti, S., Castaldelli, G., Shinn, A.P., Manera, M., Lorenzoni, M., 2012. Proliferative cell nuclear antigen (PCNA) expression in the intestine of Salmo trutta trutta naturally infected with an acanthocephalan. Parasit. Vectors 5, 198.
Dezfuli, B.S., Giari, L., Squerzanti, S., Lui, A., Lorenzoni, M., Sakalli, S., Shinn, A.P., 2011. Histological damage and inflammatory response elicited by Monobothrium wageneri (Cestoda) in the intestine of Tinca tinca (Cyprinidae). Parasit. Vectors 4, 225.
Dezfuli, B.S., Giovinazzo, G., Lui, A., Giari, L., 2008. Inflammatory response to *Dentitruncus truttae* (Acanthocephala) in the intestine of brown trout. Fish Shellfish Immunol. 24, 726–733.
Dezfuli, B.S., Lui, A., Giovinazzo, G., Boldrini, P., Giari, L., 2009. Intestinal inflammatory response of powan *Coregonus lavaretus* (Pisces) to the presence of acanthocephalan infections. Parasitology 136, 929–937.
Dezfuli, B.S., Lui, A., Pironi, F., Manera, M., Shinn, A.P., Lorenzoni, M., 2013. Cell types and structures involved in tench, *Tinca tinca* (L.), defence mechanisms against a systemic digenean infection. J. Fish. Dis. 36, 577–585.
Diconza, J., Halliday, W., 1971. Relationship of catfish serum antibodies to immunoglobulin in mucus secretion. Aust. J. Exp. Biol. 49, 512–519.
Dobson, J.T., Seibert, J., Teh, E.M., Da'as, S., Fraser, R.B., Paw, B.H., Lin, T.J., Berman, J.N., 2008. Carboxypeptidase A5 identifies a novel mast cell lineage in the zebrafish providing new insight into mast cell fate determination. Blood 112, 2969–2972.
Drzewina, A., 1905. Contribution a l'etude du tissue lymphoide des Icnthyopsides. Arch. Zool. Exp. Generale 3, 145–338.
Duff, D., 1942. The oral immunization of trout against bacterium *Salmonicida*. J. Immunol., 44.
Edholm, E.S., Bengten, E., Stafford, J.L., Sahoo, M., Taylor, E.B., Miller, N.W., Wilson, M., 2010. Identification of two IgD+ B cell populations in channel catfish, *Ictalurus punctatus*. J. Immunol. 185, 4082–4094.
Ellingsen, T., Inami, M., Gjessing, M.C., Van Nieuwenhove, K., Larsen, R., Seppola, M., Lund, V., Schroder, M.B., 2011. *Francisella noatunensis* in Atlantic cod (*Gadus morhua* L.); waterborne transmission and immune responses. Fish Shellfish Immunol. 31, 326–333.
Ellis, A., 1988. Fish Vaccination. New York, Academic Press.
Ellis, A.E., 2001. Innate host defense mechanisms of fish against viruses and bacteria. Dev. Comp. Immunol. 25, 827–839.
Esteban, M.A., Chaves-Pozo, E., Arizcun, M., Meseguer, J., Cuesta, A., 2013. Regulation of natural killer enhancing factor (NKEF) genes in teleost fish, gilthead seabream and European sea bass. Mol. Immunol. 55, 275–282.
Estensoro, I., Jung-Schroers, V., Alvarez-Pellitero, P., Steinhagen, D., Sitja-Bobadilla, A., 2013. Effects of *Enteromyxum leei* (Myxozoa) infection on gilthead sea bream (*Sparus aurata*) (Teleostei) intestinal mucus: glycoprotein profile and bacterial adhesion. Parasitol. Res. 112, 567–576.
Feng, L., Peng, Y., Wu, P., Hu, K., Jiang, W.D., Liu, Y., Jiang, J., Li, S.H., Zhou, X.Q., 2013. Threonine affects intestinal function, protein synthesis and gene expression of TOR in Jian carp (*Cyprinus carpio* var. Jian). PloS one 8, e69974.
Feng, L.N., Lu, D.Q., Bei, J.X., Chen, J.L., Liu, Y., Zhang, Y., Liu, X.C., Meng, Z.N., Wang, L., Lin, H.R., 2009. Molecular cloning and functional analysis of polymeric immunoglobulin

receptor gene in orange-spotted grouper (*Epinephelus coioides*). Comp. Biochem. Physiol. B Biochem. Mol. Biol. 154, 282–289.

Fischer, U., Koppang, E.O., Nakanishi, T., 2013. Teleost T and NK cell immunity. Fish Shellfish Immunol. 35, 197–206.

Flajnik, M.F., 2010. All GOD's creatures got dedicated mucosal immunity. Nat. Immunol. 11, 777–779.

Fleming, A., Jankowski, J., Goldsmith, P., 2010. *In vivo* analysis of gut function and disease changes in a zebrafish larvae model of inflammatory bowel disease: a feasibility study. Inflamm. Bowel Dis. 16, 1162–1172.

Fletcher, T., White, A., 1973. Antibody production in the plaice *Pleuronectes platessa* after oral and parental immunisation with *Vibrio anguillarum* antigens. Aquaculture 1, 417–428.

Fu, G.H., Bai, Z.Y., Xia, J.H., Liu, F., Liu, P., Yue, G.H., 2013. Analysis of two lysozyme genes and antimicrobial functions of their recombinant proteins in Asian seabass. PloS one 8, e79743.

Galindo-Villegas, J., Mulero, I., Garcia-Alcazar, A., Munoz, I., Penalver-Mellado, M., Streitenberger, S., Scapigliati, G., Meseguer, J., Mulero, V., 2013. Recombinant TNF alpha as oral vaccine adjuvant protects European sea bass against vibriosis: insights into the role of the CCL25/CCR9 axis. Fish Shellfish Immunol. 35, 1260–1271.

Garcia, T., Otto, K., Kjelleberg, S., Nelson, D.R., 1997. Growth of *Vibrio anguillarum* in salmon intestinal mucus. Appl. Environ. Microbiol. 63, 1034–1039.

Georgopoulou, U., Vernier, J.M., 1986. Local immunological response in the posterior intestinal segment of the rainbow trout after oral administration of macromolecules. Dev. Comp. Immunol. 10, 529–537.

German, D.P., Neuberger, D.T., Callahan, M.N., Lizardo, N.R., Evans, D.H., 2010. Feast to famine: the effects of food quality and quantity on the gut structure and function of a detritivorous catfish (Teleostei: Loricariidae). Comp. Biochem. Physiol. A Mol. Integr. Physiol. 155, 281–293.

Gomez, D., Sunyer, J.O., Salinas, I., 2013. The mucosal immune system of fish: the evolution of tolerating commensals while fighting pathogens. Fish Shellfish Immunol. 35, 1729–1739.

Grosell, M., Farrell, A., Brauner, C., 2010. The Multifunctional Gut of Fish. Amsterdam, Elsevier.

Hansen, J.D., 1997. Characterization of rainbow trout terminal deoxynucleotidyl transferase structure and expression. TdT and RAG1 co-expression define the trout primary lymphoid tissues. Immunogenetics 46, 367–375.

Hansen, J.D., Landis, E.D., Phillips, R.B., 2005. Discovery of a unique Ig heavy-chain isotype (IgT) in rainbow trout: implications for a distinctive B cell developmental pathway in teleost fish. Proc. Natl. Acad. Sci. U.S.A. A102, 6919–6924.

Hansen, J.D., Zapata, A.G., 1998. Lymphocyte development in fish and amphibians. Immunol. Rev. 166, 199–220.

Harris, J.E., 1972. The immune response of a cyprinid fish to infections of the acanthocephalan *Pomphorhynchus laevis*. Int. J. Parasitol. 2, 459–469.

Hart, S., Wrathmell, A.B., Harris, J.E., Grayson, T.H., 1988. Gut immunology in fish: a review. Dev. Comp. Immunol. 12, 453–480.

Hatten, F., Fredriksen, A., Hordvik, I., Endresen, C., 2001. Presence of IgM in cutaneous mucus, but not in gut mucus of Atlantic salmon, *Salmo salar*. Serum IgM is rapidly degraded when added to gut mucus. Fish Shellfish Immunol. 11, 257–268.

Hedrera, M.I., Galdames, J.A., Jimenez-Reyes, M.F., Reyes, A.E., Avendano-Herrera, R., Romero, J., Feijoo, C.G., 2013. Soybean meal induces intestinal inflammation in zebrafish larvae. PloS one 8, e69983.

Hill, D.A., Artis, D., 2010. Intestinal bacteria and the regulation of immune cell homeostasis. Annu. Rev. Immunol. 28, 623–667.

Holmgren, S., Olsson, C., 2009. The neuronal and endocrine regulation of gut function. In: Bernier, N.J., d.K., G.V., Farrell, A.P., Brauner, C.J. (Eds.), Fish Neuroendocrinology. Amsterdam, Academic Press, pp. 467–512.

Holopainen, R., Tapiovaara, H., Honkanen, J., 2012. Expression analysis of immune response genes in fish epithelial cells following ranavirus infection. Fish Shellfish Immunol. 32, 1095–1105.

Hoole, D., Nisan, H., 1994. Ultrastructural studies on intestinal response of carp, *Cyprinus-carpio* L., to the Pseudophyllidean tapeworm, *Bothriocephalus-acheilognathi* Yamaguti, 1934. J. Fish. Dis. 17, 623–629.

Hu, S., Yang, K., Yang, J., Li, M., Xiong, N., 2011. Critical roles of chemokine receptor CCR10 in regulating memory IgA responses in intestines. Proc. Natl. Acad. Sci. U.S.A. A108, E1035–E1044.

Huttenhuis, H.B., Grou, C.P., Taverne-Thiele, A.J., Taverne, N., Rombout, J.H., 2006a. Carp (*Cyprinus carpio* L.) innate immune factors are present before hatching. Fish Shellfish Immunol. 20, 586–596.

Huttenhuis, II.B., Huising, M.O., van der Meulen, T., van Oosterhoud, C.N., Sanchez, N.A., Taverne-Thiele, A.J., Stroband, H.W., Rombout, J.H., 2005. Rag expression identifies B and T cell lymphopoietic tissues during the development of common carp (*Cyprinus carpio*). Dev. Comp. Immunol. 29, 1033–1047.

Huttenhuis, H.B., Romano, N., Van Oosterhoud, C.N., Taverne-Thiele, A.J., Mastrolia, L., Van Muiswinkel, W.B., Rombout, J.H., 2006b. The ontogeny of mucosal immune cells in common carp (*Cyprinus carpio* L.). Anat. Embryol. 211, 19–29.

Huttenhuis, H.B., Taverne-Thiele, A.J., Grou, C.P., Bergsma, J., Saeij, J.P., Nakayasu, C., Rombout, J.H., 2006c. Ontogeny of the common carp (*Cyprinus carpio* L.) innate immune system. Dev. Comp. Immunol. 30, 557–574.

Inami, M., Taverne-Thiele, A.J., Schroder, M.B., Kiron, V., Rombout, J.H., 2009. Immunological differences in intestine and rectum of Atlantic cod (*Gadus morhua* L.). Fish Shellfish Immunol. 26, 751–759.

Ishimoto, Y., Savan, R., Endo, M., Sakai, M., 2004. Non-specific cytotoxic cell receptor (NCCRP)-1 type gene in tilapia (*Oreochromis niloticus*): its cloning and analysis. Fish Shellfish Immunol. 16, 163–172.

Jacobshagen, E., 1915. Morphologie des Spiraldarms. Anatomischer Anzeiger 48, 188–201.

Jendrysek, S., Steinhagen, D., Drommer, W., Korting, W., 1994. Carp coccidiosis intestinal histo- and cytopathology under *Goussia carpelli* infection. Dis. Aquat. Org. 20, 171–182.

Johansen, F.E., Kaetzel, C.S., 2011. Regulation of the polymeric immunoglobulin receptor and IgA transport: new advances in environmental factors that stimulate pIgR expression and its role in mucosal immunity. Mucosal Immunol. 4, 598–602.

Joosten, P.H.M., Tiemersma, E., Threels, A., CaumartinDhieux, C., Rombout, J.H.W.M., 1997. Oral vaccination of fish against *Vibrio anguillarum* using alginate microparticles. Fish Shellfish Immunol. 7, 471–485.

Jutfelt, F., 2011. The epithelial barrier function of the fish intestine. London, UK. In: Farrell, A. (Ed.), Encyclopedia of Fish Physiology. Elsevier.

Kania, P.W., Sorensen, R.R., Koch, C., Brandt, J., Kliem, A., Vitved, L., Hansen, S., Skjodt, K., 2010. Evolutionary conservation of mannan-binding lectin (MBL) in bony fish: identification, characterization and expression analysis of three bona fide collectin homologues of MBL in the rainbow trout (*Onchorhynchus mykiss*). Fish Shellfish Immunol. 29, 910–920.

Kanther, M., Rawls, J.F., 2010. Host-microbe interactions in the developing zebrafish. Curr. Opin. Immunol. 22, 10–19.

Kawano, A., Haiduk, C., Schirmer, K., Hanner, R., Lee, L., Dixon, B., Bols, N., 2011. Development of a rainbow trout intestinal epithelial cell line and its response to lipopolysaccharide. Aquacul. Nut. 17, 241–252.

Kikuchi, Y., Agathon, A., Alexander, J., Thisse, C., Waldron, S., Yelon, D., Thisse, B., Stainier, D.Y., 2001. Casanova encodes a novel Sox-related protein necessary and sufficient for early endoderm formation in zebrafish. Genes Dev. 15, 1493–1505.

Kobayashi, D., Jindo, T., Naruse, K., Takeda, H., 2006. Development of the endoderm and gut in medaka, *Oryzias latipes*. Dev. Growth Differ. 48, 283–295.

Komatsu, K., Tsutsui, S., Hino, K., Araki, K., Yoshiura, Y., Yamamoto, A., Nakamura, O., Watanabe, T., 2009. Expression profiles of cytokines released in intestinal epithelial cells of the rainbow trout, *Oncorhynchus mykiss*, in response to bacterial infection. Dev. Comp. Immunol. 33, 499–506.

Kono, T., Korenaga, H., 2013. Cytokine gene expression in CD4 positive cells of the Japanese pufferfish. PloS one 8, e66364.

Krementz, A., Chapman, G., 1975. Ultrastructure of the posterior half of intestine of the channel fish, *Ictalurus punctatus*. J. Morphol. 145, 441–482.

Kuz'mina, V., Gelman, I., 1997. Membrane linked digestion in fish. Rev. Fish. Sci. 5, 99–129.

Kvamme, B.O., Gadan, K., Finne-Fridell, F., Niklasson, L., Sundh, H., Sundell, K., Taranger, G.L., Evensen, O., 2013. Modulation of innate immune responses in Atlantic salmon by chronic hypoxia-induced stress. Fish Shellfish Immunol. 34, 55–65.

Lang, T., Hansson, G.C., Samuelsson, T., 2007. Gel-forming mucins appeared early in metazoan evolution. Proc. Natl. Acad. Sci. U.S.A. A104, 16209–16214.

Lazarus, N.H., Kunkel, E.J., Johnston, B., Wilson, E., Youngman, K.R., Butcher, E.C., 2003. A common mucosal chemokine (mucosae-associated epithelial chemokine/CCL28) selectively attracts IgA plasmablasts. J. Immunol. 170, 3799–3805.

Leino, R.L., 1974. Ultrastructure of immature, developing, and secretory rodlet cells in fish. Cell Tissue Res. 155, 367–381.

Li, J., Barreda, D.R., Zhang, Y.A., Boshra, H., Gelman, A.E., Lapatra, S., Tort, L., Sunyer, J.O., 2006. B lymphocytes from early vertebrates have potent phagocytic and microbicidal abilities. Nat. Immunol. 7, 1116–1124.

Lokesh, J., Fernandes, J.M., Korsnes, K., Bergh, O., Brinchmann, M.F., Kiron, V., 2012. Transcriptional regulation of cytokines in the intestine of Atlantic cod fed yeast derived mannan oligosaccharide or beta-glucan and challenged with *Vibrio anguillarum*. Fish Shellfish Immunol. 33, 626–631.

Lom, J., Dykova, L., 1992. Protozoan parasites of fishes. Developments in aquaculture and fisheries sciences. Elsevier, Amsterdam.

Lovoll, M., Kilvik, T., Boshra, H., Bogwald, J., Sunyer, J.O., Dalmo, R.A., 2006. Maternal transfer of complement components C3-1, C3-3, C3-4, C4, C5, C7, Bf, and Df to offspring in rainbow trout (*Oncorhynchus mykiss*). Immunogenetics 58, 168–179.

Ludwig, M., Palha, N., Torhy, C., Briolat, V., Colucci-Guyon, E., Bremont, M., Herbomel, P., Boudinot, P., Levraud, J.P., 2011. Whole-body analysis of a viral infection: vascular endothelium is a primary target of infectious hematopoietic necrosis virus in zebrafish larvae. PLoS Pathogens 7, e1001269.

Lugo-Villarino, G., Balla, K.M., Stachura, D.L., Banuelos, K., Werneck, M.B., Traver, D., 2010. Identification of dendritic antigen-presenting cells in the zebrafish. Proc. Natl. Acad. Sci. US A107, 15850–15855.

Marel, M., Adamek, M., Gonzalez, S.F., Frost, P., Rombout, J.H., Wiegertjes, G.F., Savelkoul, H.F., Steinhagen, D., 2012. Molecular cloning and expression of two beta-defensin and two mucin genes in common carp (*Cyprinus carpio* L.) and their up-regulation after beta-glucan feeding. Fish Shellfish Immunol. 32, 494–501.

Martin, E., Verlhac Trichet, V., Legrand-Frossi, C., Frippiat, J.P., 2012. Comparison between intestinal and non-mucosal immune functions of rainbow trout, *Oncorhynchus mykiss*. Fish Shellfish Immunol. 33, 1258–1268.

McConnell, R., Higginbotham, J., Shifrin, D.J., Tabb, D.L., Coffey, R.J., Tyska, M.J., 2009. The enterocyte microvillus is a vesicle-generating organelle. J. Cell Biol. 185, 1285–1298.

McDole, J.R., Wheeler, L.W., McDonald, K.G., Wang, B., Konjufca, V., Knoop, K.A., Newberry, R.D., Miller, M.J., 2012. Goblet cells deliver luminal antigen to CD103+ dendritic cells in the small intestine. Nature 483, 345–349.

McGuckin, M.A., Linden, S.K., Sutton, P., Florin, T.H., 2011. Mucin dynamics and enteric pathogens. Nat. Rev. Microbiol. 9, 265–278.

Meijer, A.H., van der Vaart, M., Spaink, H.P., 2014. Real-time imaging and genetic dissection of host-microbe interactions in zebrafish. Cellular Microbiol. 16, 39–49.

Molnar, K., 2005. Histopathological changes caused by the metacestodes of *Neogryporhynchus cheilancristrotus* (Wedl, 1855) in the gut of the gibel carp, *Carassius gibelio*. Acta. Vet. Hung. 53, 45–52.

Monte, M.M., Zou, J., Wang, T., Carrington, A., Secombes, C.J., 2011. Cloning, expression and bioactivity studies of rainbow trout (*Oncorhynchus mykiss*) interleukin 22. Cytokine 55, 62–73.

Montero, J., Ordas, M.C., Alejo, A., Gonzalez-Torres, L., Sevilla, N., Tafalla, C., 2011. CK12, a rainbow trout chemokine with lymphocyte chemo-attractant capacity associated to mucosal tissues. Mol. Immunol. 48, 1102–1113.

Mowat, A.M., Bain, C.C., 2011. Mucosal macrophages in intestinal homeostasis and inflammation. J. Innate Immun. 3, 550–564.

Mulder, I.E., Wadsworth, S., Secombes, C.J., 2007. Cytokine expression in the intestine of rainbow trout (*Oncorhynchus mykiss*) during infection with *Aeromonas salmonicida*. Fish Shellfish Immunol. 23, 747–759.

Mulero, I., Sepulcre, M.P., Meseguer, J., Garcia-Ayala, A., Mulero, V., 2007. Histamine is stored in mast cells of most evolutionarily advanced fish and regulates the fish inflammatory response. Proc. Natl. Acad. Sci. U.S.A. A104, 19434–19439.

Murray, H.M., Gallant, J.W., Douglas, S.E., 2003. Cellular localization of pleurocidin gene expression and synthesis in winter flounder gill using immunohistochemistry and *in situ* hybridization. Cell Tissue Res. 312, 197–202.

Nelson, J., Dehn, M., 2010. The GI tract in air breathing. Elsevier/Academic Press, London.

Neuhaus, H., van der Marel, M., Caspari, N., Meyer, W., Enss, M.L., Steinhagen, D., 2007. Biochemical and histochemical effects of perorally applied endotoxin on intestinal mucin glycoproteins of the common carp *Cyprinus carpio*. Dis. Aquat. Organ. 77, 17–27.

Newaj-Fyzul, A., Adesiyun, A.A., Mutani, A., Ramsubhag, A., Brunt, J., Austin, B., 2007. *Bacillus subtilis* AB1 controls *Aeromonas* infection in rainbow trout (*Oncorhynchus mykiss* Walbaum). J. Appl. Microbiol. 103, 1699–1706.

Ng, A.N., de Jong-Curtain, T.A., Mawdsley, D.J., White, S.J., Shin, J., Appel, B., Dong, P.D., Stainier, D.Y., Heath, J.K., 2005. Formation of the digestive system in zebrafish: III. Intestinal epithelium morphogenesis. Dev. Biol. 286, 114–135.

Niklasson, L., Sundh, H., Fridell, F., Taranger, G.L., Sundell, K., 2011. Disturbance of the intestinal mucosal immune system of farmed Atlantic salmon (*Salmo salar*), in response to long-term hypoxic conditions. Fish Shellfish Immunol. 31, 1072–1080.

Oehlers, S.H., Flores, M.V., Hall, C.J., Crosier, K.E., Crosier, P.S., 2012. Retinoic acid suppresses intestinal mucus production and exacerbates experimental enterocolitis. Dis. Model. Mech. 5, 457–467.

Oehlers, S.H., Flores, M.V., Hall, C.J., O'Toole, R., Swift, S., Crosier, K.E., Crosier, P.S., 2010. Expression of zebrafish cxcl8 (interleukin-8) and its receptors during development and in response to immune stimulation. Dev. Comp. Immunol. 34, 352–359.

Oehlers, S.H., Flores, M.V., Hall, C.J., Swift, S., Crosier, K.E., Crosier, P.S., 2011. The inflammatory bowel disease (IBD) susceptibility genes NOD1 and NOD2 have conserved anti-bacterial roles in zebrafish. Dis. Model. Mech. 4, 832–841.

Olsen, R., Myklebust, R., Kaino, T., Ringo, E., 1999. Lipid digestibility and ultrastructural changes in the enterocytes of Arctic char (*Salvelinus alpinus* L.) fed linseed oil and soybean lecithin. Fish Physiol. Biochem. 21, 35–44.

O'Toole, R., Von Hofsten, J., Rosqvist, R., Olsson, P.E., Wolf-Watz, H., 2004. Visualisation of zebrafish infection by GFP-labelled *Vibrio anguillarum*. Microb. Pathogen. 37, 41–46.

Page, D.M., Wittamer, V., Bertrand, J.Y., Lewis, K.L., Pratt, D.N., Delgado, N., Schale, S.E., McGue, C., Jacobsen, B.H., Doty, A., Pao, Y., Yang, H., Chi, N.C., Magor, B.G., Traver, D., 2013. An evolutionarily conserved program of B-cell development and activation in zebrafish. Blood 122, e1–e11.

Pan, C.Y., Chen, J.Y., Cheng, Y.S., Chen, C.Y., Ni, I.H., Sheen, J.F., Pan, Y.L., Kuo, C.M., 2007. Gene expression and localization of the epinecidin-1 antimicrobial peptide in the grouper (*Epinephelus coioides*), and its role in protecting fish against pathogenic infection. DNA Cell Biol. 26, 403–413.

Parra, D., Takizawa, F., Sunyer, J., 2013. Evolution of B cell immunity. Annu. Rev. Anim. Biosci. 1, 65–97.

Perez-Sanchez, J., Estensoro, I., Redondo, M.J., Calduch-Giner, J.A., Kaushik, S., Sitja-Bobadilla, A., 2013. Mucins as diagnostic and prognostic biomarkers in a fish-parasite model: transcriptional and functional analysis. PloS one 8, e65457.

Picchietti, S., Guerra, L., Bertoni, F., Randelli, E., Belardinelli, M.C., Buonocore, F., Fausto, A.M., Rombout, J.H., Scapigliati, G., Abelli, L., 2011. Intestinal T cells of *Dicentrarchus labrax* (L.): gene expression and functional studies. Fish Shellfish Immunol. 30, 609–617.

Pressley, M.E., Phelan, rIII, P.E., Witten, P.E., Mellon, M.T., Kim, C.H., 2005. Pathogenesis and inflammatory response to *Edwardsiella tarda* infection in the zebrafish. Dev. Comp. Immunol. 29, 501–513.

Rawls, J.F., Samuel, B.S., Gordon, J.I., 2004. Gnotobiotic zebrafish reveal evolutionarily conserved responses to the gut microbiota. Proc. Natl. Acad. Sci. U.S.A. A101, 4596–4601.

Redondo, M.J., Alvarez-Pellitero, P., 2010. Carbohydrate patterns in the digestive tract of *Sparus aurata* L. and *Psetta maxima* (L.) (Teleostei) parasitized by *Enteromyxum leei* and *E. scophthalmi* (Myxozoa). Parasitol. Int. 59, 445–453.

Reite, O.B., 1998. Mast cells eosinophilic granule cells of teleostean fish: a review focusing on staining properties and functional responses. Fish Shellfish Immunol. 8, 489–513.

Reite, O.B., 2005. The rodlet cells of teleostean fish: their potential role in host defence in relation to the role of mast cells/eosinophilic granule cells. Fish Shellfish Immunol. 19, 253–267.

Reite, O.B., Evensen, O., 2006. Inflammatory cells of teleostean fish: a review focusing on mast cells/eosinophilic granule cells and rodlet cells. Fish Shellfish Immunol. 20, 192–208.

Reiter, J.F., Kikuchi, Y., Stainier, D.Y., 2001. Multiple roles for GATA5 in zebrafish endoderm formation. Development 128, 125–135.

Romano, N., Caccia, E., Piergentili, R., Rossi, F., Ficca, A.G., Ceccariglia, S., Mastrolia, L., 2011. Antigen-dependent T lymphocytes (TcRbeta+) are primarily differentiated in the thymus rather than in other lymphoid tissues in sea bass (*Dicentrarchus labrax*, L.). Fish Shellfish Immunol. 30, 773–782.

Romano, N., Taverne-Thiele, J., van Maanen, J., Rombout, J., 1997. Leucocyte subpopulations in developing carp (*Cyprinus carpio* L.): immunocytochemical studies. Fish Shellfish Immunol. 7, 439–453.

Rombout, J., Bot, H., Taverne-Thiele, A., 1989. Immunological importance of the second segment of carp. II. Characterization of mucosal leukocytes. J. Fish Biol. 35, 167–178.

Rombout, J.H., Abelli, L., Picchietti, S., Scapigliati, G., Kiron, V., 2011. Teleost intestinal immunology. Fish Shellfish Immunol. 31, 616–626.

Rombout, J.H., Huttenhuis, H.B., Picchietti, S., Scapigliati, G., 2005. Phylogeny and ontogeny of fish leucocytes. Fish Shellfish Immunol. 19, 441–455.

Rombout, J.H., Joosten, P.H., Engelsma, M.Y., Vos, A.P., Taverne, N., Taverne-Thiele, J.J., 1998. Indications for a distinct putative T cell population in mucosal tissue of carp (*Cyprinus carpio* L.). Dev. Comp. Immunol. 22, 63–77.

Rombout, J.H., Lamers, C.H., Helfrich, M.H., Dekker, A., Taverne-Thiele, J.J., 1985. Uptake and transport of intact macromolecules in the intestinal epithelium of carp (*Cyprinus carpio* L.) and the possible immunological implications. Cell Tissue Res. 239, 519–530.

Rombout, J.H., Taverne-Thiele, A.J., Villena, M.I., 1993. The gut-associated lymphoid tissue (GALT) of carp (*Cyprinus carpio* L.): an immunocytochemical analysis. Dev. Comp. Immunol. 17, 55–66.

Rombout, J.H., van den Berg, A.A., 1989. Immunological importance of the second segment of carp. I. Uptake and processing of antigens by epithelial cells and macrophages. J. Fish Biol. 35, 13–22.

Rombout, J.H., van der Tuin, S.J., Yang, G., Schopman, N., Mroczek, A., Hermsen, T., Taverne-Thiele, J.J., 2008. Expression of the polymeric immunoglobulin receptor (pIgR) in mucosal tissues of common carp (*Cyprinus carpio* L.). Fish Shellfish Immunol. 24, 620–628.

Rombout, J.W., Blok, L.J., Lamers, C.H., Egberts, E., 1986. Immunization of carp (*Cyprinus carpio*) with a *Vibrio anguillarum* bacterin: indications for a common mucosal immune system. Dev. Comp. Immunol. 10, 341–351.

Round, J.L., Mazmanian, S.K., 2009. The gut microbiota shapes intestinal immune responses during health and disease. Nat. Rev. Immunol. 9, 313–323.

Roussel, P., Delmotte, P., 2004. The diversity of epithelial secreted mucins. Curr. Org. Chem. 8, 413–437.

Runft, D.L., Mitchell, K.C., Abuaita, B.H., Allen, J.P., Bajer, S., Ginsburg, K., Neely, M.N., Withey, J.H., 2014. Zebrafish as a natural host model for *Vibrio cholerae* colonization and transmission. Appl. Environ. Microbiol. 80, 1710–1717.

Ryo, S., Wijdeven, R.H., Tyagi, A., Hermsen, T., Kono, T., Karunasagar, I., Rombout, J.H., Sakai, M., Verburg-van Kemenade, B.M., Savan, R., 2010. Common carp have two subclasses of bonyfish specific antibody IgZ showing differential expression in response to infection. Dev. Comp. Immunol. 34, 1183–1190.

Salinas, I., Myklebust, R., Esteban, M.A., Olsen, R.E., Meseguer, J., Ringo, E., 2008. *In vitro* studies of *Lactobacillus delbrueckii* subsp. *lactis* in Atlantic salmon (*Salmo salar* L.) foregut: tissue responses and evidence of protection against *Aeromonas salmonicida* subsp. *salmonicida* epithelial damage. Vet. Microbiol. 128, 167–177.

Salinas, I., Zhang, Y.A., Sunyer, J.O., 2011. Mucosal immunoglobulins and B cells of teleost fish. Dev. Comp. Immunol. 35, 1346–1365.

Sanders, G.E., Batts, W.N., Winton, J.R., 2003. Susceptibility of zebrafish (*Danio rerio*) to a model pathogen, spring viremia of carp virus. Comp. Med. 53, 514–521.

Schorpp, M., Bialecki, M., Diekhoff, D., Walderich, B., Odenthal, J., Maischein, H.M., Zapata, A.G., Boehm, T., 2006. Conserved functions of Ikaros in vertebrate lymphocyte development: genetic evidence for distinct larval and adult phases of T cell development and two lineages of B cells in zebrafish. J. Immunol. 177, 2463–2476.
Schorpp, M., Wiest, W., Egger, C., Hammerschmidt, M., Schlake, T., Boehm, T., 2000. Genetic dissection of thymus development. Curr. Top Microbiol. 251, 119–124.
Schroers, V., Van der Marel, M., Steinhagen, D., 2008. Influence of carp intestinal mucus molecular size and glycosylation on bacterial adhesion. Dis. Aquat. Organ. 81, 135–142.
Shan, M., Gentile, M., Yeiser, J.R., Walland, A.C., Bornstein, V.U., Chen, K., He, B., Cassis, L., Bigas, A., Cols, M., Comerma, L., Huang, B., Blander, J.M., Xiong, H., Mayer, L., Berin, C., Augenlicht, L.H., Velcich, A., Cerutti, A., 2013. Mucus enhances gut homeostasis and oral tolerance by delivering immunoregulatory signals. Science 342, 447–453.
Shen, L., Stuge, T.B., Zhou, H., Khayat, M., Barker, K.S., Quiniou, S.M., Wilson, M., Bengten, E., Chinchar, V.G., Clem, L.W., Miller, N.W., 2002. Channel catfish cytotoxic cells: a mini-review. Dev. Comp. Immunol. 26, 141–149.
Shen, Y., Zhang, J., Xu, X., Fu, J., Li, J., 2012. Expression of complement component C7 and involvement in innate immune responses to bacteria in grass carp. Fish Shellfish Immunol. 33, 448–454.
Silphaduang, U., Noga, E.J., 2001. Peptide antibiotics in mast cells of fish. Nature 414, 268–269.
Sire, M.F., Vernier, J.M., 1995. Partial characterization of eosinophilic granule cells (EGCs) and identification of mast cells of the intestinal lamina propria in rainbow trout (*Oncorhynchus mykiss*) Biochemical and cytochemical study. Biol. Cell. 85, 35–41.
Sitja-Bobadilla, A., 2008. Fish immune response to Myxozoan parasites. Parasite 15, 420–425.
Smith, P.D., Smythies, L.E., Shen, R., Greenwell-Wild, T., Gliozzi, M., Wahl, S.M., 2011. Intestinal macrophages and response to microbial encroachment. Mucosal Immunol. 4, 31–42.
Sonnenberg, G.F., Fouser, L.A., Artis, D., 2011. Border patrol: regulation of immunity, inflammation and tissue homeostasis at barrier surfaces by IL-22. Nat. Immunol. 12, 383–390.
Steinhagen, D., Rombout, J.H., 1994. Response of Ig-positive cells to *Goussia carpelli* (Protozoa: Apicomplexa) infections in carp (*Cyprinus carpio* L.). Folia Parasitol. 41, 173–176.
Stelnhagen, D., Hespe, K., 1997. Caro coccidiosis: activity of phagocytic cells from common carp infected with *Goussia carpelli*. Dis. Aquat. Org. 31, 155–159.
Studnicka, M., Siwicki, A., 1990. The nonspecific immunological response in carp (*Cyprinus carpio* L.) during natural infection with *Eimeria subepithelial*. Bamidgeh 42, 18–21.
Sveinbjornsson, B., Olsen, R., Paulsen, S., 1996. Immunocytochemical localization of lysozyme in intestinal eosinophilic granule cells of Atlantic salmon, *Salmo salar* L. J. Fish. Dis. 19, 349–355.
Syakuri, H., Adamek, M., Brogden, G., Rakus, K.L., Matras, M., Irnazarow, I., Steinhagen, D., 2013. Intestinal barrier of carp (*Cyprinus carpio* L.) during a cyprinid herpesvirus 3-infection: molecular identification and regulation of the mRNA expression of claudin encoding genes. Fish Shellfish Immunol. 34, 305–314.
Takizawa, F., Dijkstra, J.M., Kotterba, P., Korytar, T., Kock, H., Kollner, B., Jaureguiberry, B., Nakanishi, T., Fischer, U., 2011. The expression of CD8alpha discriminates distinct T cell subsets in teleost fish. Dev. Comp. Immunol. 35, 752–763.
Tezuka, H., Abe, Y., Iwata, M., Takeuchi, H., Ishikawa, H., Matsushita, M., Shiohara, T., Akira, S., Ohteki, T., 2007. Regulation of IgA production by naturally occurring TNF/iNOS-producing dendritic cells. Nature 448, 929–933.
Thornton, D.J., Rousseau, K., McGuckin, M.A., 2008. Structure and function of the polymeric mucins in airways mucus. Ann. Rev. Physiol. 70, 459–486.

Torrecillas, S., Makol, A., Benitez-Santana, T., Caballero, M.J., Montero, D., Sweetman, J., Izquierdo, M., 2011. Reduced gut bacterial translocation in European sea bass (*Dicentrarchus labrax*) fed mannan oligosaccharides (MOS). Fish Shellfish Immunol. 30, 674–681.

Trede, N.S., Langenau, D.M., Traver, D., Look, A.T., Zon, L.I., 2004. The use of zebrafish to understand immunity. Immunity 20, 367–379.

Trede, N.S., Zon, L.I., 1998. Development of T-cells during fish embryogenesis. Dev. Comp. Immunol. 22, 253–263.

Tysnes, K.R., Jorgensen, A., Poppe, T., Midtlyng, P.J., Robertson, L.J., 2012. Preliminary experiments on use of zebrafish as a laboratory model for *Giardia duodenalis* infection. Acta Parasitol./Witold Stefanski Institute of Parasitology, Warszawa, Poland 57, 1–6.

Uematsu, S., Fujimoto, K., Jang, M.H., Yang, B.G., Jung, Y.J., Nishiyama, M., Sato, S., Tsujimura, T., Yamamoto, M., Yokota, Y., Kiyono, H., Miyasaka, M., Ishii, K.J., Akira, S., 2008. Regulation of humoral and cellular gut immunity by lamina propria dendritic cells expressing Toll-like receptor 5. Nat. Immunol. 9, 769–776.

Uran, P., Schrama, J., Rombout, J., Obach, A., Jensen, L., Koppe, W., Verreth, J., 2008. Soybean meal-induced enteritis in Atlantic salmon (*Salmo salar* L.) at different temperatures. Aquacul. Nut. 14, 324–330.

Uran, P.A., Schrama, J.W., Rombout, J.H., Taverne-Thiele, J.J., Obach, A., Koppe, W., Verreth, J.A., 2009. Time-related changes of the intestinal morphology of Atlantic salmon, *Salmo salar* L., at two different soybean meal inclusion levels. J. Fish. Dis. 32, 733–744.

Vallejo, Jr., A.N., Ellis, A.E., 1989. Ultrastructural study of the response of eosinophil granule cells to *Aeromonas salmonicida* extracellular products and histamine liberators in rainbow trout *Salmo gairdneri* Richardson. Dev. Comp. Immunol. 13, 133–148.

van der Marel, M., Pröpsting, M., Battermann, F., Jung-Schroers, V., Hübner, A., Rombout, J., Steinhagen, D., 2013. Differences between intestinal segments and soybean meal–induced changes in intestinal mucus composition of common carp *Cyprinus carpio* L. Aquacul. Nut. 20.

Vasta, G.R., Nita-Lazar, M., Giomarelli, B., Ahmed, H., Du, S., Cammarata, M., Parrinello, N., Bianchet, M.A., Amzel, L.M., 2011. Structural and functional diversity of the lectin repertoire in teleost fish: relevance to innate and adaptive immunity. Dev. Comp. Immunol. 35, 1388–1399.

Vigliano, F.A., Munoz, L., Hernandez, D., Cerutti, P., Bermudez, R., Quiroga, M.I., 2011. An immunohistochemical study of the gut neuroendocrine system in juvenile pejerrey *Odontesthes bonariensis* (Valenciennes). J. Fish Biol. 78, 901–911.

Wallace, K.N., Pack, M., 2003. Unique and conserved aspects of gut development in zebrafish. Dev. Biol. 255, 12–29.

Wanstall, S.T., Robotham, P.W., Thomas, J.S., 1986. Pathological changes induced by *Pomphorhynchus laevis* Muller (Acanthocephala) in the gut of rainbow trout *Salmo gairdneri* Richardson. Zeitschrift fur Parasitenkunde 72, 105–114.

Watanabe, Y., 1982. Intracellular digestion of horseradish peroxidase by the intestinal cells of teleost larvae and juveniles. Bull. Jap. Soc. Sci. Fish 48, 37–47.

Xia, J.H., Liu, P., Liu, F., Lin, G., Sun, F., Tu, R., Yue, G.H., 2013. Analysis of stress-responsive transcriptome in the intestine of Asian seabass (*Lates calcarifer*) using RNA-seq. DNA Res. 20, 449–460.

Xu, Z., Parra, D., Gomez, D., Salinas, I., Zhang, Y.A., von Gersdorff Jorgensen, L., Heinecke, R.D., Buchmann, K., LaPatra, S., Sunyer, J.O., 2013. Teleost skin, an ancient mucosal surface that elicits gut-like immune responses. Proc. Natl. Acad. Sci. U.S.A. 110, 13097–13102.

Yazdanbakhsh, M., Kremsner, P.G., van Ree, R., 2002. Allergy, parasites, and the hygiene hypothesis. Science 296, 490–494.

Zapata, A., 1979. Ultrastructure of the gut associated lymphoid tissue (GALT) of *Rutilus rutilus*. Morphol. Norm. Patol. Ser. 3, 23–39.

Zapata, A., Diez, B., Cejalvo, T., Gutierrez-de Frias, C., Cortes, A., 2006. Ontogeny of the immune system of fish. Fish Shellfish Immunol. 20, 126–136.

Zhang, H., Shen, B., Wu, H., Gao, L., Liu, Q., Wang, Q., Xiao, J., Zhang, Y., 2014. Th17-like immune response in fish mucosal tissues after administration of live attenuated *Vibrio anguillarum* via different vaccination routes. Fish Shellfish Immunol. 37, 229–238.

Zhang, Y.A., Salinas, I., Li, J., Parra, D., Bjork, S., Xu, Z., LaPatra, S.E., Bartholomew, J., Sunyer, J.O., 2010. IgT, a primitive immunoglobulin class specialized in mucosal immunity. Nat. Immunol. 11, 827–835.

Environmental impacts on fish mucosa

7

Henrik Sundh; Kristina S. Sundell
Fish Endocrinology Laboratory, Department of Biological and Environmental Sciences, University of Gothenburg, Gothenburg, Sweden

Chapter Outline

7.1 Introduction

Living in water, the body fluids of fish are in intimate physiological contact with the external environment across the primary barriers (i.e., the gills, skin, and gastrointestinal (GI) tract). A life in water is challenging, and different external environments constitute major physiological challenges and need to be counteracted through physiological and behavioral mechanisms. Variations in water conditions, such as dissolved oxygen (DO) levels, temperature, salinity, and pathogenic loads, will have a direct impact on these primary barriers, the epithelia, and on the internal environment (i.e., the body fluids, cells, tissues, and organs). The aqueous environment, especially marine, is also a thriving habitat for microorganisms, including both viruses and bacteria (Wilhelm and Suttle, 1999). Many of these microorganisms are pathogenic and able to infect fish. Furthermore, certain fish species go through major habitat changes during their lifecycle. One interesting example is the anadromous salmonids, which undergo marked morphological, physiological, and behavioral transitions during the parr smolt transformation to prepare for transfer from freshwater (FW) to seawater (SW). Transitional periods represent critical and often stressful events, when the fish have a reduced capacity to survive additional stressors and/or infections. The intimate contact with the external environment represents a challenge for all epithelia in their role as barriers, both in terms of osmoregulation as well as in disease resistance and preventing the entry of harmful substances. Of all the primary barriers, the intestine is the major absorptive organ for nutrients, and, because it supports a vast number of microbes, it is termed the indigenous microbiota. Microbial density of the human large intestine has been estimated to be 10^{12} bacteria per gram of luminal content (Geuking et al., 2014; Lukas et al., 2006). In fish, the bacterial density is lower, where 10^4–10^8 viable counts per gram of luminal content have been reported. Bacterial communities are frequently represented by species such as *Flavobacterium-Cytophaga, Achromobacter, Vibrio, Pseudomonas,* and *Aeromonas* (Cahill, 1990). Normally, this indigenous microflora remains harmless inside the lumen. Rather, the indigenous flora is regarded as beneficial for the host by facilitating the digestion and thereby providing the host with nutrients otherwise inaccessible (Bischoff, 2011; Jacobs et al., 2009). Further, commensal gut microbiota serve as protection against pathogenic bacteria by competing for ecological niches and other physical resources as well as by directly inhibiting growth of pathogenic bacteria (Jöborn et al., 1997). In a healthy fish with a healthy intestine, both the indigenous microbiota and potentially harmful luminal content is prevented entry to the circulation by several layers of barriers that cooperate and communicate to prevent infection. If health (in the broad definition as described in Section 7.2) is impaired, a disturbance of this balance may reduce the protective barriers and, thus, allow pathogens and other harmful substances to enter the host.

This chapter will focus on describing the physical barrier function of the intestine, the role of the tight junction (TJ), and how intestinal permeability is assessed and will also give examples of how intestinal permeability is affected and regulated by factors in the external and internal environment in relation to intestinal health.

7.2 Intestinal barrier function

The intestinal barrier, separating the luminal environment from the internal milieu, is made up of several layers of primary barrier: the extrinsic mucus barrier, the intrinsic physical epithelial barrier, and the immunological barrier (Figure 7.1). In fish, as in mammals, the mucus layer covers the epithelial cell surfaces, and the main components of this mucus layer are the secreted mucins. These mucins are continuously secreted and wash away trapped particles (Ellis, 2001; Gomez et al., 2013; Linden et al., 2008; Shephard, 1994; Sweetman et al., 2010; Torrecillas et al., 2011). In mammals, each mucin can carry in the order of 100 different carbohydrate structures, which provides a vast array of potential binding sites for microbes (Linden et al., 2008). The

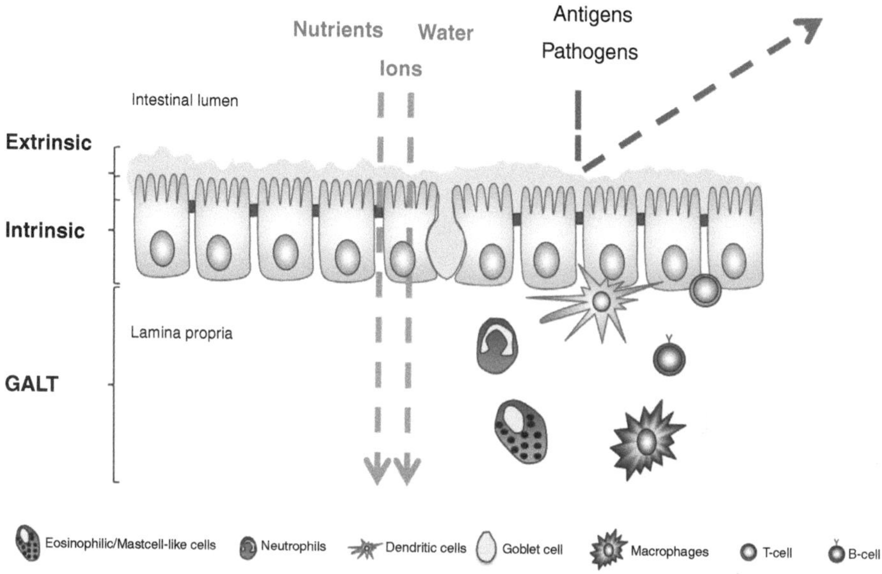

Figure 7.1 The fish intestinal barrier. The barrier is composed of a simple layer of columnar epithelial cells as well as the underlying lamina propria and muscular layer. Goblet cells, which synthesize and release mucins, the extrinsic part of the barrier, are also present.

mucus layer further contains antimicrobial and antiviral factors (Collet, 2014; Easy and Ross, 2010; Ellis, 2001; Gomez et al., 2013; Niklasson et al., 2014; Rombout et al., 2011), which actively neutralize possible intraluminal pathogens.

The epithelial barrier consists of a single-celled layer that lines the gut lumen and serves two essential and critical functions. First, it is responsible for absorption of dietary nutrients, electrolytes, and fluid from the intestinal lumen. Second, it serves as a barrier to prevent the passage of harmful substances within the intestinal lumen such as foreign antigens, pathogens, and other toxins. Thus, the intestine performs somewhat opposing tasks that demand selectivity. This selectivity is achieved and controlled at two main levels: transcellular transport through the intestinal epithelial cells (enterocytes) and a paracellular pathway between the enterocytes (Figure 7.2). Transcellular permeability reflects transport through the apical enterocyte membrane, along with transport through the cell, followed by excretion across the basolateral membrane. All three steps are usually mediated by selective transporters/carriers/channels as well as transporting proteins for ions, amino acids, peptides, sugars, and fatty acids. Paracellular permeability is mainly controlled by the cell–cell contact enforced by intercellular protein complexes situated along the lateral membrane, but is focused to the apical region of the enterocytes. The cell–cell contact is maintained by three main components: desmosomes, adherence junctions (AJs), and TJs. While AJs and desmosomes are mainly responsible for the structural cell–cell contact, the most apical protein complex (i.e., the TJs in Figure 7.3) is the main protein complex responsible for sealing intercellular space and regulating the selectivity of the paracellular pathway

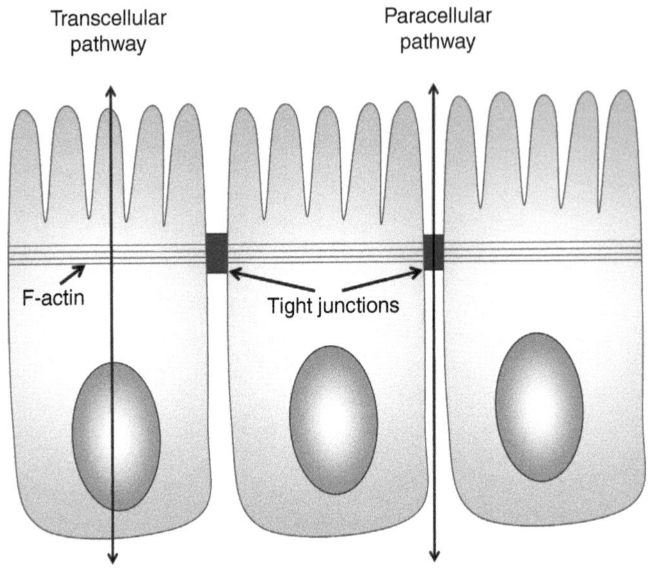

Figure 7.2 Intestinal epithelial permeability. Transcellular permeability is associated with the movement of macromolecules, ions, nutrients, and fluid through intestinal epithelial cells. Paracellular permeability is associated with movement through the lateral intercellular space between the epithelial cells and is mainly regulated by the tight junctions located towards the apical side of the lateral membranes.

(Günzel and Yu, 2013). TJs also generate a polarity to the epithelium by restricting the diffusion of lipids and proteins between the apical and basolateral membrane (Fanning et al., 1999).

Within the gut, pathogens such as viruses, bacteria, bacterial toxins, and other harmful substances that breach the first two layers will encounter the immunological barrier (i.e., the gut-associated lymphoid tissue (GALT)) (see Gomez et al., 2013; Rombout et al., 2011; and Chapter 6 for recent reviews on GALT in teleost fish).

7.2.1 The main determiner of paracellular permeability – the tight junctions

TJs, as observed on ultrathin section electron micrographs, appear as a set of fusion points between the outermost parts of the cell membrane of adjacent cells (Tsukita and Furuse, 1999). TJs constitute several physiologically regulated proteins that form the circumferential seals around adjacent epithelial cells and consist of more than 40 different proteins. Three of the main protein families found in TJs are occludins, claudins, and junction-associated membrane proteins (JAM). The claudins and occludins form the backbone of the TJ (Figure 7.3), while the JAM appear to be important for controlling the traffic of immune cells through the paracellular pathway (González-Mariscal et al., 2003). To provide a functional seal for the paracellular pathway, the TJ proteins are assembled and positioned by numerous cytosolic plaque proteins – one important

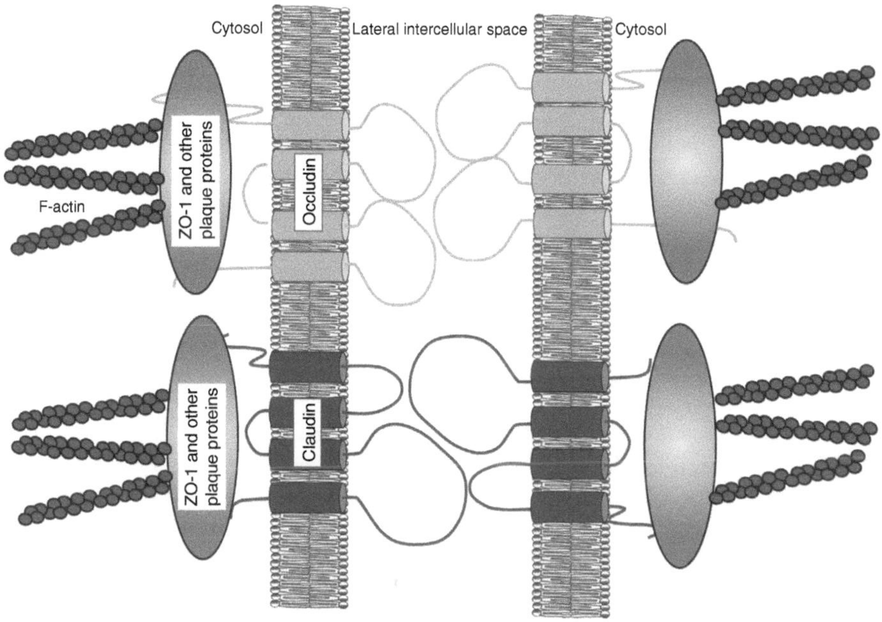

Figure 7.3 Overview of the intestinal tight junctional (TJ) complex. The intestinal epithelium consists of a single layer of polarized epithelial cells. Adjacent cells are connected by the TJ complexes, forming the rate-limiting complex of the paracellular pathway. TJ consists of transcellular proteins connected intracellularly to the F-actin cytoskeleton through a series of adaptor proteins (plaque proteins). The collection of proteins in the junctional complexes is called cytoplasmic plaques.

example being the zonula occludens proteins (ZO-1, 2, and 3). The plaque proteins, in turn, are connected to the actin-ring of the cytoskeleton, creating a continuous structure facing the apical side of the intestinal epithelium (Figure 7.3) (González-Mariscal et al., 2003; Groschwitz and Hogan, 2009; Schneeberger and Lynch, 2004).

7.2.2 The tight junctions as regulators of paracellular permeability

The permeability and selectivity of TJs towards charged and uncharged molecules is complex, described to involve the number of TJ strands, and influenced by the differential expression of the TJ proteins and temporary breaks in the TJ strands (Anderson and Van Itallie, 2009; Günzel and Yu, 2013; Van Itallie and Anderson, 2004, 2006; Van Itallie et al., 2008). One family of proteins suggested to be the main determiner of selectivity in TJ permeability is the claudins. In fact, differential claudin expression is conceived as the basis for the selective size, charge, and conductance properties of the paracellular pathway (Anderson and Van Itallie, 2009; Van Itallie and Anderson, 2004). In fish, ~63 genes encoding for claudin TJ proteins have been reported so far in 16 teleost species (reviewed in Chasiotis et al., 2012; Kolosov et al., 2013). In mammals, two main groups of claudins can be found based on their barrier-forming abilities: barrier-building claudins (claudin-1, -3, -4, -5, -6, -8, -9 -11, -14, and -19) and pore forming claudins (claudin-2, -10, -15, and 17) (Amasheh et al., 2011; Günzel and Yu, 2013). The physiological explanation behind the charge selectivity of the different claudin isoforms is that they display different numbers and types of charged amino acid residues lining the TJ pore that is formed between the adjacent cells (Anderson and Van Itallie, 2009; Günzel and Yu, 2013). These pores constitute a passageway for molecules through the paracellular pathway. Interestingly, in addition to increasing the cation permeability, claudin-2 also appears to create a paracellular water channel through the TJ (Rosenthal et al., 2010).

7.2.3 Measuring intestinal barrier function

Several techniques have been used to study the intestinal health and barrier functions in mammals as well as in fish, such as physiological measures obtained both *in vivo* and *in vitro*, histological techniques, including TEM, the use of antibodies for immunohistochemistry, immunocytochemistry, and western blots, as well as measurements of mRNA levels using qPCR. One of the most common techniques used to physiologically measure the level of intestinal barrier function is by examining *in vitro* preparations of diffusion/Ussing chambers using electrodes to measure electrical characteristics and inert marker molecules for passive diffusion (Grass and Sweetana, 1988; Ussing and Zerahn, 1951). The Ussing chambers and their equivalents have been widely used to study physiological transport and transfer mechanisms in a multitude of species and tissues (Blikslager et al., 2007; Clarke, 2009; Collie, 1985; Genz et al., 2011; Gregorio et al., 2013; Grosell et al., 2009; Jutfelt et al., 2006, 2007, 2008; Loretz, 1995; Moeser et al., 2007; Saunders et al., 2002; Sundell et al., 2003; Sundh et al., 2009, 2010, 2011; Söderholm and Perdue, 2001; Ussing and Zerahn, 1951; Wallon et al., 2008; Velin et al., 2004). When equipped with two sets of electrodes (voltage-measuring electrodes and current-creating electrodes) (reviewed in Sundell and Sundh, 2012), the Ussing chamber technique can analyze the electrical characteristics of any mounted epithelia. The three electrical parameters that can be measured are the transepithelial electrical resistance (TER), the transepithelial electrical potential, and the short-circuit current. Together they provide important information on the viability of the *in vitro* preparation, active transporting events, and the permeability of the intestinal epithelium (Sundell et al., 2003). Of these three, the TER, in leaky epithelia like the fish intestine (Loretz, 1995; Powell, 1981), is mainly reflecting paracellular permeability. A high TER is indicative of a tight epithelium for diffusion of charged molecules, which can be interpreted as a strong intestinal barrier against certain molecules or microorganisms. Paracellular permeability can also be assessed by adding uncharged inert molecules of different sizes. One such commonly used molecule is mannitol (~180 Da) (Bjarnason et al., 1995). The Ussing chamber technique is also an important tool used to study transcellular vesicular transport, during which the transport rate of, for example, bacteria, microspheres, and macromolecules like horseradish peroxidase (HRP; approx. 44 kDa) can be assessed. Steroid hormones and other easily labeled small lipophilic molecules are used to assess the passive transcellular permeability.

7.3 Intestinal barrier function and health

The continuous exposure to a sometimes harsh environment within the lumen makes the intestinal epithelium a particularly vulnerable tissue. Changes in the internal and external environment can quickly translate into changes in the intestinal barrier, which, in turn, can be related to intestinal health and, in the long run, the health and welfare of the fish. Health has been described as a pathological state of the body and brain in relation to effects of pathogens, parasites, tissue damage, or physiological disorders (Broom, 2006). Pathology, in turn, can be defined as a detrimental imbalance of molecules, cells, and functions as a result of harmful substances and/or deprivations (Broom, 2006, 2007). In this regard, environmental factors that render decreased intestinal barrier function can be defined to reduce the intestinal health as well as the general health of the fish. In line with this, intestinal health is a current topic for discussion in human medicine in which intestinal barrier function is defined as a basis for intestinal health (Bischoff, 2011; Cummings et al., 2004). Furthermore, a reduced intestinal barrier function has been implicated as one critical determinant in the predisposition as well as a consequence of disease exacerbation of intestinal inflammation and a number of gastrointestinal diseases, including inflammatory bowel disease (IBD) and food allergy (Groschwitz and Hogan, 2009; Söderholm and Perdue, 2001; Turner, 2006). This is supported by evidence from animal models of intestinal barrier dysfunction being an etiology of intestinal inflammation (Kelsall, 2008). In conclusion, intestinal barrier function is an essential factor in intestinal health as well as in the health and welfare of the fish in general.

7.4 Environmental factors affecting the intestinal barrier

7.4.1 Acute stress

Stress in mammals has a profound effect on the intestine. Both physiological stress, such as trauma, burns, and surgeries, and psychological stress can induce intestinal barrier dysfunction in mammals (Söderholm and Perdue, 2001). Acute and chronic psychological stress in mammals has been shown to lead to a decreased TER concomitant with increased intestinal permeability of small inert marker molecules (mannitol and/or Cr- EDTA) (Santos and Perdue, 2000; Santos et al., 1999; Saunders et al., 1994; Söderholm and Perdue, 2001; Velin et al., 2004) as well as to increased transfer of macromolecules and bacteria from the lumen across the intestinal epithelium (Kiliaan et al., 1998; Santos et al., 1999, 2000; Velin et al., 2004).

Compared to mammals, less is known about the effects of stress on the intestinal health of fish. However, a growing body of evidence points towards similar effects in fish as those that have been shown in mammals. The severity of stress elicited by the environment as well as its impact on the function of the primary barriers can vary with the number of stressors, their intensity, and their duration as well as their nature. Handling stress in the form of netting followed by a 4 h transportation stress resulted in goblet cell depletion and detachment of the intestinal epithelial cells from the basement membrane in the common carp (*Cyprinus carpio*), the Japanese colored carp (*Cyprinus carpio haematopterus*), the European eel (*Anguilla anguilla*), and the African catfish (*Clarias gariepinus*) (Szakolczai, 1997). Social stress resulted in flattening of the mucosal folds and loosening of the cell–cell contact between enterocytes in the European eel (Peters, 1982). Subjecting Atlantic salmon and rainbow trout to acute stress for 15 min resulted in significant changes to the ultrastructure of the intestine. This led to some damage to the TJ complexes of the proximal intestine, whereas less damage was observed in the distal intestine (Olsen et al., 2002, 2005). In contrast, subjecting Atlantic cod to the same stress protocol did not result in any damage of the TJ at the ultrastructural level (Olsen et al., 2008).

Damages to the TJ may indicate impaired intestinal barrier function. Indeed, acute stress results in an increased leakage of the paracellular marker molecule mannitol (Olsen et al., 2005, 2008). Moreover, the extrinsic mucus barrier is affected by acute stress. The bacterial content of feces increased after a 15 min acute stressor in Atlantic salmon and rainbow trout, which was suggested to be the result of stress-induced mucus secretions (Olsen et al., 2002, 2005).

7.4.2 Low-intensity chronic stress

Dissolved oxygen (DO) has been suggested to be a key limiting factor for growing Atlantic salmon in sea cages (Johansson et al., 2007) and can constitute a low intensive but long-term stressor in fish aquaculture. The size of the cages, in combination with their location in relation to ambient water currents as well as fouling on the nets, highly influences the water exchange rate and, thereby, the oxygen availability for the fish (Johansson et al., 2007). Detailed vertical mapping of the physical sea cage environment shows that DO levels can be highly variable in both space and time (Johansson et al., 2007). Apart from the variability in water flow, also season, temperature, algal production, and fish oxygen consumption are important factors that affect the final level of DO in the sea cages. Under a series of controlled experiments, subjecting Atlantic salmon to common sea cage conditions with low DO levels alone or in combination with high temperatures resulted in an induction of the primary stress response reflected as elevated plasma cortisol levels (Sundh et al., 2010). Based solely on plasma cortisol levels, the outcome of these experiments would lead to the conclusion that the allostatic load decreases with time because it was observed that the cortisol levels returned to basal values after 30–60 days, depending on the type of stressor (Sundh et al., 2010). However, the impact of the environment measured at the level of a secondary stress response, revealed impaired intestinal barrier function, which also occurred at time points when plasma cortisol levels had returned to basal levels. The detrimental effects of low DO on the intestinal barrier were more severe at higher temperatures (Sundh et al., 2010), which suggests that elevated temperature acts as an additional stressor by creating a higher allostatic load. In addition to disturbing the physical barrier, as shown by increased paracellular permeability, low DO levels and temperature were also shown to affect the immunological properties of the intestinal barrier (Niklasson et al., 2011). An increased infiltration of neutrophils and altered gene expression patterns of important pro-inflammatory and anti-inflammatory cytokines in the intestinal mucosa was demonstrated as a result of both decreased DO levels and increased temperature (Niklasson et al., 2011; Sundh et al., 2010; Sundh et al., unpublished data). An immunosuppressive effect of the stressors, suggested as interferon gamma (IFNγ), was down-regulated by low DO, and this effect was even stronger with higher water temperature. Taken together, environmental situations commonly observed in sea cages during rearing of Atlantic salmon are apparently stressful to the fish, and this leads, in addition to transient changes in the classical primary stress response parameter known as cortisol, to persistent alterations in the fish's defense system – particularly the physical barrier function of the intestine with consequences for the underlying mucosal immune system.

Regarding DO levels in the environment, not only low levels of oxygen have shown to be detrimental. Also, hyperoxygenation in the FW stage negatively affects intestinal barrier functions. The intensification of Atlantic salmon smolt production results in stocking at higher fish densities. As FW is a limited resource, water flow is reduced and, thereby, DO can be limiting. Therefore, oxygen is added to maintain adequate oxygen levels in the holding tanks (Wedemeyer, 1996). DO levels well above 100% saturation are commonly used in aquaculture in order to be able to reduce the specific water flow (EFSA, 2008). This practice can have negative impacts on other water quality parameters in terms of increased levels of metabolic wastes, such as carbon dioxide and ammonia together with decreased pH, even though the DO levels are still high (EFSA, 2008; Ellis et al., 2002; Fivelstad et al., 1999, 2004). Such an environment in the FW stage of Atlantic salmon farming has been hypothesized to be a contributing factor to the increased disease susceptibility of the fish observed after SW transfer. Studies indeed demonstrate that Atlantic salmon post-smolt have increased susceptibility to infectious pancreatic necrosis virus (IPNV) after SW transfer if they have experienced a prehistory of exposure to reduced specific water flow and hyperoxygenation in the parr stage in FW (Fridell et al., 2007; Sundh et al., 2009). Subjecting Atlantic salmon parr to hyperoxic conditions for 26 days resulted in chronically elevated plasma cortisol levels (Fridell et al., 2007). An increased allostatic load was also manifested as a disturbed intestinal barrier function, resulting in increased paracellular permeability and an increased translocation rate of *Aeromonas salmonicida* ssp. *salmonicida* (*A. salmonicida*) in the distal intestine (Sundh et al., 2009). This secondary stress response, a decreased intestinal barrier function, may be one factor responsible for the increased risk of pathogen invasion and infections after SW transfer. Moreover, the IPNV challenge *per se* served as a stressor as shown by elevated plasma levels of cortisol after IPNV co-habitant challenge (Fridell et al., 2007). In summary, the commonly used husbandry practice of hyperoxygenating FW is likely to reduce the ability of Atlantic salmon post-smolt to cope with additional stressors and represents a major risk to the welfare of the fish.

Another common husbandry stressor is the farming of fish under conditions with too high fish densities (Huntingford et al., 2006). As fish density increases, water quality parameters are affected in a complex manner, yielding decreased DO levels and increased levels of carbon dioxide, nitrates, and ammonia as well as a decreased pH (Ellis et al., 2002). Some studies have shown that high stocking density *per se* can be stressful to the fish (Adams et al., 2007; Ellis et al., 2002), whereas others have not been able to demonstrate any strong primary stress effects (Ellis et al., 2002). For instance, Atlantic salmon kept at a density of 70 kg/m^3 displayed elevated plasma cortisol levels during long time periods, whereas this was not seen in fish kept at the intermediate densities of 30 and 50 kg/m^3 (Sundh et al., unpublished data). The elevated plasma cortisol levels decreased with time, suggesting habituation. Intestinal barrier function, on the other hand, decreased in a sustained manner in response to the severity of the stress (i.e., the fish density). Again, this was observed at time points when plasma cortisol levels had been restored to basal levels. Increased fish density resulted in decreased TER as well as increased paracellular permeability to mannitol. The threshold density for mediating a decreased barrier function was between 30 and 50 kg/m^3. Additionally, local signs of inflammation in the intestinal epithelium were more evident in fish kept at 70 kg/m^3 as compared to 10 kg/m^3. This is suggested to be an effect of increased leakage of luminal content that attracts immune cells to the mucosa. Also, the expression of cytokines in the intestinal mucosa was affected by density. IFNγ was down-regulated in the 70 kg/m^3 group compared to the 10 kg/m^3 group, suggesting a suppression of the mucosal immune barrier.

7.5 Host–pathogen interactions and intestinal barrier function

Most animals have a well-developed innate defense system against pathogens. However, during the co-evolution of host and pathogen, pathogens have evolved mechanisms that can utilize the host's own defense mechanisms in order to facilitate the penetration of the barriers and infect the host. Further, epithelia, such as the intestinal mucosa, can serve as a site where pathogens are able to bind, multiply, and infect the host, which can be the case for bacterial pathogens or where viral pathogens enter the cells and initiate replication. Other pathogens may instead only use the mucosa for translocation in order to reach the circulation for distribution and infection of other tissues. For several bacterial fish pathogens spanning both gram-positive and gram-negative families, such as *Streptococcaceae, Aeromonadaceae, Campylobacteriaceae, Enterobacteriaceae, Piscirickettsiaceae,* and *Pseudomonadaceae*, impaired intestinal health is part of the characteristics of the pathology described (reviewed in Austin and Austin, 2007). Pathological signs of bacterial infection related to the intestine often include hemorrhages within the intestinal wall, lesions, congestion of mucus, and sloughing off of the epithelial cells from the intestine (Austin and Austin, 2007). In addition to bacterial pathogens, viruses that have been shown to create damage to the intestine of fish can cause similar effects on intestinal health (Sundh et al., 2009). This chapter will focus on examples of bacterial and viral fish pathogens that impair intestinal barrier function and health.

7.5.1 Bacterial pathogens

One of the most well-studied bacterial fish pathogens is *A. salmonicida*, a gram-negative bacterium that causes furunculosis. *A. salmonicida* outbreaks have had severe economical impact on the aquaculture industry and have subsequently been recognized as one of the most important bacterial diseases in both FW and marine salmonid aquaculture (Toranzo et al., 2005). The disease is named after the characteristic furuncles, such as blisters, that occur on the skin of infected fish (Cipriano and Bullock, 2001). Acute infections in salmonids are often manifested as internal hemorrhages to visceral organs. The intestine is not only used by *A. salmonicida* as an infection route in both rainbow trout and Atlantic salmon (Jutfelt et al., 2001, 2006, 2007; Ringø et al., 2009; Sundh et al., 2009), but the bacteria also creates severe damage to the intestinal epithelium. Infected fish usually stop feeding and the gut lumen, devoid of food, contains sloughed-off epithelial cells, blood, and mucus (Cipriano and Bullock, 2001). At the ultrastructural level, intestinal tissue from the pyloric ceca and proximal region/foregut exposed to *A. salmonicida* display severe damage with loss of cellular integrity and detached enterocytes in the intestinal lumen. This, in turn, exposes the intestinal basement membrane and allows pathogen access (Ringø et al., 2004, 2009). On the other hand, in the distal intestine, no loosening of the enterocytes has been observed, although severe damage to microvilli, desmosomes, and TJ complexes have been demonstrated (Ringø et al., 2004).

Vibrio anguillarum, the causative agent behind vibriosis, has been demonstrated to use the fish intestine as an infection route (Grisez et al., 1996). Further, the bacteria also cause significant alterations to the intestinal mucosa. *In vitro* exposure of the Atlantic salmon intestinal mucosa to *V. anguillarum* results in non-uniform microvilli, shortening and loss of microvilli in some areas, edema between enterocytes, serious tissue damage observed as cell debris in the intestinal lumen, protruding cells, and disintegrated tight junctions (Ringø et al., 2007). Other *Vibrio* species have also been demonstrated to impair the intestinal health (i.e., *V. harveyi* can cause severe infectious gastroenteritis in summer flounder (*Paralichthys dentatus*) (Gauger et al., 2006; Soffientino et al., 1999) and the red drum (*Sciaenops ocellatus*) (Liu et al., 2003)).

Yersinia ruckeri, the causative agent of enteric redmouth disease, mainly affects salmonids (Austin and Austin, 2007; Busch, 1978) and has been observed within the intestine shortly after *in vivo* exposure to the bacteria (Ohtani et al., 2014; Tobback et al., 2009). *Y. ruckeri* has also been demonstrated to translocate through the intestine of rainbow trout *in vitro* (Tobback et al., 2010), demonstrating the intestine as a route for infection. In rainbow trout, histopathological signs of enteric red mouth disease are hyperemia and hemorrhages throughout the intestinal mucosa. The intestinal lumen showed presence of sloughed necrotized epithelial cells and was filled with a serosanguineous yellowish liquid (Busch, 1978; Mahjoor and Akhlagi, 2012).

Piscirickettsia salmonis, an obligate intracellular gram-negative bacteria (Fryer and Hedrick, 2003), is the causative agent of piscirickettsiosis (Almendras and Fuentealba, 1997; Fryer and Hedrick, 2003). The bacterium has been reported to infect salmonid as well as non-salmonid fish (Almendras and Fuentealba, 1997). Although disease outbreaks have been reported from land-based FW facilities, disease outbreaks are also commonly observed a few weeks after transfer to sea cages (Fryer and Hedrick, 2003). This may be an indication of an intestinal route of entry when fish exposed to SW start to drink. Indeed, experimental evidence of the intestine as an entry route for *P. salmonis* has been shown for coho salmon (Smith et al., 2004).

In contrast, rainbow trout were fairly resistant to gastric intubation of the bacterium (Smith et al., 1999), suggesting that, for rainbow trout, the oral route may not be the primary route for infection. Nevertheless, rickettsiosis has a major negative impact on intestinal health, as the lamina propria of the intestine of infected fish normally shows signs of necrosis, hemorrhages, and chronic inflammation (Fryer and Hedrick, 2003).

7.5.2 Viral pathogens

Compared to bacteria, less information is available on the impact of viruses on the mucosal health of fish. This is probably not due to the fact that viral infections don't affect the GI tract, but rather that intestinal tissues are usually not sampled for diagnosis of viral diseases (Collet, 2014). Furthermore, the data that exists from a few viral infections all suggests that the intestine is an important route of infection. Infectious pancreatic necrosis (IPN) is a disease caused by the IPNV, which is a member of the animal virus genus *Aquabirnavirus* and belongs to the family *Birnavirdae*. The disease was initially a major problem in brook trout (*Salvelinus fontinalis* M.) and rainbow trout hatcheries in North America (M'Gonigle, 1941), but have subsequently also caused major concerns in Europe (Roberts and Pearson, 2005). IPNV outbreaks can occur in all life stages, but are generally conceived as being inversely linked to the age of the fish with mortality being highest in young fish and relatively scarce in older fish (Wolf, 1988).

In Atlantic salmon aquaculture, the transfer of fish from FW to SW is a particularly stressful event in the production cycle (Roberts and Pearson, 2005). During the first period after SW transfer, sudden and often high mortalities caused by IPNV can occur (Jarp et al., 1995; Roberts and Pearson, 2005; Smail et al., 1992). In salmonids suffering from an acute IPNV infection, common histopathological signs are necrosis of pancreatic acinar cells, kidney, and liver tissue (Roberts and Pearson, 2005). The IPN virions are likely to enter through the skin and gills and/or the digestive tract since clinical outbreaks can be induced by immersion challenge and do coincide with first feeding of fry (Wolf, 1988). Atlantic salmon are particularly sensitive to the IPNV virus during the first period after SW transfer (Roberts and Pearson, 2005). Data on interactions between IPNV and the intestinal epithelium of salmonid fish show that the virus can be found within the intestine early during a natural infection (Shankar and Yamamoto, 1994) as well as after an intraperitoneal injection (Swanson et al., 1982). Detailed *in vitro* studies on the intestinal epithelium demonstrate translocation of IPNV across the intestine of Atlantic salmon (Sundh et al., 2011). This indicates that the intestine is an important barrier against this virus. During an acute IPNV infection, the intestinal health is sternly reduced. Severe gut enteritis and complete sloughing of the intestinal mucosa are commonly observed in moribund post-smolts (Johansen and Sommer, 2001; M'Gonigle, 1941; McKnight and Roberts, 1976; Roberts and Pearson, 2005; Smail et al., 2006; Sundh et al., 2009; Wolf, 1988). Further, it has been suggested that the damage created in the intestine may be more acute than the necrosis of the pancreatic acinar cells (M'Gonigle, 1941; Smail et al., 1995; Wolf, 1988). IPNV infection also decreased intestinal barrier function due to increased paracellular permeability, tissue lesions as observed by transmission electron micrograph analysis, and increased translocation of *A. salmonicida* (Sundh et al., 2009). The disturbed intestinal barrier function caused by the virus may be one explanation to the increased risk of disease from secondary bacterial infections observed during acute IPNV infections (Johansen and Sommer, 2001).

Infectious salmon anemia (ISA) in Atlantic salmon (*Salmo salar* L.) is a major disease threat to the farming of Atlantic salmon worldwide (Rimstad and Mjaaland, 2002). The pathology from the ISA virus (ISAV) is characterized by circulatory disturbances, including anemia, gill pallor, ascites, liver, and spleen enlargement as well as petechial hemorrhaging of the skin and visceral organs (Evensen et al., 1991). Furthermore, the intestinal health is severely reduced. This is observed as intestinal congestion and complete sloughing of the apical region of the mucosal folds (Evensen et al., 1991; Mullins et al., 1998; Rodger et al., 1998). The route for infection is not completely known, but the gills have been suggested as the major site (Totland et al., 1996), although the intestine and skin cannot be excluded (OIE, 2014). ISAV, as well as receptors for ISAV, have been found on endothelial cells within the intestine of Atlantic salmon (Aamelfot et al., 2012), suggesting that the virus affects the intestinal barrier from the circulatory side (i.e., the serosal side). Infectious ISAV can further be found in feces (Totland et al., 1996), indicating that the virus is replicating within the intestinal tissue (Koren and Nylund, 1997).

7.6 The effect of environmental salinity on the intestinal barrier

In order to compensate for osmotically lost fluid in SW, teleost fish must extract fluid from ingested SW (Whittamore, 2012). It is well known that fish in SW have much higher drinking rates compared to FW acclimated fish (Fuentes et al., 1996; Perrott et al., 1992; Smith, 1930; Usher et al., 1988). However, water cannot be actively absorbed *per se*, therefore, the water uptake needs to be coupled to an uptake of monovalent ions (Marshall and Grosell, 2005; Smith, 1930). For stenohaline SW fish, the mechanisms involved in the solute-driven fluid transport (i.e., ion transporters, ion-channels, and co-transporters) have been extensively investigated (Grosell, 2010; Marshall and Grosell, 2005; Sundell and Sundh, 2012; Whittamore, 2012). Of equal importance among the active transport mechanisms for fluid uptake is the permeability of the epithelium. By studying anadromous salmonids capable of migrating between FW and SW, it has been shown that the barrier tightens when the fish migrate out to sea (Sundell et al., 2003; Sundell and Sundh, 2012). Two main hypotheses have been put forward regarding the physiological functions of this tightening of the paracellular pathway and are not mutually exclusive. First, the current hypothesis for fluid absorption in SW postulates a local hypertonic compartment within the lateral intercellular space (LIS) created by Na^+, K^+-ATPAses, among other processes, located at the basolateral membrane of the enterocytes (Grosell, 2010; Sundell and Sundh, 2012; Whittamore, 2012). However, in order to successfully create this hypertonic compartment, a tightening of the TJs would be beneficial since that prevents ions from leaking back into the intestinal lumen. Second, a tighter intestinal epithelium in SW acclimated fish would be beneficial as it increases barrier functions against substances in the ingested SW, which is a thriving habitat for both bacteria and viruses (Wilhelm and Suttle, 1999). Hence, the advantage of decreased paracellular permeability in SW is the reduced ability for pathogens, antigens, and other harmful substances to enter via the paracellular pathway. Thereby, the fish increases its disease resistance through a stronger intestinal barrier (Segner et al., 2012).

Increased intestinal barrier function (i.e., decreased paracellular permeability) after SW entry may seem contradictory to the increased fluid absorption. However, experimental data indicates that the permeability of water through the transcellular pathway increases in SW-acclimated salmonids (Sundell et al., 2003; Sundell and Sundh, 2012). This increased transcellular fluid permeability may be due to changes in the phospholipids constituting the lipid bilayer of the cell membrane (Seo et al., 2006; Stubbs and Smith, 1984) or by increased expression and incorporation of aquaporins (AQP) into the enterocyte membrane. Recent data on water permeability of intestine-derived lipid vesicles (Sundell and Sundh, 2012) and AQP expression in FW- and SW-acclimated Atlantic salmon suggests the AQP incorporation to be the main component (Engelund et al., 2013; Madsen et al., 2011; Tipsmark et al., 2010b).

7.7 Mediators of a decreased barrier function

7.7.1 Stress-induced barrier impairment

Corticosteroids display a major negative impact on intestinal barrier function in both fish and mammals. In rainbow trout, this has been demonstrated using slow-release cortisol implants. The treatment resulted in increased paracellular permeability to the inert marker molecule, mannitol, and concomitant with a decreased TER, clearly suggesting a decreased physical barrier function created by increased circulating levels of cortisol (Sundell and Sundh, 2012). Furthermore, Atlantic salmon receiving repeated intraperitoneal injections with cortisol down-regulated claudin-25b, a claudin isoform suggested to tighten the barrier of the TJs. The down-regulation was apparent in the proximal intestine of FW-acclimated fish and in both the proximal and distal intestine of SW-acclimated fish (Tipsmark et al., 2010a). Taken together, these results suggest that cortisol is a major regulator of intestinal paracellular permeability and barrier function in fish.

In mammals, like in fish (see Sections 7.4.1 and 7.4.2), decreased intestinal barrier function has been observed in response to environmental stress. Rats subjected to chronic environmental stress, reflected in increased circulating levels of glucocorticoid, showed a decreased intestinal barrier function (Meddings and Swain, 2000). Adrenalectomy and treatment with the glucocorticoid receptor antagonist RU486 abrogated the stress-induced reduction of intestinal barrier function (Meddings and Swain, 2000). One suggested mechanism behind the effect of corticosteroids on intestinal barrier function is a reduction of biliary production of the secretory immunoglobulin A (IgA). A major role of IgA in the intestinal lumen of mammals is to prevent adherence of bacteria onto the intestinal epithelium (Lamm, 1997). Therefore, if IgA levels decrease, luminal pathogens are able to attach to the intestinal epithelium for interaction and initiation of translocation. During this interaction between bacteria and the epithelium, intracellular signaling pathways are activated, resulting in contraction of the F-actin cytoskeleton along with widening of the TJ pores and increased intestinal permeability (Fasano and Nataro, 2004; Clayburgh et al., 2004; Spitz et al., 1994, 1995, 1996; Turner et al., 1997; Yuhan et al., 1997). In fish, the major secreted Ig in the intestine is IgT, which has been shown to coat commensal bacteria in a similar manner as that of mammalian IgA (Zhang et al., 2010), but possible effects of stress on the luminal levels of IgT in fish remain undetermined. Nevertheless, stress in salmonids has been proven to cause a reduction in the protective mucous layer, leading to increased epithelial-bacterial interaction (Olsen et al., 2002, 2005).

Another hormone released during stress in fish, as well as in mammals, is the corticotropin-releasing hormone (CRH), which mediates stress-induced abnormalities in the intestinal mucosa of mammals (Moeser et al., 2007; Santos et al., 1999; Saunders et al., 2002; Wallon et al., 2008). CRH is released from the hypothalamus during the primary stress response and plasma CRH levels are elevated also (Moeser et al., 2007). CRH can also be released locally as "immune CRH" by enteric nerves (Tsigos and Chrousos, 2002). In the experimental rat, decreased TER and increased transepithelial flux of HRP were observed after acute stress. These effects were inhibited by pretreatment with a CRH antagonist. Also, *in vitro* stimulation of intestinal segments with CRH in Ussing chambers mimicked the *in vivo* results on intestinal barrier function (Saunders et al., 2002). Interestingly, the mechanism by which CRH is suggested to increase the paracellular permeability in mammals has been linked to mucosal mast cells, which increase in number after stress. The stress effect in rats ascribed CRH was abolished in mast cell-deficient rats (Söderholm et al., 2002). Moreover, mast cells express receptors for CRH, and, by blocking these with a CRH-antagonist (Saunders et al., 2002; Wallon et al., 2008) or by administration of the mast cell stabilizer (Moeser et al., 2007), the stress effect on the intestinal barrier was attenuated. Similar to mammals, high levels of CRH can be found in the plasma of fish after acute stress (Pepels et al., 2004) and may be one of the mediators for the decreased barrier function in response to stress, also in fish. If plasma CRH levels are elevated during chronic stress or if CRH is released locally in the intestinal mucosa remains undetermined.

In the fish intestine, mast cell/eosinophilic granular cells are resident in the stratum granulosum and are highly involved in inflammatory processes (Mulero et al., 2007; Reite, 1997, 1998; Reite and Evensen, 2006). During IPNV infection, mast cells accumulate in the proximal intestine, which is known to develop acute inflammation during infection (Smail et al., 1992, 1995; Sundh et al., 2009). Mast cells also increase in number during intestinal inflammation caused by inclusion of soybean meal in the fish diet (Baeverfjord and Krogdahl, 1996; Urán et al., 2008). These intestinal inflammatory states further coincide with increased paracellular permeability (Knudsen et al., 2008; Sundh et al., 2009). The knowledge of stress-mediated mast cell recruitment and regulation in fish is scarce. One study showed that both acute and chronic stress generated a twofold increase in the number of mast cells in the gill epithelium of rainbow trout. However, in this study, the intestine was not analyzed (Holland and

Rowley, 1998). *In vitro* stimulation with lipopolysaccharide (LPS) and tumor necrosis factor alpha (TNFα) also significantly increased the number of mast cells in the gill epithelium (Holland and Rowley, 1998), suggesting that mast cell recruitment is an important mechanism in response to bacterial stress. Degranulation of mast cells has been observed in several species of salmonids after stimulation with noxious agents such as formalin-killed *A. salmonicida* or extracellular products of *A. salmonicida* and *V. salmonicida* (Powell et al., 1993a) as well as compound 48/80, a substance promoting histamine release from mast cells in mammals (Reite, 1997). An intraperitoneal injection of cortisol in brown trout (*Salmon trutta* L.) also resulted in mast cell degranulation, which provides a direct link between the primary stress response and mast cell activation in fish (Reite, 1997). Further, there is evidence for mast cell regulation by enteric nerves. Mast cells can be found in close association with nerves in the intestines of rainbow trout, and degranulation of intestinal mast cells has been observed after intraperitoneal injection of substance P (Powell et al., 1991). Interestingly, there seems to be a graded response of the mast cells dependent on position within the intestinal mucosa. Extensive degranulation was observed in the lamina propria, whereas a more moderate degranulation was found in the stratum granulosum (Powell et al., 1993b). Thus, mast cell contents are released to a higher degree in close proximity to the epithelium where these substances may act directly on barrier functions. Upon stimulation, mammalian mast cells also release tryptase, an enzyme that instantly reduces intestinal barrier function via proteinase-activated receptor 2 (PAR-2) located in the basolateral membrane (Jacob et al., 2005). These receptors mediate a redistribution of ZO-1, occludin, and perijunctional F-actin, which results in a decrease in intestinal barrier function due to decreased TER concomitant and increased transcellular permeability to HRP (Jacob et al., 2005). In fish, mast cells containing tryptase have been observed in the intestines of zebrafish (*Danio rerio*) (Dobson et al., 2008) and also in fish the mucosal mast cells release tryptase upon stimulation with compound 48/80 (Dobson et al., 2008). In Atlantic salmon, PAR-2 mRNA transcripts are abundant in the intestine and have been suggested to play a role in soybean meal-induced enteritis (Thorsen et al., 2008). However, their role in the regulation of intestinal barrier function remains available for investigation.

7.7.2 Pathogen-induced barrier impairment and the involvement of immune communication

There are several pathways through which pathogens can disrupt intestinal barrier function. Bacteria may attach to the intestinal epithelium and cause increased permeability by contracting and/or rearranging F-actin (see Section 7.7.1). Further, bacteria may also secrete toxins that directly destroy structural components of the TJ complex (Fasano and Nataro, 2004). A third pathway to disrupt intestinal barrier function is through communication with the underlying immune system. Bacterial toxins and antigens that are able to penetrate through the extrinsic and intrinsic barrier will come in contact with the GALT, resulting in a release of pro-inflammatory cytokines. Cytokines, such as TNFα and IFNγ, are important in mounting an immune response. At the same time, these may also communicate back with the epithelial barrier and affect the TJ proteins and, in the end, the intestinal permeability (Capaldo and Nusrat, 2009). Up-regulation of TNFα and IFNγ are found in the intestinal mucosa of humans suffering from IBD (Clayburgh et al., 2004), and, when these cytokines are co-cultured with mammalian intestinal cell lines, they mediate increased paracellular permeability through contraction of the F-actin cytoskeleton. This contraction is mediated by increased phosphorylation of the myosin light chain (MLC) through an up-regulation of MLC kinase (MLCK) (Turner et al., 1997). This mechanism is similar to the one observed during pathogen-induced increases in paracellular permeability (see Section 7.7.1). Besides their separate/direct effect on the paracellular permeability, TNFα and IFNγ also act synergistically in order to reduce barrier function. Other cytokines have also been reported to modulate intestinal barrier function in mammals, including interleukins (IL) and several growth factors (Capaldo and Nusrat, 2009). Apart from contraction of the F-actin, cytokines can affect intestinal permeability through a decreased expression of total TJ proteins or an internalization of the TJ proteins from the extracellular space to intracellular compartments, which leads to increased paracellular permeability (Bruewer et al., 2003, 2005; Capaldo and Nusrat, 2009; Mankertz et al., 2000). Moreover, by changing the type of claudin expressed in the TJ complex, the permeability and selectivity of the intestinal epithelium can be greatly affected.

In fish, several of the cytokines known to modulate intestinal barrier function in mammals are present (Marjara et al., 2012; Mulder et al., 2007; Niklasson et al., 2011, 2014; Reyes-Cerpa et al., 2012). The expression of these cytokines locally within the intestinal mucosal immune system is known to be affected by environmental stress (Niklasson et al., 2011), cortisol (Niklasson et al., 2014), and pathogen exposure (Kvamme et al., 2013; Niklasson et al., 2014). However, information regarding a possible cross-talk between the mucosal immune barrier and the intrinsic physical barrier (i.e., a possible effect of expressed cytokines on the intestinal physical barrier) is almost absent. One pilot study performed on rainbow trout where the intestinal epithelium was exposed to recombinant cytokines in Ussing chambers demonstrated an increase in paracellular permeability and a decrease in the physical barrier function by the cytokines IL-1β and IL-6, whereas IFNγ instead led to an increase in barrier function (Niklasson, 2013). More studies will have to be conducted in order to elucidate the cross-talk between the epithelial and immune barrier as well as the role of cytokines in intestinal health and diseases.

7.8 Concluding remarks

The intestinal epithelium of fish is faced with a complex task: providing a barrier against pathogens and harmful substances while simultaneously allowing nutrient and water absorption. For fish in SW, this task is even more complex due to the continuous ingestion of water from the environment, contributing to an increased antigen and pathogen load. Therefore, appropriate function and regulation of the intestinal barrier is essential for intestinal health as well as for the health of the whole animal. Intestinal health is maintained through cooperation between the different intestinal barriers (i.e., the intestinal epithelium in concert with secreted mucus containing antibacterial and antiviral factors and GALT). In fish, like in mammals, there is further cross-talk between the intestinal epithelium and GALT that will affect the intestinal health. As presented in the current chapter, changes in the external environment that expose the epithelia of the fish can instantly translate into changes in intestinal barrier permeability, either directly or mediated by, for example, nerves, hormones, cytokines, and pathogens. However, large gaps in knowledge remain around the underlying mechanisms of these changes in fish. The development of aquaculture demands this knowledge in order to understand how the intestinal as well as the overall health and welfare of the farmed fish can be maintained and even strengthened.

References

Aamelfot, M., Dale, O.B., Weli, S.C., Koppang, E.O., Falk, K., 2012. Expression of the infectious salmon anemia virus receptor on Atlantic salmon endothelial cells correlates with the cell tropism of the virus. J. Virol. 86, 10571–10578.

Adams, C.E., Turnbull, J.F., Bell, A., Bron, J.E., Huntingford, F.A., 2007. Multiple determinants of welfare in farmed fish: stocking density, disturbance, and aggression in Atlantic salmon (*Salmo salar*). Can. J. Fish. Aquat. Sci. 64, 336–344.

Almendras, F.E., Fuentealba, I.C., 1997. Salmonid rickettsial septicemia caused by *Piscirickettsia salmonis*: a review. Dis. Aquat. Org. 29, 137–144.

Amasheh, S., Fromm, M., Günzel, D., 2011. Claudins of intestine and nephron – a correlation of molecular tight junction structure and barrier function. Acta Physiol. (Oxf.) 201, 133–140.

Anderson, J.M., Van Itallie, C.M., 2009. Physiology and function of the tight junction. Cold Spring Harb. Perspect. Biol. 1 (2), a002584, DOI:10.1101/cshperspect.a002584.

Austin, B., Austin, D., 2007. Characteristics of the diseases. Bacterial fish pathogens – diseases of farmed and wild fish. fourth ed. Springer, Netherlands, pp. 15–46.

Baeverfjord, G., Krogdahl, A., 1996. Development and regression of soybean meal induced enteritis in Atlantic salmon, *Salmo salar* L., distal intestine: a comparison with the intestines of fasted fish. J. Fish Dis. 19, 375–387.

Bischoff, S., 2011. "Gut health": a new objective in medicine? BMC Med. 9, 24.

Bjarnason, I., MacPherson, A., Hollander, D., 1995. Intestinal permeability: an overview. Gastroenterology 108, 1566–1581.

Blikslager, A.T., Moeser, A.J., Gookin, J.L., Jones, S.L., Odle, J., 2007. Restoration of barrier function in injured intestinal mucosa. Physiol. Rev. 87, 545–564.

Broom, D.M., 2006. Behaviour and welfare in relation to pathology. Appl. Anim. Behav. Sci. 97, 73–83.

Broom, D.M., 2007. Welfare in relation to feelings, stress and health. Rev. Electr. Veterin. 8, 12B.

Bruewer, M., Luegering, A., Kucharzik, T., Parkos, C.A., Madara, J.L., Hopkins, A.M., Nusrat, A., 2003. Proinflammatory cytokines disrupt epithelial barrier function by apoptosis-independent mechanisms. J. Immunol. 171, 6164–6172.

Bruewer, M., Utech, M., Ivanov, A.I., Hopkins, A.M., Parkos, C.A., Nusrat, A., 2005. Interferon-gamma induces internalization of epithelial tight junction proteins via a macropinocytosis-like process. FASEB J. 19, 923–933.

Busch, R.A., 1978. Enteric redmouth disease (Hagerman strain). Mar. Fish. Rev. 40, 42–51.

Cahill, M., 1990. Bacterial flora of fishes: a review. Microb. Ecol. 19, 21–41.

Capaldo, C.T., Nusrat, A., 2009. Cytokine regulation of tight junctions. BBA – Biomembranes 1788, 864–871.

Chasiotis, H., Kolosov, D., Bui, P., Kelly, S.P., 2012. Tight junctions, tight junction proteins and paracellular permeability across the gill epithelium of fishes: a review. Resp. Physiol. Neurobiol. 184, 269–281.

Cipriano, C.R., Bullock, G., 2001. Furunculosis and other diseases caused by *Aeromonas salmonicida*. US Fish & Wildlife Publications Fish Dis. Leaf. 66, 1–33.

Clarke, L.L., 2009. A guide to Ussing chamber studies of mouse intestine. Am. J. Physiol. Gastr. L. 296, G1151–G1166.

Clayburgh, D.R., Shen, L., Turner, J.R., 2004. A porous defense: the leaky epithelial barrier in intestinal disease. Lab. Invest. 84, 282–291.

Collet, B., 2014. Innate immune responses of salmonid fish to viral infections. Dev. Comp. Immunol. 43, 160–173.

Collie, N.L., 1985. Intestinal nutrient transport in coho salmon (*Oncorhynchus kisutch*) and the effects of development, starvation, and seawater adaptation. J. Comp. Physiol. B. 156, 163–174.

Cummings, J.H., Antoine, J.M., Azpiroz, F., Bourdet-Sicard, R., Brandtzaeg, P., Calder, P.C., Gibson, G.R., Guarner, F., Isolauri, E., Pannemans, D., Shortt, C., Tuijtelaars, S., Watzl, B., 2004. PASSCLAIM-Gut health and immunity. Eur. J. Nutr. 43 (Suppl. 2), II118–II173.

Dobson, J.T., Seibert, J., Teh, E.M., Da'as, S., Fraser, R.B., Paw, B.H., Lin, T.-J., Berman, J.N., 2008. Carboxypeptidase A5 identifies a novel mast cell lineage in the zebrafish providing new insight into mast cell fate determination. Blood 112, 2969–2972.

Easy, R.H., Ross, N.W., 2010. Changes in Atlantic salmon *Salmo salar* mucus components following short- and long-term handling stress. J. Fish. Biol. 77, 1616–1631.

EFSA, 2008. Scientific report on animal welfare aspects of husbandry systems for farmed Atlantic salmon. Annex I EFSA J. 736, 1–121.

Ellis, A.E., 2001. Innate host defense mechanisms of fish against viruses and bacteria. Dev. Comp. Immunol. 25, 827–839.

Ellis, T., North, B., Scott, A.P., Bromage, N.R., Porter, M., Gadd, D., 2002. The relationships between stocking density and welfare in farmed rainbow trout. J. Fish Biol. 61, 493–531.

Engelund, M.B., Chauvigné, F., Christensen, B.M., Finn, R.N., Cerdà, J., Madsen, S.S., 2013. Differential expression and novel permeability properties of three aquaporin 8 paralogs from seawater-challenged Atlantic salmon smolts. J. Exp. Biol. 216, 3873–3885.

Evensen, Ø., Thorud, K.E., Olsen, Y.A., 1991. A morphological study of the gross and light microscopic lesions of infectious anaemia in Atlantic salmon (*Salmo salar*). Res. Vet. Sci. 51, 215–222.

Fanning, A.S., Mitic, L.L., Anderson, J.M., 1999. Transmembrane proteins in the tight junction barrier. J. Am. Soc. Nephrol. 10, 1337–1345.

Fasano, A., Nataro, J.P., 2004. Intestinal epithelial tight junctions as targets for enteric bacteria-derived toxins. Adv. Drug Deliv. Rev. 56, 795–807.

Fivelstad, S., Bergheim, A., Hølland, P.M., Fjermedal, A.B., 2004. Water flow requirements in the intensive production of Atlantic salmon (*Salmo salar* L.) parr-smolt at two salinity levels. Aquaculture 231, 263–277.

Fivelstad, S., Olsen, A.B., Kloften, H., Ski, H., Stefansson, S., 1999. Effects of carbon dioxide on Atlantic salmon (*Salmo salar* L.) smolts at constant pH in bicarbonate rich freshwater. Aquaculture 178, 171–187.

Fridell, F., Gadan, K., Sundh, H., Taranger, G.L., Glette, J., Olsen, R.E., Sundell, K., Evensen, Ø., 2007. Effect of hyperoxygenation and low water flow on the primary stress response and susceptibility of Atlantic salmon *Salmo salar* L. to experimental challenge with IPN virus. Aquaculture 270, 23–35.

Fryer, J.L., Hedrick, R.P., 2003. *Piscirickettsia salmonis*: a gram-negative intracellular bacterial pathogen of fish. J. Fish Dis. 26, 251–262.

Fuentes, J., Bury, N.R., Carroll, S., Eddy, F.B., 1996. Drinking in Atlantic salmon presmolts (*Salmo salar* L.) and juvenile rainbow trout (*Oncorhynchus mykiss* Walbaum) in response to cortisol and sea water challenge. Aquaculture 141, 129–137.

Gauger, E., Smolowitz, R., Uhlinger, K., Casey, J., Gómez-Chiarri, M., 2006. *Vibrio harveyi* and other bacterial pathogens in cultured summer flounder, *Paralichthys dentatus*. Aquaculture 260, 10–20.

Genz, J., Esbaugh, A.J., Grosell, M., 2011. Intestinal transport following transfer to increased salinity in an anadromous fish (*Oncorhynchus mykiss*). Comp. Biochem. Physiol. A 159, 150–158.

Geuking, M.B., Koller, Y., Rupp, S., McCoy, K.D., 2014. The interplay between the gut microbiota and the immune system. Gut Microbes 5 (3), 411–418.

Gomez, D., Sunyer, J.O., Salinas, I., 2013. The mucosal immune system of fish: the evolution of tolerating commensals while fighting pathogens. Fish Shellfish Immunol. 35, 1729–1739.

González-Mariscal, L., Betanzos, A., Nava, P., Jaramillo, B.E., 2003. Tight junction proteins. Progr. Biophys. Mol. Bio. 81, 1–44.

Grass, G.M., Sweetana, S.A., 1988. *In vitro* measurement of gastrointestinal tissue permeability using a new diffusion cell. Pharm. Res. 5, 372–376.

Gregorio, S.F., Carvalho, E.S., Encarnacao, S., Wilson, J.M., Power, D.M., Canario, A.V., Fuentes, J., 2013. Adaptation to different salinities exposes functional specialization in the intestine of the sea bream (*Sparus aurata* L.). J. Exp. Biol. 216, 470–479.

Grisez, L., Chair, M., Sorgeloos, P., Ollevier, F., 1996. Mode of infection and spread of *Vibrio anguillarum* in turbot *Scophthalmus maximus* larvae after oral challenge through live feed. Dis. Aquat. Org. 26, 181–187.

Groschwitz, K.R., Hogan, S.P., 2009. Intestinal barrier function: molecular regulation and disease pathogenesis. J. Allergy Clin. Immun. 124, 3–20, quiz 21–22.

Grosell, M., 2010. The role of the gastrointestinal tract in salt and water balance. In: Grosell, M., Farrell, A.P., Colin, J.B. (Eds.), Fish Physiology. Academic Press, San Diego, CA, pp. 135–164.

Grosell, M., Genz, J., Taylor, J.R., Perry, S.F., Gilmour, K.M., 2009. The involvement of H^+-ATPase and carbonic anhydrase in intestinal HCO_3^- secretion in seawater-acclimated rainbow trout. J. Exp. Biol. 212, 1940–1948.

Günzel, D., Yu, A.S.L., 2013. Claudins and the modulation of tight junction permeability. Physiol. Rev. 93, 525–569.

Holland, J.W., Rowley, A.F., 1998. Studies on the eosinophilic granule cells in the gills of the rainbow trout, *Oncorhynchus mykiss*. Comp. Biochem. Physiol. C 120, 321–328.

Huntingford, F.A., Adams, C., Braithwaite, V.A., Kadri, S., Pottinger, T.G., Sandø, P., Turnbull, J.F., 2006. Current issues in fish welfare. J. Fish Biol. 68, 332–372.

Jacob, C., Yang, P.-C., Darmoul, D., Amadesi, S., Saito, T., Cottrell, G.S., Coelho, A.-M., Singh, P., Grady, E.F., Perdue, M., Bunnett, N.W., 2005. Mast cell tryptase controls paracellular permeability of the intestine: role of protease activated receptor 2 and β-arrestins. J. Biol. Chem. 280, 31936–31948.

Jacobs, D.M., Gaudier, E., van Duynhoven, J., Vaughan, E.E., 2009. Non-digestible food ingredients, colonic microbiota and the impact on gut health and immunity: a role for metabolomics. Curr. Drug Metab. 10, 41–54.

Jarp, J., Gjevre, A.G., Olsen, A.B., Bruheim, T., 1995. Risk factors for furunculosis, infectious pancreatic necrosis and mortality in post-smolt of Atlantic salmon *Salmo salar* L. J. Fish Dis. 18, 67–78.

Johansen, L.H., Sommer, A.I., 2001. Infectious pancreatic necrosis virus infection in Atlantic salmon *Salmo salar* post-smolts affects the outcome of secondary infections with infectious salmon anaemia virus or *Vibrio salmonicida*. Dis. Aquat. Org. 47, 109–117.

Johansson, D., Juell, J.-E., Oppedal, F., Stiansen, J.-E., Ruohonen, K., 2007. The influence of the pycnocline and cage resistance on current flow, oxygen flux and swimming behaviour of Atlantic salmon (*Salmo salar* L.) in production cages. Aquaculture 265, 271–287.

Jutfelt, F., Olsen, R.E., Björnsson, B.T., Sundell, K., 2007. Parr-smolt transformation and dietary vegetable lipids affect intestinal nutrient uptake, barrier function and plasma cortisol levels in Atlantic salmon. Aquaculture 273, 298–311.

Jutfelt, F., Olsen, R.E., Glette, J., Ringo, E., Sundell, K., 2006. Translocation of viable *Aeromonas salmonicida* across the intestine of rainbow trout, *Oncorhynchus mykiss* (Walbaum). J. Fish Dis. 29, 255–262.

Jutfelt, F., Sundh, H., Glette, J., Mellander, L., Björnsson, B.T., Sundell, K., 2008. The involvement of *Aeromonas salmonicida* virulence factors in bacterial translocation across the rainbow trout, *Oncorhynchus mykiss* (Walbaum), intestine. J. Fish Dis. 31, 141–151.

Jöborn, A., Olsson, J.C., Westerdahl, A., Conway, P.L., Kjelleberg, S., 1997. Colonization in the fish intestinal tract and production of inhibitory substances in intestinal mucus and faecal extracts by *Carnobacterium* sp. strain K1. J. Fish Dis. 20, 383–392.

Kelsall, B.L., 2008. Innate and adaptive mechanisms to control of pathological intestinal inflammation. J. Pathol. 214, 242–259.

Kiliaan, A.J., Saunders, P.R., Bijlsma, P.B., Berin, M.C., Taminiau, J.A., Groot, J.A., Perdue, M.H., 1998. Stress stimulates transepithelial macromolecular uptake in rat jejunum. Am. J. Physiol. 275, G1037–G1044.

Knudsen, D., Jutfelt, F., Sundh, H., Sundell, K., Koppe, W., Frøkiær, H., 2008. Dietary soya saponins increase gut permeability and play a key role in the onset of soyabean-induced enteritis in Atlantic salmon (*Salmo salar* L.). Br. J. Nutr. 100, 120–129.

Kolosov, D., Bui, P., Chasiotis, H., Kelly, S.P., 2013. Claudins in teleost fishes. Tissue Barriers 1, e25391.

Koren, C.W.R., Nylund, A., 1997. Morphology and morphogenesis of infectious salmon anaemia virus replicating in the endothelium of Atlantic salmon *Salmo salar*. Dis. Aquat. Org. 29, 99–109.

Kvamme, B.O., Gadan, K., Finne-Fridell, F., Niklasson, L., Sundh, H., Sundell, K., Taranger, G.L., Evensen, O., 2013. Modulation of innate immune responses in Atlantic salmon by chronic hypoxia-induced stress. Fish Shellfish Immunol. 34, 55–65.

Lamm, M.E., 1997. Interaction of antigens and antibodies at mucosla surfaces. Annu. Rev. Microbiol. 51, 311–340.

Linden, S.K., Sutton, P., Karlsson, N.G., Korolik, V., McGuckin, M.A., 2008. Mucins in the mucosal barrier to infection. Mucosal Immun. 1, 183–197.

Liu, P.C., Chuang, W.H., Lee, K.K., 2003. Infectious gastroenteritis caused by *Vibrio harveyi* (*V. carchariae*) in cultured red drum, *Sciaenops ocellatus*. J. Appl. Ichthyol. 19, 59–61.

Loretz, C.A., 1995. Electrophysiology of ion transport in teleost intestinal cells. In: Chris, M.W., Trevor, J.S. (Eds.), Fish Physiology. Academic Press, Orlando, pp. 25–56.

Lukas, M., Bortlik, M., Maratka, Z., 2006. What is the origin of ulcerative colitis? Still more questions than answers. Postgrad. Med. J. 82, 620–625.

M'Gonigle, R.H., 1941. Acute catharral enteritis of salmonid fingerlings. Trans. Am. Fish. Soc. 70, 297–303.

Madsen, S.S., Olesen, J.H., Bedal, K., Engelund, M.B., Velasco-Santamaria, Y.M., Tipsmark, C.K., 2011. Functional characterization of water transport and cellular localization of three aquaporin paralogs in the salmonid intestine. Front. Physiol. 2, 56.

Mahjoor, A.A., Akhlagi, M., 2012. A pathological study of rainbow trout organs naturally infected with enteric red mouth disease. Asian J. Anim. Sci. 6, 147–153.

Mankertz, J., Tavalali, S., Schmitz, H., Mankertz, A., Riecken, E.O., Fromm, M., Schulzke, J.D., 2000. Expression from the human occludin promoter is affected by tumor necrosis factor α and interferon γ. J. Cell. Sci. 113, 2085–2090.

Marjara, I.S., Chikwati, E.M., Valen, E.C., Krogdahl, Å., Bakke, A.M., 2012. Transcriptional regulation of IL-17A and other inflammatory markers during the development of soybean meal-induced enteropathy in the distal intestine of Atlantic salmon (*Salmo salar* L.). Cytokine 60, 186–196.

Marshall, W.S., Grosell, M., 2005. Ion transport, osmoregulation and acid-base balance. In: Evans, D.H., Claiborne, J.B. (Eds.), The Physiology of Fishes. 3rd ed. CRC Taylor & Francis, Boca Raton, FL, pp. 177–230.

McKnight, I.J., Roberts, R.J., 1976. The pathology of infectious pancreatic necrosis. I. The sequential histopathology of the naturally ocurring condition. Br. Vet. J. 132, 76–85.

Meddings, J.B., Swain, M.G., 2000. Environmental stress-induced gastrointestinal permeability is mediated by endogenous glucocorticoids in the rat. Gastroenterology 119, 1019–1028.

Moeser, A.J., Ryan, K.A., Nighot, P.K., Blikslager, A.T., 2007. Gastrointestinal dysfunction induced by early weaning is attenuated by delayed weaning and mast cell blockade in pigs. Am. J. Physiol. Gastr. L. 293, G413–G421.

Mulder, I.E., Wadsworth, S., Secombes, C.J., 2007. Cytokine expression in the intestine of rainbow trout (*Oncorhynchus mykiss*) during infection with *Aeromonas salmonicida*. Fish Shellfish Immunol. 23, 747–759.

Mulero, I., Sepulcre, M.P., Meseguer, J., Garcia-Ayala, A., Mulero, V., 2007. Histamine is stored in mast cells of most evolutionarily advanced fish and regulates the fish inflammatory response. Proc. Natl. Acad. Sci. U.S.A. 104, 19434–19439.

Mullins, J.E., Groman, D., Wadowska, D., 1998. Infectious salmon anaemia in salt water Atlantic salmon (*Salmo salar* L.) in New Brunswick. Can. Bull. Eur. Assn. Fish. P. 18, 110–114.

Niklasson, L., 2013. Intestinal mucosal immunology of salmonids – response to stress and infection and crosstalk with the physical barrier. Ph.D. Thesis. University of Gothenburg.

Niklasson, L., Sundh, H., Fridell, F., Taranger, G.L., Sundell, K., 2011. Disturbance of the intestinal mucosal immune system of farmed Atlantic salmon (*Salmo salar*), in response to long-term hypoxic conditions. Fish Shellfish Immunol. 31, 1072–1080.

Niklasson, L., Sundh, H., Olsen, R.E., Jutfelt, F., Skjodt, K., Nilsen, T.O., Sundell, K.S., 2014. Effects of cortisol on the intestinal mucosal immune response during cohabitant challenge with IPNV in Atlantic Salmon (*Salmo salar*). PloS one 9, e94288.

Ohtani, M., Villumsen, K.R., Strom, H.K., Raida, M.K., 2014. 3D visualization of the initial *Yersinia ruckeri* infection route in rainbow trout (*Oncorhynchus mykiss*) by optical projection tomography. PloS one 9, e89672.

OIE, 2014. Manual of diagnostic tests for aquatic animals. The World Organisation for Animal Health. <http://www.oie.int/en/international-standard-setting/aquatic-manual/access-online/> (accessed 01.07.14.).

Olsen, R.E., Sundell, K., Hansen, T., Hemre, G.I., Myklebust, R., Mayhew, T.M., Ringø, E., 2002. Acute stress alters the intestinal lining of Atlantic salmon, *Salmo salar* L.: an electron microscopical study. Fish Physiol. Biochem. 26, 211–221.

Olsen, R.E., Sundell, K., Mayhew, T.M., Myklebust, R., Ringø, E., 2005. Acute stress alters intestinal function of rainbow trout, *Oncorhynchus mykiss* (Walbaum). Aquaculture 250, 480–495.

Olsen, R.E., Sundell, K., Ringø, E., Myklebust, R., Hemre, G.-I., Hansen, T., Karlsen, Ø., 2008. The acute stress response in fed and food deprived Atlantic cod, *Gadus morhua* L. Aquaculture 280, 232–241.

Pepels, P.P.L.M., van, H.H., Bonga, S.E.W., Balm, P.H.M., 2004. Corticotropin-releasing hormone in the teleost stress response: rapid appearance of the peptide in plasma of tilapia (*Oreochromis mossambicus*). J. Endocrinol. 180, 425–438.

Perrott, M.N., Grierson, C.E., Hazon, N., Balment, R.J., 1992. Drinking behavior in sea-water and fresh-water teleosts, the role of the renin-angiotensin system. Fish Physiol. Biochem. 10, 161–168.

Peters, G., 1982. The effect of stress on the stomach of the European eel, *Anguilla anguilla* L. J. Fish Biol. 21, 497–512.

Powell, D.W., 1981. Barrier function of epithelia. Am. J. Physiol. 241, G275–G288.

Powell, M.D., Briand, H.A., Wright, G.M., Burka, J.F., 1993a. Rainbow trout (*Oncorhynchus mykiss* Walbaum) intestinal eosinophilic granule cell (EGC) response to *Aeromonas salmonicida* and *Vibrio anguillarum* extracellular products. Fish Shellfish Immunol. 3, 279–289.

Powell, M.D., Wright, G.M., Burka, J.F., 1991. Degranulation of eosinophilic granule cells induced by capsaicin and substance P in the intestine of the rainbow trout (*Oncorhynchus mykiss* Walbaum). Cell Tissue Res. 266, 469–474.

Powell, M.D., Wright, G.M., Burka, J.F., 1993b. Morphological and distributional changes in the eosinophilic granule cell (EGC) population of the rainbow trout (*Oncorhynchus mykiss* Walbaum) intestine following systemic administration of capsaicin and substance P. J. Exp. Zool. 266, 19–30.

Reite, O.B., 1997. Mast cells/eosinophilic granule cells of salmonids: staining properties and responses to noxious agents. Fish Shellfish Immunol. 7, 567–584.

Reite, O.B., 1998. Mast cells/eosinophilic granule cells of teleostean fish: a review focusing on staining properties and functional responses. Fish Shellfish Immunol. 8, 489–513.

Reite, O.B., Evensen, Ø., 2006. Inflammatory cells of teleostean fish: a review focusing on mast cells/eosinophilic granule cells and rodlet cells. Fish Shellfish Immunol. 20, 192–208.

Reyes-Cerpa, S., Maisey, K., Reyes-López, F., Toro-Ascuy, D., Sandino, A.M., Imarai, M., 2012. Fish cytokines and immune response, new advances and contributions to fish biology. In: Turker, H. (Ed.), InTech, DOI: 10.5772/53504.

Rimstad, E., Mjaaland, S., 2002. Infectious salmon anaemia virus – an orthomyxovirus causing an emerging infection in Atlantic salmon. Apmis 110, 273–282.

Ringø, E., Jutfelt, F., Kanapathippillai, P., Bakken, Y., Sundell, K., Glette, J., Mayhew, T.M., Myklebust, R., Olsen, R.E., 2004. Damaging effect of the fish pathogen *Aeromonas salmonicida ssp. salmonicida* on intestinal enterocytes of Atlantic salmon (*Salmo salar* L.). Cell. Tissue Res. 318, 305–312.

Ringø, E., Løvmo, L., Kristiansen, M., Bakken, Y., Salinas, I., Myklebust, R., Olsen, R.E., Mayhew, T.M., 2009. Lactic acid bacteria vs. pathogens in the gastrointestinal tract of fish: a review. Aquacult. Res. 41 (4), 451–467.

Ringø, E., Salinas, I., Olsen, R.E., Nyhaug, A., Myklebust, R., Mayhew, T.M., 2007. Histological changes in intestine of Atlantic salmon (*Salmo salar* L.) following *in vitro* exposure to pathogenic and probiotic bacterial strains. Cell. Tissue Res. 328, 109–116.

Roberts, R.J., Pearson, M.D., 2005. Infectious pancreatic necrosis in Atlantic salmon, *Salmo salar* L. J. Fish Dis. 28, 383–390.

Rodger, H.D., Turnbull, T., Muir, F., Millar, S., Richards, R.H., 1998. Infectious salmon anaemia (ISA) in the United Kingdom. Bull. Eur. Assn. Fish. 18 (4), 115–116.

Rombout, J.H.W.M., Abelli, L., Picchietti, S., Scapigliati, G., Kiron, V., 2011. Teleost intestinal immunology. Fish Shellfish Immunol. 31, 616–626.

Rosenthal, R., Milatz, S., Krug, S.M., Oelrich, B., Schulzke, J.D., Amasheh, S., Gunzel, D., Fromm, M., 2010. Claudin-2, a component of the tight junction, forms a paracellular water channel. J. Cell Sci. 123, 1913–1921.

Santos, J., Benjamin, M., Yang, P.C., Prior, T., Perdue, M.H., 2000. Chronic stress impairs rat growth and jejunal epithelial barrier function: role of mast cells. Am. J. Physiol. Gastr. L. 278, G847–G854.

Santos, J., Perdue, M.H., 2000. Stress and neuroimmune regulation of gut mucosal function. Gut 47 (Suppl. 4), iv49–iv51, discussion iv52.

Santos, J., Saunders, P.R., Hanssen, N.P., Yang, P.C., Yates, D., Groot, J.A., Perdue, M.H., 1999. Corticotropin-releasing hormone mimics stress-induced colonic epithelial pathophysiology in the rat. Am. J. Physiol. 277, G391–G399.

Saunders, P.R., Kosecka, U., McKay, D.M., Perdue, M.H., 1994. Acute stressors stimulate ion secretion and increase epithelial permeability in rat intestine. Am. J. Physiol. Gastr. L. 267, G794–G799.

Saunders, P.R., Santos, J., Hanssen, N.P.M., Yates, D., Groot, J.A., Perdue, M.H., 2002. Physical and psychological stress in rats enhances colonic epithelial permeability via peripheral CRH. Digest. Dis. Sci. 47, 208–215.

Schneeberger, E.E., Lynch, R.D., 2004. The tight junction: a multifunctional complex. Am. J. Physiol. Cell Physiol. 286, C1213–C1228.

Segner, H., Sundh, H., Buchmann, K., Douxfils, J., Sundell, K., Mathieu, C., Ruane, N., Jutfelt, F., Toften, H., Vaughan, L., 2012. Health of farmed fish: its relation to fish welfare and its utility as welfare indicator. Fish Physiol. Biochem. 38, 85–105.

Seo, P.R., Teksin, Z.S., Kao, J.P., Polli, J.E., 2006. Lipid composition effect on permeability across PAMPA. Eur. J. Pharm. Sci. 29 (3–4), 259–268.

Shankar, K.M., Yamamoto, T., 1994. Prevalence and pathogenicity of infectious pancreatic necrosis virus (IPNV) associated with feral lake trout, *Salvelinus namaycush* (Walbaum). J. Fish Dis. 17, 461–471.

Shephard, K.L., 1994. Functions for fish mucus. Rev. Fish Biol. Fisher. 4, 401–429.

Smail, D.A., Bain, N., Bruno, D.W., King, J.A., Thompson, F., Pendrey, D.J., Morrice, S., Cunningham, C.O., 2006. Infectious pancreatic necrosis virus in Atlantic salmon, *Salmo salar* L., post-smolts in the Shetland Isles, Scotland: virus identification, histopathology, immunohistochemistry and genetic comparison with Scottish mainland isolates. J. Fish Dis. 29, 31–41.

Smail, D.A., Bruno, D.W., Dear, G., McFarlane, L.A., Ross, K., 1992. Infectious pancreatic necrosis (IPN) virus Sp serotype in farmed Atlantic salmon, *Salmo salar* L., post-smolts associated with mortality and clinical disease. J. Fish Dis. 15, 77–83.

Smail, D.A., McFarlane, L., Bruno, D.W., McVicar, A.H., 1995. The pathology of an IPN-Sp sub-type (Sh) in farmed Atlantic salmon, *Salmo salar* L., post-smolts in the Shetland Isles, Scotland. J. Fish Dis. 18, 631–638.

Smith, H.W., 1930. The absorption and excretion of water and salts by marine teleosts. Am. J. Physiol. Leg. Cont. 93, 480–505.

Smith, P.A., Pizarro, P., Ojeda, P., Contreras, J., Oyanedel, S., Larenas, J., 1999. Routes of entry of *Piscirickettsia salmonis* in rainbow trout *Oncorhynchus mykiss*. Dis. Aquat. Org. 37, 165–172.

Smith, P.A., Rojas, M.E., Guajardo, A., Contreras, J., Morales, M.A., Larenas, J., 2004. Experimental infection of coho salmon *Oncorhynchus kisutch* by exposure of skin, gills and intestine with *Piscirickettsia salmonis*. Dis. Aquat. Org. 61, 53–57.

Soffientino, B., Gwaltney, T., Nelson, D.R., Specker, J.L., Mauel, M., GÃ³mez-Chiarri, M., 1999. Infectious necrotizing enteritis and mortality caused by *Vibrio carchariae* in summer flounder *Paralichthys dentatus* during intensive culture. Dis. Aquat. Org. 38, 201–210.

Spitz, J., Hecht, G., Taveras, M., Aoys, E., Alverdy, J., 1994. The effect of dexamethasone administration on rat intestinal permeability: the role of bacterial adherence. Gastroenterology 106, 35–41.

Spitz, J., Yuhan, R., Koutsouris, A., Blatt, C., Alverdy, J., Hecht, G., 1995. Enteropathogenic *Escherichia coli* adherence to intestinal epithelial monolayers diminishes barrier function. Am. J. Physiol. 268, G374–G379.

Spitz, J.C., Ghandi, S., Taveras, M., Aoys, E., Alverdy, J.C., 1996. Characteristics of the intestinal epithelial barrier during dietary manipulation and glucocorticoid stress. Crit. Care Med. 24, 635–641.

Stubbs, C.D., Smith, A.D., 1984. The modification of mammalian membrane polyunsaturated fatty acid composition in relation to membrane fluidity and function. BBA 779, 89–137.

Sundell, K., Jutfelt, F., Agustsson, T., Olsen, R.E., Sandblom, E., Hansen, T., Björnsson, B.T., 2003. Intestinal transport mechanisms and plasma cortisol levels during normal and out-of-season parr-smolt transformation of Atlantic salmon, *Salmo salar*. Aquaculture 222, 265–285.

Sundell, K., Sundh, H., 2012. Intestinal fluid absorption in anadromous salmonids: importance of tight junctions and aquaporins. Front. Physiol. 3, 388.

Sundh, H., Calabrese, S., Jutfelt, F., Niklasson, L., Olsen, R.E., Sundell, K., 2011. Translocation of infectious pancreatic necrosis virus across the intestinal epithelium of Atlantic salmon (*Salmo salar* L.). Aquaculture 321, 85–92.

Sundh, H., Kvamme, B.O., Fridell, F., Olsen, R.E., Ellis, T., Taranger, G.L., Sundell, K., 2010. Intestinal barrier function of Atlantic salmon (*Salmo salar* L.) post smolts is reduced by common sea cage environments and suggested as a possible physiological welfare indicator. BMC Physiol. 10, 22.

Sundh, H., Olsen, R.E., Fridell, F., Gadan, K., Evensen, Ø., Glette, J., Taranger, G.L., Myklebust, R., Sundell, K., 2009. The effect of hyperoxygenation and reduced flow in fresh water and subsequent infectious pancreatic necrosis virus challenge in sea water, on the intestinal barrier integrity in Atlantic salmon, *Salmo salar* L. J. Fish Dis. 32, 687–698.

Swanson, R.N., Carlisle, J.C., Gillespie, J.H., 1982. Pathogenesis of infectious pancreatic necrosis virus infection in brook trout, *Salvelinus fontinalis* (Mitchill), following intraperitoneal injection. J. Fish Dis. 5, 449–460.

Sweetman, J.W., Torrecillas, S., Dimitroglou, A., Rider, S., Davies, S.J., Izquierdo, M.S., 2010. Enhancing the natural defences and barrier protection of aquaculture species. Aquacult. Res. 41, 345–355.

Szakolczai, J., 1997. Histopathological changes induced by environmental stress in common carp, Japanese coloured carp, European eel, and African catfish. Acta Vet. Hung. 45, 1–10.

Söderholm, J.D., Perdue, M.H., 2001. Stress and the gastrointestinal tract II. Stress and intestinal barrier function. Am. J. Physiol. Gastr. L. 280, G7–G13.

Söderholm, J.D., Yang, P.C., Ceponis, P., Vohra, A., Riddell, R., Sherman, P.M., Perdue, M.H., 2002. Chronic stress induces mast cell-dependent bacterial adherence and initiates mucosal inflammation in rat intestine. Gastroenterology 123, 1099–1108.

Thorsen, J., Lilleeng, E., Valen, E.C., Krogdahl, A., 2008. Proteinase-activated receptor-2: two potential inflammatory mediators of the gastrointestinal tract in Atlantic salmon. J. Inflamm. 5, 18.

Tipsmark, C.K., Sorensen, K.J., Hulgard, K., Madsen, S.S., 2010a. Claudin-15 and-25b expression in the intestinal tract of Atlantic salmon in response to seawater acclimation, smoltification and hormone treatment. Comp. Biochem. Physiol. A Mol. Integr. Physiol. 155, 361–370.

Tipsmark, C.K., Sorensen, K.J., Madsen, S.S., 2010b. Aquaporin expression dynamics in osmoregulatory tissues of Atlantic salmon during smoltification and seawater acclimation. J. Exp. Biol. 213, 368–379.

Tobback, E., Decostere, A., Hermans, K., Ryckaert, J., Duchateau, L., Haesebrouck, F., Chiers, K., 2009. Route of entry and tissue distribution of *Yersinia ruckeri* in experimentally infected rainbow trout *Oncorhynchus mykiss*. Dis. Aquat. Org. 84, 219–228.

Tobback, E., Hermans, K., Decostere, A., Van den Broeck, W., Haesebrouck, F., Chiers, K., 2010. Interactions of virulent and avirulent *Yersinia ruckeri* strains with isolated gill arches and intestinal explants of rainbow trout *Oncorhynchus mykiss*. Dis. Aquat. Org. 90, 175–179.

Toranzo, A.E., Magarinos, B., Romalde, J.L., 2005. A review of the main bacterial fish diseases in mariculture systems. Aquaculture 246, 37–61.

Torrecillas, S., Makol, A., Benítez-Santana, T., Caballero, M.J., Montero, D., Sweetman, J., Izquierdo, M., 2011. Reduced gut bacterial translocation in European sea bass (*Dicentrarchus labrax*) fed mannan oligosaccharides (MOS). Fish Shellfish Immunol. 30, 674–681.

Totland, G.K., Hjeltnes, B.K., Flood, P.R., 1996. Transmission of infectious salmon anaemia (ISA) through natural secretions and excretions from infected smelts of Atlantic salmon *Salmo salar* during their presymptomatic phase. Dis. Aquat. Org. 26, 25–31.

Tsigos, C., Chrousos, G.P., 2002. Hypothalamic-pituitary-adrenal axis, neuroendocrine factors and stress. J. Psychosom. Res. 53, 865–871.

Tsukita, S., Furuse, M., 1999. Occludin and claudins in tight-junction strands: leading or supporting players? Trends Cell. Biol. 9, 268–273.

Turner, J.R., 2006. Molecular basis of epithelial barrier regulation: from basic mechanisms to clinical application. Am. J. Pathol. 169, 1901–1909.

Turner, J.R., Rill, B.K., Carlson, S.L., Carnes, D., Kerner, R., Mrsny, R.J., Madara, J.L., 1997. Physiological regulation of epithelial tight junctions is associated with myosin light-chain phosphorylation. Am. J. Physiol. 273, C1378–C1385.

Urán, P.A., Schrama, J.W., Rombout, J.H.W.M., Obach, A., Jensen, L., Koppe, W., Verreth, J.A.J., 2008. Soybean meal-induced enteritis in Atlantic salmon (*Salmo salar* L.) at different temperatures. Aquacult. Nutr. 14, 324–330.

Usher, M.L., Talbot, C., Eddy, F.B., 1988. Drinking in Atlantic salmon smolts transferred to seawater and the relationship between drinking and feeding. Aquaculture 73, 237–246.

Ussing, H.H., Zerahn, K., 1951. Active transport of sodium as the source of electric current in the short-circuited isolated frog skin. Acta Physiol. Scand. 23, 110–127.

Wallon, C., Yang, P.C., Keita, Å.V., Ericson, A.C., McKay, D.M., Sherman, P.M., Perdue, M.H., Söderholm, J.D., 2008. Corticotropin-releasing hormone (CRH) regulates macromolecular permeability via mast cells in normal human colonic biopsies *in vitro*. Gu. 57, 50–58.

Van Itallie, C.M., Anderson, J.M., 2004. The molecular physiology of tight junction pores. Physiol. (Bethesda) 19, 331–338.

Van Itallie, C.M., Anderson, J.M., 2006. Claudins and epithelial paracellular transport. Annu. Rev. Physiol. 68, 403–429.

Van Itallie, C.M., Holmes, J., Bridges, A., Gookin, J.L., Coccaro, M.R., Proctor, W., Colegio, O.R., Anderson, J.M., 2008. The density of small tight junction pores varies among cell types and is increased by expression of claudin-2. J. Cell Sci. 121, 298–305.

Velin, Å.K., Ericson, A.C., Braaf, Y., Wallon, C., Söderholm, J.D., 2004. Increased antigen and bacterial uptake in follicle associated epithelium induced by chronic psychological stress in rats. Gu. 53, 494–500.

Wedemeyer, G., 1996. Physiology of Fish in Intensive Culture Systems. Chapman & Hall, New York.

Whittamore, J.M., 2012. Osmoregulation and epithelial water transport: lessons from the intestine of marine teleost fish. J. Comp. Physiol. B 182, 1–39.

Wilhelm, S.W., Suttle, C.A., 1999. Viruses and nutrient cycles in the sea. Bioscience 49, 781–788.

Wolf, K., 1988. Fish Viruses and Fish Viral Diseases. Cornell University Press, Ithaca, New York.

Yuhan, R., Koutsouris, A., Savkovic, S.D., Hecht, G., 1997. Enteropathogenic *Escherichia coli*-induced myosin light chain phosphorylation alters intestinal epithelial permeability. Gastroenterology 113, 1873–1882.

Zhang, Y.-A., Salinas, I., Li, J., Parra, D., Bjork, S., Xu, Z., LaPatra, S.E., Bartholomew, J., Sunyer, J.O., 2010. IgT, a primitive immunoglobulin class specialized in mucosal immunity. Nat. Immunol. 11, 827–835.

Nutritional impacts on fish mucosa: dietary considerations

8

Jesse Trushenski
Center for Fisheries, Aquaculture, and Aquatic Sciences, Southern Illinois University Carbondale, Illinois, USA

Chapter Outline

8.1 Introduction

The alimentary canal or gut, while functioning primarily to acquire nutrients and excrete wastes, also contributes significantly to the immunocompetence of fish. Both roles, nutritional and immunological, are important in terms of the immune system of fish. First, a fish's immune system will most certainly be compromised if it is unable to digest and absorb the energy and essential nutrients necessary for basic homeostasis, maintenance of immunologically important cells, and synthesis of various factors such as enzymes and immunoglobulins. The importance of nutritional status in determining immunocompetence cannot be overstated. Therefore, the gut's role in digestion and absorption of nutrients is relevant, albeit indirectly, to a fish's health. Second, the gut mucosa is a primary site of pathogen exclusion and immunological engagement. The interplay between the availability of essential nutrients and the function of the immune system is largely outside the scope of this chapter; thus, we will focus on the gut's second, more direct role as part of the immune system (i.e., the effect of certain dietary constituents on the competency of the gut as part of the immune system).

The gut has various attributes that inhibit pathogen translocation, including the production of mucus with antibacterial properties, the acidic nature of the lumen and/or apical surfaces of the enterocytes, rapid cell turnover, peristaltic activity, and the production of lysozyme (Ringø et al., 2004). Collectively, these constitute a range of mechanical and chemical barriers for infection. Beneficial microbes present within the gut serve as a microbiological barrier to infection, outcompeting pathogenic microbes for space and nutrients needed for proliferation or creating conditions in the gut that are inhospitable for pathogens (Kesarcodi-Watson et al., 2008). Additionally, the enterocytes exhibit substantial capacity for endocytosis, which is likely a major contributor to the gut's function

Mucosal Health in Aquaculture

as part of the immune system (i.e., antigen processing and presentation, clearance of localized infections, prevention of systemic infections, and induction of adaptive immune responses and immunological memory) (Bakke-McKellep et al., 2000). Despite these preventative mechanisms, the gut can be a site of pathogen translocation. For example, infection with *Aeromonas salmonicida* causes significant histological damage to the gut of Atlantic salmon (*Salmo salar*), suggesting that bacteria may enter the body via transcellular or paracellular pathways in the gut or by damaging enterocytes and/or dislodging them. This chapter will focus on two categories of dietary constituents, lipids and antinutritional factors, that may make such translocation events more likely and, in turn, increase susceptibility to infection and disease.

8.2 Lipids and gut health

As noted above, the gut plays many roles related to nutrition, immunity, and general fish health, but these largely relate to its ability to facilitate or prevent the exchange of endogenous and exogenous materials, including nutrients, wastes, osmolytes, and pathogens. These exchanges may occur via trans- or paracellular pathways, and the relative ease with which they occur is determined by, among other things, the nature of the epithelial membranes themselves. The functional integrity of cell membranes partially depends on their lipid and fatty acid composition. This is particularly true among poikilothermic animals that routinely alter membrane composition in order to maintain fluidity and functionality under different thermal conditions – a process commonly known as "homeoviscous adaptation" (Arts and Kohler, 2009). Given that membrane function is linked to fatty acid/lipid composition and tissue composition in fish is strongly influenced by dietary composition (Turchini et al., 2009; Trushenski and Bowzer, 2012), it is reasonable to suppose that intestinal mucosal competence and fish health may be influenced by dietary lipid and fatty acid intake. In reviewing the possible avenues by which polyunsaturated fatty acids might influence the intestinal mucosa of mammals, Donnet-Hughes and colleagues (Donnet-Hughes et al., 2001) suggested that fatty acid intake might influence gut health via mechanisms related to eicosanoid synthesis, cytokine production and reactivity of immune cells, maintenance of a tight intestinal barrier, and composition of the gut microflora. More recently, it has been suggested that the lipidome (the complete lipid profile of a cell, tissue, or organism) might be targeted and harnessed by pathogens in order to avoid detection and clearance by the immune system (van der Meer-Janssen et al., 2010). Although lipid/mucosa interactions are still not fully understood, the literature suggests there are functional relationships between lipid/fatty acid intake and gut health in vertebrates, including fish.

To perform optimally, cellular membranes must be strong but flexible. The balance between these two attributes determines how well a membrane performs in terms of permeability, endocytic processes, embedded enzyme function, and translocation of ions and other substrates (Arts and Kohler, 2009). Thus, cellular membranes must be comprised of elements that disrupt strict rigidity and confer strength as well as fluidity to the lipid bilayer. Cholesterol and phospholipids containing saturated fatty acids provide strength, particularly at warm temperatures. Conversely, phospholipids containing unsaturated fatty acids provide fluidity, particularly at cold temperatures. Long-chain polyunsaturated fatty acids (LC-PUFA) with their many double bonds and coiled or semi-coiled structures are especially relevant in this context. For example, docosahexaenoic acid (22:6n-3, DHA) is known to influence various aspects of membrane function, including membrane permeability, fusion, and elasticity as well as vesicle formation (Arts and Kohler, 2009).

The fact that the lipid and fatty acid composition of fish tissues reflects dietary intake is perhaps one of the best-documented phenomena in fish nutrition and physiology (Turchini et al., 2009; Trushenski and Bowzer, 2012). Although most research investigating tissue composition in fish is focused on edible tissues, a number of studies have reported differences in composition of the intestinal tissues and their associated properties. It is known that composition of the gut epithelium varies with function along the length of the intestine in fish. Although the levels of phospholipids, cholesterol, and proteins appear to be relatively consistent throughout the intestine of trout, membranes of the mid-intestine are reportedly more fluid and richer in unsaturated fatty acids than those of the distal intestine (Pelletier et al., 1986). Various manipulations are known to affect the lipid/fatty acid composition and, presumably, the function of the gut epithelium. For example, transferring trout from freshwater to seawater causes DHA to become enriched within the brush border tissues and fluidity of the membranes to increase (Leray et al., 1984). The same effect was induced in carp held at cold temperatures by supplementing their diet with LC-PUFA-rich fish oil (Behar et al., 1989). Feeding fish oil to channel catfish (*Ictalurus punctatus*) altered the fatty acid composition of the brush border membranes in a similar fashion, but this was associated with reduced glucose transport in comparison to feeding with a non-fish oil, stearic acid (18:0)-rich diet (Houpe et al., 1997). Conversely, accumulation of monounsaturated fatty acids (MUFA) at the expense of LC-PUFA within the gut epithelium of European seabass (*Dicentrarchus labrax*) was associated with reduced activities of various brush border enzymes (Cahu et al., 2000). Interestingly, these changes were induced not by feeding diets with different fatty acid profiles, but by feeding increasing amounts of the same lipid (fish oil), suggesting that absolute levels of lipid in the diet may also influence membrane composition and function. Although compositional analyses were not conducted, the enterocytes of gilthead seabream (*Sparus aurata*) that were fed vegetable oils exhibited a different structure than those of fish that were fed fish oil (Caballero et al., 2003). The enterocytes of fish given rapeseed, linseed, and soybean oils contained substantially more lipid droplets and exhibited altered capacities for lipoprotein synthesis, though the enterocytes otherwise appeared morphologically normal.

Few studies have investigated the relationship between lipid nutrition, membrane composition or structure, and competency of the intestinal mucosa as a pathogen barrier. However, the limited data available suggests that a functional relationship may exist. Atlantic salmon successfully completed smoltification, regardless of whether they were fed diets containing sunflower oil or fish oil (Jutfelt et al., 2007). However, basal cortisol levels suggested fish that were fed the sunflower oil diet experienced a greater degree of physiological stress during smoltification, though nutrient uptake and prevention of bacterial translocation was apparently greater in these fish.

Arctic char *Salvelinus alpinus* fed diets containing marine-origin oil, linseed oil, or soybean oil exhibited differential survival rates following challenges with *A. salmonicida*, a pathogen thought to invade primarily by disruption of the gut epithelium (Lødemel et al., 2001). In this study, fish given the plant-origin oils exhibited reduced mortality. The authors were unable to unequivocally determine the basis for greater survival among fish served soybean or, to a lesser extent, linseed oil, but suggested changes in the microfloral community and/or increased production of mucus might have reduced adherence of *A. salmonicida* to the gut epithelium and subsequent infection.

8.3 Antinutritional factors and gut health

The functional competency of the gut in preventing pathogen translocation is linked to the structural integrity of the enterocytes and supporting tissues. For many years, fish nutritionists have known that a variety of feedstuffs, particularly plant-derived ingredients, may be toxic, cause feed palatability problems, or impair nutrient utilization and growth performance because of various "antinutritional factors" (ANFs) (Tacon, 1997; Francis et al., 2001). Numerous plant-derivatives are known to contain ANFs, including meals and protein concentrates derived from various legumes, including pulses, oilseed, and sowing crops. However, soybean products are likely the most widely recognized for their ANF content, containing protease inhibitors, lectins, phytic acid, saponins, phytoestrogens, allergens, and other problematic constituents (Tacon, 1997; Francis et al., 2001). Soybean derivatives are also noteworthy for their association with the development of enteritis in fish, particularly salmonids (Refstie and Storebakken, 2001; Gatlin et al., 2007). Soy-induced enteritis, or inflammation of the gut, is commonly characterized by the widening, shortening, and occasional disruption or fusion of the intestinal villi; a reduced number of supranuclear vacuoles in the absorptive epithelium; the widening and infiltration of the lamina propria by various types of leukocytes; and elevated levels of lysozyme and IgM in the gut mucosa. It can also be accompanied by a more generalized immune response, involving increases in circulating immunoglobulins and other proteins, as well as increases in the number and activity of circulating leukocytes (Refstie and Storebakken, 2001). Soy-induced enteritis may interfere with nutrient absorption, but the loss of the gut's function as a barrier to pathogen translocation and participation in antigen recognition, processing, and presentation may be of greater importance since the signs of inflammation in soy-induced enteritis are generally restricted to the distal intestine that, more than likely, is less involved in nutrient absorption than in immunological processes (Rombout et al., 2011).

The effects of plant proteins on gut integrity appear to be largely restricted to soy derivatives. In a screening of various legume, oilseed, and cereal-derived feedstuffs, only soybean meal-fed Atlantic salmon exhibited altered gut histomorphology (Aslaksen et al., 2007). Similarly, rainbow trout (*Oncorhynchus mykiss*) that were fed lupin meal failed to exhibit signs of enteritis (Glencross et al., 2004). Since soybean-derived products can contain a variety of ANFs, it is not clear which of these is the causative agent in the development of soy-induced enteritis. Based on their effects in fish and other species, it has been suggested that trypsin inhibitors, phytoestrogens, or lectins may be responsible for soybean meal-related enteritis (Sanden et al., 2005), which is consistent with most experiments associating soybean meal with enteritis as the alcohol-extraction process most commonly used to prepare soybean meal does not remove these substances (Aslaksen et al., 2007).

Other processing strategies effectively remove some, but not all, of the ANFs that plant products contain, resulting in products that have yielded mixed results in feeding trials. Soy protein concentrate, for example, contains lower levels of phytic acid, lectins, saponins, and oligosaccharides than soybean meal. Atlantic salmon that were fed soy protein concentrate did not exhibit enteritis, however, fish given pea protein concentrate did exhibit the classic signs of inflammation and villous atrophy of the distal intestine, along with reductions in gut enzyme activities and macronutrient digestibilities (Penn et al., 2011). Both concentrates benefit from processing, which removes or neutralizes many ANFs. However, not all ANFs are addressed equally by the processing methods specific to producing each concentrate. For example, saponins are greatly reduced in soy protein concentrate during alcohol extraction of soybean meal, but there is no equivalent step to reduce saponin levels in producing pea protein concentrate. Thus, saponins are abundant in pea protein concentrate, which induces enteritis, but not in soy protein concentrate, which does not, suggesting that saponins are a likely contributor to this response in salmonids (Penn et al., 2011). However, in another study, Atlantic salmon did not develop enteritis after being fed diets supplemented with saponins or the purported ANF oligosaccharides, stachyose and raffinose, which suggests that some other component is responsible for inducing soy-related enteritis (Sorensen et al., 2011).

In an attempt to elucidate the contribution of saponins to soybean meal-induced enteritis, Bureau and colleagues (Bureau et al., 1998) fed rainbow trout and Chinook salmon (*Oncorhynchus tshawytscha*) diets containing soybean meal or soy protein concentrate supplemented with an alcohol extract of soybean meal to approximate the same level of soy-derived saponins. Both diets suppressed feed intake in Chinook salmon, but not in rainbow trout. Expectedly, histological analysis of the distal intestine of Chinook salmon revealed abnormalities consistent with reduced or absent feeding, whereas the distal intestine of rainbow trout was generally unaffected by the soybean meal or soy saponin-supplemented feeds. The distal intestine of Japanese flounder (*Paralichthys olivaceus*) was similarly affected by saponin-supplemented feeds, but it was unclear whether the enteritis observed was the result of reduced feed intake or a specific response to dietary saponin content (Chen et al., 2011).

The most significant histopathological effects of soy products appear to be primarily associated with salmonids, but there are exceptions to this generalization, and it is likely that different taxa respond differently to soy derivatives and the ANFs they contain. The distal intestines of cobia (*Rachycentron canadum*) (Romarheim et al., 2008), Egyptian sole (*Solea aegyptiaca*) (Bonaldo et al., 2006), and European seabass (Bonaldo et al., 2008) were completely unaffected by feeding soybean meal. Similarly, the intestinal integrity of hybrid striped bass (*Morone chrysops* x *M. saxatilis*) was largely unaffected by feeding soybean meal, soy protein concentrate, or soy protein isolate (Blaufuss and Trushenski, 2012; Laporte and Trushenski, 2012). Gilthead seabream exhibited only minor infiltration of leukocytes into the lamina propria of the distal intestine (Bonaldo et al., 2008). Generally, plant proteins are not considered as problematic in feeds for herbivorous or omnivorous fish, but interspecies variation is also observed among these nutritional guilds: soy-induced enteritis is virtually unknown in species such as channel catfish (Evans et al., 2005), but has been demonstrated in common carp (*Cyprinus carpio*) (Urán et al., 2008).

Although there is apparently variation in the dietary constituents that induce enteritis and how fish respond to these ANFs, the signs of diet-induced enteritis are somewhat more consistent. These include changes in the morphology and functionality of the gut, particularly the distal intestine, as well as apparent broader involvement of the immune system. For example, soybean meal-induced enteritis in Atlantic salmon and is characterized by hypertrophic or hyperanaemic mucosa, shortening of the mucosal folds, and widening and infiltration of the lamina propria by various leukocytes. These effects are accompanied by changes in mucosal enzyme activities as well as an increase in IgM. Similar morphological changes were observed in both rainbow trout and Atlantic salmon that were fed soybean meal; however, inflammatory cell infiltration was less pronounced in the former (Refstie et al., 2000). Collectively, these results suggest that element(s) of soybean meal have a toxic effect on the apical membrane of fish and may delay or otherwise interfere with the production of new enterocytes. Cellular damage coupled with a reduced ability to replace damaged enterocytes implies reduced functionality of the gut in terms of nutrient absorption and pathogen exclusion.

Mucosal IgM was elevated in the mid-intestine of Atlantic salmon that were fed both soy protein concentrate and soy molasses; IgM was also elevated in the distal intestine, but only among those fish fed with soy molasses (Krogdahl et al., 2000). Mucosal lysozyme activity was elevated in the mid- and distal intestine of fish given soy molasses. Under some circumstances, these responses might be associated with a state of increased "immunological readiness"; however, these authors considered elevated IgM and lysozyme activity as primarily a consequence of gut inflammation (Krogdahl et al., 2000). Conversely, Atlantic salmon fed with relatively low levels of soy and maize did not consistently exhibit significant changes in the cytophysiology of the gut. Fish that were fed soybean meal exhibited significantly increased enterocyte proliferation and migration of immature or proliferating cells up the villous fold, whereas fish fed maize exhibited the opposite, though this effect was observed in only a few individuals (Sanden et al., 2005). The same increase in cellular proliferation was observed in Atlantic salmon that were given soybean meal (Bakke-McKellep et al., 2007). However, the inflamed gut was further characterized by increased and widespread heat-shock protein (HSP)70 and caspase-3 immunohistochemical reactivities that indicate elevated attempts at cellular repair and apoptosis, respectively, in the soy-fed fish (Bakke-McKellep et al., 2007). Overall, these results reinforce the concept of enteritis as cellular response that attempts to compensate for the "cytotoxic" effect of some as-yet unidentified element(s) of soybean meal.

Despite exhibiting the classical signs of soybean meal-induced enteritis in the distal intestine, nutrient transport and uptake of various nutrients were not predictably altered in rainbow trout and Atlantic salmon with fed soybean meal-based feeds (Nordrum et al., 2000). However, the authors stated that their results were suggestive of increased membrane permeability in the inflamed intestinal tissues (Nordrum et al., 2000). Regardless of whether greater membrane permeability is a cause or an effect of soybean meal-induced damage to the intestinal mucosa, it raises the possibility of increased vulnerability to pathogen translocation. For example, Krogdahl and colleagues (Krogdahl et al., 2000) observed significantly greater mortality among Atlantic salmon that were fed soybean meal-based feeds following *A. salmonicida* challenge than fish that were fed a soy protein concentrate-based feed. Moreover, lower mortality was observed in fish given the soy protein concentrate-based feed than the fish given the control fish meal-based feed. Although possible mechanisms for these observations were not addressed in this work, the authors did suggest that reduced epithelial integrity of the inflamed gut may have rendered fish fed with the soybean meal-based feed more vulnerable to infection. Alternatively, the "systemic health" of Atlantic salmon may have been generally compromised by soybean meal-induced enteritis and accompanying diarrhea, which rendered them, in their weakened state, more susceptible to disease (Krogdahl et al., 2000).

Similarly, rainbow trout fed high levels (80% or more of the diet) of standard or dehulled soybean meal or soy protein concentration exhibited significantly reduced head kidney macrophage competency as measured by respiratory burst activity (Burrells et al., 1999). These changes were associated with reduced growth rates, but not with a systemic immunogenic response to soy proteins, suggesting that there may be some merit to the concept that soy-based feeds generally reduce overall fish health by affecting their nutritional status and that the immunological response to soy antigens is largely a localized event restricted to the distal intestine. Again, these effects appear to be somewhat unique to soy-derived ANF since various enzymatic and blood chemistry measures of immune function were not affected in Atlantic salmon that were fed lupin meal or hydrolyzed poultry feather meal as alternatives to fish meal, and survival following challenge with *Vibrio anguillarum* was also equivalent among these fish (Bransden et al., 2001).

The effects of soy-derived ANFs may directly influence gut integrity and the immune system of fish; however, indirect effects observed with or without the classical signs of diet-induced enteritis may also be relevant in terms of general fish health. For example, Atlantic cod (*Gadus morhua*) did not exhibit major shifts in histomorphology or enzyme activities normally associated with feeding soybean meal, but other fish fed with soybean meal did exhibit increased densities of non-adherent bacteria (transient, allochthonous) compared to adherent bacteria (indigenous, autochthonous) in the gut (Refstie et al., 2006). Additionally, the taxonomic composition of the culturable gut bacteria was also altered in cod fed with soybean meal. These effects were not apparent among fish that were fed a bio-processed, enzyme-treated soybean meal. Although these authors could not provide specific evidence regarding diet-induced differences in the fish's ability to effectively exclude pathogenic bacteria at the level of the gut mucosa, they suggested this possibility and recommended further research on this effect (Refstie et al., 2006). Conversely, in Atlantic salmon exhibiting classical soybean meal-induced enteritis, there was a significant increase in the densities of adherent bacteria in both the mid- and distal intestine, whereas non-adherent bacteria were not affected in the mid-intestine but significantly elevated in the distal intestine (Bakke-McKellep et al., 2007). These authors also reported shifts in the taxonomic composition of the gut microflora, but could not state whether these changes were a cause or effect of the observed enteritis (Bakke-McKellep et al., 2007).

8.4 Concluding remarks

The literature on the topic of certain ANFs and gut enteritis in fish is extensive; there are far fewer investigations of the effect(s) that lipid nutrition may have on intestinal integrity and function. Undoubtedly, other ANFs and nutrients may also influence gut health in fish, but, if there is research being conducted on these topics, it is not yet readily apparent in the literature. In all cases, there is a dearth of experimentation comprehensively addressing the effects dietary constituents may have on the physiological and morphological condition of the gut mucosa and, more importantly, the effects of these nutrients or antinutrients on the functional competence of the gut in terms of nutrient acquisition as well as pathogen sampling and exclusion. Studies addressing both basic and applied aspects of nutrition as it pertains to gut health are needed and encouraged.

References

Arts, M.T., Kohler, C.C., 2009. Health and condition in fish: the influence of lipids on membrane competency and immune response. In: Arts, M.T., Brett, M.T., Kainz, M.J. (Eds.), Lipids in Aquatic Ecosystems. Springer, Dordrect, pp. 237–256.

Aslaksen, M.A., Kraugerud, O.F., Penn, M., Svihus, B., Denstadli, V., Jørgensen, H.Y., Hillestad, M., Krogdahl, Å., Storebakken, T., 2007. Screening of nutrient digestibility and intestinal pathologies in Atlantic salmon, *Salmo salar*, fed diets with legumes, oilseeds, or cereals. Aquaculture 272, 541–555.

Bakke-McKellep, A.M., Press, C.M., Baeverfjord, G., Krogdahl, Å., Landsverk, T., 2000. Changes in immune and enzyme histochemical phenotypes of cells in the intestinal mucosa of Atlantic salmon, *Salmo salar* L., with soybean meal-induced enteritis. J. Fish Dis. 23, 115–127.

Bakke-McKellep, A.M., Penn, M.H., Salas, P.M., Refstie, S., Sperstad, S., Landsverk, T., Ringø, E., Krogdahl, Å., 2007. Effects of dietary soybean meal, inulin and oxytetracycline on intestinal microbiota and epithelial cell stress, apoptosis and proliferation in the teleost Atlantic salmon *(Salmo salar L.)*. Br. J. Nutr. 97, 699–713.

Behar, D., Cogan, U., Viola, S., Mokady, S., 1989. Dietary fish oil augments the function of fluidity of the intestinal brush border membrane of the carp. Lipids 24, 737–742.

Blaufuss, P., Trushenski, J.T., 2012. Exploring soy-derived alternatives to fish meal: using soy protein concentrate and soy protein isolate in hybrid striped bass (*Morone chrysops* x *M. saxatilis*) feeds. N. Am. J. Aquacult. 74, 8–19.

Bonaldo, A., Roem, A.J., Pecchini, A., Grilli, E., Gatta, P.P., 2006. Influence of dietary soybean meal levels on growth, feed utilization and gut histology of Egyptian sole (*Solea aegyptiaca*) juveniles. Aquaculture 261, 580–586.

Bonaldo, A., Roem, A.J., Fagioli, P., Pecchini, A., Cipollini, I., Gatta, P.P., 2008. Influence of dietary levels of soybean meal on the performance and gut histology of gilthead sea bream (*Sparus aurata* L.) and European sea bass *(Dicentrarchus labrax)*. Aquacult. Res. 39, 970–978.

Bransden, M.P., Carter, C.G., Nowak, B.F., 2001. Effects of dietary protein source on growth, immune function, blood chemistry and disease resistance of Atlantic salmon (*Salmo salar* L.) parr. Anim. Sci. 73, 105–113.

Bureau, D.P., Harris, A.M., Cho, C.Y., 1998. The effects of purified alcohol extracts from soy products on feed intake and growth of chinook salmon (*Oncorhynchus tshawytscha*) and rainbow trout (*Oncorhynchus mykiss*). Aquaculture 161, 27–43.

Burrells, C., Williams, P.D., Southgate, P.J., Crampton, V.O., 1999. Immunological, physiological and pathological responses of rainbow trout (*Oncorhynchus mykiss*) to increasing dietary concentrations of soybean proteins. Vet. Immunol. Immunop. 72, 277–288.

Caballero, M.J., Izquierdo, M.S., Kjørsvik, E., Montero, D., Socorro, J., Fernández, A.J., Rosenlund, G., 2003. Morphological aspects of intestinal cells from gilthead seabream (*Sparus aurata*) fed diets containing different lipid sources. Aquaculture 225, 325–340.

Cahu, C.L., Zambonino-Infante, J.L., Corraze, G., Coves, D., 2000. Dietary lipid level affects fatty acid composition and hydrolase activities of intestinal brush border membrane in seabass. Fish Physiol. Biochem. 23, 165–172.

Chen, W.C., Ai, Q., Mai, K., Xu, W., Liufu, Z., Zhang, W., Cai, Y., 2011. Effects of dietary soybean saponins on feed intake, growth performance, digestibility and intestinal structure in juvenile Japanese flounder (*Paralichthys olivaceus*). Aquaculture 318, 95–100.

Donnet-Hughes, A., Schiffrin, E.J., Turini, M.E., 2001. The intestinal mucosa as a target for dietary polyunsaturated fatty acids. Lipids 36, 1043–1052.

Evans, J.J., Pasnik, D.J., Peres, H., Lim, C., Klesius, P.H., 2005. No apparent differences in intestinal histology of channel catfish (*Ictalurus punctatus*) fed heat-treated and non-heat-treated raw soybean meal. Aquacult. Nutr. 11, 123–129.

Francis, G., Makkar, H.P.S., Becker, K., 2001. Antinutritional factors present in plant-derived alternate fish feed ingredients and their effects in fish. Aquaculture 199, 197–227.

Gatlin, D.M., Barrows, F.T., Brown, P., Dabrowski, K., Gaylord, T.G., Hardy, R.W., Herman, E., Hu, G., Krogdahl, Å., Nelson, R., Overturf, K., Rust, M., Sealey, W., Skonberg, D., Souza, E.J., Stone, D., Wilson, R., Wurtele, E., 2007. Expanding the utilization of sustainable plant products in aquafeeds: a review. Aquacult. Res. 38, 551–579.

Glencross, B., Evans, D., Hawkins, W., Jones, B., 2004. Evaluation of dietary inclusion of yellow lupin (*Lupinus luteus*) kernel meal on the growth, feed utilization and tissue histology of rainbow trout (*Oncorhynchus mykiss*). Aquaculture 235, 411–422.

Houpe, K.L., Malo, C., Buddington, R.K., 1997. Dietary lipid and intestinal brush border membrane phospholipid fatty acid composition and glucose transport of channel catfish. Physiol. Zool. 70, 230–236.

Jutfelt, F., Olsen, R.E., Björnsson, B.T., Sundell, K., 2007. Parr-smolt transformation and dietary vegetable lipids affect intestinal nutrient uptake, barrier function and plasma cortisol levels in Atlantic salmon. Aquaculture 273, 298–311.

Kesarcodi-Watson, A., Kaspar, H., Lategan, M.J., Gibson, L., 2008. Probiotics in aquaculture: the need, principles and mechanisms of action and screening processes. Aquaculture 274, 1–14.

Krogdahl, Å., Bakke-McKellep, A.M., Røed, K.H., Baeverfjord, G., 2000. Feeding Atlantic salmon *Salmo salar* L. soybean products: effects on disease resistance (furunculosis), and lysozyme and IgM levels in the intestinal mucosa. Aquacult. Nutr. 6, 77–84.

Laporte, J., Trushenski, J.T., 2012. Production performance, stress tolerance, and intestinal integrity of sunshine bass fed increasing levels of soybean meal. J. Anim. Physiol. Nutr. 96, 513–526.

Leray, C., Chapelle, S., Duportail, G., Florentz, Al., 1984. Changes in fluidity and 22: 6(n-3) content in phospholipids of trout intestinal brush border membrane as related to environmental salinity. Biochimica et Biophysica Acta Biomembranes 778, 233–238.

Lødemel, J.B., Mayhew, T.M., Myklebust, R., Olsen, R.E., Espelid, S., Ringø, E., 2001. Effect of three dietary oils on disease susceptibility in Arctic charr (*Salvelinus alpinus* L.) during cohabitant challenge with *Aeromonas salmonicida* ssp. *Salmonicida*. Aquacult. Res. 32, 935–945.

Nordrum, S., Bakke-McKellep, A.M., Krogdahl, Å., Buddington, R.K., 2000. Effects of soybean meal and salinity on intestinal transport of nutrients in Atlantic salmon (*Salmo salar* L.) and rainbow trout (*Oncorhynchus mykiss*). Comp. Biochem. Phys. B 125, 317–335.

Pelletier, X., Duportail, G., Leray, C., 1986. Isolation and characterization of brush border membrane from trout intestine, regional differences. Biochimica et Biophysica Acta Biomembranes 856, 267–273.

Penn, M.H., Bendiksen, E.Å., Campbell, P., Krogdahl, Å., 2011. High level of dietary pea protein concentrate induces enteropathy in Atlantic salmon (*Salmo salar* L.). Aquaculture 310, 267–273.

Refstie, S., Korsøen, Ø.J., Storebakken, T., Baeverfjord, G., Lein, I., Roem, A.J., 2000. Differing nutritional responses to dietary soybean meal in rainbow trout (*Oncorhynchus mykiss*) and Atlantic salmon (*Salmo salar*). Aquaculture 190, 49–63.

Refstie, S., Landsverk, T., Bakke-McKellep, A.M., Ringø, E., Sundby, A., Shearer, K.D., Krogdahl, Å., 2006. Digestive capacity, intestinal morphology, and microflora of 1-year and 2-year old Atlantic cod (*Gadus morhua*) fed standard or bioprocessed soybean meal. Aquaculture 261, 269–284.

Refstie, S., Storebakken, T., 2001. Vegetable protein sources for carnivorous fish: potential and challenges. Rec. Adv. Anim. Nutr. Aust. 13, 195–203.

Ringø, E., Jutfelt, F., Kanapathippillai, P., Bakken, Y., Sundell, K., Glette, J., Mayhew, T.M., Myklebust, R., Olsen, R.E., 2004. Damaging effect of the fish pathogen *Aeromonas salmonicida* ssp. *Salmonicida* on intestinal enterocytes of Atlantic salmon (Salmo salar L.). Cell Tissue Res. 318, 305–311.

Romarheim, O.H., Zhang, C., Penn, M., Liu, Y.-J., Tian, L.-X., Skrede, A., Krogdahl, Å., Storebakken, T., 2008. Growth and intestinal morphology in cobia (*Rachycentron canadum*) fed extruded diets with two types of soybean meal partly replacing fish meal. Aquacult. Nutr. 14, 174–180.

Rombout, J.H.W.M., Abelli, L., Picchietti, S., Scapigliati, G., Kiron, V., 2011. Teleost intestinal immunology. Fish Shellfish Immunol. 31, 616–626.

Sanden, M., Berntssen, M.H.G., Krogdahl, Å., Hemre, G.-I., Bakke-McKellep, A.M., 2005. An examination of the intestinal tract of Atlantic salmon, *Salmo salar* L., parr fed different varieties of soy and maize. J. Fish Dis. 28, 317–330.

Sørensen, M., Penn, M., El-Mowafi, A., Storebakken, T., Chunfang, C., Øverland, M., Krogdahl, Å., 2011. Effect of stachyose, raffinose and soya-saponins supplementation on nutrient digestibility, digestive enzymes, gut morphology and growth performance in Atlantic salmon (*Salmo salar* L.). Aquaculture 314, 145–152.

Tacon, A.G.J., 1997. Fishmeal replacers: review of antinutrients within oilseeds and pulses – a limiting factor for the aquafeed Green Revolution? In: Tacon, A.G.J., Basurco, B. (Eds.), Feeding Tomorrow's Fish. International Centre for Advanced Mediterranean Agronomic Studies, Paris, pp. 153–182.

Trushenski, J.T., Bowzer, J.C., 2012. Having your omega 3 fatty acids and eating them, too: strategies to ensure and improve the long-chain polyunsaturated fatty acid content of farm-raised fish. In: De Meester, F., Watson, R.R., Zibadi, S. (Eds.), Sustainable Long Chain Omega-3 Fatty Acids in Cardiovascular and Mental Health. Springer, New York, pp. 319–340.

Turchini, G.M., Torstensen, B.E., Ng, W.-K., 2009. Fish oil replacement in finfish nutrition. Rev. Aquacult. 1, 10–57.

Urán, P.A., Gonçalves, A.A., Taverne-Thiele, J.J., Schrama, J.W., Verreth, J.A.J., Rombout, H.W.M., 2008. Soybean meal induces intestinal inflammation in common carp (*Cyprinus carpio* L.). Fish Shellfish Immunol. 25, 751–760.

van der Meer-Janssen, Y.P.M., van Galen, J., Batenburg, J.J., Helms, B., 2010. Lipids in host-pathogen interactions: pathogens exploit the complexity of the host cell lipidome. Prog. Lipid Res. 49, 1–26.

Nutritional impacts on fish mucosa: immunostimulants, pre- and probiotics

9

Christopher Marlowe A. Caipang; Carlo C. Lazado***
*School of Applied Science, Temasek Polytechnic, Singapore
**Aquaculture Genomics Research Unit, Faculty of Biosciences and Aquaculture, University of Nordland, Bodø, Norway

Chapter Outline

9.1 Background

Fish live in aquatic environments that provide an ideal medium for the growth of various kinds of microorganisms. These conditions pose additional challenges to the mucosal immune system of aquatic vertebrates in comparison with their terrestrial counterparts. As a consequence, some of the principles of mammalian mucosal immunity may not be necessarily applicable to aquatic vertebrates. The gut, the skin, and the gills are the main mucosal surfaces and immune barriers of teleosts. Lower vertebrates, including cartilaginous and teleost fish, are the oldest animals that possess an adaptive immune system including antibodies, B cells, and T cells (Flajnik and Kasahara, 2010). In addition, teleost fish are the most primitive vertebrates where antibodies that are specific to mucosal surfaces have been well characterized (Zhang et al., 2010). These large and multifunctional surfaces are the sites where the innate and adaptive immune systems initially cooperate during the evolution of vertebrates to allow "good" while avoiding "bad" microorganisms (Gomez et al., 2013).

Fish skin is considered as the primary barrier that provides the physical and chemical protection in association with its mucus. The latter is composed of glycoproteins, proteoglycans, and proteins. The mucus constitutes a layer that exists as an interface between the fish and the environment (Dalmo et al., 1997). Diverse antimicrobial factors that are found in the mucus prevent the colonization of the integument by potentially harmful microorganisms (Alexander and Ingram, 1992; Ruangsri et al., 2010).

Fish gills are multifunctional in nature and act as a respiratory organ. They are also involved in the immune defense through the mucosa-associated lymphoid tissues that harbor macrophages, neutrophils, lymphocytes, and mast cells/eosinophilic granulocytes (Pratap and Wendelaar Bonga, 1993; Reite and Evensen, 2006). Lymphoid cell aggregations, including T cells, are similar to those that are described in mammalian mucosa. These cells are found in the interbranchial septum at the base of the gill filaments, suggesting their involvement in the immune response during gill infections (Haugarvoll et al., 2008).

The gastrointestinal tract (GIT) is an organ with several functions in nutrition and in immunity. The organization of the gut-associated lymphoid system of teleost intestine is not as complex compared with mammals, and has a more diffused pattern (Rombout et al., 2011).

The gut mucosa is rich in immune cells such as lymphocytes, plasma cells, eosinophilic (mast cell-like) granulocytes, and macrophages and can elicit local responses (Press and Evensen, 1999). The GIT mucosal surface is a natural interface where the intestinal microbiota and antigens cross-talk with the host (Montalto et al., 2009). Commensals or pathogenic bacteria are in direct contact with the gut mucosa and the gut-associated lymphoid tissue (GALT) has the ability to distinguish between the two kinds of bacteria and eventually initiate either tolerance or an immune response towards that bacteria.

The major portals of entry that pathogens can penetrate fish include the gills, intestines and the skin (Baudin Laurencin and Germon, 1987). Recently, in the case of infectious hemapoietic necrosis virus (IHNV), the virus can also enter the fish via the fin bases (Harmache et al., 2006). The mucosal immune system in fish includes the above-mentioned tissues and presents the primary barrier to ward off pathogen invasion. These tissues are in direct contact with the external environment; thus, exposed to potential pathogens. They mediate the innate and adaptive responses to potential invaders and also function to limit the intensity of activation to avoid tissue damage. In mammals, the mucosal immune system apparently functions independently from systemic immunity (Holmgren and Czerkinsky, 2005). In teleost fish, the gills and intestinal epithelium, like the mammalian mucosal epithelium, are functionally diverse.

While the gill epithelium, together with its mucus layer, acts as an important physical barrier (Press and Evensen, 1999), there is no evidence of lymphoid tissue architecture similar to the mammalian GALT such as the Peyer's patches. However, the teleost gut contains important populations of leukocytes (Press and Evensen, 1999) and there is sufficient evidence to show the presence of a functional cutaneous innate and adaptive immunity in fish (Schluter et al., 1999; Ellis, 2001).

In the mucosa of the intestines, the immune-stimulating (IS) component of fish diets often contain molecules such as pathogen-associated molecular patterns (PAMPs) that interact with a diverse set of cellular receptors known as pattern recognition receptors (PRRs). Upon contact of the PAMPs with the PRRs, specific cellular responses are elicited, which leads to the initiation of an immune response to pathogenic organisms (Sirard et al., 2006). As such, immunostimulation via enteric formulation aims to induce a PAMP-PRR host response and to increase the activity of the immune system over a definite period of time. This approach aims to avoid a general induction of the immune response that would not be beneficial to the organism.

The concept of maintaining the health of fish through the best possible nutrition is well accepted in modern aquaculture. Scientific evidence clearly indicates that dietary nutrients as well as additives have the ability to stimulate the immune system and to protect the fish from pathogenic diseases. Despite these findings, the supporting information is scarce as compared to the knowledge on terrestrial animals. As feeds for aquaculture evolve, there will be an increasing number of "functional feeds" on the market; thus, fish farmers will have difficulty in deciding on the appropriate choice of feed for their fish. Therefore, it is important to determine the bioavailability and functionality of the active ingredients that are incorporated in the feeds in order to present the true value of the feeds that are being given to fish.

9.2 Immunostimulants

Aquaculture has grown rapidly for food production in the last few decades. Several commercial fish species have been cultured intensively in various aquaculture systems such as ponds, cages, or tanks. The culture of the fish at high densities adversely affects the health of the fish in a stressful environment and in the presence of potential infectious diseases (Sakai, 1999). Outbreaks of infectious diseases are major constraints in the development of aquaculture. The occurrences of such outbreaks in different areas take place due to the uncontrolled movement of live aquatic animals resulting in the transfer of pathogenic organisms among these areas (Jadhav et al., 2006). Antibiotics and chemotherapeutics have been used to prevent or control bacterial infections in aquaculture for a number of years (Sakai, 1999). Unfortunately, the use of antibiotics for treatment is not successful and sustainable due to increase in antibiotic-resistant bacteria, negative effects on the indigenous microflora of the fish (Misra et al., 2006), and the accumulation of antibiotic residues in fish tissue and the environment causing human and animal health issues. Vaccination is an effective prophylactic treatment for infectious diseases in fish during the culture period, but the process of doing so could be very expensive and stressful to the fish. A single vaccine is effective against only a specific type of pathogen, thus, which limits the effectiveness of that particular vaccine for a wide range of pathogens due to the complex antigenic structure (Ardo et al., 2008). Therefore, there is a need to look for alternative techniques for disease prevention, which are at the same time environmentally friendly and highly effective.

The manipulation of the immune response in aquatic organisms by diet is a commonly accepted practice in many intensive aquaculture systems. Diets that contain immunostimulants are mostly utilized in aquaculture to enhance the resistance of the cultured species against pathogenic diseases. Previously, these diets were thought to act primarily on the innate immune system by enhancing the activity of phagocytic cells (Sakai, 1999); however, a more generic definition has been advanced by Bricknell and Dalmo (2005), suggesting to include the full potential of the immune response and its corresponding cellular players.

An immunostimulant is a naturally occurring substance that has a modulatory effect upon the immune system. The term has been interchangeably used with immunomodulator, adjuvant and biological response modifier (Ganguly et al., 2010). Sakai (1999) indicated that immunostimulants could be grouped depending on their sources; bacterial, algae-derived, animal-derived, nutritional factors and hormones/cytokines. This subgrouping changed the concept that immunostimulants instead are divided according to their modes of actions. Previously, an immunostimulant was defined based upon its activity on the mononuclear phagocytic system only (Seljelid, 1990). However, due to recent discoveries of the pattern recognition receptors (PPRs) of phagocytic cells, the former definition of an immunostimulant has been changed based on the different PPRs and the immune cells that bring about the varied immune responses depending on the types of ligands that the PPRs interact with. According to Bricknell and Dalmo (2005), an immunostimulant is "a naturally occurring compound that modulates the immune system by increasing the resistance of the host against diseases that in most cases are caused by pathogens." Immunostimulants have been used as feed additives for several years in aquaculture, and yeast β-glucan might be the one that has the longest track record. β-glucans are widespread in nature and have been characterized in microorganisms, algae, fungi, and plants (Volman et al., 2008). The chemical structure of β-glucan varies depending on the molecular weight and degree of branching. For example, β-glucan from yeast contains a particular carbohydrate with glucose and mannose residues and is a major constituent in the cell membrane.

To this end, diet additives with immune-stimulating ability form a diverse range of bioactive compounds ranging from synthetic chemicals such as levamisole, an anthelminthic used to treat nematode infections in mammals (Keiser and Utzinger, 2008), bacterial lipopolysaccharides (Guttvik et al., 2002), nucleotides (Carrington and Secombes, 2006; Li and Gatlin, 2006), a range of polysaccharides, animal and plant extracts, specific dietary nutrients such as vitamin C, and certain hormones and cytokines (Sakai, 1999). However, commercial immunostimulant diets are mainly limited to the addition of β1-3 and β1-6 glucans (Ringø et al., 2012).

The following are the more commonly used immunostimulants in aquaculture:

9.2.1 Synthetic chemicals

A well-known synthetic chemical that is used as an immunostimulant in fish and shellfish is levamisole. This chemical is an antihelminthic compound that is used to treat nematode infections in humans and in animals. It can stimulate immune responses *in vitro*. Levamisole enhanced phagocytic activity, NBT reaction, and increased antibody-producing cells. Oral administration of levamisole increased the number of leukocytes as well as lysozyme activities in serum (Siwicki, 1989). However, no differences were found in the levels of hematocrit or immunoglobulin using levamisole in rainbow trout (Ispir and Dorucu, 2005). Findlay et al. (2000) recommended the application of levamisole as an immunostimulant in fish, and it was observed that rainbow trout following exposure to a bath treatment containing 5, 10, 25 μg/mL levamisole for a 2 h period showed resistance to *Yersinia ruckeri* (Ispir, 2009).

9.2.2 Bacterial derivatives

There are several components of both gram-positive and gram-negative bacteria that have been tested as immunostimulants for fish in aquaculture. These include the following.

9.2.2.1 LPS (lipopolysaccharide)

LPS is a cell wall component of gram-negative bacteria. This substance can stimulate the proliferation of B cells and enhance macrophage phagocytic activity in red seabream, Pagrus major (Salati et al., 1987). It can also trigger the increased production of macrophage-activating factor in goldfish lymphocytes (Neumann et al., 1995). It was reported that LPS is effective in preventing *A. hydrophila* infections and in stimulating the innate immune response of rainbow trout (Nya and Austin, 2010). These substances are very potent even in very low doses and may occur as contaminants in bacterin preparations and used in fish immunizing programs.

9.2.2.2 Whole bacterial cells

Vibrio anguillarum bacterin (inactivated whole cell vaccine) is the most successful vaccine for salmonid fish, administered through injection, oral, and immersion methods (Sakai, 1999). Immunostimulation of *V. anguillarum* bacterin was observed in fish and shellfish. Norqvist et al. (1989) reported that vaccination of rainbow trout with attenuated *V. anguillarum* stimulates protection against *Aeromonas salmonicida* challenge.

9.2.3 Polysaccharides

The most common derivatives from polysaccharides that are popularly used as immunostimulants are the following.

9.2.3.1 Glucans

Glucans include diverse glucose polymers that differ in the position of glycosidic bonds, which can be short or long, branched or unbranched, alpha or beta isomers, and soluble or particulate (Goodridge et al., 2009). They are high molecular-weight substances composed of glucose as building blocks, usually isolated from cell walls of bacteria, mushrooms, algae, cereal grains, yeast, and fungi (Zekovic and Kwiatowski, 2005). Glucans in general comprise a wide variety of substances that are commonly found in nature including cellulose, glycogen, and starch, most of which do not interact with the immune system. Pharmacologically, they are classified as biological response modifiers (BRM). The common feature of immunomodulatory glucans is a chain of glucose residues linked by β-1,3-linkages, also called beta-glucans. Of the different β-glucans, the products known as β-1,3/1,6-glucans, derived from baker's yeast, are suggested to be the most potent immune-system enhancers (Ringø et al., 2012). β-1,3/1,6-glucans are characterized by the presence of side-chains that are attached to the backbone that radiate outward like branches on a tree.

The frequency and nature of the side-chains strongly affect the ability of the glucan to mediate binding to surface receptors on the target cells; thus, influencing the effectiveness of the glucan as an immunostimulant (Ringø et al., 2012). A number of reports showed that dietary administration of β-glucan increases resistance of fish against infection. Selvaraj et al. (2005) reported that highest antibody titer against *A. hydrophila* injected with β-glucan (100–1000 μg glucans/fish). In addition, Robertsen et al. (1990) recorded that intraperitoneal injection of β-glucan prepared from cell walls of *Saccharomyces cerevisiae* injected in Atlantic salmon showed increased resistance to *V. anguillarum*, *V. salmonicida*, and *Y. ruckeri*.

9.2.3.2 Chitin and chitosan

Chitin is a polysaccharide that constitutes the principal component of exoskeletons of crustaceans and insects as well as cell walls of select fungi (Sakai, 1999). This substance enhances macrophage activity and provides resistance from certain bacteria (Kawakami et al., 1998). Also, brook trout, *Salvelinus fontinalis*, were significantly protected from *A. salmonicida* infection when injected with or immersed in chitosan solution (Anderson and Siwicki, 1994).

9.2.4 Animal and plant extracts

Various animal and plant extracts have been tested as immunostimulants in fish by incorporating these additives in the feed.

9.2.4.1 Animal extracts

An extract from the marine tunicate, *Ecteinascida turbinata* (Ete) enhanced the phagocytosis and increased survival of eel following experimental challenge with *A. hydrophila* (Davis and Hayasaka, 1984). In addition, rainbow trout injected with the glycoprotein fraction of the water extract from abalone, *Haliotis discus hannai* (Hde), showed increased survival along with enhanced phagocytic activities during infection with *Vibrio anguillarum* (Sakai et al., 1991).

9.2.4.2 Plant extracts

Some immunostimulants cannot be used because of various disadvantages, such as high cost and limited effectiveness upon parenteral administration. Numerous plants have, on the other hand, long been used in traditional medicine for the treatment and control of several diseases (Duke, 1987). Herbs have little side effects, are easily degradable, and are abundantly available in farm areas, thus, numerous studies have been done to investigate the effects of these different plant products on the immune responses and to determine the protective abilities of these plant products against pathogenic agents in fish and shellfish (Harikrishnan et al., 2011).

Medicinal plants contain a number of bioactive compounds, e.g., glycyrrhizin (GL) and its aglycon glycyrrhetic acid (GA), liquiritin (LQ), liquiritin apioside (LA), isoliquiritin (IL), and glabridin (GLAB) and also contain several active components, including polysaccharides, alkaloids, and/or flavonoids (Cinatl et al., 2003). *Astragalus membranaceus* and *Lonicera japonica* extracts can be used as immunostimulants to enhance immune response and disease resistance of cultured fish species (Ardo et al., 2008). The herbal immunostimulants such as *Emblica officinalis*, *Cynodon dactylon*, and *Adathoda vasica* improved the immune system and reduced microbial infection in the goldfish, *Carassius auratus* (Minomol, 2005) and similar work was also carried out by Magdelin (2005) on another ornamental fish, *Poecilia sphenops*, using herbal immunostimulants. Nile tilapia showed enhanced phagocytic activity after treatment with *Astragalus* extract for one week (Yin et al., 2006; Ardo et al., 2008). Dugenci et al. (2003) documented that ginger extract was highly effective in enhancing phagocytic and extracellular burst activity of white blood cells in rainbow trout.

9.2.5 Nutritional factors

Vitamins and minerals are micronutrients that can affect disease resistance. However, there are controversies whether or not these nutritional factors fit into the latest definition of immunostimulants (Sakai, 1999; Suchner et al., 2000). Ringø et al (2012) did not include these nutritional factors in their latest review because vitamins and minerals enhance the immune system by providing substrates and serving as cofactors that are necessary for the immune system to work properly rather than modulating the immune responses. No definite consensus has been reached on this subject, and to make the topic wider in scope, the authors have included nutritional factors, particularly vitamins C and E as immunostimulants.

9.2.5.1 Vitamin C

Vitamin C or ascorbic acid is one of the powerful reducing agents available to cells by serving as a cofactor for the incorporation of molecular oxygen into various substrates (Englard and Seifter, 1986). Vitamin C is involved in several physiological functions including growth, development, reproduction, wound healing, response to stressors, and possibly lipid metabolism through its action on carnitine synthesis when given to the fish through dietary administration. Because vitamin C is a cofactor in many biological processes including collagen synthesis and cellular functions related to neuromodulation, hormone, and immunity, there have been a number of studies that were conducted in fish to determine the effects of this vitamin on the immune responses particularly in salmonids and catfish (Dabrowski, 2000). From an immunological perspective, it is interesting to note that vitamin C concentrations are high in the head kidney, the spleen, and the leucocytes of fish (Gabaudan and Verlhac, 2001). Therefore, it is likely that the cells of the immune system rely on this vitamin for achieving protection during pathogen invasion. It has been observed by Tewary and Patra (2008) that higher levels of dietary vitamin C significantly increased protection against *A. hydrophila* infections in fish.

9.2.5.2 Vitamin E

Vitamin E compounds (tocopherols) are the major chain-breaking antioxidants. They help in the maintenance of inter- and intracellular homeostasis of labile metabolites such as oxidizable vitamins and unsaturated fatty acids (Halver, 2002). Inadequate amounts of dietary vitamin E would result in nonspecific cell degenerative conditions. Erythrocytes exhibited greater fragility when there is inadequate level of Vitamin E in the diet (Kiron et al., 1994). The free radical quenching ability of vitamin E enables it to protect the polyunsaturated fatty acids (PUFA) of membrane phospholipids from the single oxygen that is produced during the oxidation process. As a therapeutic nutrient, high dietary vitamin E has been shown to increase lymphocyte counts, stimulate cytotoxic activity of cells, and enhance phagocytosis and mitogen responsiveness in mammals (Watson, 1998). Further, it is presumed to be involved in disease prevention by preventing the production of infection-induced tissue prostaglandins and by regulating cytokine production (Watson, 1998). Vitamin E can enhance specific and cell-mediated immunity against infection in Japanese flounder, *Paralichthys olivaceus* (Villegas et al., 2006) and macrophage phagocytosis in channel catfish, *Ictalurus punctatus* (Wise et al., 1993) and turbot, *Scopthalamus maximus* (Pulsford et al., 1995).

9.2.6 Hormones

9.2.6.1 Growth hormone (GH)

GH directly affects immunocompetent cells such as macrophages, lymphocytes, and NK cells (Sakai, 1999). In fish, exogenous growth hormone (GH) has mitogenic activity on lymphocytes and activates NK cells and production of superoxide anions of leukocytes (Sakai et al., 1996b).

9.2.6.2 Prolactin

Prolactin also directly affects immunocompetent cells like macrophages, lymphocytes, and NK cells. It can enhance the production of superoxide anions of leukocytes. Sakai et al. (1996a) demonstrated that prolactin increased the level of production of superoxide anion in the leukocytes of rainbow trout.

9.2.6.3 Lactoferrin

This hormone consists of a single peptide chain with molecular weight of approximately 87,000 Da and possesses 2 Fe-binding sites per molecule; this considered to be the most popular physiological fluids of mammals (Sakai, 1999).

9.2.7 Cytokines

These are polypeptides or glycoproteins that act as modulators in the immune system. Cytokines may be useful as powerful immunostimulants if their structures can be identified and recombinant molecules are prepared. A recombinant interferon-like has been produced from Japanese flounder, *Paralichthys olivaceus*, and this recombinant hormone inhibited the replication of a virus *in vitro* (Tamai et al., 1993).

9.2.8 Algal derivatives

9.2.8.1 Laminaran

Laminaran is a β (1, 6)-branched β (1, 3)-D-glucan, a major component in sublittoral brown algae, e.g., *Phaeophyceae*. Almost all β-(1, 3) D-glucans display poor water solubility, which makes them more difficult to handle than the aqueous soluble laminaria. Laminaran, which is obtained from *Laminaria hyperhorea*, has an immunomodulatory effect on immune system as well.

9.2.8.2 Alginic acid

Alginic acid or alginates are capsular polysaccharides in soil bacteria or as constituents of cell walls of brown algae (*Phaeophyceae*). They are a family of linear unbranched polysaccharides with (1→4) linked β-D-mannuronic acid and α-L-guluronic acid residues in different ratios (Gombotz and Wee, 1998). Usually they are extracted from seaweeds (*Macrocystis pyrifera, Ascophyllum nodosum*, or different types of Laminaria), though bacteria of genera *Pseudomonas* and zotobacter also produce these substances. The application of alginates in feeds, for larval rearing or for during the grow-out phase, benefits the fish by stimulating the innate immune system. Various types of alginates have been found to improve disease resistance in fish.

9.2.9 Dietary oligonucleotides

These substances are not strictly immunostimulants by definition but provide a dietary supplement that allows improved resistance during invasion of a pathogen (Ringø et al., 2012). Dietary nucleotides are considered nonessential due to the high rates of their *de novo* synthesis (e.g., RNA and DNA) that takes place in the human body, compared to the actual intake (Grimble and Westwood, 2001). Cosgrove (1998) has described nucleotides as "ubiquitous intracellular compounds that are involved in the vital cell function and metabolism – as nucleic acids, in biosynthetic pathways, in transferring chemical energy, as co-enzyme components and as biological regulators."

The relationship between dietary nucleotides and immune functions has been reviewed by Gil (2002). Dietary oligonucleotides influence lymphocyte activation and proliferation, enhance phagocytic activity, influence immunoglobulin responses during the early life stages, and augment production of cytokines, particularly in the intestine. In addition, Li and Gatlin (2006) discussed the influence of dietary oligonucleotides on the innate and adaptive immunity in fish and have pointed out that the dietary oligonucleotides could support lymphoid tissues that have limited *de novo* synthesizing capacity. The benefits of dietary nucleotides has been demonstrated in both marine and freshwater fish.

9.3 Prebiotics

9.3.1 The prebiotic concept

The prebiotic concept was introduced by Gibson and Roberfroid in 1995 to describe nondigestible food ingredients that selectively stimulate the growth and/or the metabolism of beneficial bacterial community in the gut, thus improving host well-being and health (Ganguly et al., 2013; Gibson and Roberfroid, 1995). Some people often regard prebiotics and probiotics to be the same. Though both are agents that can promote health and improve the well-being of an organism, there are different aspects by which prebiotics can be technically differentiated from probiotics. First, the use of prebiotics as feed additives does not require particular precautions and authorization (Gatesoupe, 2005). Second, prebiotics unlike probiotics are not “microorganisms” (though some are microorganism-derived), thus having less influence on the environment (Yousefian and Amiri, 2009). This aspect is a challenge with the use of probiotics because safety is a major concern in employing microbial intervention strategies both for the host and the associated organisms of its rearing environment. During the initial introduction of the concept, prebiotics were characterized by substances capable of stimulating the *Bifidobacteria* and *Lactobacilli* populations, the known beneficial microbial communities of human gastrointestinal tract (Gatesoupe, 2005). Besides in human (Gibson and Roberfroid, 1995; Manning and Gibson, 2004; Rastall, 2004), the shifting of intestinal microbial communities particularly the dominance of *Bifidobacterium* spp. and *Lactobacillus* spp. populations following prebiotic administration have been documented in poultry (Stanley et al., 2012; Patterson and Burkholder, 2003) and pigs (Berge and Wierup, 2012; Konstantinov et al., 2004; Smiricky-Tjardes et al., 2003a). The promotion of these bacterial communities is considered a beneficial effect because the by-products they produce during the fermentation of prebiotics play a major role in improving host health (Choque-Delgado et al., 2011). Prebiotics are also known as functional saccharides by serving as energy sources to the commensal bacteria during fermentation in the intestinal tract (Roberfroid, 1993).

In principle, any carbohydrate that enters the colon can be potentially considered as prebiotics (O’Sullivan et al., 2010). This is one of the reasons why “prebiotic” properties have been attributed loosely to many substances without taking into consideration if they have indeed fulfilled the defined criteria to be regarded as one. In order for a particular compound to be considered as prebiotics, it needs to pass the three major considerations (Gibson et al., 2004). These scientific requirements are patterned on mammalian models but may be applied to fish as well. At present, no specific requirements are available for "fish prebiotics" and the human-based requirements serve a purpose in fish and in other animals thus remained a widely accepted qualification criteria. A substance is qualified as prebiotics if it resists gastric acidity, enzymatic hydrolysis, and gastrointestinal absorption; is fermented by the intestinal microflora; and selectively stimulates the growth and/or activity of intestinal bacteria associated with health and well-being.

Many substances have been regarded as prebiotics but only a few have been fully demonstrated qualifying the above-mentioned criteria. Only three carbohydrate types are accepted as true prebiotics to date: inulin and oligofructose, galactooligosaccharides, and lactulose (Kolida and Gibson, 2008).

9.3.2 Common prebiotics in aquaculture

9.3.2.1 Fructooligosaccharides (FOS)

Fructooligosaccharides (FOS) are oligosaccharides that occur naturally in plants such as onion, chicory, garlic, asparagus, banana, artichoke, among many others (Sabater-Molina et al., 2009). This group of nondigestible carbohydrate represents one of the major classes of bifidogenic (capable of stimulating the *Bifidobacterium* spp.) oligosaccharides (Murphy, 2001; Rivero-Urgell and Santamaria-Orleans, 2001). The structural component of FOS is composed of short-chain oligomers of monosaccharide units containing kestose, nystose, and 1-β-fructofuranosyl nystose in which fructosyl units are bound by β-(2→1) position of sucrose with the last one attached to a terminal glucose moiety (Ganaie et al., 2014). The presence of terminal glucose unit linked by β-(2→1) glycosidic bonds in the chain of fructose units made this compound nondigestible by human digestive enzymes that are known to be specific for α-glycosidic bonds (Teitelbaum and Walker, 2002). The valuable prebiotic property of FOS is characterized by the metabolic transformation aided by the cell-associated β-fructofuranosidases of the beneficial bacterial population in the gut, which eventually liberate monomeric fructose molecules that are then transported into the bacterial cell (Perrin et al., 2001). Consequently, the metabolic products selectively support the growth and activity of beneficial bacterial community in the gastrointestinal tract of animals leading to an improved gut health.

9.3.2.2 Mannan oligosaccharides (MOS)

The majority of the mannan oligosaccharides (MOS)-based products that are used in aquaculture species are derived from the outer cell wall of yeast (*S. cerevisiae*) that is present in a complex formation (Torrecillas et al., 2014). The main constituents of the outer cell wall are mannan polymers with α-(1→6) and α-(1→2) bonds or to a lesser extent α-(1→3) bounded side chains (Kogan and Kocher, 2007). One of the distinguishing features that differentiate MOS from other prebiotics is that mannose sugar could interfere with the colonization of pathogen by serving as a blocking agent in intestinal cells. It has been shown that the adherence of quite a number of pathogenic microbes to the enterocyte cell wall is a prerequisite for the onset of infection (Gibbons and Van Houte, 1975); therefore, the capability of prebiotics in interfering this process is considered a beneficial property. MOS act as high affinity ligands, offering a competitive binding site for bacteria (Ofek et al., 1977). The mannose-specific Type-1 fimbriae typified by most pathogenic bacteria is essential in the adsorbtion of these pathogens to the MOS instead of attaching to intestinal epithelial cells, which then pass through the intestinal tract without colonization (Ferket et al., 2002). MOSs are also capable of triggering potent innate immune responses from the host animal. The mannose receptor (MR) that is present in macrophages and endothelial cell subsets serves an endocytic receptor capable of recognizing both self-glycoproteins and microbial glycans (Ringø et al., 2014). In the presence of MOS, intracellular signaling cascades can be induced in dendritic cells by mannose-containing ligands through MR leading to stimulated production of pro-inflammatory cytokines (Song et al., 2014). MOSs have been assigned as nutricines as well on the principle that they are not direct nutrients either for intestinal microbiota or for the host, but potentially have a positive effect on the health and performance of farm animals (Adams, 2001).

9.3.2.3 Short-chain fructooligosaccharides (scFOS)

Short-chain fructooligosaccharides occur in a number of plants such as onions, Jerusalem artichokes, asparagus, wheat, rye, and garlic. Onion has the highest content of scFOSs, ranging from 25–40% (dry matter basis) (Clevenger et al., 1988). scFOS are produced either from sucrose by transfructosylation with fructosyltransferases (β-fructofuranosidase, EC 3.2.1.26 or β-d-fructosyltransferase, EC 2.4.1.9) or from inulin by controlled enzymatic hydrolysis (Vega-Paulino and Zúniga-Hansen, 2012). As similar to most prebiotics, these substances promote the dominance of beneficial gastrointestinal bacteria and stimulate their metabolic activity (Huebner et al., 2007), thereby, suppressing potentially pathogenic bacteria (Roberfroid et al., 1998). They are fermented by resident bacteria into short-chain fatty acids (i.e., acetate, propionate, and butyrate), lactic acid, carbon dioxide, and hydrogen (Philippeau et al., 2010; Smiricky-Tjardes et al., 2003a; Smiricky-Tjardes et al., 2003b). Interestingly, they are fermented only by a limited number of microorganisms including Bacteroides and Bifidibacteria family (Philippeau et al., 2010; Hidaka et al. 1986; Smiricky-Tjardes et al., 2003a; Smiricky-Tjardes et al., 2003b).

9.3.2.4 Galactooligosaccharide (GOS)

Galactooligosaccharides are also regarded as bifidogenic prebiotics (Bouhnik et al., 1997; Ito et al., 1990). The commercial form of galactooligosaccharides is produced from lactose using glycosyltransferase activity of the enzyme β-galactosidase (Nilsson, 1988); a GOS constitutes around 2–20 molecules of galactose and glucose (Yang and Silva, 1995). Indigestibility and stability to hydrolysis from digestive enzymes of GOS have been demonstrated, making them as ideal prebiotics. Recently, GOS was distinctively defined as "a mixture of those substances produced from lactose, comprising between 2 and 8 saccharide units, with one of these units being a terminal glucose and the remaining saccharide units being galactose and disaccharides comprising 2 units of galactose" (Tzortzis and Vulevic, 2009).

9.3.2.5 Arabinoxylan-oligosaccharide (AXOS)

One of the newest candidate prebiotics in fish is the oligosaccharide class of arabinoxylan-oligosaccharide (AXOS) (Song et al., 2014). Arabinoxylan (AX) is a major component of the cell walls of wheat and rye with a linear backbone of (1→4)-linked β-D-xylopyranose units (Damen et al., 2012). The prebiotic forms of AXOS are enzymatic fragmentation products of arabinoxylans (AX) and they are obtained by chemical extraction of AX from cereal grains or bran followed by enzymatic hydrolysis of the extracted AX by specific AX-degrading enzymes. The fragmentation process is a key step in preparing different AXOS with varying degree of polymerization (DP) and arabinose to xylose ratio (DS) (Swennen et al., 2005, 2006). At present, the production of AXOS is only performed under laboratory and pilot scales (Damen et al., 2012). Though AXOS meet all the criteria to be considered as prebiotics (Broekaert et al., 2011), data in fish and in other farm animals are relatively scarce. The beneficial potential of AXOS is not only limited to their influence in the microbial ecosystem in the gut (Courtin et al., 2008; Van Craeyveld et al., 2008; Van Laere et al., 2000) as they are also capable of modulating the immunological responses of the host (Monobe et al., 2008).

9.3.2.6 Isomaltooligosaccharide (IMO)

Isomaltooligosaccharide (IMO) is enzymatically processed from starch as a mixture of α-(1→6) linked glucosides, such as isolmaltose, isolmatotriose, panose, and isomaltotetraose (Kaneko et al., 1995). There is a major concern on classifying IMOs as prebiotics because of their digestibility in the gastrointestinal tract and only IMOs with high degrees of polymerization, for instance, isomaltotetraose and larger oligomers, are considered indigestible. Nevertheless, they have been demonstrated to have bifidogenic properties in the human gut (Kaneko et al., 1994). In rats, increased *Lactobacillus* numbers have been observed following IMO intake (Ketabi et al., 2011). The application of IMO as prebiotics in fish is still under a laboratory-scale perspective.

9.3.2.7 Inulin

Fructans are all naturally occurring plant oligo- and polysaccharides in which one or more fructosyl-fructose linkages comprise the majority of glycosidic bonds; hence, they are primarily polymers of fructose units (Kelly, 2008). Inulin is a generic term that covers all linear fructans with β-(2→1) fructosyl-fructose glycosidic bonds (Roberfroid, 2007). Inulin is most commonly extracted from chicory roots (*Cichorium intybus*) using a hot water diffusion process (Niness, 1999). The fructosyl-fructose linkages always occur as β-(2→1) in inulin while the fructosyl-glucose linkage is β-(2↔1) (Roberfriod, 2007). Inulin can withstand enzymatic digestion in the human gastrointestinal tract due to the β-(2→1) bonds, but not in the colon where β-fructosidase-producing bacteria can hydrolyze this bond (Makras et al., 2005). Inulin is bifidogenic and a minimal dose appears to be needed to produce such effects (Kelly, 2008).

9.3.3 Mechanisms of prebiotic actions

In general, our understanding of the mechanisms by which prebiotics confer benefits to fish is mainly based on human findings. The general prebiotic concept is the same but the underlying mechanisms may vary between fish and human. It is important to highlight that variations may exist because of the – (i) differences in the rearing environment, wherein environmental factors have significant influence on the intestinal microflora of fish; (ii) differences in the diversity, physiology, and biochemistry of the gastrointestinal microflora between fish and human; and (iii) differences on the physiological activities (e.g., enzymes) of the teleost and human gastrointestinal tract. Several studies have already been conducted describing potential prebiotics and their beneficial properties in a number of tropical and cold-water aquaculture species. Research in fish has significantly progressed in recent years but there remains much to be explored in future studies, particularly on the mechanisms of prebiotic actions. The review papers by Song et al. (2014), Merrifield et al. (2010), Ringø et al. (2010), Yousefian and Amiri (2009) and Burr et al. (2005), though exhaustive, mainly dealt on the different prebiotics used in aquaculture and their effects, and the underlying mechanisms are barely explored. Nevertheless, Torrecillas et al. (2014) collated all studies on MOS in fish and provided possible mechanisms that may be involved in the associated improvement of health and growth following dietary supplementation. In their integrative analysis, they have proposed that the primary mode of action of MOS in fish could be the reinforcement of the intestinal integrity and functionality, together with the stimulation of immune system.

Three possible mechanisms of prebiotic actions in fish are discussed and this is based on the collated major findings in numerous fish species available at present. A general concept of immunostimulation by prebiotics is provided in this section and their relevance in mucosal immunity is discretely discussed in Section 9.6.

9.3.3.1 Selective stimulation of gastrointestinal microorganisms

The gastrointestinal tract of fish is composed of resident (autochthonous) and transient populations (allocthonous) of microbial communities. These microorganisms are oftentimes regarded as an "extra organ" of the fish because of their significant role in the development, homeostasis, and protection of the gastrointestinal tract (O'Hara and Shanahan, 2006). Microbial manipulations for fish health improvement may be characterized into two main strategic concepts: (i) augmentation, wherein the beneficial microorganisms are introduced to fish to improve their microbiological makeup; and (ii) stimulation, where microorganisms or ingredients are offered to modulate the activities of the beneficial microbial communities. The two strategies may be used conjunctionally for a better result, though it is often that only one of two is highlighted in a research study. The use of prebiotics lies on the second strategic concept. Along this line, one fundamental question may arise: Will the introduction of these compounds in fish also stimulate the activity of pathogens that may be present? In fact, many opportunistic bacteria are capable of utilizing a wide range of carbohydrates (Gatesoupe, 2005). The above posed question may be expounded in two viewpoints. First, pathogenic microorganisms are highly specialized and typified by a complex metabolism; hence, they are very unlikely to benefit from the prebiotics. On the other hand, the continuous supply of the substrate in the intestine may create a risk that the pathogens could acquire the ability to use either the native compound or its degraded products (Denev et al., 2009). This dilemma should be taken into consideration in selecting candidate prebiotics for fish.

Majority of the known prebiotics are considered "bifidogenic." The capability of compounds in stimulating the growth and metabolism of the members of the *Bifidobacterium* family has been one of the defining features of commonly known prebiotics. Lactic acid bacteria (particularly those belonging to the genera *Streptococcus*, *Leuconostoc*, *Lactobacillus*, and *Carnobacterium*) are present in the normal microbiota of the gastrointestinal tract in healthy fish. Nevertheless, their presence is highly influenced by nutritional and environmental factors such as dietary polyunsaturated fatty acids, chromic oxide, stress, and salinity (Ringø and Gatesoupe, 1998). The presence of *Bifidobacteria* in the gastrointestinal tract of fish is still debatable. To the best of our knowledge, only one study had described their presence in the gastrointestinal tract of teleosts. Vlková et al. (2012) described bifidobacterial communities in the digestive tract of some freshwater fish, namely, Cyprinus *carpio, Oncorhynchus mykiss, Carassius auratus, Tinca tinca, Perca fluviatilis, Rutilus rutilus, Scardinius erythrophthalmus, Oreochromis niloticus*, and *Squalius cephalus*. They isolated *Bifidobacterium longum, B. dentium, B. asteroids*, and an isolate not identified at the species level. Therefore, the word "bifidogenic" should be used with caution when describing prebiotics employed in fish, especially those that have been attributed to such properties in humans. We are proposing that the conjoined word "micro-stimulant" may be used instead in describing these compounds used in fish that display a "bifidogenic" property that was initially described in humans.

One of the earliest "prebiotics-related" studies in fish demonstrated that supplementation of linoleic acid in Arctic charr diets increased the total viable counts of the intestinal microbiota by 10-fold (Ringø, 1993a). Besides linoleic acid, polyunsaturated fatty acids of the *n*-3 and *n*-6 series were also capable of altering the microbial population, especially the stimulation of facultative anaerobic LAB, *Carnobacterium* spp. (Ringø et al., 1998). An *in vitro* screening strategy for prebiotics in fish that are capable of stimulating the growth of probiotic bacteria was developed by Rurangwa et al. (2009). They showed that selected bacteria are able to ferment and grow on the prebiotic carbohydrates but in a substrate dependent manner. From culture-based methods on determining microbial changes in the intestine of fish, the current studies are tapping molecular-based techniques for more discriminating approaches. 16S rRNA gene sequencing analysis was used to identify changes in the hindgut of Arctic charr following inulin administration (Ringø et al., 2006). It was shown that prebiotic administration facilitated the dominance of gram-positive bacteria of the genera *Staphylococcus, Streptococcus, Carnobacterium,* and *Bacillus.* Using denaturing gradient gel electrophoresis (DGGE) analysis in determining microbial diversity alterations in the intestine of hybrid striped bass (*Morone chrysops*×*Morone saxatilis*) following prebiotic feeding, different prebiotic treatments (i.e., GroBiotic®-A, MOS, GOS, and inulin) produced dissimilar types of microbial community fingerprints as compared to the control group (Burr et al., 2010). The same molecular approach was used in a study on Siberian sturgeon (*Acipenser baerii*) wherein LAB and *Clostridium* sp. were shown to be stimulated following supplementation of AXOS with a high degree of polymerization in the diets (Geraylou et al., 2012). In a sister study, which used a dose-dependent prebiotic supplementation approach, it was observed that the abundance of *Lactobacillus* spp. and *Lactococcus lactis* was greater in groups fed supplements in a low dose but a higher AXOS polymerization degree as revealed by 454 pyrosequencing (Geraylou et al., 2013). This dose-dependent effect of prebiotic administration was also observed in stellate sturgeon (*Acipenser stellatus*) fed with FOS, wherein the low dose displayed significantly higher levels of presumptive LAB than the control and the high-dose group (Akrami et al., 2013).

9.3.3.2 Prebiotics as immunostimulants

The immune system of the fish is an intricate network composed of genes and their proteins, and cells that play a significant role in protecting the fish from stressors and pathogens. The concept of nutritional modulation for preventive health care primarily lies on the capability of a number of compounds in boosting the immune system of the fish; hence, more potent responses may be effectuated in the presence of pathogens. Prebiotics have been demonstrated to possess the capability of modulating the immune system either by direct or indirect mechanisms. The direct immunostimulatory properties of prebiotics may be explained when the prebiotic ligands interact with their associated receptors (pattern recognition receptors; PRR) such as β-glucan and dectin-1 receptors present in macrophages (Brown et al., 2002). A down-stream process will occur when the ligand-receptor interaction activates signal transduction molecules such as NF-kB, which stimulate a number of immune cells (Yadav and Schorey, 2002). In another perspective, immune responses could be triggered when the saccharides interact with PRRs in the form of microbe associated molecular patterns (MAMPs) such as teichoic acid, peptidoglycan glycosylated protein, or the capsular polysaccharide of bacteria (Bron et al., 2012) (see recent review of Song et al., 2014). It has to be pointed out that, even though prebiotics are capable of stimulating the immune system of fish, having an immunostimulatory activity should not be a prerequisite for a prebiotic candidate to be considered as one. A prebiotic is not necessarily an immunostimulant, and vice versa (Song et al., 2014). Besides their influence on mucosal immunity as discussed later below, prebiotics have been demonstrated to predominantly influence lysozyme, phagocytic, and respiratory burst activities in fish.

Lysozyme is one of the major immune defenses in fish. It protects the organisms from bacterial pathogens by hydrolyzing the 1, 4-β-linkages between *N*-acetyl-D-glucosamine and *N*-acetylmuramic acid in peptidoglycan heteropolymers of bacterial cell walls (Alexander and Ingram, 1992; Chipman and Sharon, 1969). Several studies have shown that FOS administration can significantly influence lysozyme activity in fish. In caspian roach (*Rutilus rutilus*) fry, all tested dietary levels (i.e., 10, 20, or 30 g/kg) of FOS significantly enhanced lysozyme activity (Soleimani et al. 2012). The improvement of lysozyme activity has also been demonstrated in Japanese flounder (*Paralichthys olivaceus*) (Ye et al., 2011) and stellate sturgeon (*Acipenser stellatus*) (Akrami et al., 2013). Specifically in stellate sturgeon, the lower dose (10 g/kg) elicited a significant improvement on lysozyme activity than the high dose (20 g/kg). Stimulation of lysozyme activity following prebiotic administration was also observed in fish fed with MOS such as Japanese flounder (Ye et al., 2011) and European sea bass (*Dicentrarchus labrax*) (Torrecillas et al., 2011).

Another fundamental defense mechanism of fish is phagocytosis wherein immune cells such as neutrophils, monocytes, and macrophages ingest large particles (micro-organisms, intact cells, macro-molecules, or cellular debris). Following ingestion, the immune cells release degradative enzymes (i.e., proteases, nucleases, phosphatases, esterases, and lipases) and antimicrobial peptides (i.e., neutrophilic peptides and basic proteins), which aid in the destruction of the particle (e.g., pathogen).

Feeding trials of candidate prebiotics in fish revealed that fish phagocytosis could be modulated by these substances. The improvement of phagocytic activity was observed in rainbow trout (Rodriguez-Estrada et al., 2009, 2013) and European sea bass (Torrecillas et al., 2011) fed with MOS. In the two sister studies in Siberian sturgeon, dietary administration of AXOS influenced the phagocytic activity both at short (Geraylou et al., 2013) and extended (Geraylou et al., 2012) periods of feeding. In addition, it was shown that a more significant effect was noted in AXOS with high degree of polymerization.

Reactive oxygen species (e.g., superoxide anion, hydrogen peroxide) collectively describes a number of reactive molecules and free radicals derived from molecular oxygen and they are used by the phagocytic cells to kill or degrade engulfed materials, particularly pathogens. Respiratory burst is the stimulated production of reactive oxygen species by phagocytic cells due to the increased consumption of oxygen by these cells (Babior et al., 1973). There is no concrete evidence supporting the role of prebiotics in the respiratory burst activity of fish; however, their influence is manifested in some recent studies. For example, in gilthead seabream, a significant improvement of leukocyte respiratory burst activity was observed following dietary administration of inulin (Cerezuela et al., 2012a). On the other hand, whole-blood neutrophil oxidative radical production decreased significantly in Atlantic salmon fed with MOS (Grisdale-Helland et al., 2008). A decreased respiratory burst activity was also observed in Siberian sturgeon fed with AXOS (Geraylou et al., 2013). These conflicting observations present the need for more studies elucidating the immune-related functions of prebiotics on the ROS defense system of fish.

9.3.3.3 Growth promoters

Growth is one of the tangible parameters in assessing the success of fish culture. There are several factors affecting fish growth but nutrition remains as one of the significant contributors. Dietary manipulation has been a customary practice and the search for growth promoters is oftentimes the focal strategy. Traditionally, the aquaculture industry relied heavily on the use of synthetic substances such as antibiotics and steroid hormones as growth promoters. The introduction of the prebiotic concept in aquaculture opened opportunities in exploring these substances as sustainable alternatives, similar to preceding studies in swine (Thacker, 2013) and poultry animals (Huyghebaert et al., 2011), which demonstrated their growth-promoting potential. Even though prebiotics have been regarded as a sustainable growth-promoting alternative, studies discussing their potential were mostly inconclusive. There is a high degree of variability observed amongst species on different prebiotic candidates. This suggests the possibility that growth-promoting properties of prebiotics in fish have complex underlying mechanisms that may be stochastic in nature and highly influenced by the maturity of the physiological status of the host. Nevertheless, the disparities among results should be viewed positively by the aquaculture scientists in understanding this aspect of prebiotic actions in fish in future studies.

Despite the challenges surmounting the potential of prebiotics as growth promoters in fish, numerous studies have provided positive baseline information for the advancement of their use as a sustainable growth-promoting alternative in aquaculture. MOS, FOS, and GOS were separately incorporated into the fish meal-based diets of Atlantic salmon (*Salmo salar*). Though growth parameters were not significantly influenced, the authors highlighted the tendencies in feed efficiency and energy retention to be affected by prebiotic treatments (Grisdale Helland et al., 2008). The soybean meal-based diets improved nutrient and energy digestibility in red drum (*Sciaenops ocellatus*), especially when they were supplemented with prebiotics (i.e., GroBiotic-A, MOS, GOS, and inulin) (Burr et al., 2008). The commercial prebiotic Immunogen® was supplemented at varying levels into the diets of common carp (*Cyprinus carpio*) fingerlings. Though weight gain was not significantly influenced, both feed efficiency ratio and protein efficiency ratio were significantly elevated with increasing Immunogen levels in the diet (Ebrahimi et al., 2012). Similar results on improved feed efficiency with unaffected growth in the prebiotic-fed group were also demonstrated in hybrid striped bass fed with a commercial prebiotic GroBiotic-A (Li and Gatlin, 2004). Favorable influence on feed conversion was also observed in rainbow trout following dietary supplementation of a commercial prebiotic mixture Profeed® (Řehulka et al., 2011). A commercial form of MOS, Bio-MOS, which was incorporated into the diets of gilthead seabream (*Sparus aurata*) also elicited feed conversion improvement as well. It was shown that apparent digestibility values for protein, carbohydrate, and energy was affected by the dietary inclusion and may be attributed with the observed growth enhancement (Gültepe et al., 2011). Two commercial prebiotics named Immunoster and Immunowall were tested in a low-dose–high-dose strategy for their growth-promoting potential in juvenile beluga (*Huso huso*). Dietary inclusion improved the growth performance of the fish and higher final weight was observed in the low-dose group (Ta'ati et al., 2011). The same tendency of having a more favorable effect on a lower prebiotic dose was observed in the same fish species fed with MOS (Razeghi Mansour et al., 2012).

9.4 Probiotics

9.4.1 Beneficial microorganisms as health-promoting agents

Antonie Van Leeuwenhoek (1632–1723) was one of the first scientists who observed microorganisms under a microscope. His pioneering researches on the life forms that were not visible to the naked eye gave him the distinction of the "Father of Microbiology." His works laid the foundations of our current knowledge on microorganisms and their importance on the daily lives of mankind.

Traditionally, humans perceived microorganisms in a negative standpoint albeit their relevance in many processes. Humans used to believe that the sole purpose of microorganisms was to cause harm. The word "microorganism" had become synonymous to "diseases," "bad bacteria," "pathogen," among many others. As human knowledge proceeded in understanding biological phenomenon in different perspectives, that notion was ceded particularly with the development of biotherapies and utilization of functional bacteria in the late nineteenth century (Escherich, 1885).

The concept of probiotics was first introduced in 1907 by the Russian Nobel laureate Elie Metchnikoff who was working at the Pasteur Institute in Paris (Metchnikoff, 1907). His key hypothesis was that lactic acid bacteria (LAB) were capable of promoting longevity through their offered health benefits. In his concept of "intestinal auto-intoxication," he suggested that aging could be suppressed by modifying the gut microbiota and by replacing proteolytic microbes such as *Clostridium* that produce putrefactive metabolites like phenols, indoles, and ammonia from the digestion of proteins by "useful microbes." He also observed that Bulgarian peasants and those living in the Russian Steppes who were largely dependent on milk fermented by LAB ("Bulgarian Bacillus"; later named *Lactobacillus bulgaricus*) had higher lifespan (Vaughan, 1965).

The first *Bifidobacterium* isolate was described by Henry Tissier and presently it is one of the commonly used probiotics (Tissier, 1900). The bacterium was from a breast-fed infant and he named it *Bacillus bifidus communis* (later renamed *Bifidobacterium bifidum*). He described that *Bifidobacteria* dominated the gut microflora of breast-fed infants approximately 3 days postpartum in contrast to bottle-fed neonates, which predominantly contained *B. acidophilus*. He further claimed that successive administration of *Bifidobacteria* to infants suffering from diarrhea would displace the proteolytic bacteria that cause the disease; therefore, microbial intervention was regarded as a cure. The first non-LAB probiotics was described by the German professor Alfred Nissle who isolated a nonpathogenic strain of *Escherichia coli* from the feces of a First World War soldier who did not develop enterocolitis during the outbreak of shigellosis (Nissle, 1918). Interestingly, this description was made even before the discovery of penicillin by Sir Alexander Fleming.

In an experiment of Herter and Kendall (1908), they showed that *L. bulgaricus* failed to establish a population in the human gut, yet other changes in the gut microflora were still observed. In two sister studies by Rettger and Cheplin (1920a, 1920b), they reported that feeding of lactose to rats or humans resulted to a transformation of the intestinal microflora, particularly the predominance of *Acidophilus* and *Bifidus* type cultures, which were regarded as beneficial microbial populations. Preventive health through functional microbial interventions had become a key driving force for a Japanese researcher Minoru Shirota. He was able to isolate and characterize a *Lactobacillus* strain that was later named *Lactobacillus casei* strain Shirota capable of surviving the passage through the harsh conditions of the gastrointestinal tract. This has led to the establishment of a company producing fermented dairy product called Yakult, as we know today (Yakult, 1998).

Indeed, the trailblazing postulate of Metchnikoff has provided considerable foundation on the application and benefits of probiotics as beneficial microorganisms. For over several decades, probiotics are being used to promote human well-being and alleviate health issues. It was only in the last 15 years that their relevance in animal husbandry, including fish, had generated substantial research and applications (Chaucheyras-Durand and Durand, 2010).

9.4.2 The dynamic contemporary perspective of probiotics

The word "probiotics" was connoted from the Latin word "pro" means "for" and Greek word "bios" meaning "life" (Zivkovic, 1999). The conjugated word of "probiotics" that stands "for life" is in line with the pioneering observation of Metchnikoff that described this group of microorganisms as promoters of longevity. It is believed that Kollath proposed the word in 1953 to denote all organic and inorganic food complexes, in contrast to the harmful antibiotics (Kollath, 1953). In some papers the term is attributed to Lilley and Stillwell (1965), who described them as substances secreted by one microorganism, which stimulated the growth of another and as a modification of the original word "probiotika."

The definition of probiotics has expanded and diversified through the years, accommodating the staggering number of observations published. Sperti (1971) modified the concept by describing it as "tissue extracts that stimulate microbial growth." Under the context of microbial feed/food supplement, Parker described probiotics in 1974 as "organisms and substances that contribute to intestinal microbial balance" (Parker, 1974). The definition of Parker had become the standard that was used in describing probiotics under a feed supplement perspective, not until Dr. Roy Fuller made a substantial update and revision in 1989. The definition of Fuller (1989) described probiotics as "… a live microbial feed supplement which beneficially affects the host animal by improving microbial balance." Fuller's definition was essentially a modification of the observations in protozoans producing substances that stimulated other protozoans where Lilley and Stillwell (1965) derived their initial description. The definition of Fuller was one of the first definitions that transcended the application of probiotics from human to their relevance in other animals. With that, it has become the widely referred definition of probiotics both in human and animal applications. The definition of Fuller did not discretely specify whether probiotics should be single or mixed populations, thus a slight modification was introduced by Havenaar and Huis (1992) stating, "monocultures or mixed cultures of microorganisms applied to animals or humans, that benefit the host by improving properties of indigenous microflora."

The application of probiotics in other animals has prompted researchers to revisit the definition and introduce amendments that would reflect the requirements and peculiarities of the host species. The foundation of probiotic research is mainly based on a terrestrial perspective, on humans to be specific. Aquaculture presents several caveats to the traditional human-derived situation: (i) unlike humans, fish live in water and are characterized by close contact to their very dynamic environment; (ii) physiological differences exist between fish and human particularly on the points of digestion and immunity; (iii) the mode of delivery may not be by dietary administration alone, as addition to the rearing water and using live feed vectors are possible alternatives. In the early 2000s, Verschuere and colleagues provided a very lengthy yet encompassing definition that states, "probiotic is a live microbial adjunct which has a beneficial effect on the host by modifying the host-associated or ambient microbial community, by ensuring improved use of the feed and enhancing its nutritional value, by enhancing the host response towards diseases, or by improving the quality of its ambient environment" (Verschuere et al., 2000). Though this definition presented many aspects that the terrestrial-based definition was lacking especially the peculiarities of the aquatic environment, one area was not dealt with and this was on microbial viability. Even the group of experts commissioned by the Joint Food and Agriculture Organization of the United Nations/World Health Organization (FAO/WHO) in 2001 did not consider the importance of this issue as they stated that probiotics are live microorganisms, which, when consumed in adequate amounts, confer a health benefit for the host (FAO/WHO, 2002). However, it was earlier reported in mammalian models that probiotics may not necessarily be alive to confer beneficial effects to the host because even components of the microbial cells could provide benefits (Salminen et al., 1999). This was also supported by several reports in fish that the viability of a number of probiotic candidates did not serve as a limiting factor of their beneficial actions (Díaz-Rosales et al., 2006; Lazado and Caipang, 2014a; Lazado et al., 2010a; Pan et al., 2008; Salinas et al., 2006). This viability issue has a practical relevance when probiotics are incorporated in fish diets that are prepared under relatively elevated temperatures than the physiological temperature range of most microbial candidates.

Probiotics administration has been at the forefront of being a key and viable disease-control alternative for a sustainable aquaculture, though the community does not have a unified definition of probiotics at present. Why should there be a commonly accepted and unified definition in aquaculture? A working definition of probiotics from an aquaculture point of view eliminates ambiguity on the term being used and to acknowledge that physiological differences between organisms exist (Lazado and Caipang, 2014b). The issue on having a working definition in aquaculture was raised by two research groups, namely those working on salmonids (Merrifield et al., 2010) and Atlantic cod (Lazado and Caipang, 2014b). In this chapter, probiotics are referred to as live or dead, or even a component of microorganisms that act under different modes of action in conferring beneficial effects to the host or to its environment.

9.4.3 Probiotic microorganisms used in aquaculture species

The overwhelming number of candidate probiotics in fish raises an important question: What is the best probiotic microorganism for fish? The straightforward answer is NONE. There may never be a universally accepted and applicable probiotic microorganism because "probiotic action" is not only about the intrinsic beneficial properties of a microorganism. It also involves the host and its responses, and a number of environmental factors (Lazado and Caipang, 2014b, 2014c). The unending quest of probiotic microorganisms should not be regarded as searching for the best probiotics but rather on looking for the best option for a specific intention.

Many of the failures in probiotic research can be attributed to the selection of inappropriate microorganisms (Gomez-Gil et al., 2000). A number of selection outlines have been proposed on identifying and characterizing a microorganisms for its consideration as a probiotic (Balcázar et al., 2006a; Verschuere et al., 2000). At present, there is no standard protocol in the selection of probiotics in fish and oftentimes it is on a country to country basis. In addition, each probiotic researcher in fish has his/her personal selection criteria and the inclination of the strategy frequently depends on the intended use and desired probiotic properties. According to FAO/WHO, the development of commercial probiotics requires their unequivocal taxonomic identification, as well as their well-documented *in vitro* and *in vivo* functions and safety assessment (FAO/WHO, 2006). A system was proposed by the European Food Safety Agency (EFSA) on the pre-market safety assessment of microorganisms used in food/feed and the production of food/feed additives leading to a Qualified Presumption of Safety (QPS) status (EC, 2003; EFSA, 2007, 2011). A multidimensional qualification is included in the QPS approach particularly that the safety assessment of a defined taxonomic group may be made based on establishing taxonomic identity, body of knowledge, possible pathogenicity, and commercial end use.

The selection of probiotic microorganisms in fish may be divided into four core criteria: safety, technological, functional, and physiological aspects (Figure 9.1). Each

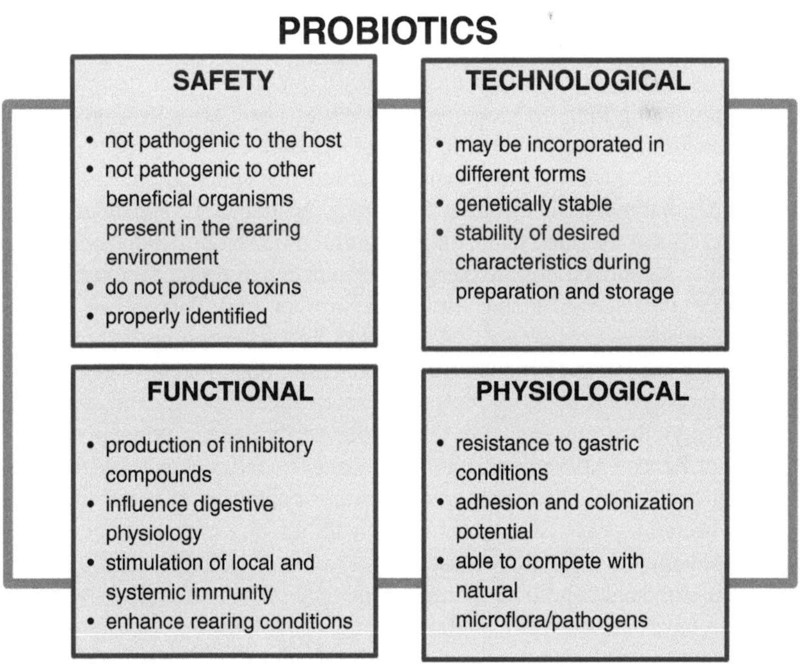

Figure 9.1 The four core criteria in the selection of probiotics for fish. A candidate probiotics must comply with all the four major criteria but compliance to all specific guidelines of each criterion, though ideal, is not necessary. Nevertheless, a multifaceted and multifunctional probiotics is most desired.

criterion enumerates specific requirements though a candidate may not necessarily comply with all of these. Nevertheless, the compliance to the majority of these specifications is ideal and definitely a bargaining chip. In fact, the majority of probiotic researchers in fish desire that candidate microorganisms for aquaculture use need to be multifaceted and multifunctional.

9.4.3.1 Terrestrial and commercial probiotics

The first described probiotics and the most widely studied are from the lactic acid bacteria family – a group of rod and cocci gram-positive, acid-tolerant microorganisms (Ljungh and Wadström, 2006). Intensive research particularly in human applications have been conducted with the members of the genera *Lactobacillus* and *Bifidobacterium*. The longest known and proven health benefits and safe use of probiotic bacteria for human consumption is documented for *Lactobacillus casei* Shirota strain (Shirota et al., 1966).

A great percentage of probiotics research in fish utilized LAB of terrestrial origin. The popularity of LAB as probiotics in fish could be because: (i) they were generally regarded as safe; (ii) their probiotic actions were well characterized; (iii) their taxonomic identity was verified and established; and (iv) they were readily available (Lazado and Caipang, 2014b). These qualities of LAB comply with the mentioned criteria on safety, technological, functional, and physiological aspects to be considered as probiotics. This group of microorganisms share common metabolic and physiological characteristics that are considered of immense importance. For instance, they are capable of producing inhibitory compounds such as lactic acid, hydrogen peroxide, diacetyl, acetaldehyde, and bacteriocin (Zapata and Lara-Flores, 2013).

Several probiotic products have been authorized for human applications and they are available in the market in different forms (e.g., lyophilized, supplement capsules, functional food). On the other hand, only a handful of probiotic products for aquaculture are legally authorized despite the growing number of probiotic microorganisms identified and characterized in and for fish. At present, only Bactocell®, a probiotic culture of *Pediococcus acidilactici* CNCM MA18/5 M is the only authorized probiotic for aquaculture use in the European Union. This probiotic product offers stability of gut microflora and contributes to improved performance, survival, and consequently, an increase in yield (Lellamand). In China, one of the widely popular commercial probiotics is Effective Microorganisms (EM) from Dr. Teruo Higa's EM Technology of Japan (Qi et al., 2009). This probiotic mixture is composed of beneficial and non-pathogenic bacteria, yeasts, and *Actinomyces* with a major advertised benefit of degrading environmental and culture wastes.

Under experimental conditions, some commercial probiotics that are marketed for other animals have been utilized as well in fish. LEVUCELL® SB is a natural and well-documented live yeast *Saccharomyces cerevisiae boulardii* (CNCM I-1079) that was primarily intended for swine. It was delivered through rotifers during pre- and post-hatch stages of Atlantic cod but it promoted high larval mortality (Lauzon et al., 2010). Calsporin® is a spore-forming probiotic that contains *Bacillus subtilis* C-3102, which had been tested in tilapia hybrid (*Oreochromis niloticus* ♀ × *Oreochromis aureus* ♂)

and resulted to the modulation of some immune parameters (He et al., 2013). Though Calsporin is an EU-registered product, its authorized use is for piglets and chickens. The famous human probiotic drink Yakult® was also explored in fish as well. Though the results were not significant when compared with the observed effects in human, administration increased the protein content of the mucus in *Poecilopsis gracilis* (Hernandez et al., 2010).

9.4.3.2 Host-derived probiotics

The microbiota constitutes an important component of the overall biological makeup of an organism, including fish. On the course of exploring new probiotic microorganisms, the attention was directed to the commensal microorganisms of the host. Several host-derived candidate probiotics have been characterized both from cold-water (Lazado et al., 2010c; Brunt et al., 2007; Spanggaard et al., 2001; Robertson et al., 2000; Gildberg and Mikkelsen, 1998; Jöborn et al., 1997) and warm-water fish species (Lara-Flores and Olvera-Novoa, 2013; Chantharasophon et al., 2011; Ghosh et al., 2007; Kumar et al., 2006). Their probiotic activities range from inhibition of pathogens to nutritional influence.

There are two fundamental principles on the exploration of host microorganisms as probiotics (Lazado and Caipang, 2014b). First, there may never be a single probiotic microorganism that could be used in all host species. The physiological peculiarities of every organism and the influence of environmental factors play a significant role in the beneficial actions of microorganisms. Second, it is widely recognized that microorganisms perform at optimum conditions in their natural environment. However, there is no definite indication that candidate probiotics isolated from the host or from their ambient environment perform better than those of terrestrial origin or from a very different environment (Verschuere et al., 2000). Nevertheless, the issues on the influence of physico-chemical factors on probiotic properties may be excluded if the candidate microorganisms are naturally thriving in the environment of their intended application.

Host-derived candidate probiotics are frequently isolated from the gastrointestinal tract of fish. The digestive tract of vertebrates is colonized by complex assemblages of microorganisms (Ringø et al., 2010). With the amount of microorganisms present, the gut is regarded as a biological basin for candidate probiotics (Lazado and Caipang, 2014b). The microbial community in the gut is also constantly exposed to variations in the environment; hence, they develop unique biochemical and physiological competence for survival that can be utilized for beneficial use. Two resident bacteria of the gastrointestinal tract of Atlantic cod, named GP21 (*Pseudomonas* sp.) and GP12 (*Pyschrobacter* sp.), were profiled for their beneficial properties and results indicated that they could be good candidate probiotics. They were shown to possess many remarkable probiotic properties such as the production of inhibitory metabolites (Lazado et al., 2010c), interference of pathogens (Lazado et al., 2010c, 2011), contribution to digestion (Lazado et al., 2012), and modulation of immune responses (Lazado and Caipang, 2014a, 2014d; Ruangsri et al., 2013; Lazado et al., 2010a, 2010b). In another study, four bacteria isolated from the gastroinstestinal tract of Atlantic cod (*Psychrobacter* sp. [GP11], *Shewanella* sp. [GS11], *Photobacterium* sp. [GP31],) and *Vibrio* sp. [GV11]) were also demonstrated to be potential probiotics with antagonistic and immunomodulatory properties. Interestingly, antagonistic activity of GS11 towards both test bacterial pathogens (*Listonella anguillarum* and *Aeromonas salmonicida*) was higher at 20 °C than at 13 °C (Caipang et al., 2010). Two criteria were used by Fjellheim et al. (2010) in the selection of host-derived probiotics: from the (i) dominant intestinal microflora; and from the (ii) pool with inhibitory activity against pathogens. Putative probiotics had been selected from the dominant population (*Vibrio* and two different strains of *Microbacterium*) and antagonistic group (*Ruegeria* and *Pseudoalteromonas*) and were proposed to be suitable in developing a multi-strain probiotic with complementary beneficial properties. An endospore-forming, gram-positive bacterium identified as *Bacillus subtilis* was isolated from the intestine of rainbow trout (Newaj-Fyzul et al., 2007). Probiotic feeding significantly reduced cumulative mortalities after challenge with *Aeromonas* sp. regardless of dietary incorporation strategies (i.e., whole, sonicated, formalized cells or cell-free supernatant). The results of Newaj-Fyzul et al. (2007) as supported by two sister studies on heat-inactivation of host-derived candidate probiotics (Lazado and Caipang, 2014d; Lazado et al. 2010a) suggest a possibility that probiotic properties of host-derived microorganisms may be independent of inclusion or delivery form, but this needs to be proven with additional functional studies.

The LAB also inhabit the gastrointestinal tract of fish and their presence, though with great variability, has been prospected for probiotics development. With their beneficial properties identified in mammalian models, attempts have been made in increasing the population of *Lactobacillus* and *Carnobacterium* in the gastrointestinal tract of fish by manipulating abiotic factors that greatly influence these bacterial communities (Ringø et al., 1998; Ringø, 1993b). A *Carnobacterium* sp. that was isolated from the intestine of Atlantic salmon had been proposed as potential probiotics for salmonids. It was demonstrated to possess a wide range of antagonistic activity against a number of salmonid pathogens *in vitro* and was able to colonize the gastrointestinal tract (Robertson et al., 2000; Jöborn et al., 1997). *In vivo* trials showed that exposure of fish to this bacteria indicated protection against *Aeromonas salmonicida, Vibrio ordalii*, and *Yersinia ruckeri* but not with *V. anguillarum* (Robertson et al., 2000). Five members of LAB family identified as *Enterococcus faecium, E. durans, Leuconostoc* sp., *Streptococcus* sp. I, and *Streptococcus* sp. II were isolated from the intestinal tract of Nile tilapia (*Oreochromis niloticus*). It was demonstrated that fish offered with isocaloric diets with the identified LAB had significantly higher growth and feeding performance than the group fed with commercial probiotic that is mainly constituted of *S. faecium* and *Lactobacillus acidophilus* (Lara-Flores and Olvera-Novoa, 2013).

9.4.4 Modes of actions of probiotics

9.4.4.1 Production of inhibitory compounds

Inhibitory activity has been the mode of action that is widely characterized in a probiotic candidate for fish. However, there is no universal rule that a probiotic candidate should produce inhibitory substances in order to be considered as one. The expansion of the probiotic definition is in itself an indication that the mechanism of probiotic action is not limited to the production of inhibitory substances alone. Nevertheless, the inclination observed on most probiotic studies in fish towards the production of inhibitory substances may have sprung from the active initiative of looking for a sustainable alternative for antibiotics in aquaculture.

Some of the inhibitory metabolites that are produced by candidate probiotics are antibiotics, bacteriocins, siderophores, enzymes (i.e., lysozymes, proteases), and/or hydrogen peroxide, along with modification of the intestinal pH due to the generation of organic acids (Verschuere et al., 2000). In particular, bacteriocins are ribosomally synthesized antibacterial compounds produced by LAB, which are bactericidal against other organisms, mostly by closely related bacteria (Riley and Wertz, 2002). A typical bacteriocin contains a toxin (bacteriocin) gene, an immunity gene (which confers resistance to the aforementioned toxin), and a lysis gene, which encodes a protein that aids in toxin release from the producing cell (Chavan and Riley, 2007). LAB isolates from the gut of tilapia had higher antagonistic activity from extra cellular protein (ECP), putatively bacteriocin compared to the intracellular protein (ICP) against *A. hydrophila* (Vijayabaskar and Somasundaram, 2008). In addition, inhibitory genes such as nicin and enterocin are found in the genome of these isolates. Inhibitory activity of the extracellular supernatant was also identified in GP21 (*Pseudomonas* sp.) and GP12 (*Psychrobacter* sp.), candidate probiotics from the intestinal microbiota of Atlantic cod (Lazado et al., 2010c). Siderophores are low-molecular weight ferric ion-specific chelating agents produced by bacteria that can dissolve precipitated iron and use it for growth, thereby making it unavailable for their competitors (Nielands, 1981). Some pathogens such as *V. anguillarum* have a high iron requirement for virulence and probiotics that can outcompete for iron acquisition by this pathogen are regarded as beneficial candidates. The siderophore-producing ability of a potential probiotic bacterium has been linked to its antagonistic activity (Lazado et al., 2010c) and the protection obtained during a pathogen challenge experiment (Gatesoupe, 1997).

The plate assay in determining antagonistic activity has been a very common practice in commencing a probiotic selection strategy. This approach is still relevant, but one must acknowledge that antagonism in a natural environment is a complex scenario. The antagonism that is observed *in vitro* may not be translated to actual inhibition *in vivo*. There are several factors (e.g., temperature, salinity, pH) that could immensely influence the antagonistic activity of a candidate probiotic (Caipang et al., 2010; Lazado et al., 2010c) and these should be considered especially in extrapolating and making comparative deductions between the results from *in vitro* and *in vivo* studies.

9.4.4.2 Interference of pathogen adhesion

Virulence of many fish pathogens is initiated by their adhesion on mucosal surfaces that enables them to deliver virulent factors and disrupt microbial equilibrium. Bacterial interference is the ability of one microorganism to protect its host against a neighboring or invading microbial pathogen by interfering with its adhesion and toxic effects (Reid et al., 2001). This form of antagonism is typified by a number of probiotics used in human and aquaculture species. There are different strategies identified in the adhesion of microorganisms to attachment sites such as passive forces, electrostatic interactions, hydrophobic, steric forces, lipoteichoic acids, adhesions and specific structures of adhesion (Salyers and Whitt, 2002). A significant advantage of competitive exclusion based on enhanced attachment is that unlike antibiotics, the factors that inhibit pathogen binding do not necessarily kill the pathogen, thereby exerting less selective pressure on the pathogen to evolve resistance (Reid et al., 2001).

The use of mucus and intestinal epithelial cell cultures represent widely used *in vitro* models in demonstrating the adhesion potential of candidate probiotics and their capability of interfering the adhesion of pathogens. It was demonstrated by Balcázar et al. (2007) that LAB probiotic candidate could competitively exclude the adhesion of fish pathogens such as *A. salmonicida* and *V. anguillarum* on the mucus of rainbow trout and the production of antagonistic compounds contributed significantly in the observed suppression of pathogen growth. Host-derived candidate probiotics were also demonstrated to be capable of displacing fish pathogens using *in vitro* mucus models (Vine et al., 2004). Earlier studies on understanding adhesion and interference potential of probiotics employed human intestinal epithelial cell lines. There is one major technical issue on this strategy. Human cell lines for studies on fish probiotics are improper as it does not provide a "close to" natural substratum for their adhesion (Lazado et al., 2011; Pan et al., 2008). Primary intestinal epithelial cell cultures of Chinese drums (*Miichthys miiuy*) were used in demonstrating the adhesion potential of *Clostridium butyricum*, a soil isolate, and their capability of interfering *A. hydrophila* and *V. anguillarum* adhesion. In a different approach, Lazado et al. (2011) showed that host-derived probiotics displayed adhesion specificity on primary intestinal epithelial cells that were isolated from the different regions of Atlantic cod intestine. Furthermore, the observed mode of interference could be by exclusion, competition, or displacement, and probiotics could reduce cell damage during pathogenic infection by lowering caspase-3 and lactate dehydrogenase activities.

9.4.4.3 Influence on digestive physiology

The spectrum of enzymatic activities characterized by most microorganisms is one of the reasons to explore the potential of probiotics from a nutritional perspective. The digestive enzymatic physiology is affected by ingested feed ingredients and the improvement of fish performance and growth is oftentimes the gauge of maximal utilization (Bolasina et al., 2006; Shan et al., 2008). Fish have endogenous and exogenous digestive enzymes and probiotics are primarily considered as exogenous contributors. Exogenous contribution by probiotics could be further categorized as direct, indirect, or a combination of both. Direct exogenous contribution is when probiotics produce enzymes that directly act as a key agent in the digestion of the feed ingredients. On the other hand, indirect exogenous contribution could be attributed to the promotion of beneficial bacteria by the probiotics in the gastrointestinal tract that subsequently stimulates their enzymatic activities. In most cases, probiotics act as a direct and indirect exogenous contributor of digestive enzymes. Many of the probiotics tested in fish are capable of producing enzymes such as amylase, cellulase, protease, chitinase, to name a few, that are important enzymes in utilizing the components of the feeds that are commonly offered.

In a study in Atlantic cod, dietary administration of host-derived probiotics influenced the digestive capacity of the host by modulating the enzymatic activities, particularly amylase and cellulase in the different regions of the intestine (Lazado et al., 2012). In another cold-water fish Arctic charr, some microorganisms such as *Agrobacterium* sp., *Pseudomonas* sp., *Brevibacterium* sp., *Microbacterium* sp., and *Staphylococcus* sp. may also contribute to nutritional processes in the gastrointestinal tract (Ringø et al., 1995). Significant increases in protease and lipase activities were observed in rohu, *Labeo rohita*, fed with either *B. subtilis*, *L. lactis*, or *S. cerevisiae.* The increase in digestive enzymes corresponds to the influences on protein efficiency ratio, nutrient retention, and digestibility (Mohapatra et al., 2012a). The biogenic effect is one of the claimed health benefits of fermented functional foods such as probiotics in humans. The biogenic properties are provided from the microbial production of bioactive metabolites such as certain vitamins, bioactive peptides, organic acids, or fatty acids during fermentation (Stanton et al., 2005). This aspect in the nutritional relevance of probiotic applications in fish is barely explored. However, in a recent study, it was shown that the changes in the liver and enterocyte linolenic and linoleic acid levels were related to the dietary administration of *Shewanella baltica* Pdp13 in the diet (Tapia-Paniagua et al., 2014).

9.4.4.4 Influence on water quality

Probiotics are not only capable of modulating host physiology and the associated microbiota for improved health and welfare, but they could also influence the rearing water as an indirect beneficial effect. The quality of the rearing water has a significant impact in fish and the physico-chemical parameters should be at the levels that promote health and sustainability. Probiotics capable of modifying and improving water quality are generally called "water probiotics" (Venkateswara, 2007). The capability of probiotics in modifying the quality of the rearing water has advanced their functions as not just feed supplements, but also as water additives (Moriarty, 1998). The number of discoveries published in recent years has prompted the incorporation of this concept into the definition of probiotics in aquaculture that had been previously too focused on being feed supplements.

The most common water probiotics are from the genus *Bacillus*. Being gram-positive bacteria, *Bacillus* are more efficient in converting organic matter back to CO_2 than most of the gram-negative bacteria, which convert a greater percentage of organic carbon to bacterial biomass or slime (Stanier et al., 1963). The use of probiotics as water quality modifiers are mostly performed in production systems involving Penaied species. Nevertheless, there are studies demonstrating the improvement of water quality in a fish rearing system following probiotic administration. Besides the influence on growth performance and innate immunity of olive flounder, the supplementation of *Bacillus* spp. into the rearing water significantly decreased ammonia concentration and fish mortality (Cha et al., 2013). Incorporation of *Bacillus* spp. could also reduce high concentrations of nitrogen in a raceway-system in trout farms (Maillard et al., 2005). Other than *Bacillus* spp., there are other bacteria that could be used as water probiotics. For example, strains of *Azotobacter* and *Azospirillum* were used as water probiotics for *Oreochromis niloticus* (Sayeda et al., 2011). The single inoculation of *Azotobacter* bacteria was the most effective strategy because mixed culture (*Azotobacter* and *Azospirillum*) resulted in severe histopathological lesions in fish even though some improvements in water quality were observed.

9.4.4.5 Immunomodulation

Probiotics had been initially applied in fish on a collective basis that these microorganisms act as a direct inhibitor of pathogens that pose a great concern for fish health. There is substantial evidence indicating that the multifaceted benefits of probiotics could be extended to being modulators of immune system. This concept may overlap with immunostimulants because probiotics may be categorically considered as immunostimulatory agents. However, it has to be pointed out that not all immunostimulants are probiotics, and vice versa. Another fundamental distinction of probiotics and immunostimulants is that the former may have additional beneficial actions other than immunostimulation following administration. This feature is a leverage if the strategic purpose of administering health-promoting compounds is not only targeted to one physiological component. For example, dietary administration of host-derived probiotics in Atlantic cod significantly improved the digestive enzymatic physiology (Lazado et al., 2012) and both intestinal and humoral immunity of the host (Lazado and Caipang, unpublished). In another study, it was shown that besides acting as growth promoters, *Bacillus subtilis* VSG1 administered in combination with *Lactobacillus plantarum* VSG3 or/and *Pseudomonas aeruginosa* VSG2 influenced a number of immune parameters leading to an improved resistance following a pathogen challenge (Giri et al., 2014). These examples show that both host-derived and non-host probiotics are capable of influencing the immune system of the host fish. Further, the influence of dietary probiotic administration on host immunity could be local or/and systemic in nature.

Dietary administration of probiotics in fish influences humoral defenses such as lysozyme, bactericidin, complement, myeloperoxidase, antiprotease, phosphatase, superoxide dismutase, catalase, among many others. Probiotics could also increase the number and improve the activities of many immune cells particularly erythrocytes, granulocytes, macrophages, and lymphocytes. In particular, respiratory burst and phagocytic activities are the commonly assayed parameters in determining the effects of probiotics on cellular immunity. The immunomodulatory action following probiotic feeding is also reflected in the transcriptional profiles of antibacterial, cytokines, oxidative stress genes, to name a few, of the host especially in immune-related organs/tissues (see reviews of Lazado and Caipang, 2014a, 2014b, 2014c; Nayak, 2010). One of the major indicators in determining the potency of the probiotics-induced modulation of the immune system is the improved resistance after a pathogen challenge. Even though it is possible to draw scientific conclusions from the increase/decrease of the immune parameters following dietary feeding, the immunostimulatory properties of probiotics could be well substantiated if a feeding experiment is followed by a pathogen challenge or stress exposure test.

9.5 Dietary administration of immunostimulants and their effects on mucosal immunity and disease resistance

A large number of reviews have been published during the past few years concerning the advantages of immunostimulants in fish and the immune system (Gannam and Schrock, 1999; Sakai, 1999; Bricknell and Dalmo, 2005; Harikrishnan et al., 2011; Ringø et al., 2012). Besides genetic and environmental factors, the nutritional status of the fish is considered to be a major aspect that influences the immune response and modulates the resistance to infection. From a number of published studies in fish, it can be deduced that most of the studies done on immunonutrition have been largely based on single nutrients using a wide array of humoral and cellular immune markers and disease challenge models. Kiron (2012) suggests a number of experimental approaches on how to assess the performance of these additives in fish. First, the approach should cover a wide range of responses in the fish, i.e., from a whole fish response to the tissue or cellular level and at the mechanistic level. This approach can be attained using pathogen challenges using mortality as an end point. Another approach is to measure the production of specific antibodies in response to vaccination, after subjecting the fish to different dietary treatments. Though this is an integrated measure, which is an indication of both immune function and vaccine efficacy, determination of antibody production is not frequently employed in fish nutrition studies. Lastly, *in vitro* assessments are done following the prescribed feed regime in order to determine the immune responses of the host. The *in vitro* studies are mainly done using primary cells that are harvested from the immune-related organs including the head kidney, the spleen, the liver or the intestines of the fish that were fed different dietary treatments.

Oral administration of immunostimulants has already been reported for glucans, lactoferrin, levamisole, and chitosan (Harikrishnan et al., 2011). The oral administration of these immunostimulants results in enhancement of leucocyte function and protection against infectious diseases such as furunculosis, vibriosis, and streptococcosis. Several types of β-glucans have been tested in terms of their efficacy in modulating the immune responses of fish and shellfish and how these compounds provided protection to the host following experimental challenge of pathogens including bacteria, viruses, and parasites (Ringø et al., 2012). While the effects of immunostimulants on the systemic immune responses (both humoral and adaptive) have been studied extensively, very few studies have been done to elucidate the effects of these various immune-stimulating compunds on mucosal immunity of the fish, particularly during oral administration. The number of published papers along this aspect of fish immunity account for less than 20% of the total publications done on immunostimulants and fish immunity. Table 9.1 shows the effects of these different kinds of immunostimulants on the mucosal immune system of the fish, including the gut- (GALT), skin- (SALT), and

Table 9.1 Effects of dietary administration of immunostimulants in the mucosa-associated lymphoid tissues (MALT) of the fish

MALT	Kind of immuno-stimulant*	Name of immu-nostimulant	Application dose	Fish species	Age of fish**	Observations†	References
Gut-associated lymphoid tissues (GALT)	• Polysaccharide	β-1,3 and β-1,6 yeast glucan	0, 500, 1000 mg/kg	Salmon, *Salmo salar*	Larvae	‖effect on gut health	Refstie et al., 2010
	• Polysaccharide	High M-alginate	Powdered diet	Atlantic cod, *Gadus morhua*		↑ uptake of 125 I-labelled molecule in the gastrointestinal tract	Vollstad et al., 2006
	• Plant derivatives/ extracts	Soybean meal	20% replacement of fishmeal	Atlantic salmon, *S. salar*	Juveniles	Inflammation in distal intestine; transcriptional upregulation of immune-related genes; downregulation of genes related to metabolic and digestive processes	Sahlmann et al., 2013
		Soybean extracts and derivatives	Various dosages	Atlantic salmon, *S. salar*	Juveniles	Enteritis in distal intestine; ↑ levels of lysozyme and IgM in mid and distal intestinal mucosa	Krogdahl et al., 2000
Skin-associated lymphoid tissues (SALT)	• Polysaccharide	β-Glucan	Immersion (25 mg/L)	Atlantic halibut, *Hippoglossus hippoglossus*	Larvae	Absorbed in the skin	Strand and Dalmo, 1997
	• Polysaccharide	β-1,3 and β-1,6 yeast glucan	0, 500, 1000 mg/kg	Salmon, *S. salar*	Juveniles	↓ lice infestation in skin	Refstie et al., 2010
Gill-associated lymphoid tissues	• Polysaccharide	β-Glucan	Oral (0.1%)	Seabass, *Dicentrarchus labrax*		↑ heat shock protein (HSP) expression in gills	Bagni et al., 2005
	• Polysaccharide	Ergosan	Diet (0.5%)	Seabass, *D. labrax*		↑ heat shock protein (HSP) expression in gills	Bagni et al., 2005

* Chemical agents, bacterial/yeast components, polysaccharides, animal or plant extracts, nutritional factors and cytokines.
** Larval/juvenile.

gill-associated lymphoid tissues (GIALT). Among the immunostimulants, the effects of β-glucans on mucosal immunity in fish have been demonstrated to a certain extent, e.g., increased uptake of some molecules (Vollstad et al., 2006) or these can be absorbed by the skin in fish larvae (Strand and Dalmo, 1997). Glucans can also help in the reduction of sea lice infestations in Atlantic salmon (Refstie et al., 2010), and can also lead to increased transcription of heat shock proteins in the gills of some fish species (Bagni et al., 2005). However, not all immunostimulants have a positive effect on the mucosal immunity in fish. Krogdahl et al. (2000) and Sahlmann et al. (2013) showed that when Atlantic salmon were fed with diets containing soybean extracts or derivatives, the fish had enteritis at the distal intestines as well as decreased expression of metabolism- and digestion-related genes after prolonged feeding of these plant products.

While few studies have been done on the effects during oral administration of immunostimulants to the mucosal immunity in fish, the reverse is true for the protective effects of these substances during pathogen challenge. In most studies dealing with immunostimulants, the efficiency of these substances was assessed using pathogen challenge following feeding. Table 9.2 shows the different kinds of immunostimulants in fish and their known protective effects against various pathogens. The commonly used immunostimulants in fish were the glucans, bacterial/yeast components, and plant extracts/derivatives. These compounds have been used in a wide range of fish species and were found to protect the fish from bacterial pathogens including *Aeromonas hydrophila, A. salmonicida, Edwardsiella ictaluri, E. tarda, Mycobacterium marinum, Photoacterium damselae, Streptococcus agalactiae, S. iniae, Vibrio alginolyticus, V. anguillarum*, and *V. harveyi*, among others.

Given the importance of mucosal immunity on the defense of the fish against pathogens, the role of these immunostimulants especially during feeding is very critical. A generalized representation as to how dietary administration of immunostimulants affects growth and resistance of fish against pathogens is shown in Figure 9.2. Various types of immunostimulants, when incorporated in the feeds, likely trigger the various components of the mucosal immunity in fish. Depending on the type of the immunostimulant, the immune responses that are involved in mucosal immunity are modulated in such a way that the systemic immune system of the fish is also affected, which in turn provides resistance and protection of the fish against the invading pathogens. Moreover, some of these immunostimulants are also growth factors, and when combined in the feed, could also result in positive effects on the growth of the fish.

9.6 Dietary administration of prebiotics and their effects on mucosal immunity

9.6.1 Effects of prebiotics on gut-associated lymphoid tissues (GALT)

The concept underlying the use of prebiotics is an apparent reason why their influences on GALT are well documented as compared to the two other mucosal tissues (Figure 9.3). The amount of contemporary evidence indicates that prebiotics primarily

Table 9.2 **Effects of dietary administration of immunostimulants on the resistance of the fish against pathogens**

Pathogen	Kind of immunostimulant*	Name of immunostimulant	Application dose	Fish species	Age of fish**	Observations†	References
Aeromonas hydrophila	• Polysaccharide	Glucan	0.1%	Rohu, *Labeo rohita*	Juveniles	↑ protection	Sahoo and Mukherjee, 2001
	• Polysaccharide	Glucan	Oral delivery	Asian catfish, *Clarias batrachus*	Juveniles	↑ protection	Kumari and Sahoo, 2006
	• Polysaccharide	Macroguard	0.5, 1, and 2 g/kg	Tench, *Tinca tinca*	Juveniles	↑ protection at higher inclusion levels	Siwicki et al., 2010
	• Bacterial/yeast components	Whole yeast, *Saccharomyces cerevisiae*	0.25, 0.5, 1, 2, and 5 g/kg	Nile tilapia, *Oreochromis niloticus*	Juveniles	↑ protection	Abdel-Tawwab et al., 2008
	• Bacterial/yeast components	Autolyzed yeast/cell wall	2% autolyzed yeast; 0.3% cell wall	Nile tilapia, *O. niloticus*	Juveniles	↑ protection	Reque et al., 2010
	• Bacterial/yeast components	*Debaryomyces hansenii*	10^6 yeast cells g^{-1}	Leopard grouper, *Mycteroperca rosacea*	Juveniles	↑ resistance	Reyes-Becerril et al., 2011
	• Bacterial/yeast components	PHB-HV from *Bacillus thuringiensis*	1, 3, and 5%	Tilapia, *O. mossambicus*	Juveniles	↑ protection	Suguna et al., 2014
	• Plant components and/or extracts	Green tea, *Camellia sinensis*	0.125, 0.25, 0.5, 1, and 2 g/kg	Nile tilapia, *O. niloticus*	Juveniles	↑ resistance	Abdel-Tawwab et al., 2010
	• Hormones	Bovine lactoferrin	50, 100, 200 mg/kg	Catfish, *C. batrachus*	Juveniles	↑ resistance	Kumari et al., 2003
	• Nutritional factors	Vitamin C	500 mg/kg	Rohu, *L. rohita*	Juveniles	↑ protection	Sahoo and Mukherjee, 2003
	• Plant components and/or extracts	Leaves of *Eclipta alba*	0.01, 0.1, and 1%	Tilapia, *O. mossambicus*	Juveniles	↑ protection	Radu et al., 2003
	• Plant components and/or extracts	Seeds of *Achyranthes aspera*	0.05, 0.1, 0.5%	Rohu, *L. rohita*	Juveniles	↑ protection	Rao et al., 2006
	• Plant components and/or extracts	Extracts of *Allium sativum*	0.05, 0.1, 0.5, and 1 g	Rainbow trout, *Oncorhynchus mykiss*	Juveniles	↑ protection	Nya and Austin, 2009

Pathogen	Kind of immunostimulant*	Name of immunostimulant	Application dose	Fish species	Age of fish**	Observations[†]	References
	• Plant components and/or extracts	Kernel of *Mangifera indica*	1, 5, and 10 g	Rohu, *L. rohita*	Juveniles	↑ protection	Sahu et al., 2007
	• Plant components and/or extracts	Chloroform extract of seeds from *Nyctanthes arbortristis*	0.01, 0.1, and 1%	Tilapia, *O. mossambicus*	Juveniles	↑ protection	Kirubakaran et al., 2010
	• Plant components and/or extracts	Aqueous extracts of *Viscum album*	0.1, 0.5, and 1%	Eel, *Anguilla japonica*	Juveniles	↑ protection	Yin et al., 2008
	• Plant components and/or extracts	Leaves of *Withania somnifera*	1, 2, and 3%	Rohu, *L. rohita*	Juveniles	↑ protection	Sharma et al., 2010
Aeromonas salmonicida	• Polysaccharide	Macroguard	Oral delivery	Trout, *O. mykiss*	Juveniles	↑ resistance	Siwicki et al., 1994
	• Plant components and/or extracts	Soybean products	Oral delivery	Atlantic salmon, *S. salar*	Juveniles	↓ protection	Krogdahl et al., 2000
Edwardsiella ictaluri	• Polysaccharide	Glucan	Oral delivery	Channel catfish, *Ictalurus punctatus*	Juveniles	‖ resistance	Duncan and Klesius, 1996
E. tarda	• Plant components and/or extracts	Fruits of *Eleutherococcus senticosus*	3 and 7%	Flounder, *Paralichthys olivaceus*	Juveniles	↑ protection	Won et al., 2008
Mycobacterium marinum	• Bacterial/yeast components	*S. cerevisiae*	1 and 2%	Hybrid striped bass, *Morone chrysops* female × *M. saxatilis* male	Juveniles	‖ resistance	Li and Gatlin, 2005
Photobacterium damselae	• Plant components and/or extracts	Leaves of *Porphyridium cruentum*	10 g	Sole, *Solea senegalensis*	Juveniles	↑ protection	Díaz-Rosales et al., 2008
Streptococcus agalactiae	• Plant components and/or extracts	Aqueous extract from leaves of *Cinnamomum verum*	0.5, 1, and 1.5%	Nile tilapia, *O. niloticus*	Juveniles	↑ protection	Rattanachaikunsopon and Phumkhachorn, 2010

(Continued)

Table 9.2 Effects of dietary administration of immunostimulants on the resistance of the fish against pathogens (*cont.*)

Pathogen	Kind of immunostimulant*	Name of immunostimulant	Application dose	Fish species	Age of fish**	Observations†	References
Streptococcus iniae	• Polysaccharide	Glucan	Oral delivery; 0.1%	Hybrid striped bass, *Morone chrysops* female × *M. saxatilis* male	Juveniles	‖ resistance	Jaramillo and Gatlin, 2004
	• Polysaccharide	Glucan	100 and 200 mg/kg	Nile tilapia, *O. niloticus*	Juveniles	↑ resistance	Whittington et al., 2005
	• Polysaccharide	Glucan	Oral administration	Red-tail black shark, *Epalzeorhynchos bicolor*	Juveniles	↑ resistance	Russo et al., 2006
	• Bacterial/yeast components	*S. cerevisiae*	1 and 2%	Hybrid striped bass, *Morone chrysops* female × *M. saxatilis* male	Juveniles	↑ resistance	Li and Gatlin, 2004
	• Plant components and/or extracts	Ethanol/methanolic extracts of the leaves from *Rosmarinus officinalis*	Various ratios	Tilapia, *Oreochromis* sp.	Juveniles	↑ resistance	Abutbul et al., 2004
Vibrio alginolyticus	• Polysaccharide	β-Glucan from mushroom	0.1 and 0.2%	Grouper, *Epinephelus coioides*	Juveniles	↑ protection	Chang et al., 2013
V. anguillarum	• Plant components and/or extracts	Fruits of *E. senticosus*	3 and 7%	Flounder, *P. olivaceus*	Juveniles	↑ protection	Won et al., 2008
V. harveyi	• Polysaccharide	Chitosan	3 and 6 g/kg	*Rachycentron canadum*	Juveniles	↑ protection	Geng et al., 2011

* Chemical agents, bacterial/yeast components, polysaccharides, animal or plant extracts, nutritional factors and cytokines.
** Larval/juvenile.
† (↑) increased; (↓) decreased; (‖) no effect.

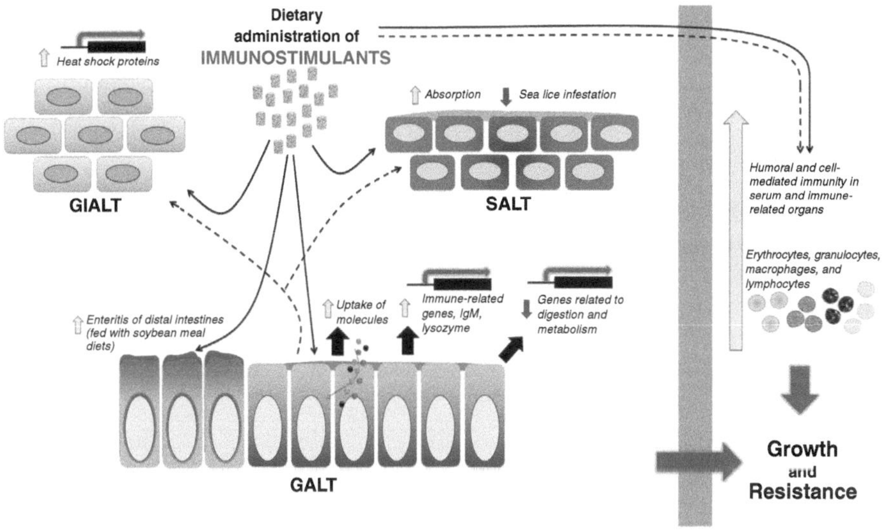

Figure 9.2 Immunological influences of immunostimulants on the mucosa-associated lymphatic tissues (MALT) of the fish. The influence of dietary administration may be by direct (arrow with solid line) and indirect (arrow with dashed-line) mechanism. Besides the MALT, the systemic immunity is also influenced by immunostimulants. The gray block represents the link in the influence of the dietary administration of immunostimulants between mucosal and systemic immunity that is largely unknown. The modulation of immune is indicated by either upward (light gray [yellow in the web version]) or downward (dark gray [red in the web version]) pointing arrow.

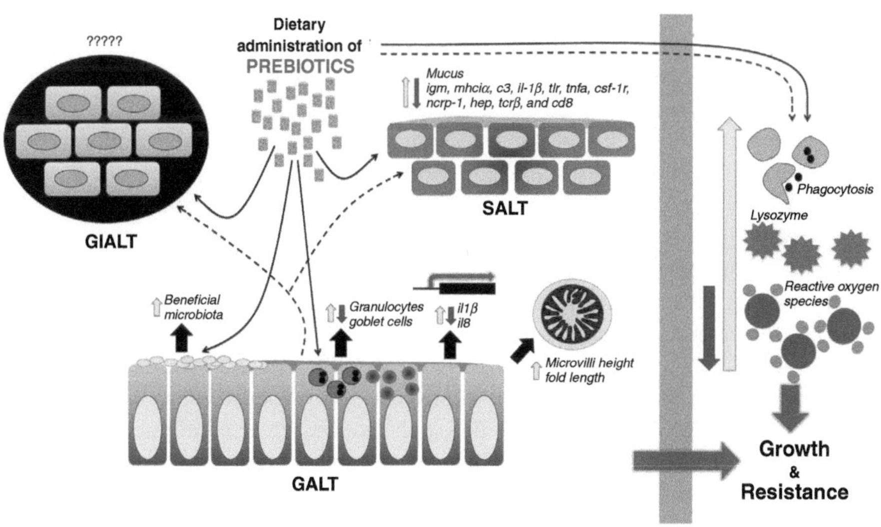

Figure 9.3 Immunological influences of prebiotics on the mucosa-associated lymphatic tissues (MALT) of the fish. The block circle of the GIALT represents that no studies have been done at the moment. Kindly refer to the caption of Figure 9.2 for additional explanation.

act on GALT of most host fish. However, the exploration on the beneficial features of these substances should not be limited to the GALT. It is also interesting to point out that although effects of prebiotics is mostly focused on the gut, only a small fraction of these studies have discussed the probiotic-induced changes in the GALT compared with what have been done on the associated microorganisms.

The effect on intestinal morphology is one of the significant influences of dietary prebiotics in the GALT. The improvement of gut protection particularly the stimulation of immune cells is a common positive effect of dietary MOS in fish. For instance, the number of mucin-secreting cells (goblet cells) in both the proximal intestine and distal intestine increased significantly following MOS feeding in European sea bass (Torrecillas et al., 2011). An expansion of the lamina propia (contained infiltrated eosinophilic granulocytes) was also observed as a consequence of prebiotic feeding. Each of the following prebiotics were tested on red drum (*Sciaenops ocellatus*): fructooligosaccharides (FOS) in the form of inulin, galactooligosaccharides (GOS), Bio-MOS®, containing mannan oligosaccharides (MOS) derived from yeast, and Previda™ containing galacto-gluco-mannans from hemicellulose extract. It was observed that microvilli heights in pyloric caeca, proximal and mid-intestine were significantly increased in fish group fed with prebiotics (Zhou et al., 2010). In a different but similar study, four different probiotics (i.e., fructo-oligosaccharide, Bio-MOS, transgalacto-oligosaccharide, and GroBiotic-A) were administered individually to the diets of juvenile hybrid striped bass (*Morone chrysops* × *M. saxatilis*) and red drum (*Sciaenops ocellatus*). Prebiotic inclusion significantly increased the length of folds and the height of both enterocyte and microvilli (Anguiano et al., 2013). These gut morphological changes were similarly observed in channel catfish (*Ictalurus punctatus*) fed with yeast polysaccharide. The dietary supplementation increased the height of intestinal fold and the thickness of muscular layers in the intestine and improved the number of goblet cells (Zhu et al., 2012). Intestinal cytokines are also affected by prebiotic feeding in fish. It was demonstrated in Atlantic cod fed with yeast-derived mannan oligosaccharide that the transcript level of *il1β* in the posterior intestine and rectum of post-challenge fish was significantly higher than that of pre-challenge fish, whereas the difference in *il8* transcripts was only observed in the rectum (Lokesh et al., 2012). Interestingly, some negative effects on intestinal morphology were observed when gilthead seabream were fed with inulin and *B. subtilis*. Different signs of edema and inflammation were observed in the mentioned compounds/microorganism when administered individually or in combination. The presence of vacuolated cytoplasm in enterocytes and reduction in the number of goblet cells are some of the remarkable histological alterations observed (Cerezuela et al., 2013a). This is one of the few studies discussing the negative impacts of prebiotics/synbiotics feeding in intestinal morphology of fish. Though this study may be perceived in a negative standpoint, the results actually supported the previous report of the same research group that the increase in immune parameters following the dietary administration of the same substance/microorganisms did not correlate with disease resistance (Cerezuela et al., 2012b). Further, these results indicate that prebiotic property should not be extrapolated between species and actual effect should be primarily demonstrated before claiming its potential use with only a reference from another host fish.

9.6.2 *Effects of prebiotics on skin-associated lymphoid tissues (SALT)*

Unlike in GALT, there are only few studies in fish documenting the effects of prebiotic feeding on skin-associated lymphoid tissues or SALT. MOS is the prebiotics with multiple studies supporting its capability in eliciting immune responses on SALT. Dietary administration of 0.4% Bio-Mos for 12 weeks in rainbow trout revealed a remarkable increase in the skin mucus weight (Rodrigues-Estrada et al., 2008). However, this influence on skin mucus was not corroborated by a recent study in European sea bass where it employed the same incorporation concentration and feeding duration of Bio-Mos (Torrecillas et al., 2011). These conflicting results revealed a significant practical concern that prebiotic actions may be influenced by host species. Though it was not a strictly pure prebiotic research when inulin was administered with *Debaryomyces hansenii* L2 to *Sparus aurata*, it was shown that the transcript levels of immune-related genes such as *igm*, *mhciα*, *mhciiα*, *c3*, *il-1β*, *tlr*, *tnfα*, *csf-1r*, *nccrp-1*, *hep*, *tcrβ*, and *cd8* were modulated in the skin (Tapia-Paniagua et al., 2011). These changes coincided with the modulation in the mRNA levels of these genes in the head kidney and the intestine as well the alteration of the intestinal microbiota.

9.6.3 *Effects of prebiotics on gill-associated lymphoid tissues (GIALT)*

To the best of our knowledge, there are no studies available discussing the effects of dietary administration of prebiotics, of any kind, on fish gill-associated lymphoid tissues (GIALT). Though the chances that dietary incorporated prebiotics get in contact with the gills are almost nil, there is a possibility that GIALT may also be affected by prebiotic feeding through an indirect mechanism of immunostimulation.

9.7 Dietary administration of probiotics and their effects on mucosal immunity

9.7.1 *Effects of probiotics on gut-associated lymphoid tissues (GALT)*

There are several methods in delivering probiotics to fish and dietary incorporation remains to be the most popular strategy. There is no unequivocal acceptance that dietary administration is the best delivery method in evoking the most effective benefits from probiotics. The choice of the most suitable delivery method may depend on several factors such as the physiological characteristics of the probiotics, the host species, and the expected probiotic actions. Dietary administration is by far the most efficient method when probiotics are expected to boost the immune defenses of gut-associated lymphoid tissues or GALT. The chances are high that probiotics directly interact with the GALT when administered orally than by addition to rearing water, for instance.

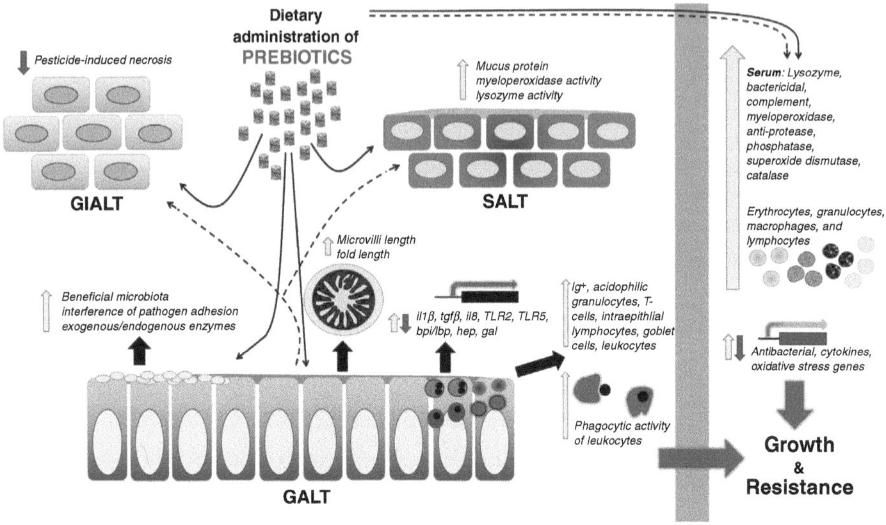

Figure 9.4 Immunological influences of probiotics on the mucosa-associated lymphatic tissues (MALT) of the fish. Kindly refer to the caption of Figure 9.2 for explanation.

Histological and molecular approaches have significantly shed light on the influences of probiotics on fish GALT (Figure 9.4). Probiotics could improve the cellular immune repertoire of GALT either by increasing their numbers or by improving their defense-related activities, but they could also act in both mechanisms at the same time. There was an elevated population of Ig^{+} and acidophilic granulocytes when terrestrial-derived *Lactobacillus fructivorans* (AS17B) and *Lactobacillus plantarum* were delivered to seabream using live feed vectors (Picchietti et al., 2007). When host-derived *Lactobacillus delbrueckii* ssp. *delbrueckii* (AS13B) was administered live to developing sea bass, a significant increase was observed in the density of T-cells and acidophilic granulocytes in the intestinal mucosa besides the decrease in the transcript levels of pro-inflammatory cytokines. This was the first study in fish to have reported probiotic-induced changes on T-cell activity (Picchietti et al., 2009). The increase in the number of immune-related cells particularly on the population of intraepithelial lymphocytes and acidophilic granulocytes following probiotic feeding (human-derived probionts; *Lactobacillus rhamnosus* GG) was also observed in tilapia (Pirarat et al., 2011). Bactocell, the first commercially available probiotic mixture to be accredited for aquaculture use in the EU, has been reported in several studies of their capacity in influencing the cellular components of the GALT. The number of intestinal intraepithelial leukocytes of tilapia and Atlantic salmon increased significantly after Bactocell feeding. In addition, substantial increments on goblet cell population and structural changes in villi as typified by increase in length and fold length were also noted in the mentioned fish species as well as in rainbow trout (Standen et al., 2012; Cerezuela et al., 2012a; Merrifield et al., 2010).

Though increases in numbers and morphological changes may indicate positive benefits from probiotic administration, these changes could be well substantiated by

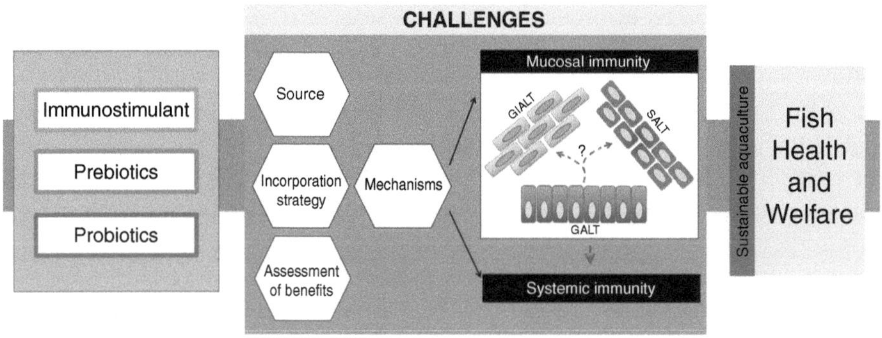

Figure 9.5 Paradigm of present status and future perspective in the application of immunostimulants, prebiotics, and probiotics in fish. These three sustainable alternatives are regarded with great importance as health-promoting agents in aquaculture. Several benefits have already been documented both from cold-water and temperate fish species. Despite the immense potential, they are restricted with several challenges particularly on the sources; incorporation strategy to meet large-scale preparation and maximum conferment of benefits; assessment of benefits for scientifically sound comparison; and most importantly, their mechanisms of actions that are mostly speculative and products of extrapolation from human studies. One of the benefits that has generated significant attention in the last years is their capability of modulating the immune system of fish. They are capable of modulating both the systemic and mucosal immunity. Their influence on the mucosal immunity especially on the GALT, GIALT, and SALT and the interactions within these mucosal tissues are fragmentary. Though positive changes have been observed following the dietary inclusion of these health-promoting agents, there is still much to be explored particularly on the exact mechanisms by which they confer their benefits. Furthering our understanding will lead to a more well-defined approach in promoting fish health and welfare for a sustainable aquaculture.

determining the influence of probiotics on the physiological and biochemical activities of these immune cells. In fact, the increase in number of these immune cells may not necessarily equate to potent immunological responses. Phagocytic and respiratory burst activities are usually affected by probiotic feeding but these stimulated activities are oftentimes determined in immune cells of the blood and head kidney and not from GALT. Nevertheless, feeding of rainbow trout with *L. lactis* subsp. *lactis* revealed a significant increase in the phagocytosis of live *A. salmonicida* by the intestinal leukocytes (Balcázar et al., 2006b).

Another mode by which probiotics influence GALT is through transcriptional modulation of immune-related genes. The changes in the mRNA levels following dietary administration suggest that probiotics may be priming the molecular immune repertoire of intestinal mucosa for a better response. In particular, the genes in the GALT that have been shown to be modulated by probiotics are primarily involved in the cytokine network. Dietary administration of *Bacillus subtilis* C-3102 in hybrid tilapia resulted to the modulation of *il-1b*, *tgf-β*, and *tnf-α* transcript levels in the gut (He et al., 2013). Besides cytokines (e.g., *il8*), genes related to cytoskeleton, junction complexes, and transport proteins in the intestine of gilthead seabream were remarkably influenced by probiotic diets (Cerezuela et al., 2013b). In a recent gene expression study, it was suggested that MyD88-independent TLR2 signaling may have a key role in the modulation of gut immunity by probiotics. The feeding of *Psychrobacter* sp. SE6 in grouper *Epinephelus coioides* resulted to the up-regulation of TLR2 and TLR5, adaptor MyD88, and cytokines (i.e., IL-1β, IL-8 and TGF-β1) in fish fed the viable form, whereas elevated expression of TLR2, but not MyD88 and cytokines, was observed in fish fed the heat-inactivated form of the bacteria (Sun et al., 2014). Live host-derived probiotics were administered through the diets in Atlantic cod and explicit differential regulation of immune-related genes was observed in the gut and the transcriptional variations were segment- and sampling-point dependent (Lazado et al., unpublished). It was further revealed that dietary administration of host-derived probiotics elicited stronger immune responses in the gut than in the blood, suggesting that these probiotics are more potent regulators of local than systemic immunity.

The relevance of histological and molecular changes in the gut upon the dietary applications of probiotics could be confirmed by the improvement of resistance against pathogens. The currently available studies on the influences of probiotics on the fish GALT are primarily devoted to profiling the changes by histo-morphological, biochemical, and molecular approaches. Only a handful studies have correlated the changes observed during probiotic feeding with the resistance of the host in the presence of a pathogen. This area could be explored in the subsequent studies as it will expand the knowledge and application potential of probiotics as immunostimulatory agents. For example, the resistance of rainbow trout against *Lactococcus garvieae*, the main agent of lactococcosis, was significantly improved when fed with *Lactobacillus plantarum*. Associated to this protection was the significant modulation of *il-10*, *il-8*, and *igt* gene expression in the intestine of probiotic-fed fish after *L. garvieae* infection, suggesting that *Lb. plantarum* can stimulate the immune response of rainbow trout in the presence of a pathogen (Pérez-Sánchez et al., 2011).

9.7.2 Effects of probiotics on skin-associated lymphoid tissues (SALT)

There are only few studies in fish that have explored the influence of probiotics on the skin-associated lymphoid tissues or SALT. This profile is similar with the observation on the application of prebiotics. The changes in the skin mucosa associated to probiotic feeding primarily focused on the mucous lining of the SALT. The skin mucus is an important first line of defense in teleost as it contains numerous immune factors significant in protecting the fish against pathogens and stressors. In this regard, probiotics capable of bolstering this defense system are regarded as ideal beneficial agents. To the best of our knowledge, no studies have been conducted describing morphological alterations or transcriptional changes in the skin following probiotic feeding. Nonetheless, an *in vitro* study in Atlantic cod had shown that probiotics were able to modulate the transcription of immune-related genes and protect the epidermal skin cells during pathogenic infection (Lazado et al., 2014d).

The first demonstration that probiotics can protect fish against surface infections was reported by Pieters et al. (2008). In their study, *Aeromonas bestiarum* and

Ichthyophthirius multifiliis skin infections in rainbow trout could be alleviated by dietary administration of GC2 (*Aeromonas sobria*) and BA211 (*Brochothrix thermosphacta*). The protection could be due to the stimulated innate immunity (i.e., GC2 promoted higher phagocytic activity, whereas probiotic BA211 resulted to enhanced respiratory burst activity) but the epidermal mucus total protein concentration could not be reliably used as an indicator because of extremely variable values. *Bacillus amyloliquefaciens* FPTB16 previously isolated from a fermented fishery product influenced the lytic activities of the skin mucus in catla *Catla catla*. The skin mucus of the probiotic-fed group showed higher myeloperoxidase activity, lysozyme activity, and total protein content. The enhanced resistance of catla to *Edwardsiella tarda* could be partly attributed to the remarkable changes in these parameters in the skin mucus (Das et al., 2013). Besides resistance to bacterial pathogen, an improved resistance to stress was also observed in Porthole livebearer *Poeciliopsis gracilis* fed with cells of *Lactobacillus casei*. Associated with this improved stress resistance was the significant increase of protein content in the skin mucus. It was not clear though on what mechanisms do these changes to mitigate the effects of air exposure-induced stress (Hernandez et al., 2010).

9.7.3 Effects of probiotics on gill-associated lymphoid tissues (GIALT)

Little is known on the effects of dietary administration of probiotics on the gill-associated lymphoid tissues or GIALT in fish. Unlike in prebiotics, there are studies available on the effects of probiotics on GIALT, though relatively lesser than those discussing the influences on GALT and SALT. An interesting study in *Labeo rohita* demonstrated the mitigation of gill-related necrotic effects of the pesticide fenvalerate by probiotic feeding (Mohapatra et al., 2012b). The best effect was observed when probiotics were administered in a multi-species bacterial mixture. In another study, it was observed that the transcript level of antimicrobial peptide defensin (defb) coding gene was significantly regulated in the gills of Atlantic cod. However, the administration strategy was through the rearing water and not through diets (Ruangsri et al., 2014). In future studies, it would be compelling to explore the capability of probiotic administration in influencing, particularly, stimulating the gill-associated lymphoid tissues of fish, because it is not just an important mucosal immune organ but the site of initial infection in some fish pathogens such as *Vibrio anguillarum* and atypical *Aeromonas salmonicida*. We can hypothesize that the dietary administration of probiotics could act through direct and indirect mechanisms in the gills of the fish. An indirect mechanism could be probable when probiotics are ingested through the diets and elicit immune responses from the GALT. The immune-related signals from the elicited responses will then be transmitted to the GIALT, hence, prompting immune responses as well. On the other hand, it could also be a direct mechanism because of the possibility that probiotics in the diet may be diffused and suspended in the rearing water. Being a structure that is in constant contact with the rearing water, the gills may be exposed to the probiotics that may eventually provoke immune responses.

9.8 Concluding remarks

Preventive health care by dietary manipulation has become one of the focal strategies of contemporary aquaculture. The acceptance of the aquaculture industry with this sustainable approach is reflected on the number of publications on the health benefits of candidate agents and several of them are now readily available in the market. These agents have been regarded to be natural, environmentally friendly, and safe. These discoveries are welcomed with optimism as the industry is drifting away from the use of synthetic compounds, antibiotics in particular, as disease control agents that pose negative consequences on the host fish as well as to the environment. Despite the very encompassing nature of the strategy, the focus has been on the use of immunostimulants, prebiotics, and probiotics for fish (Figure 9.5). Several benefits have been attributed to these substances/microorganisms and indeed they have shown that they could be ideal agents that promote fish health and welfare.

The development of immnunostimulants, prebiotics, and probiotics is challenged with some key issues that should be addressed in order for them to completely prosper as alternative agents. There are countless opportunities where to look for these substances/microorganisms but the discovery is oftentimes stochastic. Therefore, the sources of the substances/microorganisms should be well defined because it is important for marketing when it reaches commercial scale production in the future. The incorporation strategy should be considered as well. The biochemical or physiological requirements of the incorporated agents must be known as they have consequential effects on the conferment of benefits. Trials should be conducted on what is the most ideal incorporation strategy (e.g., viable or nonviable; pure or crude extract; formulated diets or live vectors) of each agent for a particular host species. Another important aspect is on the assessment of benefits following exposure to these substances/ microorganisms. The failure of comparative analysis often lies on the differing techniques used in assessing the effects of these agents. A multi-perspective approach in determining the benefits is also highly encouraged. Several biochemical and molecular techniques are widely available and they should be utilized maximally. In addition, challenge or stress experiment should ideally follow every dietary administration of these agents to substantiate the claim of being health promoters. One of the principal challenges that is of most significance in the present discussion is the mechanisms by which these agents confer their benefits. Reference to the observed mechanisms in human is not entirely unacceptable but extrapolation should be cautiously made as two host species have biological and physiological peculiarities. Most of the studies in fish usually discussed these agents in a cause-effect paradigm and the underlying mechanisms are often products of speculation. Their effects on the immune system have generated considerable attention with the hypothesis that boosting the immune system prepares the organisms to mount potent responses when it is under danger. Studies have shown that these substances trigger systemic immune responses; however, their influences on the mucosal immune system in fish are largely unknown. The mucosal immunity of fish has been explored in greater depth in the last years and it holds a special importance in the immune defense system of teleost.

Bridging the current knowledge and looking into possibilities to address the challenges is important for the advancement of these health-promoting agents in aquaculture. Fish health and welfare is a major defining factor in a sustainable aquaculture. Immunostimulants, prebiotics, and probiotics offer sustainable alternatives but must be understood in multitudinal contexts in order that their use and beneficial features are fully maximized.

Acknowledgments

The authors would like to thank their respective institutions for the support provided during the writing of this book chapter.

References

Abdel-Tawwab, M., Abdel-Rahman, A.M., Ismael, N.E.M., 2008. Evaluation of commercial live baker's yeast, *Saccharomyces cerevisiae* as growth and immunity promoter for fry Nile tilapia. *Oreochromis niloticus* (L.) challenged in situ with *Aeromonas hydrophila*. Aquaculture 280, 185–189.

Abdel-Tawwab, M., Ahmad, M.H., Seden, M.E.A., Sakr, S.F.M., 2010. Use of green tea, *Camellia sinensis* L., in practical diet for growth and protection of Nile tilapia, *Oreochromis niloticus* (L.), against *Aeromonas hydrophila* infection. J. World Aquacult. Soc. 41, 208–213.

Abutbul, S., Golan-Goldhirsh, A., Brazani, O., Zilberg, D., 2004. Use of *Rosmarinus officinalis* as a treatment against *Streptococcus iniae* in tilapia (*Oreochromis* sp.). Aquaculture 238, 97–105.

Adams, C.A., 2001. The role of nutricines in health and total nutrition. Proc. Aus. Poult. Sci. Sym. 12, 17–24.

Akrami, R., Iri, Y., Khoshbavar Rostami, H., Razeghi Mansour, M., 2013. Effect of dietary supplementation of fructooligosaccharide (FOS) on growth performance, survival. *Lactobacillus* bacterial population and hemato-immunological parameters of stellate sturgeon (*Acipenser stellatus*) juvenile. Fish Shellfish Immunol. 35, 1235–1239.

Alexander, J.B., Ingram, G.A., 1992. Noncellular nonspecific defense mechanisms of fish. Ann. Rev. Fish. Dis. 2, 249–280.

Anderson, D.P., Siwicki, A.K., 1994. Duration of protection against aeromona salmonicida in brook trout immunostimulated with glucan or chitosan by injection or immersion. Prog. Fish Culturist 56, 258–261.

Anguiano, M., Pohlenz, C., Buentello, A., Gatlin, D.M., 2013. The effects of prebiotics on the digestive enzymes and gut histomorphology of red drum (*Sciaenops ocellatus*) and hybrid striped bass (*Morone chrysops* × *M. saxatilis*). Br. J. Nutr. 109, 623–629.

Ardo, L., Yin, G., Xu, P., Váradi, L., Szigeti, G., Jeney, Z., Jeney, G., 2008. Chinese herbs (*Astragalus membranaceus* and *Lonicera japonica*) and boron enhance the non-specific immune response of Nile tilapia (*Oreochromis niloticus*) and resistance against *Aeromonas hydrophila*. Aquaculture 275, 26–33.

Babior, B.M., Kipnes, R.S., Curnutte, J.T., 1973. The productions by leukocytes of superoxide; a potential bactericidal agent. J. Clin. Invest. 52, 741.

Bagni, M., Romano, N., Finoia, M.G., Abelli, L., Scapigliati, G., et al.,2005. Short and long-term effects of a dietary yeast beta-glucan (Macrogard) and alginic acid (Ergosan) preparation on immune response in sea bass (*Dicentrarchus labrax*). Fish Shellfish Immunol. 18, 311–325.

Balcázar, J.L., de Blas, I., Ruiz-Zarzuela, I., Cunningham, D., Vendrell, D., Múzquiz, J.L., 2006a. The role of probiotics in aquaculture. Vet. Microbiol. 114, 173–186.

Balcázar, J.L., Vendrell, D., de Blas, I., Ruiz-Zarzuela, I., Gironés, O., Muzquiz, J.L., 2006b. Immune modulation by probiotic strains: quantification of phagocytosis of *Aeromonas salmonicida* by leukocytes isolated from gut of rainbow trout (*Oncorhynchus mykiss*) using a radiolabelling assay. Comp. Immunol. Microbiol. Infect. Dis. 29, e335–e343.

Balcázar, J.L., Vendrell, D., de Blas, I., Ruiz-Zarzuela, I., Gironés, O., Múzquiz, J.L., 2007. In vitro competitive adhesion and production of antagonistic compounds by lactic acid bacteria against fish pathogens. Vet. Microbiol 122, 373–380.

Baudin Laurencin, F., Germon, E., 1987. Experimental infection of rainbow trout, *Salmo gairdneri* R., by dipping in suspensions of *Vibrio anguillarum*: ways of bacterial penetration; influence of temperature and salinity. Aquaculture 67, 203–205.

Berge, A.C., Wierup, M., 2012. Nutritional strategies to combat *Salmonella* in mono-gastric food animal production. Animal 6, 557–564.

Bieklecka, M., Biedraycka, E., Majkowska, A., Juskiewcz, J., Wróbewska, M., 2002. Effect of nondigestible oligosaccharide on gut micro-ecosystems in rats. Food Res. Intl. 35, 139–144.

Bolasina, S., Perez, A., Yamashita, Y., 2006. Digestive enzymes activity during ontogenetic development and effect of starvation in Japanese flounder (*Paralichthys olivaceus*). Aquaculture 252, 503–515.

Bouhnik, Y., Flourie, B., Agay-Abensour, D., Pochart, P., Gramet, G., Durand, M., Rambaud, J.-C., 1997. Administration of transgalactooligosaccharides increases fecal bifidobacteria and modifies colonic fermentation metabolism in healthy humans. J. Nutr. 127, 444–448.

Bricknell, I., Dalmo, R.A., 2005. The use of immunostimulants in fish larval aquaculture. Fish Shellfish Immunol. 19, 457–472.

Broekaert, W.F., Courtin, C.M., Verbeke, K., Van de Wiele, T., Verstraete, W., Delcour, J.A., 2011. Prebiotic and other health-related effects of cereal-derived arabinoxylans, arabinoxylan-oligosaccharides and xylooligosaccharides. Crit. Rev. Food Sci. Nutr. 51, 178–194.

Bron, P.A., van Baarlen, P., Kleerebezem, M., 2012. Emerging molecular insights into the interaction between probiotics and the host intestinal mucosa. Nat. Rev. Microbiol. 10, e66–e78.

Brown, G.D., Taylor, P.R., Reid, D.M., Willment, J.A., Williams, D.L., Martinez Pomares, L., et al.,2002. Dectin-1 is a major b-glucan receptor on macrophages. J. Exp. Med. 196, 407e12.

Brunt, J., Newaj-Fyzul, A., Austin, B., 2007. The development of probiotics for the control of multiple bacterial diseases of rainbow trout, *Oncorhynchus mykiss* (Walbaum). J. Fish Dis. 30, 573–579.

Burr, G., Gatlin, III, D., Ricke, S., 2005. Microbial ecology of the gastrointestinal tract of fish and the potential application of prebiotics and probiotics in Finnish aquaculture. J. World Aquacult. Soc. 36, 425–435.

Burr, G., Gatlin, D.M., Hume, M., 2008. Effects of the prebiotics GroBiotic®-A and inulin on the intestinal microbiota of red drum, *Sciaenops ocellatus*. J. World Aquacult. Soc. 40, 440–449.

Burr, G., Gatlin, D.M., Hume, M., 2009. Effects of the prebiotics GroBiotic®-A and inulin on the intestinal microbiota of red drum. *Sciaenops ocellatus*. J. World Aquacult. Soc. 40, 440–449.

Burr, G., Hume, M., Ricke, S., Nisbet, D., Gatlin, III, D., 2010. *In vitro* and *in vivo* evaluation of the prebiotics GroBiotic®-A, Inulin, mannanoligosaccharide, and galactooligosaccharide on the digestive microbiota and performance of hybrid striped bass (*Morone chrysops* × *Morone saxatilis*). Microb. Ecol. 59, 187–198.

Caipang, C.M.A., Brinchmann, M.F., Kiron, V., 2010. Antagonistic activity of bacterial isolates from intestinalmicrobiota of Atlantic cod, *Gadus morhua*, and an investigation of their immunomodulatory capabilities. Aquacult. Res. 41, 249–256.

Carrington, A.C., Secombes, C.J., 2006. A review of CpGs and their relevance to aquaculture. Vet. Immunol. Immunopathol. 112, 87–101.

Cerezuela, R., Fumanal, M., Tapia-Paniagua, S.T., Meseguer, J., Moriñigo, M.T., Esteban, M.T., 2013a. Changes in intestinal morphology and microbiota caused by dietary administration of inulin and *Bacillus subtilis* in gilthead sea bream (*Sparus aurata* L.) specimens. Fish Shellfish Immunol. 34, 1063–1070.

Cerezuela, R., Meseguer, J., Esteban, M.Á., 2013b. Effects of dietary inulin, *Bacillus subtilis* and microalgae on intestinal gene expression in gilthead seabream (*Sparus aurata* L.). Fish Shellfish Immunol. 34, 843e8.

Cerezuela, R., Fumanal, M., Tapia-Paniagua, S.T., Meseguer, J., Morinigo, M.A., Esteban, M.A., 2012a. Histological alterations and microbial ecology of the intestine in gilthead seabream (*Sparus aurata* L.) fed dietary probiotics and microalgae. Cell Tissue Res. 350, 477e89.

Cerezuela, R., Guardiola, F.A., Meseguer, J., Esteban, M.Á., 2012b. Increases in immune parameters by inulin and *Bacillus subtilis* dietary administration to gilthead seabream (*Sparus aurata* L.) did not correlate with disease resistance to *Photobacterium damselae*. Fish Shellfish Immunol. 32, 1032–1040.

Cha, J.-H., Rahimnejad, S., Yang, S.-Y., Kim, K.-W., Lee, K.-J., 2013. Evaluations of *Bacillus* spp. as dietary additives on growth performance, innate immunity and disease resistance of olive flounder (*Paralichthys olivaceus*) against *Streptococcus iniae* and as water additives. Aquaculture, 402–403, 50-57.

Chang, C.F., Su, M.S., Chen, H.Y., Liao, I.C., 2003. Dietary β-1, 3-glucan effectively improves immunity and survival of *Penaeus monodon* challenged with white spot syndrome virus. Fish Shellfish Immunol. 15, 297–310.

Chantharasophon, K., Warong, T., Mapatsa, P., Leelavatcharamas, V., 2011. High potential probiotic *Bacillus* species from gastro-intestinal tract of Nile tilapia (*Oreochromis niloticus*). Biotechnology 10, 498–505.

Chaucheyras-Durand, F., Durand, H., 2010. Probiotics in animal nutrition and health. Benef. Microb. 1, 3–9.

Chavan, M.A., Riley, M.A., 2007. Molecular evolution of bacteriocins in Gram-negative bacteria. In: Riley, M.A., Chavan, M.A. (Eds.), Bacteriocins: Ecology, Evolution. Springer, Heidelberg, Germany, pp. 5–18, ISBN 3-540-36603-2.

Cheplin, H.A., Rettger, L.F., 1920. Studies on the transformation of the intestinal flora, with special reference to the implantation of *Bacillus acidophilus*, II. Feeding experiments of man. Proc. Natl. Acad. Sci. U.S.A. 6, 704–705.

Chipman, D.M., Sharon, N., 1969. Mechanism of lysozyme action. Science 165, 454–465.

Choque-Delgado, G.T., Tamashiro, W.M.S.C., Maróstica-Júnior, M.R., Moreno, Y.M.F., Pastore, G.M., 2011. The putative effects of prebiotics as immunomodulatory agents. Food Res. Int. 43, 1231–1236.

Cinatl, J., Morgenstern, B., Bauer, G., Chandra, P., Rabenau, H., Doerr, H.W., 2003. Glycyrrhizin, an active component of liquorice roots, and replication of SARS associated coronavirus. Lancet 361, 2045–2046.

Clevenger, M.A., Turnbull, D., Moue, H., Enomoto, M., Allen, J.A., Henderson, L.M., et al.,1988. Toxicological evaluation of neosugar: genotoxicity, carcinogenicity and chronic toxicology. J. Am. Col. Toxicol. 7, 643–662.

Cosgrove, M., 1998. Nucleotides. Nutrition 14, 748–751.

Courtin, C.M., Broekaert, W.F., Swennen, K., Lescroart, O., Onagbesan, O., Buyse, J., et al.,2008. Dietary inclusion of wheat bran arabinoxylooligosaccharides induces beneficial nutritional effects in chickens. Cereal Chem. 85, 607–613.

Dabrowski, K. (Ed.), 2000. Ascorbic Acid in Aquatic Organisms. CRC Press LLC, Boca Raton, FL.

Dalmo, R.A., Ingebrigtsen, K., Bøgwald, J., 1997. Non-specific defence mechanisms in fish, with particular reference to the reticuloendothelial system (RES). J. Fish Dis. 20, 241–273.

Damen, B., Pollet, A., Dornez, E., Broekaert, W.F., Haesendonck, I.V., Trogh, I., Arnaut, F., Delcour, J.A., Courtin, C.M., 2012. Xylanase-mediated in situ production of arabinoxylan oligosaccharides with prebiotic potential in whole meal breads and breads enriched with arabinoxylan rich materials. Food Chem. 131, 111–118.

Das, B.K., Debnath, C.D., Patnaik, P., Swain, D.K., Kumar, K., et al.,2009. Effect of β-glucan on immunity and survival of early stage of *Anabas testudineus* (Bloch). Fish Shellfish Immunol. 27, 678–683.

Das, A., Nakhro, K., Chowdhury, S., Kamilya, D., 2013. Effects of potential probiotic *Bacillus amyloliquifaciens* FPTB16 on systemic and cutaneous mucosal immune responses and disease resistance of catla (*Catla catla*). Fish Shellfish Immunol. 35, 1547e53.

Davis, J.F., Hayasaka, S.S., 1984. The enhancement of resistance of the American eel, *Anguilla rostrata* Le Sueur, to a pathogenic bacterium *Aeromonas hydrophila*, by an extract of the tunicate *Ecteinascidia turbinata*. J. Fish Dis. 7, 311–316.

Denev, S., Staykov, Y., Moutafchieva, R., Beev, G., 2009. Microbial ecology of the gastrointestinal tract of fish and the potential application of probiotics and prebiotics in finfish aquaculture. Int. Aquat. Res. 1, 1–29.

Díaz-Rosales, P., Chabrillón, M., Abdala, R.T., Figueroa, F.L., Balebona, M.C., Moriñigo, M.A., 2008. Effect of dietary administration of *Porphyridium cruentum* on the respiratory burst activity of sole, *Solea senegalensis* (Kaup), phagocytes. J. Fish Dis. 31, 489–495.

Díaz-Rosales, P., Salinas, I., Rodríguez, A., Cuesta, A., Chabrillón, M., Balebona, M.C., Moriñigo, M.A., Esteban, M.Á., Meseguer, J., 2006. Gilthead seabream (*Sparus aurata* L.) innate immune response after dietary administration of heat-inactivated potential probiotics. Fish Shellfish Immunol. 20, 482–492.

Duke, J.A., 1987. CRC Handbook of Medicinal Herbs, 5th ed. CRC Press, Boca Raton, FL.

Duncan, P.L., Klesius, P.H., 1996. Dietary immunostimulants enhance nonspecific immune response in channel catfish but not resistance to *Edwardsiella ictaluri*. J Aquat. Anim. Health 8, 241–248.

Dugenci, S.K., Arda, N., Candan, A., 2003. Some medicinal plants as immunostimulant for fish. J. Ethnopharmacol. 88, 99–106.

Dügenci, S.K., Arda, N., Candan, A., 2003. Some medicinal plants as immunostimulants for fish. J. Ethnopharmacol. 88, 99–106.

Ebrahimi, G.H., Ouraji, H., Khalesi, M.K., Sudagar, M., Barari, A., Zarei Dangesaraki, M., Jani Khalili, K.H., 2012. Effects of a prebiotic, Immunogen®, on feed utilization, body composition, immunity and resistance to *Aeromonas hydrophila* infection in the common carp *Cyprinus carpio* (Linnaeus) fingerlings. J. Anim. Physiol. Anim. Nutr. 6, 591–599.

EC, 2003. On a generic approach to the safety assessment of microorganisms used in feed/food and feed/food production – a working paper open for comment. <http://ec.europa.eu/food/fs/sc/scf/out178_en.pdf website>.

EFSA, 2007. Introduction of a Qualified Presumption of Safety (QPS) approach for assessment of selected microorganisms referred to EFSA. EFSA J. 587, 1–16.

EFSA, 2011. Maintenance of the list of QPS biological agents intentionally added to food and feed (2011 update). EFSA J. 9, 1–82.

Ellis, A.E., 2001. Innate host defense mechanisms of fish against viruses and bacteria. Dev. Comp. Immunol. 25, 827–839.

Englard, S., Seifter, S., 1986. The biochemical functions of ascorbic acid. Annu. Rev. Nutr. 6, 365–406.

Engstad, R.E., Robertsen, B., Frivold, E., 1992. Yeast glucan induces increase in lysozyme and complement-mediated haemolytic activity in Atlantic salmon blood. Fish Shellfish Immunol. 2, 287–297.

Escherich, T., 1885. Die Darmbakterien des Neugeborenen und Säuglinge. Fortschr. Med. 3, 515–522.

FAO/WHO. 2002. Guideline for the evaluation of probiotics in food. Joint FAO/WHO Working Group Report. London, Ontario, Canada, April 30 and May 1, 2002.

FAO/WHO, 2006. Probiotics in food. Health and nutritional properties and guidelines for evaluation. FAO Food Nutr. Pap. 85, 1–50.

Ferket, P.R., Parks, C.W., Grimes, J.L., 2002. Benefits of dietary antibiotic and mannanoligosaccharide supplementation for poultry. Multi-State Poultry Meeting May 14–16, 2002.

Findlay, V.L., Zilberg, D., Munday, B.L., 2000. Evaluation of levamisole as a treatment for amoebic gill disease of Atlantic salmon, *Salmo salar* L. J. Fish Dis. 23, 193–198.

Fjellheim, A.J., Klinkenberg, G., Skjermo, J., Aasen, I.M., Vadstein, O., 2010. Selection of candidate probionts by two different screening strategies from Atlantic cod (*Gadus morhua* L.) larvae. Vet. Microbiol. 144, 153–159.

Flajnik, M.F., Kasahara, M., 2010. Origin and evolution of the adaptive immune system: genetic events and selective pressures. Nat. Rev. Genet. 11, 47–59.

Fuller, R., 1989. Probiotics in man and animals. J. Appl. Bacteriol. 66, 365–378.

Gabaudan, J., Verlhac, V., 2001. Critical review of the requirements of ascorbic acid in cold and cool water fishes (salmonids, percids, plecoglossids, and flatfishes). In: Dabrowski, K. (Ed.), Ascorbic Acid in Aquatic Organisms. CRC Press LLC, Boca Raton, FL, pp. 33–48.

Gabrielsen, B.O., Austreng, E., 1998. Growth, product quality and immune status of Atlantic salmon, *Salmo salar* L., fed wet feed with alginate. Aquacult. Res. 29, 397–401.

Ganaie, M.A., Lateef, A., Gupta, U.S., 2014. Enzymatic trends of fructooligosaccharides production by microorganisms. Appl. Biochem. Biotechnol. 172, 2143–2159.

Ganguly, S., Chandra Dora, K., Sarkar, S., Chowdhury, S., 2013. Supplementation of prebiotics in fish feed: a review. Rev. Fish Biol. Fish. 23, 195–199.

Ganguly, S., Paul, I., Mukhopadhayay, S.K., 2010. Application and effectiveness of immunostimulants, probiotics, and prebiotics in aquaculture: a review. Israeli J. Aquacult. Bamidgeh 62, 130–138.

Gannam, A.L., Schrock, R.M., 1999. Immunostimulants in fish diets. J. Appl. Aquacult. 9, 53–89.

Gatesoupe, F.J., 1997. Siderophore production and probiotic effect of *Vibrio* sp., associated with turbot larvae, *Scophthalmus maximus*. Aquat. Living Resour. 10, 239–282.

Gatesoupe, F.J., 2005. Probiotics and prebiotics for fish culture, at the parting of the ways. Aqua Feeds Formulation Beyond 2, 3–5.

Geng, X., Dong, X.H., Tan, B.P., Yang, Q.H., Chi, S.Y., Liu, H.Y., et al.,2011. Effects of dietary chitosan and *Bacillus subtilis* on the growth performance, nonspecific immunity and disease resistance of cobia, *Rachycentron canadum*. Fish Shellfish Immunol. 31, 400–406.

Geraylou, Z., Souffreau, C., Rurangwa, E.M., de, G.E., Spanier, K.I., Courtin, C.M., Delcour, J.A., Buyse, J., Ollevier, F., 2013. Prebiotic effects of arabinoxylan oligosaccharides on juvenile Siberian sturgeon (*Acipenser baerii*) with emphasis on the modulation of the gut microbiota using 454 pyrosequencing. FEMS Microbiol. Ecol. 86, 357–371.

Geraylou, Z., Souffreau, C., Rurangwa, E., D'Hondt, S., Callewaert, L., Courtin, C.M., Delcour, J.A., Buyse, J.F., Ollevier, F., 2012. Effects of arabinoxylan-oligosaccharides (AXOS) on juvenile Siberian sturgeon (*Acipenser baerii*) performance, immune responses and gastrointestinal microbial community. Fish Shellfish Immunol. 33, 718–724.

Ghosh, S., Sinha, A., Sahu, C., 2007. Isolation of putative probionts from the intestines of Indian major carps. Israeli J. Aquacult. Bamidgeh 59, 127–132.

Gibbons, R.J., Van Houte, J., 1975. Bacterial adherance in oral microbial ecology. Ann. Rev. Microbiol. 29, 19–44.

Gibson, G.R., Roberfroid, M.B., 1995. Dietary modulationof the human colonic microbiota: introducing the concept of prebiotics. J. Nutr. 125, 1401–1412.

Gibson, G.R., Probert, H.M., Van Loo, J., Rastall, R.A., Roberfroid, M.B., 2004. Dietary manipulation of human colonic microbiota: updating the concept of prebiotics. Nutr. Res. Rev. 17, 259–275.

Gil, A., 2002. Modulation of the immune response mediated by dietary nucleotides. Eur. J. Clin. Nutr. 56, S1–S4.

Gildberg, A., Mikkelsen, H., 1998. Effects of supplementing the feed to Atlantic cod (*Gadus morhua*) fry with lactic acid bacteria and immuno-stimulating peptides during a challenge trial with *Vibrio anguillarum*. Aquaculture 167, 103–113.

Gioacchini, G., Lombardo, F., Avella, M.A., Olivotto, I., Carnevali, O., 2010. Welfare improvements using algínico acid in rainbow trout (*Oncorhynchus mykiss*) juveniles. Chem. Ecol. 26, 111–121.

Giri, S.S., Sukumaran, V., Sen, S.S., Jena, P.K., 2014. Effects of dietary supplementation of potential probiotic *Bacillus subtilis* VSG1 singularly or in combination with *Lactobacillus plantarum* VSG3 or/and *Pseudomonas aeruginosa* VSG2 on the growth, immunity and disease resistance of *Labeo rohita*. Aquacult. Nutr. 20 (2), 163–171.

Gombotz, W.R., Wee, S., 1998. Protein release from alginate matrices. Adv. Drug Del. Rev. 31, 267–285.

Gomez, D., Sunyer, J.O., Salinas, I., 2013. The mucosal immune system of fish: the evolution of tolerating commensals while fighting pathogens. Fish Shellfish Immunol. 35, 1729–1739.

Gomez-Gil, B., Roque, A., Turnbull, J.F., 2000. The use and selection of probiotic bacteria for use in the culture of larval aquatic organisms. Aquaculture 19, 259–270.

Goodridge, H.S., Wolf, A.J., Underhill, D.M., 2009. β-Glucan recognition by the innate immune system. Immunol. Rev. 230, 38–50.

Grimble, G.K., Westwood, O.M.R., 2001. Nucleotides as immunomodulators in clinical nutrition. Curr. Op. Clin. Nutr. Metabolic Care 4, 57–64.

Grisdale-Helland, B., Helland, S.J., Gatlin, III, D.M., 2008. The effects of dietary supplementation with mannanoligosaccharide, fructooligosaccharide or galactooligosaccharide on the growth and feed utilization of Atlantic salmon (*Salmo salar*). Aquaculture 283, 163–167.

Guttvik, A., Paulsen, B., Dalmo, R.A., Espelid, S., Lund, V., Bøgwald, J., 2002. Oral administration of lipopolysaccharide to Atlantic salmon (*Salmo salar* L.) fry. Uptake, distribution, influence on growth and immune stimulation. Aquaculture 214, 35–53.

Gültepe, N., Salnur, S., Hos¸su, B., Hisar, O., 2011. Dietary supplementation with mannanoligosaccharides (MOS) from Bio-Mos enhances growth parameters and digestive capacity of gilthead sea bream (*Sparus aurata*). Aquacult. Nutr. 17, 482–487.

Halver, J.E., 2002. The vitamins. In: Halver, J.E., Hardy, R.W. (Eds.), Fish Nutrition. Academic Press, California, pp. 62–141.
Harikrishnan, R., Balasundaram, C., Heo MS, 2011. Impact of plant products on innate and adaptive immune system of cultured finfish and shellfish. Aquaculture 317, 1–15.
Harmache, A., Leberre, M., Droineau, S., Giovannini, M., Bremont, M., 2006. Bioluminescence imaging of live infected salmonids reveals that the fin bases are the major portal of entry for *Novirhabdovirus*. J. Virol. 80, 3655–3659.
Haugarvoll, E., Bjerkås, I., Nowak, B.F., Hordvik, I., Koppang, E.O., 2008. Identification and characterization of a novel intraepithelial lymphoid tissue in the gills of Atlantic salmon. J. Anat. 213, 202–209.
Havenaar, R., Huis, I., 1992. Wood, B.J.B. (Ed.), The Lactic Acid Bacteria in Health and Disease, vol. 1, Elsevier, New York, NY.
He, S., Zhang, Y., Xu, L., Yang, Y., Marubashi, T., Zhou, Z., et al.,2013. Effects of dietary *Bacillus subtilis* C-3102 on the production, intestinal cytokine expression and autochthonous bacteria of hybrid tilapia *Oreochromis niloticus* ♀ × *Oreochromis aureus* ♂. Aquaculture, e412–e413, 125e30.
Hernandez, L.H.H., Barrera, T.C., Mejia, J.C., Mejia, G.C., Del Carmen, M., Dosta, M., et al.,2010. Effects of the commercial probiotic *Lactobacillus casei* on the growth, protein content of skin mucus and stress resistance of juveniles of the Porthole livebearer *Poecilopsis gracilis* (Poecilidae). Aquacult. Nutr. 16, 407e11.
Herter, C.A., Kendall, A.I., 1908. An observation on the fate of *B. bulgaricus* in the digestive tract of a monkey. J. Bacteriol. 5, 293–302.
Hidaka, H., Eida, T., Tarizawa, T., Tokunaga, T., Tashiro, Y., 1986. Effects of fructo-oligosaccharide on intestinal flora and human health. Bifidodact. Microflora J. 5, 37–50.
Holmgren, J., Czerkinsky, C., 2005. Mucosal immunity and vaccines. Nat. Med. 11, S45–S53.
Huebner, J., Wehling, R.L., Hutkins, R.W., 2007. Functional activity of commercial prebiotics. Intl. Dairy J. 17, 770–775.
Huyghebaert, G., Ducatelle, R., Immerseel, F.V., 2011. An update on alternatives to antimicrobial growth promoters for broilers. Vet. J. 187, 182–188.
Ispir, U., 2009. Prophylactic effect of levamisole on rainbow trout (*Oncorhynchus mykiss*) against *Yersinia ruckeri* Pesq. Vet. Bras. 29, 700–702.
Ispir, U., Dorucu, M., 2005. A study on the effects of levamisole on the immune system of rainbow trout (*Oncorhynchus mykiss* Walbaum). Turk. J. Vet. Anim. Sci. 29, 1169–1176.
Ito, M., Deguchi, Y., Miyamori, A., Matsumoto, K., Kikuchi, H., Kobayashi, Y., Yajiama, T., Kan, T., 1990. Effects of administration of galactooligosaccharides on human faecal microflora, stool weight and abdominal sensation. Microb. Ecol. Health Dis. 3, 285–292.
Jadhav, V.S., Khan, S.I., Girkar, M.M., Gitte, M.J., 2006. The role of immunostimulants in fish and shrimp aquaculture. Aquacult. Asia XI 3, 24–27.
Jaramillo, F., Gatlin, D.M., 2004. Comparison of purified and practical diets supplemented with or without beta-glucan and selenium on resistance of hybrid striped bass *Morone chrysops* female × *M. saxatilis* male to *Streptococcus iniae* infection. J. World Aquacult. Soc. 35, 245–252.
Jöborn, A., Olsson, J.C., Westerdahl, A., Conway, P.L., Kjelleberg, S., 1997. Colonization in the fish intestinal tract and production of inhibitory substances in intestinal mucus and faecal extracts by *Carnobacterium* sp. strain K1. J. Fish Dis. 20, 383–392.
Kaneko, T., et al.,1994. Effects of isomaltooligosaccharides with different degrees of polymerization on human fecal bifidobacteria. Biosci. Biotechnol. Biochem. 58, 2288–2290.
Kaneko, T., Yokoyama, A., Suzuki, M., 1995. Digestibility characteristics of isomaltooligosaccharides in comparison with several saccharides using the rat jejunum loop method. Biosci. Biotechnol. Biochem. 59, 1190–1194.

Kawakami, H., Shinohara, N., Sakai, M., 1998. The non-specific immunostimulation and adjuvant effects of *Vibrio anguillarum* bacterin, M-glucan, chitin or Freund's complete adjuvant in yellowtail *Seriola quinqueradiata* to *Pasteurella piscicida* infection. Fish Pathol. 33, 287–292.

Keiser, J., Utzinger, J., 2008. Efficacy of current drugs against soil-transmitted helminth infections: systematic review and meta-analysis. JAMA 299, 1937–1948.

Kelly, G., 2008. Inulin-type prebiotics – a review: part I. Altern. Med. Rev. 13, 315–329.

Ketabi, A., Dieleman, L.A., Gaenzle, M.G., 2011. Influence of isomalto-oligosaccharides on intestinal microbiota in rats. J. Appl. Microbiol. 110, 1297–1306.

Kiron, V., 2012. Fish immune system and its nutritional modulation for preventive health care. Anim. Feed Sci. Technol. 173, 111–133.

Kiron, V., Takeuchi, T., Watanabe, T., 1994. The osmotic fragility of erythrocytes in rainbow trout under different dietary fatty acid status. Fish Sci. 60, 93–95.

Kirubakaran, C.J.W., Alexander, C.P., Dinakaran, M.R., 2010. Enhancement of nonspecific immune responses and disease resistance on oral administration of *Nyctanthes arbortristis* seed extract in *Oreochromis mossambicus* (Peters). Aquacult. Res. 41, 1630–1639.

Kogan, G., Kocher, A., 2007. Role of yeast cell wall polysaccharides in pig nutrition and health protection. Livest. Sci. 109, 161–165.

Kolida, S., Gibson, G.R., 2008. The prebiotic effect: review of experimental and human data. In: Gibson, G.R., Roberfroid, M. (Eds.), Handbook of Prebiotics. CRC Press, Boca Raton, FL, pp. 69–93.

Kollath, W., 1953. Ernährung und Zahnsystem. Deutsch. Zahnaerzt. Z. 8, 7–16.

Konstantinov, S., Awati, A., Smidt, H., Williams, B., Akkermans, A., de Vos, W., 2004. Specific response of a novel and abundant *Lactobacillus amylovorus*-like phylotype to dietary prebiotics in the guts of weaning piglets. Appl. Environ. Microbiol. 70, 3821–3830.

Krogdahl, A.E., Bakke-Mckellep, A.M., Roed, K.H., Baeverfjord, G., 2000. Feeding Atlantic salmon *Salmo salar* L. soybean products: effects on disease resistance (furunculosis), and lysozyme and IgM levels in the intestinal mucosa. Aquacult. Nutr. 6, 77–84.

Kumar, R., Mukherjee, S.C., Prasad, K.P., Pal, A.K., 2006. Evaluation of *Bacillus subtilis* as a probiotic to Indian major carp *Labeo rohita* (Ham). Aquacult. Res. 37, 1215–1221.

Kumari, J., Sahoo, P.K., 2006. Dietary immunostimulants influence specific immune response and resistance of healthy and immunocompromised Asian catfish *Clarias batrachus* to *Aeromonas hydrophila* infection. Dis. Aquacult. Org. 70, 63–70.

Kumari, J., Swain, T., Sahoo, P.K., 2003. Dietary bovine lactoferrin induces changes in immunity level and disease resistance in Asian catfish *Clarias batrachus*. Vet. Immunol. Immunopathol. 94, 1–9.

Lara-Flores, M., Olvera-Novoa, M.A., 2013. The use of lactic acid bacteria isolated from intestinal tract of Nile tilapia (*Oreochromis niloticus*), as growth promoters in fish fed low protein diets. Latin Am. J. Aquat. Res. 41, 490–497.

Lauzon, H.L., Gudmundsdottir, S., Petursdottir, S.K., Reynisson, E., Steinarsson, A., Oddgeirsson, M., Bjornsdottir, R., Gudmundsdottir, B.K., 2010. Microbiota of Atlantic cod (*Gadus morhua* L.) rearing systems at pre- and post-hatch stages and the effect of different treatments. J. Appl. Microbiol. 109, 1775–1789.

Lazado, C.C., Caipang, C.M.A., 2014a. Bacterial viability differentially influences the immunomodulatory capabilities of potential host-derived probiotics in the intestinal epithelial cells of Atlantic cod *Gadus morhua*. J. Appl. Microbiol. 116, 990–998.

Lazado, C.C., Caipang, C.M.A., 2014b. Atlantic cod in the dynamic probiotics research in aquaculture. Aquaculture, 424–425, 53–62.

Lazado, C.C., Caipang, C.M.A., 2014c. Mucosal immunity and probiotics in fish. Fish Shellfish Immunol. 39, 78–89.

Lazado, C.C., Caipang, C.M.A., 2014d. Probiotics–pathogen interactions elicit differential regulation of cutaneous immune responses in epidermal cells of Atlantic cod *Gadus morhua*. Fish Shellfish Immunol. 36, 113–119.

Lazado, C.C., Caipang, C.M.A., Gallage, S., Brinchmann, M.F., Kiron, V., 2010a. Expression profiles of genes associated with immune response and oxidative stress in Atlantic cod, *Gadus morhua* head kidney leukocytes modulated by live and heat-inactivated intestinal bacteria. Comp. Biochem. Physiol. B 155, 249–255.

Lazado, C.C., Caipang, C.M.A., Gallage, S., Brinchmann, M.F., Kiron, V., 2010b. Responses of Atlantic cod *Gadus morhua* head kidney leukocytes to phytase produced by gastrointestinal-derived bacteria. Fish Physiol. Biochem. 36, 883–891.

Lazado, C.C., Caipang, C.M.A., Rajan, B., Brinchmann, M.F., Kiron, V., 2010c. Characterization of GP21 and GP12: two potential probiotic bacteria isolated from the gastrointestinal tract of Atlantic cod. Probiotics Antimicrob. Proteins 2, 134.

Lazado, C.C., Caipang, C.M.A., Brinchmann, M.F., Kiron, V., 2011. *In vitro* adherence of two candidate probiotics from Atlantic cod and their interference with the adhesion of two pathogenic bacteria. Vet. Microbiol. 148, 252–259.

Lazado, C.C., Caipang, C.M.A., Kiron, V., 2012. Enzymes from the gut bacteria of Atlantic cod, *Gadus morhua* and their influence on intestinal enzyme activity. Aquacult. Nutr. 18, 423–431.

Li, P., Gatlin, D.M., 2004. Dietary brewer's yeast and the prebiotic GroBiotic™ AE influence growth performance, immune responses and resistance of hybrid striped bass (*Morone chrysops* × *M. saxatilis*) to *Streptococcus iniae* infection. Aquaculture 231, 445–456.

Li, P., Gatlin, D.M., 2005. Evaluation of the prebiotic GroBiotic®-A and brewer's yeast as dietary supplements for sub-adult hybrid striped bass (*Morone chrysops* × *M. saxatilis*) challenged in situ with *Mycobacterium marinum*. Aquaculture 248, 197–2005.

Li, P., Gatlin, D.M., 2006. Nucleotide nutrition in fish: current knowledge and future applications. Aquaculture 251, 141–152.

Lilley, D.M., Stillwell, R.J., 1965. Probiotics: growth promoting factors produced by microorganisms. Science 147, 747–748.

Ljungh, A.L., Wadström, T., 2006. Lactic acid bacteria as probiotics. Curr. Issues Intest. Microbiol. 7, 73–89.

Lokesh, J., Fernandes, J.M.O., Korsnes, K., Bergh, Ø., Brinchmann, M.F., Kiron, V., 2012. Transcriptional regulation of cytokines in the intestine of Atlantic cod fed yeast derived mannan oligosaccharide or β-Glucan and challenged with Vibrio anguillarum. Fish Shellfish Immunol. 33, 626–631.

Magdelin, S.M. 2005. Culture of ornamental fish, Black molly (*Poecilia sphenops*) using medicinal plants having immunostimulant characteristics. M.Phil. dissertation. Manonmaniam Sundaranar University, India.

Maillard, V.M., Boardman, G.D., Nyland, J.E., Kuhn, D.D., 2005. Water quality and sludge characterization at raceway-system trout farms. Aquacult. Eng. 33, 271–284.

Makras, L., Van Acker, G., De Vuyst, L., 2005. *Lactobacillus paracasei* subsp. *paracasei* 8700:2 degrades inulin-types fructan exhibiting different degrees of polymerization. Appl. Environ. Microbiol. 71, 6531–6537.

Manning, T.S., Gibson, G.R., 2004. Prebiotics – Best Practice & Research. Clin. Gastroenterol. 18, 287–298.

Merrifield, D.L., Harper, G.M., Dimitroglou, A., Ringø, E., Davies, S.J., 2010. Possible influence of probiotic adhesion to intestinal mucosa on the activity and morphology of rainbow trout (*Oncorhynchus mykiss*) enterocytes. Aquacult. Res. 41, 1268e72.

Metchnikoff, E.CT In the prolongation of life, 1907. In: Chalmers, M. (Ed.), Optimistic Studies. William Heinemann, London.

Minomol, M., 2005. Culture of gold fish *Carassius auratus* using medicinal plants having immunostimulant characteristics. M.Phil Dissertation. M. Sundaranar University, India.
Mitsuoka, T., Hidaka, H., Eida, T., 1987. Effect of fructo-oligosaccharides on intestinal microflora. Die Nahrung 31, 427–436.
Mohapatra, S., Chakraborty, T., Prusty, A.K., Das, P., Paniprasad, K., Mohanta, K.N., 2012a. Use of different microbial probiotics in the diet of rohu, *Labeo rohita* fingerlings: effects on growth, nutrient digestibility and retention, digestive enzyme activities and intestinal microflora. Aquacult. Nutr. 18, 1–11.
Mohapatra, S., Chakraborty, T., Prusty, A.K., Kumar, K., Pani Prasad, K., Mohanta, K.N., 2012b. Fenvalerate induced stress mitigation by dietary supplementation of multispecies probiotic mixture in a tropical freshwater fish, *Labeo rohita* (Hamilton). Pestic. Biochem. Physiol. 104, e28–e37.
Monobe, M., Maeda-Yamamoto, M., Matsuoka, Y., Kaneko, A., Hiramoto, S., 2008. Immunostimulating activity and molecular weight dependence of an arabinoxylan derived from wheat bran. J. Jpn. Soc. Food Sci. Technol./Nippon Shokuhin Kagaku Kogaku Kaishi 55, 245–249.
Montalto, M., D'Onofrio, F., Gallo, A., Cazzato, A., Gasbarrini, G., 2009. Intestinal microbiota and its functions. Dig. Liver Dis. 3 (Suppl.), 30–34.
Moriarty, D.J.W., 1998. Control of luminous *Vibrio* sp. penaeid aquaculture ponds. Aquaculture 164, 351–358.
Murphy, O., 2001. Non-polyol low-digestible carbohydrates: food applications and functional benefits. Brit. J. Nutr. 1, 53.
Nayak, S.K., 2010. Probiotics and immunity: a fish perspective. Fish Shellfish Immunol. 29, 2–14.
Neumann, N.F., Fagan, D., Belosevic, M., 1995. Macrophage activating factors secreted by mitogen stimulated goldfish kidney leucocytes synergies with bacterial lipopolysaccharide to induce nitric oxideproduction in teleost macrophages. Dev. Comp. Immunol. 19, 475–482.
Newaj-Fyzul, A., Adesiyun, A.A., Mutani, A., Ramsubhag, A., Brunt, J., Austin, B., 2007. Bacillus subtilis AB1 controls *Aeromonas* infection in rainbow trout (*Oncorhynchus mykiss* Walbaum). J. Appl. Microbiol. 103, 1699–1706.
Nilsson, K.G., 1988. Enzymatic synthesis of oligosaccharides. Trends Biotechnol. 6, 256–264.
Niness, K.R., 1999. Inulin and oligofructose: what are they? J. Nutr. 129, S1402–S1406.
Nissle, A., 1918. Die antagonistische Behandlung chronischer Darmstörungen mit Colibakterien. Med. Klin. 2, 29–30.
Norqvist, A., Hagstrom, A., Wolf-Watz, H., 1989. Protection of rainbow trout against vibriosis and furunculosis by the use of attenuated strains of *Vibrio anguillarum*. Appl. Environ. Microbiol. 55, 1400–1405.
Nya, E., Austin, B., 2009. Use of dietary ginger, Zingiber officinale 1219 Roscoe, as an immunostimulant to control *Aeromonas hydrophila* infections in rainbow trout, *Oncorhynchus mykiss* (Walbaum). J Fish Dis 32, 971–977.
Nya, E.J., Austin, B., 2010. Use of bacterial lipopolysaccharide (LPS) as an immunostimulant for the control of *Aeromonas hydrophilla* infections in rainbow trout, *Oncorhynchus mykiss* (Walbaum). J. Fish Dis. 32, 971–977.
Ofek, I., Mirelman, D., Sharon, N., 1977. Adherance of *Escherichia coli* to human mucosal cells mediated by mannose receptors. Nature 265, 623–625.
O'Hara, A.M., Shanahan, F., 2006. The gut flora as a forgotten organ. EMBO Rep. 7, 688e93.
O'Sullivan, L., Murphy, B., McLoughlin, P., Duggan, P., Lawlor, P.G., Hughes, H., Gardiner, G.E., 2010. Prebiotics from marine macroalgae for human and animal health applications. Mar. Drugs 8, 2038–2064.

Pan, X., Wu, T., Song, Z., Tang, H., Zhao, Z., 2008. Immune responses and enhanced disease resistance in Chinese drum, *Miichthys miiuy* (Basilewsky), after oral administration of live or dead cells of *Clostridium butyrium* CB2. J. Fish Dis. 31, 679–686.

Parker, R.B., 1974. Probiotics, the other half of the antibiotics story. Anim. Nutr. Health 29, 4–8.

Patterson, J.A., Burkholder, K.M., 2003. Application of prebiotics and probiotics in poultry production. Poultry Sci. 82, 627–631.

Pérez-Sánchez, T., Balcázar, J.L., Merrifield, D.L., Carnevali, O., Gioacchini, G., de Blas, I., Ruiz-Zarzuela, I., 2011. Expression of immune-related genes in rainbow trout (*Oncorhynchus mykiss*) induced by probiotic bacteria during *Lactococcus garvieae* infection. Fish Shellfish Immunol. 31, 196–201.

Perrin, S., Warchol, M., Grill, J.P., Schneider, F., 2001. Fermentations of fructo-oligosaccharides and their components by *Bifidobacterium* infantis ATCC 15697 on batch culture in semi-synthetic medium. J. Appl. Microbiol. 90, 859–865.

Philippeau, C., Respondek, F., Julliand, V., 2010. *In vitro* effects of fructo-oligosaccharides on bacterial concentration and fermentation profiles in veal calf ileal contents. Anim. Feed Sci. Technol. 162, 83–90.

Picchietti, S., Mazzini, M., Taddei, A.R., Renna, R., Fausto, A.M., Mulero, V., et al.,2007. Effects of administration of probiotic strains on GALT of larval gilthead seabream: immunohistochemical and ultrastructural studies. Fish Shellfish Immunol. 22, e57–e67.

Picchietti, S., Fausto, A.M., Randelli, E., Carnevali, O., Taddei, A.R., Buonocore, F., Scapigliati, G., Abelli, L., 2009. Early treatment with *Lactobacillus delbrueckii* strain induces an increase in intestinal T-cells and granulocytes and modulates immune-related genes of larval *Dicentrarchus labrax* (L). Fish Shellfish Immunol. 26, 368–376.

Pieters, N., Brunt, J., Austin, B., Lyndon, A.R., 2008. Efficacy of in-feed probiotics against *Aeromonas bestiarum* and *Ichthyophthirius multifiliis* skin infections in rainbow trout (*Oncorhynchus mykiss* Walbaum). J Appl. Microbiol. 105, 723–732.

Pirarat, N., Pinpimai, K., Endo, M., Katagiri, T., Ponpornpisit, A., Chansue, N., et al.,2011. Modulation of intestinal morphology and immunity in Nile tilapia (*Oreochromis niloticus*) by *Lactobacillus rhamnosus* GG. Res. Vet. Sci. 91, e92e7.

Pratap, H.B., Wendelaar Bonga, S.E., 1993. Effect of ambient and dietary cadmium on pavement cells, chloride cells, and Na+/K+-ATPase activity in the gills of the freshwater teleost *Oreochromis mossambicus* at normal and high calcium levels in the ambient water. Aquat. Toxicol. 26, 133–149.

Press, C.M., Evensen, Ø., 1999. The morphology of the immune system in teleost fishes. Fish Shellfish Immunol. 9, 309–318.

Pulsford, A.L., Crampe, M., Langston, A., Glynn, P.J., 1995. Modulatory effects of disease, stress, copper, TBT and vitamin E on the immune system of flatfish. Fish Shellfish. Immunol. 5, 631–643.

Qi, Z., Zhang, X.-H., Boon, N., Bossier, P., 2009. Probiotics in aquaculture of China – current state, problems and prospect. Aquaculture 290, 15–21.

Radu, S., Ahmad, H., Ling, F.H., Reezal, A., 2003. Prevalence and resistance to antibiotics for *Aeromonas* species from retail fish in Malaysia. Int. J. Food Microbiol. 81, 261–266.

Rao, Y.V., Das, B.K., Jyotrymayee, J., Chakrabarti, R., 2006. Effect of *Achyranthes aspera.* on the immunity and survival of the *Labeo rohita*. Fish Shellfish Immunol. 20, 263–273.

Rastall, R.A., 2004. Bacteria in the gut: friends and foes and how to alter the balance. J. Nutr. 134, 2022S–2026S.

Rattanachaikunsopon, P., Phumkhachorn, P., 2009. Prophylactic effect of *Andrographis paniculata* extracts against *Streptococcus agalactiae* infection in Nile tilapia (*Oreochromis niloticus*). J. Biosci. Bioeng. 107, 579–582.

Razeghi Mansour, M., Akrami, R., Ghobadi, S.H., Amani Denji, K., Ezatrahimi, N., Gharaei, A., 2012. Effect of dietary mannan oligosaccharide (MOS) on growth performance, survival, body composition, and some hematological parameters in giant sturgeon juvenile (*Huso huso* Linnaeus, 1754). Fish Physiol. Biochem. 38, 829–835.

Refstie, S., Baeverfjord, G., Seim, R.P., Elvebø, O., 2010. Effects of dietary yeast cell wall β-glucans and MOS on performance, gut health, and salmon lice resistance in Atlantic salmon (*Salmo salar*) fed sunflower and soybean meal. Aquaculture 305, 109–116.

Řehulka, J., Minařík, B., Cink, D., Žalák, J., 2011. Prebiotic effect of fructooligosaccharides on growth and physiological state of rainbow trout, Oncorhynchus mykiss (Walbaum). Acta Univ. Agric. Silviculturae Mendelianae Brunensis 59, 227–236.

Reid, G., Howard, J., Gan, B.S., 2001. Can bacterial interference prevent infection? Trends Microbiol. 9, 424–428.

Reite, O.B., Evensen, O., 2006. Inflammatory cells of teleostean fish: s review focusing on mast cells/eosinophilic granule cells and rodlet cells. Fish Shellfish Immunol. 20, 192–208.

Rettger, L.F., Cheplin, H.A., 1920a. The transformation of the intestinal flora, with special reference to the implantation of *Bacillus acidophilus*. I. Feeding experiments with albino rats. Proc. Natl. Acad. Sci. U.S.A. 6, 423–426.

Rettger, L.F., Cheplin, H.A., 1920b. The transformation of the intestinal flora, with special reference to the implantation of *Bacillus acidophilus*. II. Feeding experiments on man. Proc. Natl. Acad. Sci. U.S.A. 6, 704–705.

Reque, V.R., de Moraes, J.R.E., de Andrade Belo, M.A., de Moraes, F.R., 2010. Inflammation induced by inactivated *Aeromonas hydrophila* in Nile tilapia fed diets supplemented with *Saccharomyces cerevisiae*. Aquaculture 300, 37–42.

Reyes-Becerril, M., Tovar-Ramirez, D., Ascenico-valle, F., Civera-Cerecedo, R., Gracia-lopez, V., et al.,2011. Effects of dietary supplementation with probiotic live yeast *Debaryomyces hansenii* on the immune and antioxidant systems of leooard grouper *Mycteroperca rosacea* infected with *Aeromonas hydrophila*. Aquacult. Res. 42, 1676–1686.

Riley, M.A., Wertz, J.E., 2002. Bacteriocins: evolution, ecology, and application. Annu. Rev. Microbiol. 56, 117–137.

Ringø, E., 1993a. Does dietary linoleic acid affect intestinal microflora in Artic charr, *Salvelinus alpinus* (L.). Aquacult. Fish. Manage. 24, 133–135.

Ringø, E., 1993b. The effect of chromic oxide Cr_2O_3 on aerobic bacterial populations associated with the epithelial mucosa of Arctic charr, *Salvelinus alpinus* (L.). Can. J. Microbiol. 39, 1169–1173.

Ringø, E., Bendiksen, H.R., Gausen, S.J., Sundsfjord, A., Olsen, R.E., 1998. The effect of dietary fatty acids on lactic acid bacteria associated with the epithelial mucosa and from faecalia of Arctic charr, *Salvelinus alpinus* (L.). J. Appl. Microbiol. 85, 855–864.

Ringø, E., Dimitroglou, A., Hoseinifar, S.H., Davies, S.J., 2014. Prebiotics in finfish: an update. In: Merrifield, D.L., Ringø, E. (Eds.), Aquaculture Nutrition: Gut Health, Probiotics and Prebiotics. Wiley-Blackwell Publishing, Oxford, UK, pp. 360–400.

Ringø, E., Gatesoupe, F.J., 1998. Lactic acid bacteria in fish: a review. Aquaculture 160, 177–203.

Ringø, E., Olsen, J.E., Vecino, J.L.G., Wadsworth, S., Song, S.-Y., 2012. Use of immunostimulants and nucleotides in aquaculture: a review. J. Marine Sci. Res. Dev. 2, 1.

Ringø, E., Olsen, R.E., Gifstad, T., Dalmo, R.A., Amlund, H., Hemre, G.-I., Bakke, A.M., 2010. Prebiotics in aquaculture: a review. Aquacult. Nutr. 16, 117–136.

Ringø, E., Sperstad, S., Myklebust, R., Mayhew, T.M., Olsen, R.E., 2006. The effect of dietary inulin on aerobic bacteria associated with hindgut of Arctic charr (*Salvelinus alpinus* L.). Aquacult. Res. 37, 891–897.

Ringø, E., Strøm, E., Tabacheck, J., 1995. Intestinal microflora of salmonids: a review. Aquacult. Res. 26, 773–789.

Rivero-Urgell, M., Santamaria-Orleans, A., 2001. Oligosaccharides: application in infant food. Early Hum. Dev. 65, S43–S52.

Roberfroid, M.B., 1993. Dietary fiber, inulin, and oligofructose: a review comparing their physiological effects. Crit. Rev. Food Sci. Nutr. 33, 103–148.

Roberfroid, M., 2007. Prebiotics: the concept revisited. J. Nutr. 137, 830S–837S.

Roberfroid, M.B., Van Loo, J.A.E., Gibson, G.R., 1998. The bifidogenic nature of chicory inulin and its hydrolysis products. J. Nutr. 128, 11–19.

Robertsen, B., Rørstad, G., Engstad, R., Raa, J., 1990. Enhancement of non-specific disease resistance in Atlantic salmon, *Salmo salar* L., by a glucan from *Saccharomyces cerevisiae* cell walls. J. Fish Dis. 13, 391–400.

Robertson, P.A.W., O'Dowd, C., Burrells, C., Williams, P., Austin, B., 2000. Use of *Carnobacterium* sp. as a probiotic for Atlantic salmon (*Salmo salar* L.) and rainbow trout (*Oncorhynchus mykiss*, Walbaum). Aquaculture 185, 235–243.

Rodriguez-Estrada, U., Satoh, S., Haga, Y., Fushimi, H., Sweetman, J., 2013. Effects of inactivated *Enterococcus faecalis* and mannan oligosaccharide and their combination on growth, immunity, and disease protection in rainbow trout. N. Am. J. Aquacult. 75, 416–428.

Rodrigues-Estrada, U., Satoh, S., Haga, Y., Fushimi, H., Sweetman, J., 2008. Studies of the effects of mannan-oligosaccharides, *Enterococcus faecalis*, and poly hydrobutyric acid as immune stimulant and growth promoting ingredients in rainbow trout diets. 5th World Fisheries Congress, Yokohama, Japan, p. 158, Abstract 2d-1-5.

Rombout, J.H., Abelli, L., Picchietti, S., Scapigliati, G., Kiron, V., 2011. Teleost intestinal immunology. Fish Shellfish Immunol. 31, 616–626.

Ruangsri, J., Fernandes, J.M.O., Brinchmann, M., Kiron, V., 2010. Antimicrobial activity in the tissues of Atlantic cod (*Gadus morhua* L.). Fish Shellfish Immunol. 28, 879–886.

Ruangsri, J., Lokesh, J., Fernandes, J.M.O., Kiron, V., 2014. Transcriptional regulation of antimicrobial peptides in mucosal tissues of Atlantic cod *Gadus morhua* L. in response to different stimuli. Aquacult. Res. 45, 1893–1905.

Rurangwa, E., Laranja, J.L., Van Houdt, R., Delaedt, Y., Geraylou, Z., Van De Wiele, T., Van Loo, J., Van Craeyveld, V., Courtin, C.M., Delcour, J.A., Ollevier, F., 2009. Selected non-digestible carbohydrates and prebiotics support the growth of probiotic fish bacteria mono-cultures *in vitro*. J. Appl. Microbiol. 106, 932–940.

Russo, R., Yanong, R.P.E., Mitchell, H., 2006. Dietary beta-glucans and nucleotides enhance resistance of red-tail black shark (*Epalzeorhynchos bicolor*, fam. Cyprinidae) to *Streptococcus iniae* infection. J. World Aquacult. Soc. 37, 298–306.

Sahlmann,C.,Sutherland,B.J.G.,Kortner,T.M.,Koop,B.F.,Krogdahl,Å.,Bakke,A.M.,2013.Early response of gene expression in the distal intestine of Atlantic salmon (*Salmo salar* L.) during the development of soybean meal induced enteritis. Fish Shellfish Immunol. 34, 599–609.

Sahoo, P.K., Mukherjee, S.C., 2001. Effect of dietary β-1, 3 glucan on immune responses and disease resistance of healthy and aflatoxin B1-induced immunocompromised rohu (*Labeo rohita* Hamilton). Fish Shellfish Immunol. 11, 683–695.

Sahoo, P.K., Mukherjee, S.C., 2003. Immunomodulation by dietary vitamin C in healthy and aflatoxin B1-induced immunocompromised rohu (*Labeo rohita*). Comp. Immunol. Micro. Inf. Dis. 26, 65–76.

Sahu, S., Das, B.K., Pradhan, J., Mohapatra, B.C., Mishra, B.K., Sarangi, N., 2007. Effect of *Mangifera indica* as feed additive on immunity and resistance to *Aeromonas hydrophila* in *Labeo rohita* fingerlings. Fish Shellfish Immunol. 23, 109–118.

Sakai, M., Kobayashi, M., Kawauchi, H., 1996a. *In vitro* activation of fish phagocytic cells by GH, prolactin and somatolactin. J. Endocrinol. 151, 113–118.
Sakai, M., Kobayashi, M., Kawauchi, H., 1996b. Mitogenic effects of growth hormone and prolactin on chum salmon *Oncorhynchus keta* leucocytes *in vitro*. Vet. Immunol. Immunopathol. 53, 185–189.
Sakai, M., 1999. Current research status of fish immunostimulants. Aquaculture 172, 63–92.
Sakai, M., Kamiya, H., Atusta, S., Kobayashi, M., 1991. Immunodulatory effects on rainbow trout, *Oncorhynchus mykiss*, injected with the extract of abalone, *Haliotis discus hannai*. J. Appl. Ichthyol. 7, 54–59.
Salati, F., Hamaguchi, M., Kusuda, R., 1987. Immune response of red sea bream to *Edwardsiella tarda* antigens. Fish Pathol. 22, 93–98.
Salinas, I., Díaz-Rosales, P., Cuesta, A., Meseguer, J., Chabrillón, M., Moriñigo, M.A., Esteban, M.A., 2006. Effect of heat-inactivated fish and non-fish derived probiotics on the innate immune parameters of a teleost fish (*Sparus aurata* L.). Vet. Immunol. Immunopathol. 111, 279–286.
Salminen, S., Ouwehand, A., Benno, Y., Lee, Y.-K., 1999. Probiotics: how should they be defined? Trends Food Sci. Technol. 10, 107–110.
Salyers, A.A., Whitt, D.D., 2002. Bacterial Pathogenesis: A Molecular Approach. ASM Press, Washington D.C..
Sayeda, M.A., Mohamed, I.A.W., Wafaa, T.A., 2011. Evaluation of Azotobacter and Azospirillum biofertilizers as a probiotics in *Oreochromis niloticus* aquaculture. J. Fish Aquat. Sci. 6, 535–544.
Schluter, S.F., Bernstein, R.M., Bernstein, H., Marchalonis, J.J., 1999. 'Big Bang' emergence of the combinatorial immune system. Dev. Comp. Immunol. 23, 107–111.
Seljelid, R., 1990. Immunomodulators – medicine for the 90-ies? In: Wadström, T. et al., (Ed.), Workshop on Pathogenesis of Wound and Biomaterial-Associated Infections. Aug. 30–Sep. 01, 1989. Springer Verlag, New York, pp. 107–113.
Selvaraj, V., Sampath, K., Sekar, V., 2005. Administration of yeast glucan enhances survival and some non-specific and specific immune parameters in carp (*Cyprinus carpio*) infected with *Aeromonas hydrophila*. Fish Shellfish Immunol. 19, 293–306.
Shan, S., Xiao, Z., Huang, W., Dou, S., 2008. Effect of photoperiod on growth, mortality and digestive enzymes in miiuy croaker larvae and juveniles. Aquaculture 281, 70–76.
Sharma, A., Deo, A.D., Riteshkumar, S.T., Chanu, T.I., Das, A., 2010. Effect of *Withania somnifera* (L. Dunal) root as feed additive on immunological parameters and disease resistance to *Aeromonas hydrophila* in *Labeo rohita* (Hamilton) fingerlings. Fish Shellfish Immunol. 29, 508–512.
Shirota, M., Aso, K., Iwabuchi, A., 1966. Studies on intestinal microflora. 1. Its constitution in healthy infants and the effect of oral administration of *L. acidophilus* strain Shirota. Nippon Saikingaku Zasshi. 21, 274–283.
Sirard, J.C., Bayardo, M., Didierlaurent, A., 2006. Pathogen-specific TLR signaling in mucosa: mutual contribution of microbial TLR agonists and virulence factors. Eur. J. Immunol. 36, 260–263.
Siwicki, A.K., 1989. Immunostimulating influence of levamisole on non-specific immunity in carp (*Cyprinus carpio*). Dev. Comp. Immunol. 13, 87–91.
Siwicki, A.K., Anderson, D.P., Rumsey, G.L., 1994. Dietary intake of immunostimulants by rainbow trout affects non-specific immunity and protection against furunculosis. Vet. Immunol. Immunopathol. 41, 125–139.
Siwicki, A.K., Zakes, Z., Terech-Majewska, E., Kazun, K., Lepa, A., et al.,2010. Dietary macrogard reduces *Aeromonas hydrophila* mortality in tench (*Tinca tinca*) through the activation of cellular and humoral defence mechanisms. Rev. Fish. Biol. Fish. 20, 435–439.

Smiricky-Tjardes, M., Grieshop, C., Flickinger, E., Bauer, L., Fahey, Jr., G., 2003. Dietary galactooligosaccharides affect ileal and total-tract nutrient digestibility, ileal and fecal bacterial concentrations, and ileal fermentative characteristics of growing pigs. J. Anim. Sci. 81, 2535–2545.

Smiricky-Tjardes, M.R., Flickinger, E.A., Grieshop, C.M., Bauer, L.L., Murphy, M.R., Fahey, Jr., G.C., 2003b. *In vitro* fermentation characteristics of selected oligosaccharides by swine fecal microflora. J. Anim. Sci. 81, 2505–2514.

Soleimani, N., Hoseinifar, S.H., Merrifield, D.L., Barati, M., Abadi, Z.H., 2012. Dietary supplementation of fructooligosaccharide (FOS) improves the innate immune response, stress resistance, digestive enzyme activities and growth performance of Caspian roach (*Rutilus rutilus*) fry. Fish Shellfish Immunol. 32, 316–321.

Song, S.K., Beck, B.R., Kim, D., Park, J., Kim, J., Kim, H.D., Ringø, E., 2014. Prebiotics as immunostimulants in aquaculture: a review. Fish Shellfish Immunol. 40, 40–48.

Spanggaard, B., Huber, I., Nielsen, J., Sick, E.B., Pipper, C.B., Martinussen, T., Slierendrecht, W.J., Gram, L., 2001. The probiotic potential against vibriosis of the indigenous microflora of rainbow trout. Environ. Microbiol. 3, 755–765.

Sperti, G.S., 1971. Probiotics. Avi Publishing, West Point, MS.

Standen, B.T., Rawling, M.D., Davies, S.J., Castex, M., Foey, A., Gioacchini, G., et al.,2012. Probiotic *Pediococcus acidilactici* modulates both localised intestinal- and peripheral-immunity in tilapia (*Oreochromis niloticus*). Fish Shellfish Immunol. 35, 1097–1104.

Stanier, R.Y., Doudoroff, M., Adelberg, E.A., 1963. The Microbial World. Prentice-Hall Inc, Englewood Cliffs, NJ.

Stanley, D., Denman, S.E., Hughes, R.J., Geier, M.S., Crowley, T.M., Chen, H., Haring, V.R., Moore, R.J., 2012. Intestinal microbiota associated with differential feed conversion efficiency in chickens. Appl. Microbiol. Biotechnol. 96, 1361–1369.

Stanton, C., Ross, R.P., Fitzgerald, G.F., Van Sinderen, D., 2005. Fermented functional foods based on probiotics and their biogenic metabolites. Curr. Opin. Biotechnol. 16, 198–203.

Strand, H.K., Dalmo, R.A., 1997. Absorption of immunomodulating β(1,3)-glucan in yolk sac larvae of Atlantic halibut, *Hippoglossus hippoglossus* (L.). J. Fish Dis. 20, 41–49.

Suchner, U., Kuhn, K.S., Fürst, P., 2000. The scientific basis of immunonutrition. Proc. Nutr. Soc. 59, 553–563.

Suguna, P., Binuramesh, C., Abirami, P., Saranya, P.V., Poornima, K., Rajeswari, V., Shenbagarathai, R., 2014. Immunostimulation by polyhydroxybutyrate hydroxyvalerate (PHB-HV) from *Bacillus thuringiensis* 1492 in *Oreochromis mossambicus*. Fish Shellfish Immunol. 36, 90–97.

Swennen, M.K., Courtin, C.M., Lindemans, G.C.J.E., Delcour, J.A., 2006. Large-scale production and characterization of wheat bran arabinoxylooligosaccharides. J. Sci. Food Agric. 86, 1722–1731.

Swennen, M.K., Courtin, C.M., Van der Bruggen, B., Vandecasteele, C., Delcour, J.A., 2005. Ultrafiltration and ethanol precipitation for isolation of arabinoxylooligosaccharides with different structures. Carbohydr. Polym. 62, 283–292.

Sun, Y.-Z., Xia, H.-Q., Yang, H.-L., Wang, Y.-L., Zou, W.-C., 2014. TLR2 signaling may play a key role in the probiotic modulation of intestinal microbiota in grouper *Epinephelus coioides*. Aquaculture 430, 1–7.

Tamai, T., Shirahata, S., Noguchi, T., Sato, N., Kimura, S., Murakami, H., 1993. Cloning and expression of flatfish *Paralichthys olivaceus* interferon cDNA. Biochem. Biophys. Acta 1174, 182–186.

Tapia-Paniagua, S.T., Díaz-Rosales, P., García de la Banda, I., Lobo, C., Clavijo, E., Balebona, M.C., Moriñigo, M.A., 2014. Modulation of certain liver fatty acids in Solea senegalensis is influenced by the dietary administration of probiotic microorganisms. Aquaculture, 424–425, 234–238.

Tapia-Paniagua, S.T., Reyes-Becerril, M., Ascencio-Valle, F., Esteban, M.A., Clavijo, E., Balebona, M.C., Moriñigo, M.A., 2011. Modulation of the intestinal microbiota and immune system of farmed *Sparus aurata* by the administration of the yeast *Debaryomyces hansenii* L2 in conjunction with inulin. J. Aquac. Res. Dev. Issue SPEC. 1, 012.

Ta'ati, R., Soltani, M., Bahmani, M., Zamini, A.A., 2011. Effects of the prebiotics Immunoster and Immunowall on growth performance of juvenile beluga (Huso huso). J. Appl. Ichthyol. 27, 796–798.

Teitelbaum, J.E., Walker, W.A., 2002. Nutritional impact of pre-and probiotics as protective gastrointestinal organisms. Ann. Rev. Nutr. 22.1, 107–138.

Tewary, A., Patra, B.C., 2008. Use of vitamin C as an immunostimulant – effect on growth, nutritional quality, and immune response of *Labeo rohita* (Ham.). Fish Physiol. Biochem. 34, 251–259.

Thacker, P.A., 2013. Alternatives to antibiotics as growth promoters for use in swine production: a review. J. Anim. Sci. Biotechnol. 4, 35.

Tissier, H. 1900. Recherchers sur la flora intestinale normale et pathologique du nourisson. Thesis. University of Paris, Paris, France.

Thompson, K.D., Cachos, A., Inglis, V., 1995. Immunomodulating effects of glucans and oxytetracycline in rainbow trout, Oncorhynchus mykiss, on serum lysozyme and protection. Shariff, M., Subasighe, R.P., Arthur, J.R. (Eds.), Diseases in Asian Aquaculture, Vol. 11, Fish health Section, Asian Fisheries Society, Manila, Philippines, pp. 433–439.

Torrecillas, S., Montero, D., Izquierdo, M., 2014. Improved health and growth of fish fed mannan oligosaccharides: potential mode of action. Fish Shellfish Immunol. 36, 525–544.

Torrecillas, S., Makol, A., Benítez-Santana, T., Caballero, M.J., Montero, D., Sweetman, J., et al.,2011. Reduced gut bacterial translocation in European sea bass (*Dicentrarchus labrax*) fed mannan oligosaccharides (MOS). Fish Shellfish Immunol. 30, 674–681.

Tzortzis, G., Vulevic, J., 2009. Galacto-oligosaccharide prebiotics. In: Charalampopoulos, D, Rastall, RA (Eds.), Prebiotics and Probiotics Science and Technology. Springer, New York, pp. 207–244.

Van Craeyveld, V., Swennen, K., Dornez, E., Van de Wiele, T., Marzorati, M., Verstraete, W., et al.,2008. Structurally different wheat-derived arabinoxylooligosaccharides have different prebiotic and fermentation properties in rats. J. Nutr. 138, 2348–2355.

Van Laere, K.M.J., Hartemink, R., Bosveld, M., Schols, H.A., Voragen, A.G.J., 2000. Fermentation of plant cell wall derived polysaccharides by intestinal bacteria. J. Agric. Food Chem. 48, 1644–1652.

Vaughan, R.B., 1965. The romantic rationalist: a study of Elie Metchnikoff. Med. Hist. 9, 201–215.

Vega-Paulino, R.J., Zúniga-Hansen, M.E., 2012. Potential application of commercial enzyme preparations for industrial production of short-chain fructooligosaccharides. J. Mol. Catal. B Enzym. 76, 44–51.

Venkateswara, A.R., 2007. Bioremediation to restore the health of aquaculture. Pond Ecosyst. Hyderabad, 1–12, 500.082.

Verschuere, L., Rombaut, G., Sorgeloos, P., Verstraete, W., 2000. Probiotic bacteria as biological control agents in aquaculture. Microbiol. Mol. Biol. Rev. 64, 655–671.

Vijayabaskar, P., Somasundaram, S.T., 2008. Isolation of bacteriocin producing lactic acid bacteria from fish gut and probiotic activity against common fresh water fish pathogen *Aeromonas hydrophila*. Biotechnology 7, 124–128.

Villegas, J.G., Fukada, H., Masumoto, T., Hosokawa, H., 2006. Effect of dietary immunostimulants on some innate immune responses and disease resistance against *Edwardsiella tarda* infection in Japanese flounder (*Paralichthys olivaceus*). Aquacult. Sci. 54, 153–162.

Vine, N.G., Leukes, W.D., Kaiser, H., Daya, S., Baxter, J., Hecht, T., 2004. Competition for attachment of aquaculture candidate probiotic and pathogenic bacteria on fish intestinal mucus. J. Fish Dis. 27, 319–326.

Vlková, E., Kalous, L., Bunešová, V., Rylková, K., Světlíková, R., Rada, V., 2012. Occurrence of bifidobacteria and lactobacilli in digestive tract of some freshwater fishes. Biologia 67 (2), 411–416.

Vollstad, D., Bøgwald, J., Gaserød, O., Dalmo, R.A., 2006. Influence of high-M alginate on the growth and survival of Atlantic cod (*Gadus morhua* L.) and spotted wolffish (*Anarhichas minor* Olafsen) fry. Fish Shellfish Immunol. 20, 548–561.

Volman, J.J., Ramakers, J.D., Plat, J., 2008. Dietary modulation of immune function by β-glucans. Physiol. Behav. 94, 276–284.

Watson, R.R., 1998. Vitamin E and the immune system. In: Peter, J.D. (Ed.), Encyclopedia of Immunology. Elsevier, Oxford, pp. 2500–2501.

Whittington, R., Lim, C., Klesius, P.H., 2005. Effect of dietary β-glucan levels on the growth response and efficacy of *Streptococcus iniae* vaccine in Nile tilapia, *Oreochromis niloticus*. Aquaculture 248, 217–225.

Wise, D.J., Tomasso, J.R., Gatlin, III, D.M., Bai, S.C., Blazer, V.S., 1993. Effects of dietary selenium and vitamin E on red blood cell peroxidation, glutathione peroxidase activity, and macrophage superoxideanion production in channel catfish. J. Aquat. Anim. Health 5, 177–182.

Won, K.M., Kim, P.K., Lee, S.H., Park, S.I., 2008. Effect of the residuum extract of Siberian ginseng *Eleutherococcus senticosus* on non-specific immunity in olive flounder *Paralichthys olivaceus*. Fish. Sci. 74, 635–641.

Yadav, M., Schorey, J.S., 2002. The β-glucan receptor dectin-1 functions together with TLR2 to mediate macrophage activation by mycobacteria. Blood 108, 3168e75.

Yang, S.T., Silva, E.M., 1995. Novel products and new technologies for use of a familiar carbohydrate, milk lactose. J. Dairy Sci. 78, 2541–2562.

Yakult, 1998. Central Institute for Microbiological Research, Lactobacillus Cases Strain Shirota. Yakult Honsha Co. Ltd, Tokyo, Japan.

Ye, J.D., Wang, K., Li, F.D., Sun, Y.Z., 2011. Single or combined effects of fructo- and mannan oligosaccharide supplements and *Bacillus clausii* on the growth, feed utilization, body composition, digestive enzyme activity, innate immune response and lipid metabolism of Japanese flounder *Paralichthys olivaceus*. Aquacult. Nutr. 17, e902–e911.

Yin, G., Ardo, L., Jeney, Z., Xu, P., Jeney, G., 2008. Chinese herbs (*Lonicera japonica* and *Ganoderma lucidum*) enhance non-specific immune response of tilapia, *Oreochromis niloticus*, and protection against *Aeromonas hydrophila*. In: Bondad-Reantaso, M.G., Mohan, C.V., Crumlish, M., Subasinghe, R.P. (Eds.), Diseases in Asian Aquaculture VI. Fish Health Section, Asian Fisheries Society, Manila, Philippines, pp. 269–282.

Yin, G., Jency, G., Racz, T., Xu, P., Jun, X., Jency, Z., 2006. Effect of two Chinese herbs (*Astragalus radix* and *Scutellaria radix*) on non specific immune response of tilapia, *Oreochromis niloticus*. Aquaculture 253, 39–47.

Yousefian, M., Amiri, M.S., 2009. A review of the use of prebiotic in aquaculture for fish and shrimp. Afr. J. Biotechnol. 8, 7313–7318.

Zapata, A., Lara-Flores, M., 2013. Antimicrobial activities of lactic acid bacteria strains isolated from Nile tilapia intestine (*Oreochromis niloticus*). J. Biol. Life Sci. 4, 164–171.

Zekovic, D.B., Kwiatowski, S., 2005. Natural and modified (1->3)-beta-D-glucans in health promotion and disease alleviation. Crit. Rev. Biotechnol. 25, 205–230.

Zhang, Y.A., Salinas, I., Li, J., Parra, D., Bjork, S., Xu, Z., et al.,2010. IgT, a primitive immunoglobulin class specialized in mucosal immunity. Nat. Immunol. 11, 827–835.

Zhou, Q.-C., Buentello, J.A., Gatlin, D.M., 2010. Effects of dietary prebiotics on growth performance, immune response and intestinal morphology of red drum (*Sciaenops ocellatus*). Aquaculture 309, 253–257.

Zhu, H., Liu, H., Yan, J., Wang, R., Liu, L., 2012. Effect of yeast polysaccharide on some hematologic parameter and gut morphology in channel catfish (*Ictalurus punctatus*). Fish Physiol. Biochem. 38, 1441–1447.

Zivkovic, R., 1999. Probiotics of microbes against microbes. Acta Med. Croatica 53, 23–28.

The fish microbiome and its interactions with mucosal tissues

10

Daniel L. Merrifield; Ana Rodiles
School of Biological Sciences, Plymouth University, Plymouth, United Kingdom

Chapter Outline

10.1 Introduction

The earliest studies of the microbial communities associated with fish date back to the late 1920s (Harrison, 1929; Reed and Spence, 1929). Since these pioneering investigations, much research effort has been dedicated to describing the microbial communities present on, and in, teleost fish. These communities have historically been termed, collectively, as the "microflora" or "microbiota" but more recently the term "microbiome" has emerged. The skin, gills, and gastrointestinal (GI) tract are recognized as the major pathways for pathogen entry in fish (Wilson and Laurent, 2002; Ringø et al., 2007; Bøgwald and Dalmo, 2014), and as such, the majority of studies have focused on the microbial communities associated with these regions (with a bias towards the GI tract), as well as the microbial communities associated with fish eggs. Early studies utilized a variety of culture media to enumerate bacterial levels and used phenotypic and biochemical characteristics for identification of isolates. The limitations of such approaches have become apparent in the last two decades with the realization that the majority of the community components are largely uncultivable using laboratory protocols (see Figure 10.1 for examples of the cultivability of GI microbes). Latterly, studies adopted 16S rRNA sequencing as the gold standard for isolate identification and used the variability in the 16S rRNA to characterize the composition of total bacterial (and archaeal, to a far lesser extent) communities via culture-independent means.

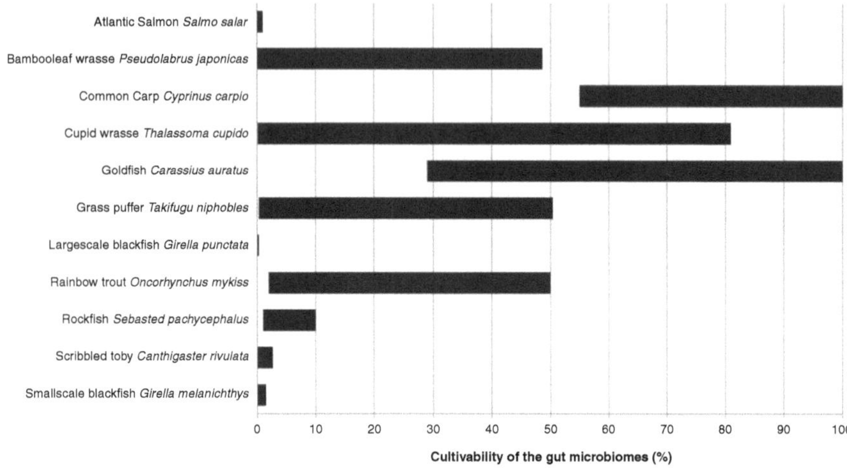

Figure 10.1 Reported cultivability of the gut microbiomes of fish species. Readers with an interest are referred to the review of Zhou et al. (2014), which provides details of the original studies and the culture conditions used.

The communities present on the skin, gills, and in the GI tract are key components of the host mucosal barrier defenses (as described in the earlier chapters of this book). Through competition for adhesion sites and nutrients they may limit or reduce the abundance of pathogens. They may also antagonize pathogens via the production of various compounds such as organic acids, siderophores, bacteriocins, H_2O_2, and various antimicrobial peptides. Despite this, these communities contain opportunistic pathogens that can infect the host as secondary pathogens or infect immunocompromized hosts, and may also contain low levels of primary pathogens, which are suppressed under normal conditions, by the antagonistic actions of the commensal/symbiotic microbes and the host's localized immunity. Clearly the presence of such communities in intimate contact with the host can influence the development and functionality of the host mucosa. Beyond the mechanisms of pathogen adhesion, and the subsequent mucosal inflammatory responses and possible mucosal translocation, very little is known of the complicated process of cross-talk between the fish host and its microbiome. Much of our understanding of this relationship is inferred from mammals, and to a lesser extent derived from a small number of germ-free and gnotobiotic studies in fish. This chapter presents a review of our knowledge on fish (Teleostei) microbiomes in terms of composition and function, and their relationship with the host mucosa.

10.2 Ontology of the fish microbiome

The glycoproteinaceous nature of the fish chorion is well suited for bacterial adhesion and colonization (Hansen and Olafsen, 1999). The microbial community present on the embryo, or the eggs prior to fertilization, is termed the "epibiota." The surrounding water typically harbors rich microbial communities that either come into contact with eggs/embryos inadvertently due to fluidic movements or via microbial chemotactic actions. Fish embryos secrete low molecular weight organic compounds across the chorion, which can establish a gradient, particularly in static aqueous environments, which may attract microbes capable of utilizing the secreted compounds. A number of studies have investigated the communities associated with eggs and embryos, but these have typically focused on characterizing potential pathogens, rather than elucidating the identity of the commensal or mutualistic communities.

Such pathogens in early developmental stages include members of the Vibrionaceae, *Flexibacter ovolyticus*, *Flavobacterium columnare*, *Pseudoalteromonas piscicida*, and *Saprolegnia* species, as described in detail elsewhere (for reviews see Olafsen, 2001; Hansen and Olafsen, 1999). Some pathogens, such as *Flexibacter ovolyticus*, may dissolve the chorion and zona radiata via enzymatic means. Microbial overgrowth by other species (e.g., *Saprolegnia*) can cause mortalities by hypoxia. Although the adaptive immune system is not functional at this stage, fish embryos are not defenseless against pathogens. Immunoglobulins, lectins, and lysozyme have been identified in fish eggs, and subsequently egg extracts exhibit bactericidal activity (Hansen and Olafsen, 1999). The epibiota itself will contain mutualistic and commensal species, which are also likely to provide a barrier function, via competition and antagonism against potential pathogens. Comprehensive information is not available on the microbial communities associated with fish eggs and embryos, but a recent study used various molecular methods to undertake a meta-taxonomic analysis of Atlantic salmon *Salmo salar* eyed eggs (i.e., embryos) (Liu et al., 2014). This study revealed highly diverse fungal, oomycete, and bacterial communities, and the presence of three archaeal operational taxonomic units (OTUs). The fungal communities of healthy eggs were dominated by *Ascomycota* which in turn was dominated by *Microdochium*, but *Spirosphaera* and *Saccharicola* were also present. Although *Microdochium* were also dominant in diseased (saprolegniosis) eggs, significant differences in the community were detected: reads assigned to the *Microdochium* and *Mortierella* genera were more abundant in diseased samples, and *Chytriomyces* reads were unique to the diseased egg samples. A total 31,278 bacterial OTUs were identified, *Proteobacteria* comprised 44% of the reads, 9% belonged to the *Bacteroidetes*, 12% to the *Actinobacteria*, and 24% belonged to the *Firmicutes*. A number of OTUs belonging to the *Actinobacteria*, that is, *Streptomycetaceae*, *Microbacteriaceae*, and *Micrococcaceae*, were exclusively present in healthy samples. *Oomycete* communities consisted of *Saprolegnia*, *Achlya*, and *Aphanomyces*; *Saprolegnia* reads were recorded from all egg samples and accounted for $\geq 50\%$ of the *Oomycete* clones in both diseased and healthy samples. This study demonstrated a correlation in the occurrence of saprolegniosis and the abundance of specific bacterial communities; a high richness and abundance of commensal *Actinobacteria* reduced the incidence of saprolegniosis, demonstrating epibiota barrier function, and *in vivo* assays revealed that the genus *Frondihabitans* (Family *Microbacteriaceae*) inhibited *Saprolegnia* attachment to salmon eggs.

Given the likely physical contact of larvae with the external surfaces of the egg during hatching, and the close proximity after hatching, the epibiota may later participate the colonization of the larvae along with microbial communities present in the water column and those associated with first feeds (Llewellyn et al., 2014). Furthermore, larvae may ingest egg debris and therefore influence the GI microbial community (Olafsen, 2001).

10.3 Microbiota associated with the skin

Research on the microbiota associated with the skin of fish species dates back to the 1920s. This early research was conducted to determine the role of microbes in fish spoilage and as such microbial counts, and identification of isolates, were carried out on skin epidermal samples, fish muscle, and epidermal "slime" (i.e., mucus) (Harrison, 1929; Reed and Spence, 1929; Stewart, 1932).

The mucous layer of the epithelium provides a mechanical and chemical protective barrier against external environments and pathogenic organisms. As such, the epidermal mucus contains immunoglobulins, defensins, lysozyme, lectin-like agglutinins, and a variety of antimicrobial peptides that provides a broad spectrum of antimicrobial activity. In addition, due to its viscous nature mucus can bind and trap microbes and the high mucus secretion rates can effectively remove microbes from the epidermal surfaces.

However, the mucous coat may also be an adhesion site for microbial species and many species are well adapted to evading or resisting the immunological components of fish mucus (Ringø and Holzapfel, 2000). Epidermal mucus components can be metabolized by some mucous-dwelling microbes in a mutualistic relationship between the fish and cutaneous microbiota. Indeed, part of the multifunctionality of the epidermal mucus is due to its microbial content (Sar and Rosenberg, 1987); it has been demonstrated that the skin microbiota can interfere with pathogen colonization (Olsson et al., 1992; Ringø and Olsen, 1999; Olafsen, 2001) by antagonistic activity and competition for adhesion sites and/or nutrients (Balcazar et al., 2007; Pérez-Sánchez et al., 2011a).

Accurate determination of the abundance of microbes on the skin of fish is challenging. First, it is difficult to avoid contamination of the epidermal tissues during the capture and handling of the fish when conducting sampling. Second, a major issue is the standardization of the precise sampling site on the skin; the precise epidermal location is not always described in research papers and it is not unreasonable, given the observations in mammals, to speculate that there may be variations in the microbial communities present on different locations of the body surface. Third, defining microbial abundance per unit is not straightforward and a consistent method of standardization has not been implemented universally, which makes comparisons across experiments difficult. Some studies have presented abundance per surface area of skin (either by taking skin scrapes or sampling epidermal tissue), some studies have reported counts on the basis of weight (either of skin or mucus) and other studies have washed mucus from the whole surface of the fish (i.e., submergence of whole fish in a known volume of diluent and used agitation to remove the mucus from the epidermal surfaces). For the determination of relative abundance of microbial community components, where determination of absolute abundance is not the objective, surface swabs have been used. It is therefore very difficult to compare quantitative data across studies, fish species, and body regions, but comparisons made on a CFU per gram basis reveal that microbial abundance on the skin is typically several orders of magnitude lower than that of the GI tract.

The abundance of aerobes exceeds that of anaerobes. The aerobic heterotrophic bacterial populations on the surface of fish are usually of a similar order of magnitude to the surrounding water (Shewan, 1961; Skjermo and Vadstein, 1993; Nedoluha and Westhoff, 1997), but the composition of the skin microbiota of healthy fish is different to that of the rearing water; the microbial richness can be higher in fish cutaneous mucus, as reported for whiting *Merlangius merlangus* and Atlantic salmon (Smith et al., 2007; Landeira-Dabarca et al., 2013). Typically the bacterial populations on fish skin are in the range of 10^2 to 10^4 CFU cm^{-2} (as reviewed by Austin, 2002). Levels in this range have been reported for Atlantic salmon (Horsley, 1973; Landeira-Dabarca et al., 2013), striped bass *Morone saxatilis* (Nedoluha and Westhoff, 1995, 1997), gray mullet *Mugil cephalus*, sand whiting *Sillago ciliato*, flathead *Platycephalus fiscus* (Gillespie and Macrae, 1975), brown trout *Salmo trutta*, pike *Esox lucius*, and rainbow trout *Oncorhynchus mykiss* (Gonzalez et al., 1999). When standardized by weight, aerobic heterotrophic bacterial levels of 10^1–10^7 CFU/g have been reported on rainbow trout skin (Diler et al., 2000) and 10^3 CFU/g reported on Atlantic mackerel *Scomber scombrus* skin (Svanevik and Lunestad, 2011).

Several groups of microorganisms are typically reported to be components of fish skin microbiome, even though the fish hosts live in diverse environments (Gram and Ringø, 2005; Figure 10.2); these include *Proteobacteria* (*Pseudomonadales*, *Enterobacteriales*, *Aeromonadales*, *Burkholderiales*, *Vibrionales*, *Rhizobiales*, *Rhodospirillales*, *Alteromonadales*, *Rickettsiales*, *Caulobacterales*, *Xanthomonadales*, *Neisseriales*, *Sphingomonadales*), *Actinobacteria* (*Actinomycetales*), *Firmicutes* (*Bacillales*, *Lactobacillales*, *Clostridiales*) and *Bacteriodetes* (*Bacteriodales*, *Flavobacteriales*, *Cytophagales*, *Sphingobacteriales*). Gram and Ringø (2005) suggested that the skin microbiome of warm water species may contain higher abundances of *Bacillus*, *Micrococcus*, and *Enterobacteriaceae*. Similarities in the adherent actinomycetal community between the skin of different hosts have been reported that suggests that these may be common fish skin microbes (Wang et al., 2010). *Proteobacteria* (dominated by the *Gammaproteobacteria*) is often the most abundant phyla reported on the skin of marine fish (Larsen et al., 2013). These generalizations may not be true for all fish species and are largely based on reports of cultivable bacterial species.

The majority of information available on the skin microbiota of fish pertains to the bacterial components; however, some information is available for *Fungi*. Fungal levels on the skin of Atlantic salmon have been observed at 10^2–10^3 CFU/ml, accounting for 2.3% of the cultivable aerobic heterotrophic microbial load, with bacteria comprising the remaining 97.7% (Landeira-Dabarca et al., 2013). Yeast have been identified as a minor component of the striped bass skin microbiota (Nedoluha and Westhoff, 1997) and have also been detected on the skin of gibel carp *Carassius auratus gibelio* and bluntnose black bream *Megalobrama amblycephala* (Wang et al., 2010). Using PCR-DGGE the relative abundance of fungal OTUs on the skin of gibel carp belonging to the *Ascomycota* was 57%, 19% were *Basidiomycota*, 9% were *Haplosporidia*, 3%

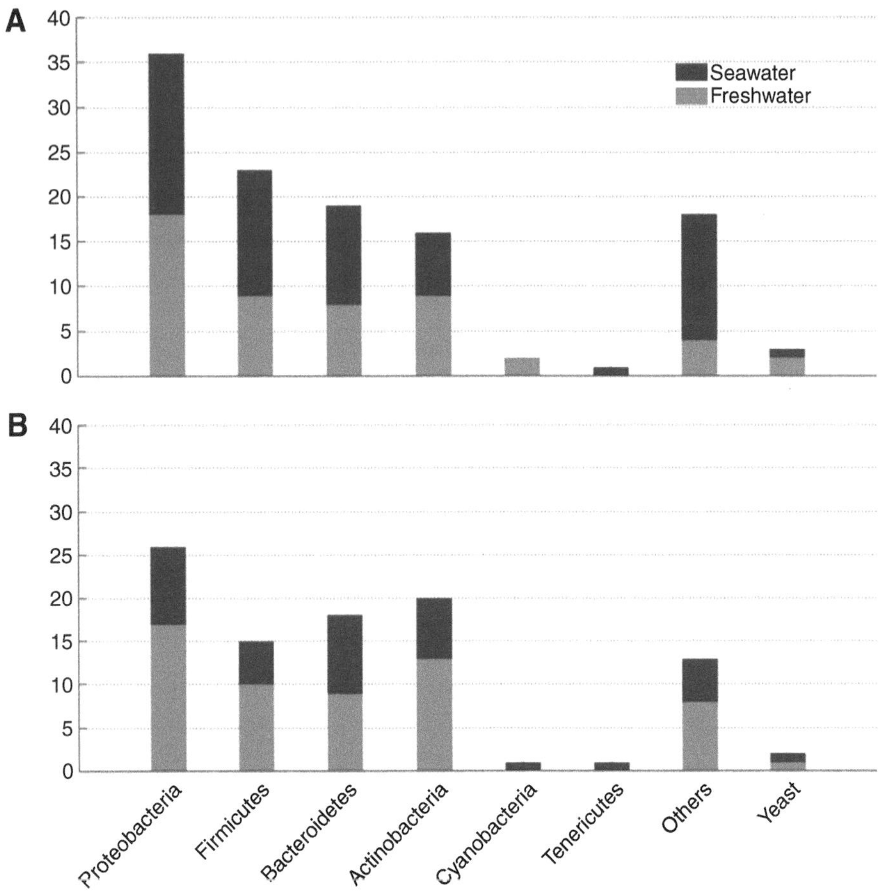

Figure 10.2 The number of studies which have reported the presence of bacterial and yeast phyla on the (A) skin and (B) gills of fresh and marine water fish species. A total of 36 research articles from skin and 26 research articles from gills are represented.

were *Choanozoa*, 5% were *Magnoliophyta*, and 7% were unidentified *Fungi* (Wang et al., 2010). On the skin of bluntnose black bream 87% of the fungal OTUs were identified as *Ascomycota*, 2% were *Basidiomycota*, 2% were *Haplosporidia*, and 9% were *Magnoliophyta*.

A number of factors have been reported to affect the skin microbiome composition or abundance (Table 10.1). For example, significant differences of epidermal mucous bacterial levels have been observed between unfed Atlantic salmon, Atlantic salmon fed a commercial diet, Atlantic salmon fed a diet of macroinvertebrates, and Atlantic salmon fed a diet containing antibiotics (Landeira-Dabarca et al., 2013). Fungal levels were also affected by diet and starvation in this study. It is perhaps not surprising that the skin microbial communities can be affected by diet since it is well known that the diet can influence the composition, volume, and turnover levels of fish epidermal

Table 10.1 Overview of factors reported to influence the composition of the microbiomes of fish

Factors		Details	Microbiome region
Dietary factors	Dietary form	Pelleted *vs.* natural diet	GI, skin
	Trophic level		GI
	Food deprivation	Fed *vs.* unfed fish	GI, skin
	Dietary lipid	Lipid levels, lipid sources	GI
	Protein sources	Plant derived proteins, yeast protein concentrates, insect meals	GI
	Carbohydrates	Plant-derived carbohydrates, chitin	GI
	Feed additives	Probiotics	GI
		Prebiotics	GI
		Antibiotics/disinfectants	Eggs, GI, skin
		Phytobiotics	GI
		Immunostimulants	GI
Environmental factors	Water salinity		GI
	Water quality		Eggs, skin, GI, gills
	Toxicants	Metal nanoparticles, heavy metals	GI
	Seasonality		GI, gills
	Temperature		GI
	Wild *vs.* farmed fish		GI
Other	Genetics	Different fish families within a species, transgenic individuals	GI, gills, skin
	Hierarchy/stress	Dominant *vs.* subordinant individuals	GI
	Stocking density		GI

Adapted from Romero et al. (2014).

mucus (Church et al., 2009; Esteban, 2012). The differences in fungal community composition observed between fish species, such as the comparison between blunt-nose black bream and gibel carp reared in the same ponds (Wang et al., 2010), is indicative of a host selective pressure that shapes the skin microbiome.

It is hoped that our knowledge of the skin microbiome will expand in the coming years with the application of quantitative culture independent techniques. Recently the first metagenomics study using next generation sequencing (NGS) of the fish skin microbiome was conducted on the Western mosquitofish *Gambusia affinis* (Leonard et al., 2014). The authors isolated the skin microbial community by vortexing whole fish in PBS containing Tween® 20. The authors reported that this sampling process was sufficient to account for 99.9% of the cultivable community, but unfortunately no validation information was presented with respect to the noncultivable community. Nonetheless, useful data was presented via the construction of comprehensive 16S rRNA libraries; reads assigned to the *Gammaproteobacteria* were the most abundant (accounting for 30% of the reads), followed by *Betaproteobacteria* (25%), *Sphingobacteria* (16%), *Clostridia* (10%), *Alphaproteobacteria* (8%), and *Flavobacteria* (6%). At the genus level, most reads were unidentified (31%), followed by *Acinetobacter* (17%), *Sphingomonas* (16%), *Acidovorax* (9%), *Enhydrobacter* (7%), *Aquabacterium* (7%), and *Myroides* (4%). These values should be interpreted with caution; a direct correlation of reads with cellular abundance cannot be made easily since bacterial cells often contain multiple copies of the 16S rRNA gene, and members of the *Proteobacteria* typically contain high numbers of 16S rRNA copies.

10.4 Microbiota associated with the gills

There remains a paucity of comprehensive information on the microbial communities associated with fish gills but investigations on both marine and freshwater fishes have demonstrated that the gills support high populations of a wide range of bacterial genera (Trust, 1975; Horsley, 1977; Nieto et al., 1984; Mudarris and Austin, 1988; Nedoluha and Westhoff, 1995; Ringø and Holzapfel, 2000). Moreover, the presence of a nonpathogenic microbiota with antibacterial properties on the mucosal surface of the gills has been reported (Ringø and Holzapfel, 2000; Kanno et al., 1989; Svendsen et al., 1999). It has been suggested however, that due to the continuous water current passing over the gills, that this organ represents a difficult habitat for microbes and that microbial colonization is restricted to protected areas, such as clefts between pharyngeal arches and lamellae (Mudarris and Austin, 1988). Nevertheless, the cultivable microbial communities on the gills are typically of the same order or higher than those present on the skin, and of the same order or lower than those reported in the GI tract. Bacterial populations up to 10^6 CFU/g of gill tissue have been reported (Trust, 1975); with aerobic bacterial levels in the range of 10^3–10^6 CFU/g of gill filaments reported for Atlantic salmon, turbot *Scophthalmus maximus*, striped bass, Nile tilapia *Oreochromis niloticus*, brown trout, pike, Atlantic mackerel, and rainbow trout.

Several studies have reported that the microbiota diversity of fish gills is lower than that of fish skin (Mudarris and Austin, 1988; Horsley, 1973; Kapetanovic et al., 2006; Wang et al., 2010). Culture-based studies have demonstrated that the main microbial components of the gills of Atlantic salmon, rainbow trout, turbot, striped bass, and Nile tilapia were similar to the surrounding water (Horsley, 1977; Nieto et al., 1984; Mudarris and Austin, 1988; Nedoluha and Westhoff, 1997; Al-Harbi and Uddin, 2005). The bacterial community from the gills of striped bass have been reported to be more similar to the bacterial communities of the rearing water than the intestinal bacterial community (Nedoluha and Westhoff, 1997) and the microbial community profiles of the gibel carp and bluntnose black bream are more similar to the skin communities than the rearing water communities (Wang et al., 2010).

Several groups of microorganism are typically reported to be components of the microbiomes of fish gills, even though the fish hosts live in diverse environments (Gram and Ringø, 2005; Figure 10.2); these include Proteobacteria (*Pseudomonadales*, *Enterobacteriales*, *Aeromonadales*, *Vibrionales*, *Alteromonadales*, *Rhizobiales*, *Burkholderiales*, *Pasteurellales*, *Caulobacterales*, *Xanthomonadales*), Actinobacteria (*Actinomycetales*), Firmicutes (*Bacillales*, *Lactobacillales*, *Erysipelotrichales*), and Bacteroidetes (*Flavobacteriales*, *Bacteriodales*).

Fungi have been identified on the gills of gibel carp, bluntnose black bream, striped bass, rainbow trout, stone flounder *Kareius bicoloratus*, and turbot (Nedoluha and Westhoff, 1997; Gram and Ringø, 2005; Spanggaard et al., 2001). The fungal OTUs on the gills of gibel carp were identified as *Ascomycota* (accounting for 71% of the relative abundance as determined by the their DGGE band intensities relative to the intensities of all DGGE bands), *Basidiomycota* (8%), *Haplosporidia* (8%), *Magnoliophyta* (9%), and 3% of the fungal OTUs could not be identified (Wang et al., 2010). On the gills of bluntnose black bream, 42% of the fungal relative abundance was attributed to the *Ascomycota*, 6% were *Basidiomycota*, 15% were *Haplosporidia*, 29% were *Magnoliophyta*, and 8% could not be identified (Wang et al., 2010). A comparison of the fungal gill microbiota of bluntnose black bream and gibel carp reared in the same ponds revealed differences in community composition, particularly evident in the abundance of the *Ascomycota*, which indicates a host selective pressure that can influence the composition of the gill microbiome (Wang et al., 2010).

Cahill (1990) suggested that stress factors including poor water quality, temperature changes, nutritional deficiencies, overcrowding, trauma, parasitism, or primary viral infections could affect the microbiota of the gills and skin. Supporting evidence has since emerged which demonstrate that seasonality (Al-Harbi and Uddin, 2007) and poor water quality (Masouleh et al., 2006) are factors that influence the gill microbiota (Table 10.1).

10.5 The gut microbiomes of fish

The gut microbiomes of fish are well studied in comparison to the communities present on fish eggs, skin, and gills; however, they remain only partly described and their influence on the host remains poorly understood. Since the early studies on the gut microbiota of fish, over half a century ago, the sophistication and sensitivity of the methods available to study these microbial populations have increased considerably. Early studies relied on the use of media to cultivate microbes for the determination of microbial abundance and identification. However, it has become increasingly clear that such approaches are insufficient given that the microbial communities in the fish gut are inherently low in cultivability; the cultivability of communities in the intestine of many fish species can be as low as <0.1% (Figure 10.1; Zhou et al., 2014). In the last decade, therefore, culture independent approaches, typically based on the variability of the 16S rRNA gene, have become more common. Clone libraries, and more recently NGS libraries, have been used to identify the microbiota composition, fingerprinting methods such as DGGE have been used to investigated microbial community

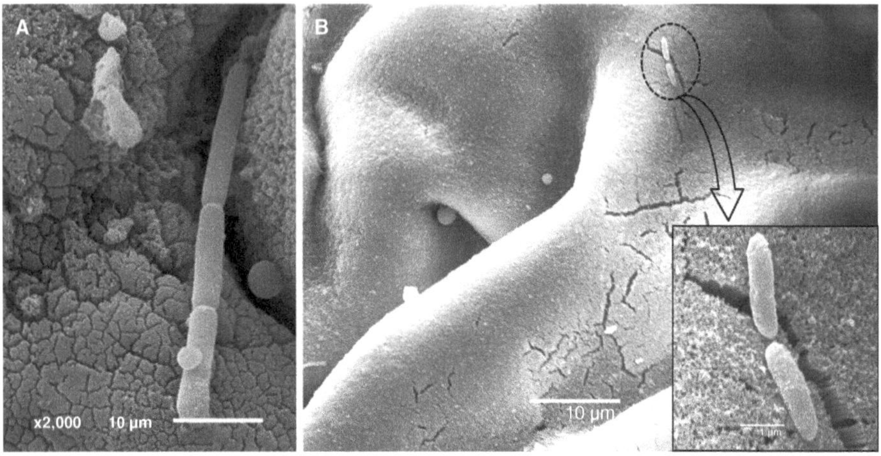

Figure 10.3 Scanning electron micrographs of the proximal intestine of Senegalese sole (*Solea senegalensis*) showing rod-shaped cells (belonging to the *Bacteria* or *Archaea*) in close association with the brush border. Scale bars: (A) and (B) = 10 μm, (B) inset = 1 μm.

structure and diversity and quantitative real-time PCR (qPCR) or fluorescent *in situ* hybridization (FISH) have been used to determine the abundance of particular taxa or total microbial levels (Zhou et al., 2014). These approaches have provided useful information on microbial composition and the factors that influence these communities.

The vertebrate gut contains a complex consortium of microbes which play critical roles in the development and health of the host at both a localized and systemic level. This community consists of viruses, protozoa, yeast and members of the *Archaea* and *Bacteria*; these microbes can be subcategorized into one of two groups, depending on their location and residence within the GI tract. One group, the allochthonous microbiota, passes through the lumen with food or digesta and are largely transient, and the other group, the autochthonous microbiota, lives in close proximity to the host on the mucosa, or in the mucus layer, and are potentially resident communities (Figure 10.3).

10.5.1 Microbial composition

Few studies have investigated the viral components of the gut microbiota of fish. It is likely however that viruses are common components of the microbiome, particularly in marine species, as the oceans are estimated to contain 10^{30} virus particles in totality (Suttle, 2007), and can contain over 10^8 particles per ml (Bergh et al., 1989). Given the abundance of bacteria present in the fish GI tract it is not unreasonable to speculate that bacteriophages may be common components of the GI microbiota. *Vibrio parahaemolyticus* bacteriophages have been isolated from digestive tracts of Mexican fish from Puerto Progreso (Bastías et al., 2010), but there remains a paucity of information on this subject. Recent observations in terrestrial vertebrates suggest that bacteriophages may influence the bacterial composition of the mammalian gut by predation (Thingstad et al., 2008; Rodriguez-Valera et al., 2009) – the so-called kill the winner hypothesis, but it remains to be seen if this also occurs in fish. The extent to which these viruses may influence the host mucosa, either directly via interactions with host cell receptors (e.g., TLRs 3, 7, 8, 9, 21, and 22), or indirectly via modulation of the bacterial communities interacting with the host mucosa, warrants further investigation.

Archaea are common components of the gut microbiota of mammals, particularly ruminants, where methanogens are symbionts that play important roles in carbohydrate fermentation (Flint et al., 2008; Pimentel et al., 2012; St-Pierre and Wright, 2013). Information on the archaeal communities associated with the fish gut is scarce, but *Archaea* have been detected in fecal or intestinal samples of European flounder *Platichthys flesus* (van der Maarel et al., 1998, 1999), gray mullet (van der Maarel et al., 1998, 1999), gilthead seabream *Sparus aurata* (Kormas et al., 2014), and grass carp *Ctenopharyngodon idella* (Ni et al., 2014; Xia et al., 2014). Although information is not available for archaeal abundance, the archaeal diversity appears considerably lower than that of the bacterial communities in the fish GI tract (Li et al., 2014; Ni et al., 2014). For example, metagenomic sequencing revealed that the grass carp microbiome contained 1112 bacterial phylotypes and only 116 *Archaea* phylotypes (Ni et al., 2014). The Archaea detected in the gut of fish thus far are members of the phyla *Euryarchaeota*, *Nanoarchaeota*, *Thaumarchaeota*, *Korarchaeota*, or are unidentified archaeal clones. In contrast however, no Archaea products were detected in two spotted red snapper *Lutjanus bohar*, whitecheek surgeonfish *Acanthurus nigricans*, daisy parrotfish *Chlorurus sordidus*, or zebra-perch sea chub *Hermosilla azurea* (Fidopiastis et al., 2006; Smriga et al., 2010) when using Archaea targeted approaches. No information is presently available on archaeal functionality or their impacts on host mucosal responses but the majority of archaeal OTUs detected in the seabream gut were anaerobic methanotrophs (Kormas et al., 2014).

Protozoa have been commonly reported in a number of fish species, some of which have been detected in the GI tract (Grim and Clemments, 1996; Grim, 2006; Grim et al., 2002; Li et al., 2009; Merrifield et al., 2011). Identification of these organisms is difficult but *Balantidium* and *Paracichlidotherus* have been reported to inhabit the intestines of several surgeonfish species (Family Acanthuridae) (Grim and Clemments, 1996; Grim et al., 2002; Grim, 2006). There remains a paucity of information on protozoan abundance in the GI tract of fish, but flagellated protozoan levels of up to 10^6 cells per gram of digesta have been reported in the hindgut of herring cale *Olisthops cyanomelas* (Clements, 1991). Further research is required to expand our knowledge on the abundance of protozoans in the fish GI tract and to elucidate their impact on the host mucosa and their possible contribution to host nutrition.

Yeasts are components of the microbiota of the fish GI tract. Typically the yeast identified from the fish GI tract belong to the *Ascomycota* or *Basidiomycota* (for reviews see Gatesoupe (2007) and Romero et al. (2014)). *Metschnikowia zobelii*, *Candida tropicalis*, and *Trichosporon cutaneum* are reportedly the dominant yeasts in some marine fish species and *Debaryomyces hansenii*, *Candida* spp., *Saccharomyces cerevisiae*, and *Leucosporidium* spp. have been reported as the dominant yeasts in the rainbow trout intestine. *Rhodotorula* (red yeast) have also been identified in the gut of a number of marine and freshwater fish, including European plaice *Pleuronectes platessa* (Andlid et al., 1995), European flounder (Andlid et al., 1995), bluefish *Pomatomus saltatrix* (Newman et al., 1972), rainbow trout (Andlid et al., 1995; Aubin et al., 2005) and various tropical-island, estuarine and coastal fish species (Roth et al., 1962; Bruce and Morris, 1973). According to Gatesoupe (2007), the common presence of yeasts in fish mucus may generally be considered as commensalism, in spite of the reported cases of pathological infections of immunocompromized fish, which are mainly due to opportunistic strains. The abundance of yeast communities is highly variable, with some studies reporting no detectable levels whilst others report levels as high as 10^7 CFU/g of intestinal content (Ohwada et al., 1980; Sakata et al., 1993). Even though the levels are often considerably lower than those reported for bacteria, due to their large size (with some exceptions, such as *Epulopiscium* spp., yeast cells in the GI tract of fish tend to be considerably larger than bacterial cells) and the fact that they are a rich source of bioactive substances (e.g., β-glucans, MOS, nucleotides, etc.), yeast are likely to be important components of the community with implications towards host mucosal function. Indeed, β-glucans and MOS are well-documented immunostimulants and prebiotics, respectively, which have been demonstrated to modulate the cytokine gene expression profiles, mucosal leucocyte populations, and/or goblet cell abundance in fish mucosal tissues (Dalmo and Bøgwald, 2008; Merrifield et al., 2010; Dimitroglou et al., 2011; Ringø et al., 2014; Chapter 8).

In terms of abundance, *Bacteria* are typically the dominant microbes present in the GI tract of fish. As such, and given the often easier methods for their study, far more information is available on these microbes than the other microbial components of the GI tract. The bacterial communities in the GI tracts of fish are diverse, comprising 100s–1000s of OTUs, and are present in levels of up to log 11 cells per gram of fecal material (Zhou et al., 2014). Although these communities are complex and are influenced by a number of factors, species from the phyla *Proteobacteria*, *Firmicutes*, *Actinobacteria*, *Bacteroidetes*, *Fusobacteria*, and *Tenericutes* are commonly reported to be amongst the most dominant members present in the GI tracts of fish species (Nayak 2010; Llewellyn et al., 2014; Romero et al., 2014). There is some information available in regards to the factors that influence these communities, their functionality, and why these communities are of importance to the host.

10.5.2 Factors affecting the gut microbiome

Studies have suggested that the microbial communities in the GI tract of fish can: (1) evolve over time, that is, they can vary across different fish sizes/life stages (Navarrete et al., 2010; Merrifield and Rodiles unpublished), (2) vary between individuals within a species (Navarrete et al., 2010; Ni et al., 2014), (3) differ within the different GI tract locations (Fidopiastis et al., 2006; Navarrete et al., 2009; Xing et al., 2013; Al-Hisnawi et al., 2014), and (4) differ with seasonality (Al-Harbi and Uddin 2004; Hagi et al., 2004; Hovda et al., 2011). A general rule of thumb, which may not be true for all species, appears to be that the GI microbiota increases in complexity and diversity with increasing host herbivory (Ward et al., 2009). A number of factors that can affect the level, stability, composition, and/or diversity of these communities have been described (refer to Table 10.1). A meta-analysis of environmental and ecological factors associated with twenty-five 16S rRNA libraries derived from the GI tracts of freshwater and marine fish species revealed that salinity and trophic level shape the composition of fish gut bacteria (Sullam et al., 2012). An in-depth discussion of these factors is beyond the scope of this chapter, but readers with an interest are referred to the review of Romero et al. (2014).

Despite the growing list of factors that have been identified as influencing the gut microbiomes of fish, a core microbiota is likely to exist. This has been demonstrated in a number of fish species. For example, in zebrafish *Danio rerio* reared at different laboratories in the United States and India, 21 OTUs from the total of 127–178 OTUs identified per cohort, were common to zebrafish at all three rearing facilities (Roeselers et al., 2011). These core components were dominated by *Proteobacteria* and to a lesser extent *Fusobacteria*. It was recently reported that rainbow trout possess a large core intestinal microbiota that may persist following alterations in diet and rearing density (Wong et al., 2014). This core community consisted of 52 bacterial lineages and was dominated by members of the class *Bacilli*, followed by members of the *Alphaproteobacteria* and *Gammaproteobacteria*. Further, the comparison of the gut microbiomes of wild and reared individuals of the same species display a great deal of similarity and common community components (Roeselers et al., 2011; Kormas et al., 2014; Rodiles, Waines, Saoud and Merrifield, unpublished date).

This core microbiota is likely to be shaped by the host selection pressures present within the GI tract, with the large differences in GI tract morphology, host genetics, rearing environment, and diet between different fish species, providing distinctive habitats that are exploited by microbes well adapted to these unique conditions. Rawls et al. (2007) demonstrated the effect of this host selection pressure by conducting fecal transplant studies between mice *Mus musculus* and zebrafish. The community composition when transplanted from the zebrafish to mice, and vice versa, clearly shifted towards a composition reflecting the community typical of the recipient host species, as opposed to remaining consistent with that of the donor.

10.5.3 Functionality of the gut microbiota

Compared to microbial composition and abundance, microbial functionality in the fish gut is poorly understood. It is however accepted that the GI microbiome plays important roles in aiding host digestion. Many early studies identified that gut microbes from fish were capable of producing various digestive enzymes that have led to the conclusion that these communities are likely to contribute to the hosts' digestive function (for review see: Ray et al., 2012). It is likely that the production of enzymes that are not produced by the host (e.g., β-glucanases, carbohydrases, cellulases, and chitinases) may be of particular importance to herbivorous and detritivorous fish species. The production of vitamins by fish gut microbes has also been reported. For example, *Cetobacterium somerae* is known to produce abundant amounts of vitamin B12 (cobalamin), and this organism is commonly present in the GI tract of a number of fish species (Tsuchiya et al., 2008). Its contribution to the vitamin B12 requirements of the host is inferred not only by the bacterium's high abundance and production of vitamin B12, but also by the fact that various fish species in which the bacterium is present in the GI tract, such as Nile tilapia and common carp *Cyprinus carpio*, have no dietary vitamin B12 requirement, whereas species in which the bacteria is not commonly present, such as channel catfish *Ictalurus punctatus* and Japanese eel *Anguilla japonica*, have a requirement for dietary vitamin B12 (Tsuchiya et al., 2008; NRC, 2011; Romero et al., 2014). Fermentation of dietary fiber by the GI microbiota leads to the production of various short-chain fatty acids (SCFAs); high acetate (along with smaller quantities of propionate and butyrate) levels have been detected in the hindgut sections of herbivorous fish species (Clements and Choat, 1995; Mountfort et al., 2002). SCFAs can be utilized directly by the enterocytes as an energy source and can also be transported across the intestine to the vascular system with turnover rates comparable to those reported in herbivorous mammals (Mountfort et al., 2002). SCFAs contribute considerably to the host energy requirements of herbivorous mammals and it is not unreasonable to speculate that this could also be the case for some herbivorous fish species. In addition, the production of SCFAs reduces intestinal pH, which can make the environment less favorable to some potential pathogens, and also increases the solubility of minerals potentially making them more easily absorbed.

The Human Microbiome Project (Human Microbiome Project Consortium, 2012) recently reported interesting findings when comparing the bacterial composition (i.e., abundance of phylogenetic groups) of the human microbiome (in multiple body sites) with the metabolic capacity of the microbiome. It was clear that although the bacterial composition varied greatly between individuals (and indeed, body sites) the metabolic pathways varied to a lesser degree, being more stable across individuals. This leads to the theory that the microbiome activity could be more important than the microbiome phylogenetic composition. Since many bacterial strains share similar metabolic capacity, or share common metabolic pathways, it may matter less which bacteria are present, and more that the bacterial functions and activities are occurring, irrespective of which bacteria are executing them. By extrapolation, this might also be the case for the nonbacterial components of the microbiome. Although this theory is rather speculative, and of course there will be some microbial species that break this rule (i.e., there may be core microbes essential for certain functions that cannot be replaced by other microbes, and the presence of pathogens is likely never desirable for the host), this theory is gaining traction in this field in mammals. Whether this is also the case in fish remains to be seen, however, a recent study in turbot provides some interesting information in the context of bacterial abundance and functional analysis using metagenomics combined with 16S rRNA gene sequence analyses (Xing et al., 2013). To the authors' knowledge, this is the first such study published on the fish microbiome, and although the study was not designed to correlate the stability of bacterial functionality in comparison to bacterial composition, interesting data were presented providing fundamental information on the functions of the microbiome in the turbot GI tract. The analyses revealed that many metabolic subsystems were dominant in the turbot GI metagenome and in comparison to other gut metagenomes (striped bass, mammals, chicken, and termites), quorum sensing and biofilm formation were abundant in the turbot GI metagenome. Additionally, iron acquisition and metabolism were more abundant in the turbot GI metagenome when compared with the striped bass gut metagenome, suggesting that differences in metabolic potential may occur in marine and freshwater fish GI microbiomes. These genes were predominantly found in species within the *Vibrio* genus, which are commonly reported to in the GI tract of marine fish species.

10.6 Microbiome–mucosa interactions

Beyond the described nutritional functions of the GI microbiota, the microbiome is also recognized as a key component of mucosal barrier function, providing competition and antagonism against pathogens (as described in the earlier chapters of this book), but the mechanisms in which this is mediated, and the importance of the community to the host mucosal development, immune response and function has only received attention in recent years. Most of the information available has focused on pathogens and pathogenesis, with only limited studies available on the cross-talk between the components of the *normal* microbiome and the fish mucosa.

Germ-free or gnotobiotic models have provided fundamental information on the relevance of these communities on vertebrate hosts, and specifically, several zebrafish studies have shed light on this in the fish context. Zebrafish larvae reared in germ-free environments, with no microbial interactions, fail to develop correctly (Bates et al., 2006; Rawls et al., 2007). The GI tract fails to differentiate properly and the intestine displays: reduced levels of enteroendocrine cells and goblet cells, a lack of brush border intestinal alkaline phosphatase (IAP) activity (an enzyme involved in mucosal tolerance due to its ability to detoxify bacterial lipopolysaccharide (LPS) endotoxins), reduced epithelial cell turnover rates, immature patterns of glycans are expressed on the enterocytes and a loss of epidermal integrity develops (Rawls et al., 2004; Bates et al., 2006). These characteristics ultimately lead to a failure of the intestine to uptake protein macromolecules. Further, 212 genes in the GI tract were regulated by the presence or absence of the microbial communities; these genes were involved in numerous processes including immunity (e.g., homologs of mammalian *Saa1*, *Crp*, *C3*, and *Socs3*), nutrition (e.g., homologs of several mammalian genes involved in lipid metabolism, *Cpt1a*, *Ctp1b*, and *Fbp1*), cell division and DNA replication (e.g., multiple mini-chromosome maintenance genes and *Pcna*) (Rawls et al., 2004). These changes in phenotype however could be reversed with the reintroduction of the microbiota at 3 or 6 days post-fertilization (Rawls et al., 2004).

Host-microbe cross-talk at the mucosal interface is a complex process that determines the nature of the subsequent host-microbe relationship. The mechanisms involved in mammals are partly described, and a number of key molecules have been identified. Some of these molecules and processes, or their analogous counterparts, have been identified in fish. Recognition of the microbe occurs by pattern recognition receptors (PRRs), of which the toll-like receptors (TLRs) have received most attention. TLRs-1, 2, 4, 5, 9, 14, and 21 are involved in the recognition of bacterial pathogen associated molecular patterns (PAMPs). TLR activation initiates a complex molecular cascade, including various adaptor molecules (Myd88 is likely to be the most important, but Mal, TRIF, TRAM, and SARM have also been identified in fish) and the transcription factor NFκB, which results in the production of pro-inflammatory cytokines (e.g. IL-1β, IL-8, and TNFα). The regulatory molecules DIGIRR and Tollip, which can act to prevent TLR signaling to avoid an excessive inflammatory response, have also been identified in fish. In the absence of pathogenic stimuli the anti-inflammatory TGF-β and IL-10 are expressed, which act to maintain mucosal tolerance. Readers are referred to Chapter 5, Foey and Picchietti (2014) for reviews of inflammatory pathways.

IgT (also known as IgZ), an immunoglobulin isotype that is analogous to IgA in mammals, is a specialized teleost mucosal antibody (Zhang et al., 2010). It is resistant to the often harsh environmental conditions associated with mucus (as is particularly the case in the GI tract) and can be secreted via PIgRs present on epithelial cells into mucus coatings (Zhang et al., 2011; Foey and Picchietti, 2014; Chapter 5). IgT has been detected in a number of teleosts and has been identified in skin mucus, gill mucus, intestinal mucus, and the pyloric caeaca. The expression of IgT mRNA in the fish intestine has been observed to increase in response to the presence of various microbes, typically in studies assessing host-probiotic and host-pathogen interactions (Pérez-Sánchez et al., 2011b; Abid et al., 2012). Little is known about its interaction with the *normal* microbiome of fish in the mucus and on the epithelial mucosa. In mammals a large component of the gut microbiome is bound to IgA and similarly this has been observed to be the case for rainbow trout gut luminal bacteria, in which nearly half of the community were IgT coated (Zhang et al., 2010). This process helps to reduce the attachment of microbes to the mucosa, thus maintaining homeostasis by limiting mucosal interactions with too many, or unfavorable, microbes; a process known as immune exclusion. The importance of this process is highlighted in humans by the fact 3–5 grams of IgA is secreted into the human GI tract each day (Conley and Delacroix, 1987).

IAP is also in important molecule involved in regulating mucosal tolerance. IAP detoxifies LPS by lipid A dephosphorylation and has been reported to prevent inflammation in the zebrafish gut (Bates et al., 2007; Lallès 2010). IAP production is induced during the establishment of the GI microbiome and zebrafish lacking IAP display a lack of intestinal neutrophils and increased sensitivity, and elevated mortality levels, when exposed to LPS (Bates et al., 2006). Bates et al. (2006) described a homeostatic feedback loop in which IAP prevents excessive TLR stimulation and therefore reduces *Tnf* expression to limit intestinal inflammation and promote tolerance to the GI microbiota.

The host-microbe cross-talk is more complicated than merely detecting the presence of microbe-associated molecular patterns (MAMPs) or microbial metabolites. For instance, exposure of germ-free reared zebrafish to heat killed bacterial preparations or bacterial LPS was not sufficient to reverse some of the characteristics of germ-free reared phenotypes (Bates et al., 2006). Using germ-free and mono-associated zebrafish, Rawls et al. (2007) investigated microbiota-zebrafish interactions and reported that *Pseudomonas aeruginosa* lacking flagella (flagella contain flagellin, MAMPs recognized by TLR5) were unable to interact with host and non-motile mutants expressing flagella showed very limited interactions. In contrast, wild-type (i.e., motile, flagella containing) *Pseudomonas aeruginosa* stimulated inflammatory signals (i.e., *Saa* and *Mpo*) in zebrafish that were not expressed in response to the mutant strains. The authors suggested that flagella-driven motility promoted interactions between the bacterium and the host mucosal epithelium, leading to the detection and monitoring of luminal and mucous antigens (including flagella) by the host. These studies indicate an active participation of bacteria which drives host responses.

Teleosts have evolved a suite of mechanisms to maintain mucosal tolerance towards commensal and symbiotic microbes whilst simultaneously maintaining responsiveness towards pathogens. These processes are partly described, and include the production of IgT, IAP, antimicrobial peptides, anti-inflammatory cytokines, and a number of regulatory molecules that act to prevent excessive inflammatory responses. This is a complex process and further research is required to improve our understanding of host-microbe interactions at the mucosal interface.

10.7 Future research

The literature available to date has focused heavily on the bacterial components of the microbiome, and predominantly those present in the GI tract. Future research efforts must focus more attention on the microbial communities present on fish eggs/embryos, and on the gills, skin, and fins. These studies must also seek to expand our knowledge of the *Archaea*, protozoa, yeasts, and viruses. We must also look beyond mere microbial abundance and embrace the approach currently being applied in mammalian microbiome research: assessment of microbial functionality. With the ever decreasing cost of reagents and sequencing platforms, and the expansion of bioinformatics tools and databases, it is expected that metagenomic and metatranscriptomic approaches will become the foundation of fish microbiome research in the coming years, and with it a wealth of knowledge on the microbiomes of fish will be revealed. The molecular mechanisms involved in the cross-talk between the fish host and its microbiome, which helps maintain homeostasis, particularly in the GI tract, must be further explored. Fundamental information on the *normal* microbiome, must also be accompanied by comprehensive applied research to reveal the extent of microbial modulation of feed additives such as probiotics and prebiotics, and their impacts on the host mucosa.

References

Abid, A., Bradley, G., Davies, S.J., Castex, M., Carnevali, O., Goacchini, G., Merrifield, D.L., 2012. Influence of Dietary *Pediococcus acidilactici* on Health and the Microbial Communities of Rainbow Trout (*Oncorhynchus mykiss* Walbaum). Society for Applied Microbiology Summer Meeting, Edinburgh, UK, 2nd–5th July.

Al-Hisnawi, A., Ringø, E., Davies, S.J., Waines, P., Bradley, G., Merrifield, D.L., 2014. First report on the autochthonous gut microbiota of brown trout (*Salmo trutta* Linnaeus). Aquacult. Res. Early View, DOI: 10.1111/are.12451.

Al-Harbi, A., Uddin, N., 2004. Seasonal variation in the intestinal bacterial flora of hybrid tilapia (*Oreochromis niloticus* × *Oreochromis aureus*) cultured in earthen ponds in Saudi Arabia. Aquaculture 229 (1–4), 37–44.

Al-Harbi, A., Uddin, N., 2005. Bacterial diversity of tilapia (*Oreochromis niloticus*) cultured in brackish water in Saudi Arabia. Aquaculture 250, 566–572.

Al-Harbi, A., Uddin, N., 2007. Seasonal trends in gill bacterial flora of hybrid tilapia, *Oreochromis niloticus* x *O. aureus*. J. Appl. Aquacult. 19 (1), 61–70.

Andlid, T., Juárez, R.V., Gustafsson, L., 1995. Yeast colonizing the intestine of rainbow trout (*Salmo gairdneri*) and turbot (*Scophtalmus maximus*). Microb. Ecol. 30, 321–334.

Aubin, J., Gatesoupe, F.J., Labbé, L., Lebrun, L., 2005. Trial of probiotics to prevent the vertebral column compression syndrome in rainbow trout (*Oncorhynchus mykiss* Walbaum). Aquac. Res. 36, 758–767.

Austin, B., 2002. The bacterial microflora of fish revised. Review article. Scient. World J. 6, 931–945.

Balcazar, J.L., Vendrell, D., De Blas, I., Ruiz-Zarzuela, I., Girones, O., Muzquiz, J.L., 2007. *In Vitro* competitive adhesion and production of antagonistic compounds by lactic acid bacteria against fish pathogens. Vet. Microbiol. 122, 373–380.

Bastías, R., Higuera, G., Sierralta, W., Espejo, R.T., 2010. A new group of cosmopolitan bacteriophages induce a carrier state in the pandemic strain of *Vibrio parahaemolyticus*. Environ. Microbiol. 12 (4), 990–1000.

Bates, J.M., Mittge, E., Kuhlman, J., Baden, K.N., Cheesman, S.E., Guillemin, K., 2006. Distinct signals from the microbiota promote different aspects of zebrafish gut differentiation. Dev. Biol. 297 (2), 374–386.

Bates, J.M., Akerlund, J., Mittge, E., Guillemin, K., 2007. Intestinal alkaline phosphatase detoxifies lipopolysaccharide and prevents inflammation in response to the gut microbiota. Cell Host Microbe 2 (6), 371–382.

Bøgwald, Dalmo, 2014. In: Merrifield, D.L., Ringø, E. (Eds.), Gastrointestinal pathogenesis in aquatic animals. Wiley, London, pp. 53–74.

Bruce, J., Morris, E.O., 1973. Psychrophilic yeasts isolated from marine fish. Antonie van Leeuwenhoek 39, 331–339.

Cahill, M.M., 1990. Bacterial flora of fishes: a review. Microb. Ecol. 19 (1), 21–41.

Church, M.R., Ebersole, J.L., Rensmeyer, K.M., Couture, R.B., Barrows, F.T., Noakes, D.L.G., 2009. Mucus: a new tissue fraction for rapid determination of fish diet switching using stable isotope analysis. Can. J. Fish. Aquat. Sci. 66, 1–5.

Clements, K.D., 1991. Endosymbiotic communities of two herbivorous labroid fishes *Odax cyanomelas* and *O. pullus*. Marine Biology 109 (2), 223–229.

Clements, K.D., Choat, J.H., 1995. Fermentation in tropical marine herbivorous fish. Physiol. Zool 68, 355–378.

Committee on the Nutrient Requirements of Fish and Shrimp; National Research Council, 2011. Nutrient requirements of fish and shrimp. National Academy Press, Washington, D.C., p. 360 ISBN 9780309163385.

Conley, M.E., Delacroix, D.L., 1987. Intravascular and mucosal immunoglobulin A: two separate but related systems of immune defense? Ann. Intern. Med. 106, 892–899.

Dalmo, R.A., Bogwald, J., 2008. B-glucans as conductors of immune symphonies. Fish Shellfish Immunol. 25 (4), 384–396.

Diler, O., Altun, S., Calikusu, F., Diler, A., 2000. A study on qualitative and quantitative bacterial flora of the rainbow trout (*Oncorhynchus mykiss*) living in different fish farms. Turk. J. Vet. Anim. Sci. 24, 251–259.

Dimitroglou, A., Merrifield, D.L., Carnevali, O., Picchietti, S., Avella, M., Daniels, C.L., Güroy, D., Davies, S.J., 2011. Microbial manipulations to improve fish health and production – a Mediterranean perspective. Fish Shellfish Immunol. 30, 1–16.

Esteban, M.A., 2012. Review article An overview of the immunological defenses in fish skin. ISRN Immunol. 853470, 29.

Fidopiastis, P.M., Bezdek, Æ.D.J., Horn, M.H., Kandel, Æ.J.S., 2006. Characterizing the resident, fermentative microbial consortium in the hindgut of the temperate-zone herbivorous fish *Hermosilla azurea* (Teleostei: Kyphosidae). Marine Biol. 148, 631–642.

Flint, H.J., Bayer, E.A., Rincon, M.T., Lamed, R., White, B.A., 2008. Polysaccharide utilization by gut bacteria: potential for new insights from genomic analysis. Nat. Rev. Microbiol. 6, 121–131, doi:10. 1038/nrmicro1817.

Gatesoupe, F.-J., 2007. Live yeasts in the gut: natural occurrence, dietary introduction, and their effects on fish health and development. Aquaculture 267 (1–4), 20–30.

Gillespie, N.C., Macrae, I.C., 1975. The bacterial flora of some Queensland fish and its ability to cause spoilage. J. Appl. Bacteriol. 39, 91–100.

Gonzalez, C.J., Lopez-Diaz, T.M., Garcia-Lopez, M.L., Prieto, M., Otero, A., 1999. Bacterial microflora of wild brown trout (*Salmo trutta*), wild pike (*Esox lucius*), and aquacultured rainbow trout (*Oncorhynchus mykiss*). J. Food Protect. 62, 1270–1277.

Gram, Ringø, 2005. Prospects of fish probiotics. In: Holzapfel, W., Naughton, P. (Eds.), Microbial ecology in growing animals. Elsevier, London, pp. 379–451.

Grim, J.N., 2006. Food vacuole contents in the ciliate, *Balantidium jocularum* (Balantididae), a symbiont in the intestine of the surgeonfish *Naso tonganus* (Acanthuridae). J. Eukaryot. Microbiol. 53 (4), 269–274.

Grim, J.N., Clemments, K.D., 1996. Description of a new species of opalinid by light-microscopy, SEM and TEM – protoopalina-polykineta, n-sp from the intestines of the surgeonfish, *Acanthurus nigrofuscus* surface-features, kinetal organization, vesicles, and endocytobionts. Eur. J. Protistol. 32 (1), 81–89, 1996.

Grim, J.N., Clements, K.D., Byfield, T., 2002. New species of *Balantidium* and *Paracichlidotherus* (Ciliophora) inhabiting the intestines of four surgeonfish species from the Tuvalu Islands, Pacific Ocean. J. Eukaryot. Microbiol. 49, 146–153.

Hagi, T., Tanaka, D., Iwamura, Y., Hoshino, T., 2004. Diversity and seasonal changes in lactic acid bacteria in the intestinal tract of cultured freshwater fish. Aquaculture 234 (1–4), 335–346.

Hansen, G.H., Olafsen, J.A., 1999. Bacterial interactions in early life stages of marine cold water fish. Microb. Ecol. 38 (1), 1–26.

Harrison, F.C., 1929. The discoloration of halibut. Can. J. Res. 1, 214–239.

Horsley, R.W., 1973. The bacterial flora of the Atlantic salmon (*Salmo salar* L.) in relation to its environment. J. Appl. Bacteriol. 36, 377–386.

Hovda, M.B., Fontanillas, Ramon, McGurk, C., Obach, A., Rosnes, J.T., 2011. Seasonal variations in the intestinal microbiota of farmed Atlantic salmon (*Salmo salar* L). Aquacult. Res. 43, 154–159.

Human Microbiome Project Consortium, 2012. Structure, function and diversity of the healthy human microbiome. Nature 486, 207–214.

Kanno, T., Nakai, T., Muroga, K., 1989. Mode of transmission of vibriosis among ayu *Plecoglossus altivelis*. J. Aqua. Anim. Health 1, 2–6.

Kapetanovic, D., Kurtovic, B., Vardic, I., Valic, D., Teskeredzic, Z., Teskeredzic, E., 2006. Preliminary studies on bacterial diversity of cultured bluefin tuna *Thunnus thynnus* from the Adriatic Sea. Aquacult. Res. 37, 1265–1266.

Kormas, K.A., Meziti, A., Mente, E., Frentzos, A., 2014. Dietary differences are reflected on the gut prokaryotic community structure of wild and commercially reared sea bream (*Sparus aurata*). MicrobiologyOpen, 3(5), 718–728.

Landeira-Dabarca, A., Sieiro, C., Alvarez, M., 2013. Change in food ingestion induces rapid shifts in the diversity of microbiota associated with cutaneous mucus of Atlantic salmon *Salmo salar*. J. Fish Biol. 82, 893–906.

Lallès, J.P., 2010. Intestinal alkaline phosphatase: multiple biological roles in maintenance of intestinal homeostasis and modulation by diet. Nutr. Rev. 68 (6), 323–332.

Leonard, A.B., Carlson, J.M., Bishoffl, D.E., Sendelbach, S.I., Yun, S.B., Ramzanali, S., Manage, A.B.W., Hyde, E.R., Petrosino, J.F., Primm, T.P., 2014. The skin microbiome of *Gambusia affinis* is defined and selective. Adv. Microbiol. 4, 335–343.

Li, M., Wang, C., Wang, J., Li, A., Gong, X., Ma, H., 2009. Redescription of *Balantidium polyvacuolum* Li 1963 (Class: Litostomatea) inhabiting the intestines of Xenocyprinae fishes in Hubei, China. Parasitol. Res. 106, 177–182.

Li, H., Zhong, Q., Wirth, S., Wang, W., Hao, Y., Wu, S., Zou, H., Li, W., Wang G. 2014. Diversity of autochthonous bacterial communities in the intestinal mucosa of grass carp (*Ctenopharyngodon idellus*) (Valenciennes) determined by culture-dependent and culture independent techniques. Aquac. Res., early view DOI: 10.1111/are.12391.

Liu, Y., de Bruijn, I., Jack, A.L.H., Drynan, K., van den Berg, A.H., Thoen, E., Sandoval-Sierra, V., Skaar, I., van West, P., Diéguez-Uribeondo, J., van der Voort, M., Mendes, R., Mazzola, M., Raaijmakers, J.M., 2014. Deciphering microbial landscapes of fish eggs to mitigate emerging diseases. ISME J., 8, 1–13.

Llewellyn, M.S., Boutin, S., Hoseinifar, S.H., Derome, N., 2014. Teleost microbiomes: the state of the art in their characterization, manipulation and importance in aquaculture and fisheries. Front. Microbiol., 5, article 207.

Masouleh, S.A.S., Sharifpour, I., Arani, A.S., 2006. The aerobic bacterial flora of hatchery reared Caspian Sea sturgeon fingerlings. J. Appl. Ichthyol. 22, 261–264.

Merrifield, D.L., Dimitroglou, A., Foey, A., Davies, S.J., Baker, R.T.M., Bogwald, J., Castex, M., Ringø, E., 2010. The current status and future focus of probiotic and prebiotic applications for salmonids. Aquaculture 302, 1–18.

Merrifield, D.L., Harper, G., Mustafa, S., Carnevali, O., Picchietti, S., Davies, S.J., 2011. Effect of dietary alginic acid on juvenile tilapia (*Oreochromis niloticus*) intestinal microbial balance, intestinal histology and growth performance. Cell Tissue Res. 344, 135–146.

Mountfort, Douglas, O., Campbell, J., Clements, Kendall, D., 2002. Hindgut fermentation in three species of marine herbivorous fish. Society 68 (3), 1374–1380.

Mudarris, M., Austin, B., 1988. Quantitative and qualitative studies of the bacterial microflora of turbot, *Scophthalmus maximus* L., gills. J. Fish Biol. 32, 223–229.

Nayak, S.K., 2010. Role of gastrointestinal microbiota in fish. Aquacult. Res. 41, 1553–1573.

Navarrete, P., Espejo, R.T., Romero, J., 2009. Molecular analysis of microbiota along the digestive tract of juvenile Atlantic salmon (*Salmo salar* L.). Microb. Ecol. 57 (3), 550–561.

Nedoluha, P.C., Westhoff, D., 1995. Microbiological analysis of Stripped bass (*Morone saxatilis*) grown in flow-through tanks. Food Protect. 58, 1363–1368.

Nedoluha, P.C., Westhoff, D., 1997. Microbiological analysis of striped bass (*Morone saxatilis*) grown in a three aquaculture system. Food Microbiol. 14, 255–264.

Newman, Jr., J.T., Cosenza, B.J., Buck, J.D., 1972. Aerobic Microflora of the bluefish (*Pomatomus saltatrix*) intestine. J. Fish. Res. Board Can. 29 (3), 333–336.

Ni, J., Yan, Q., Yu, Y., Zhang, T., 2014. Factors influencing the grass carp gut microbiome and its effect on metabolism. FEMS Microbiol. Ecol. 87 (3), 704–714.

Nieto, T.P., Toranzo, A.E., Barja, J.L., 1984. Comparison between the bacterial flora associated with fingerling rainbow trout cultured in two different hatcheries in the north-west of Spain. Aquaculture 42, 193–206.

Ohwada, K., Tabor, P.S., Colwell, R.R., 1980. Species composition and barotolerance of gut microflora of deep-sea benthic macrofauna collected at various depths in the Atlantic Ocean. Appl. Environ. Microbiol. 40, 746–755.

Olafsen, J., 2001. Interactions between fish larvae and bacteria in marine aquaculture. Aquaculture 200 (1–2), 223–247.

Olsson, J.C., Westerdahl, A., Conway, P.L., Kjelleberg, S., 1992. Intestinal colonization potential of turbot (*Scophthalmus maximus*) – and dab (*Limanda limanda*)-associated bacteria with inhibitory effects against *Vibrio anguillarum*. Appl. Environ. Microbiol. 58, 551–556.

Pérez-Sánchez, T., Balcázar, J.L., García, Y., Halaihel, N., Vendrell, D., de Blas, I., Merrifield, D.L., Ruiz-Zarzuela, I., 2011a. Identification and characterization of lactic acid bacteria isolated from rainbow trout *Oncorhynchus mykiss* (Walbaum) with inhibitory activity against *Lactococcus garvieae*. J. Fish Dis. 34, 499–507.

Pérez-Sánchez, T., Balcázar, J.L., Merrifield, D.L., Carnevali, O., Gioacchini, G., de Blas, I., Ruiz-Zarzuela, I., 2011b. Expression of immune-related genes in rainbow trout (*Oncorhynchus mykiss*) induced by probiotic bacteria during *Lactococcus garvieae* infection. Fish Shellfish Immunol. 31, 196–201.

Pimentel, M.P., Gunsalus, R.S., Rao, S.C., Zhang, H., 2012. Methanogens in human health and disease. Am. J. Gastroenterol. Suppl. 1, 28–33, doi: 10. 1038/ajgsup. 2012.6.

Rawls, J.F., Mahowald, M.A., Goodman, A.L., Trent, C.M., Gordon, J.I., 2007. *In vivo* imaging and genetic analysis link bacterial motility and symbiosis in the zebrafish gut. Proc. Natl. Acad. Sci. U.S.A. 104, 7622–7627.

Rawls, J.F., Samuel, B.S., Gordon, J.I., 2004. Gnotobiotic zebrafish reveal evolutionarily conserved responses to the gut microbiota. PNAS 101, 4596–4601.

Ray, A.K., Ghosh, K., Ringø, E., 2012. Enzyme-producing bacteria isolated from fish gut: a review. Aquacult. Nutr. 18, 465–492.

Reed, G.M., Spence, C.M., 1929. The intestinal and slime flora of the haddock: a preliminary note. Contrib. Canadian. Biol. Fish. N. S. 4, 257–264.

Ringø, E., Dimitroglou, A., Hoseinifar, S.H., Davies, S.J., 2014. Prebiotics in finfish: an update. In: Merrifield, D.L., Ringø, E. (Eds.), In: Aquaculture Nutrition: Gut Health, Probiotics and Prebiotics. Wiley, London, pp. 360–394.

Ringø, E., Holzapfel, W., 2000. Identification and characterization of carnobacteria associated with the gills of Atlantic salmon (*Salmo salar L.)*. Syst. Appl. M. 23 (4), 523–527.

Ringø, E., Olsen, R.E., 1999. The effect of diet on aerobic bacterial flora associated with intestine of Arctic charr (*Salvelinus alpinus* L.). J. Appl. Microbiol. 86, 22–28.

Roeselers, G., Mittge, E.K., Stephens, W.Z., Parichy, D.M., Cavanaugh, C.M., Guillemin, K., Rawls, J.F., 2011. Evidence for a core gut microbiota in the zebrafish. ISME J., 1–14.

Rodriguez-Valera, F., Martin-Cuadrado, A.-B., Rodriguez-Brito, B., Pa, L., Thingstad, T.F., Rohwer, F., Mira, A., 2009. Explaining microbial population genomics through phage predation. Nat. Rev. Microbiol. **7**, 828–836, doi:10.1038/nrmicro2235.

Romero, J., Ringø, E., Merrifield, D.L., 2014. The gut microbiota of fish. In: Merrifield, D.L., Ringø, E. (Eds.), In: Aquaculture Nutrition: Gut Health, Probiotics and Prebiotics. Wiley, London, pp. 75–100.

Roth, Jr., F.J., Ahearn, D.G., Fell, J.W., Meyers, S.P., Meyer, S.A., 1962. Ecology and taxonomy of yeasts isolated from various marine substrates. Limnol. Oceanogr. 7, 178–185.

Sar, N., Rosenberg, E., 1987. Fish skin bacteria – colonial and cellular hydrophobicity. Mar. Ecol. 13, 193–202.

Sakata, T., Oshiro, T., Teshima, S.I., 1993. Characteristics and fatty acid composition of yeast isolated from the intestines of rainbow trout *Oncorhynchus mykiss*. Mem. Fac. Fish. Kagoshima Univ. 42, 51–59.

Shewan, J.M., 1961. The microbiology of sea-water fish. Borgstrom, G. (Ed.), Fish as Food, vol. 1, Academic Press, New York, pp. 487–560.

Skjermo, J., Vadstein, O., 1993. The effect of microalgae on skin and gut bacterial flora of halibut larvae. In: Reinertsen, H., Dahle, L.A., Jørgensen, L., Tvinnereim, K. (Eds.), Fish Farming Technology. A.A. Ž. Balkema Publishers, Rotterdam, pp. 61–67.

Smith, C.J., Danilowicz, B.S., Meijer, W.G., 2007. Characterization of the bacterial community associated with the surface and mucus layer of whiting (*Merlangius merlangus*). FEMS Microbiol. Ecol. 62, 90–97.

Smriga, S., Sandin, S. a., Azam, F., 2010. Abundance, diversity, and activity of microbial assemblages associated with coral reef fish guts and feces. FEMS Microbiol. Ecol. 73 (1), 31–42.

Spanggaard, B., Huber, I., Nielsen, J., Sick, E.B., Pipper, C.B., Martinussen, T., Slierendrecht, W.J., Gram, L., 2001. The probiotic potential against vibriosis of the indigenous microflora of rainbow trout. Environ. Microbiol. 3 (12), 755–765.

St-Pierre, B., Wright, A.D.G., 2013. Diversity of gut methanogens in herbivorous animals. Animal 7, 49–56.

Stewart, M.M., 1932. The bacterial flora of the slime and intestinal contents of the haddock (*Gadus aeglefinus*). J. Mar. Biol. Assoc. U. K. 18, 35–50.

Sullam, K.E., Essinger, S.D., Lozupone, C.A., O'Connor, M.P., Rosen, G.L., Knight, R., Kilham, S.S., Russell, J.A., 2012. Environmental and ecological factors that shape the gut bacterial communities of fish: a meta-analysis. Mol. Ecol. 21 (13), .

Suttle, C.A., 2007. Marine viruses major players in the global ecosystem. Nat. Rev. Microbiol. 5, 801–812.

Svanevik, C.S., Lunestad, B.T., 2011. Characterisation of the microbiota of Atlantic mackerel (*Scomber scombrus*). Int. J. Food Microbiol. 151, 164–170.

Thingstad, T.F., Bratbak, G., Heldal, M., 2008. Aquatic phage ecology. In: Abedon, S.T. (Ed.), Bacteriophage Ecology. Cambridge University Press, Cambridge, pp. 251–280.

Trust, T.J., 1975. Bacteria associated with the gills of salmonid fishes in freshwater. J. Appl. Bacteriol. 38, 225–233.

Tsuchiya, C., Sakata, T., Sugita, H., 2008. Novel ecological niche of *Cetobacterium somerae*, an anaerobic bacterium in the intestinal tracts of freshwater fish. Lett. Appl. Microbiol. 46 (1), 43–48.

van der Maarel, M.J.E.C., Artz, R.R.E., Haanstra, R., Forney, L.J., 1998. Association of marine Archaea with the digestive tracts of two marine fish species. Appl. Environ. Microbiol. 64, 2894–2898.

van der Maarel, M.J., Sprenger, W., Haanstra, R., Forney, L.J., 1999. Detection of methanogenic Archaea in seawater particles and the digestive tract of a marine fish species. FEMS Microbiol. Lett. 173 (1), 189–194.

Wang, W., Zhou, Z., He, S., Liu, Y., Cao, Y., Shi, P., Yao, B., Ringø, E., 2010. Identification of the adherent microbiota on the gills and skin of poly-cultured gibel carp (*Carassius auratus gibelio*) and bluntnose black bream (*Megalobrama amblycephala* Yih). Aquacult. Res. 41, e72–e83.

Ward, R.D., Hanner, R., Hebert, P.D.N., 2009. The campaign to DNA barcode all fishes, FISH-BOL. J. Fish Biol. 74 (2), 329–356.

Wilson, J. M., Laurent, P. 2002. Fish gill morphology: inside out. J. Exp. Zool. 293 (3), 192–213.

Wong, S., Waldrop, T., Summerfelt, S., Davidson, J., Barrows, F., Kenney, P.B., Welch, T., Wiens, G.D., Snekvik, K., Rawls, J.F., Good, C., 2014. Aquacultured rainbow trout (*Oncorhynchus mykiss*) possess a large core intestinal microbiota that is resistant to variation in diet and rearing density. Appl. Environ. Microbiol. 79 (16), 4974–4984.

Xia, J.H., Lin, G., Fu, G.H., Wan, Z.Y., Lee, M., Wang, L., Liu, X.J., Yue, G.H., 2014. The intestinal microbiome of fish under starvation. BMC Genom. 15, 266, doi:10.1186/1471-2164-15-266.

Xing, M., Hou, Z., Yuan, J., Liu, Y., Qu, Y., Liu, B., 2013. Taxonomic and functional metagenomic profiling of gastrointestinal tract microbiome of the farmed adult turbot (*Scophthalmus maximus*). FEMS Microbiol. Ecol. 86 (3), 432–443.

Zhang, Y.A., Salinas, I., Li, J., Parra, D., Bjork, S., Xu, Z., LaPatra, S.E., Bartholomew, J., Sunyer, J.O., 2010. IgT, a primitive immunoglobulin class specialized in mucosal immunity. Nat. Immunol. 11 (9), 827–835.

Zhang, Y.A., Salinas, I., Sunyer, J.O., 2011. Recent findings on the structure and function of teleost IgT. Fish Shellfish Immunol. 31 (5), 627–634.

Zhou, Z., Yao, B., Romero, J., Waines, P., Ringø, E., Emery, M., Liles, M.R., Merrifield, D.L., 2014. Methodological approaches used to assess fish gastrointestinal communities. In: Merrifield, D.L., Ringø (Eds.), Aquaculture Nutrition: Gut Health, Probiotics and Prebiotics. Wiley, London, pp. 101–127.

Mucosal vaccines

11

Esteban Soto; Matt J. Griffin**; Jaime A. Tobar*[†]
[*]Department of Biomedical Sciences, Ross University School of Veterinary Medicine, West Farms, St. Kitts, West Indies
[**]Thad Cochran National Warmwater Aquaculture Center, Aquatic Research and Diagnostic Laboratory, College of Veterinary Medicine, Mississippi State University, Stoneville, Mississippi, USA
[†]Investigación y Desarrollo Biológicos, Laboratorio Centrovet, Santiago, Chile

Chapter Outline

11.1 Introduction

Today, aquaculture is recognized as the fastest-growing animal food-producing sector in the world. Global production of fish reached an impressive 52.5 million tons in 2008, almost doubling its production in 8 years (Table 11.1) (FAO, 2010). With wild

Table 11.1 **Global production of fish in 2008 according to FAO (2010)**

Area	Tons	United States ($)
Europe	2.5 million	9.4 billion
Asia-Pacific	46.6 million	77 billion
North America	644,000	1.6 billion
Latin America and the Caribbean	1.76 million	7.2 billion
Sub-Saharan Africa	239,000	665 million
East and North Africa	910,000	2.1 billion

fisheries declining and an expected global population of 9 billion by 2050, aquaculture has become an important source of revenue for developing countries and a great source of high-quality protein worldwide. Globally, fish currently represent approximately 16.6% of animal protein supply and 6.5% of all protein for human consumption (FAO, 2012). Recent models project global fish markets to increase from 154 million tons in 2011 to 186 million tons in the year 2030. Aquaculture is projected to supply over 60% of fish destined for direct human consumption by 2030 (World Bank, 2013). However, advancements and increased intensification are frequently hampered by epizootic or enzootic infectious and noninfectious diseases.

Aquaculture covers a wide range of aquatic environments, from freshwater to brackish or marine waters at a variety of temperatures. In addition, there is tremendous diversity in the types of production systems as well as aquatic species, which includes fish, crustaceans, mollusks, and seaweed. Intensification, together with a need for greater production while reducing time to harvest, has resulted in an increase in incidences of stress and higher transmission rates of infectious agents. Increased dissemination and transmission efficiency of pathogens in water, coupled with the high stocking densities used in large-scale commercial aquaculture, facilitates rapid spread of pathogens within populations of farmed fish. Moreover, poor management and inadequate records can result in suboptimal water quality, low levels of dissolved oxygen, poor biosafety measures, and deficient nutrition programs, all of which can result in additional stressors to fish.

Stress has long been recognized as one of the main causes of immunosuppression in terrestrial and aquatic animals, resulting in an increased susceptibility to classical and emerging infectious agents. The most common causative agents of infectious diseases in aquaculture are bacteria (~55%), followed by viruses (~23%), parasites (~19%), and fungi (~3%) (Kibenge et al., 2012). A large amount of work has been devoted to improving aquaculture practices and avoiding disease outbreaks. Improved biosecurity, disease surveillance, and prophylactic practices are key for a successful health management program. Over the last century, the discovery and subsequent application of antibiotics and other chemotherapeutants in food animal production has played an integral role in reducing economic losses attributed to outbreaks of bacterial diseases in fish. At present, the proper use of antibiotics and parasiticides can be highly effective to ameliorate losses during disease outbreaks. However, once the effectiveness of antimicrobials was demonstrated, their increased use resulted in increased selective pressures on natural populations of bacteria, leading to the emergence of bacterial strains that were resistant to a wide range of antibiotics. This is especially true in the poultry, swine, and aquaculture industries. Although a simplification of the issue by reducing the need for antibiotics is a possibility, vaccines may reduce the prevalence and impede the development of antimicrobial resistant bacterial strains. Moreover, repeated use of some antimicrobial compounds can suppress fish immune systems and antibiotic residues present in fish tissues destined for human consumption and can be a health risk (Rijkers et al., 1980). In addition, antibiotics are not effective against viral diseases, and no antivirals are currently used in aquaculture.

As most antimicrobials are delivered in the form of medicated feeds, several factors need to be considered when using chemotherapeutants in aquaculture. Namely, the cost of medication, the method of delivery, the feasibility of incorporating therapeutants with feed, and any associated palatability issues. In addition, the efficacy of delivery, especially in periods of disease-induced inappetence, must be considered since animals that won't eat will not be treated. However, there are only three antimicrobial feed additives currently approved by the United States Food and Drug Administration for use in aquaculture. Most likely, the reason aquaculture has so few chemotherapeutic options is due to the minimal return on investment. There is limited incentive to develop new antimicrobial molecules specifically for use in aquatic animals. The front end costs to cover the basic research as well as the significant legal and industrial development required to bring a new compound to market are high, which weighs heavily against the drug manufacturer's bottom line. In addition, with growing public sentiment against the use of antibiotics in food animal production, it is unlikely that there will be any new antimicrobial compounds developed in the near future.

A substantial body of peer-reviewed documents provides solid evidence of the efficiency of vaccination in the aquaculture industry. This is especially true for intensive farming systems, as effective vaccines have been one of the most important attributing factors in successful aquaculture production (Brudeseth et al., 2013). A good example is the salmon industry, where vaccines have been applied for over 30 years and have been shown over time to be a realistic alternative to antibiotics. For example, in the Norwegian salmon industry, vaccination dropped the use of antimicrobials from 50,000 kg/year to less than 2,000 kg/year in the 10-year period ranging from 1987–1997 (Sommerset et al., 2005).

The ideal vaccine should provide protection for individuals if administered before exposure, or, in cases where disease occurs in vaccinated individuals, the disease should be milder than in the naïve cohorts. The vaccine should be stable, economically sound, easy to produce and administer, and capable of inducing a strong, long-lasting protective immunity. In addition, the vaccine should prevent carrier formation, be safe for fish and humans, be environmentally friendly, produce minimal or no side effects, protect the immunized, but also reduce disease among unimmunized individuals through "indirect effects" or "herd immunity" (Salgado-Miranda et al., 2013). Moreover, it should be licensed or registered in the country or region that will be used, preferably where the pathogen has been diagnosed and is endemic. Lastly, vaccinated and naturally infected animals should be easily differentiated in order to facilitate diagnostic and control or contingency strategies against the disease. Currently there are vaccines available for more than 17 species of fish in more than 40 countries protecting against over 20 bacterial and 6 viral diseases (Brudeseth et al., 2013).

There are costs associated with vaccination because immunization programs require funding for infrastructure (i.e., cold-chain maintenance) and vaccine purchase as well as a well-trained staff for vaccine application. However, the mortality and morbidity prevented by vaccination translates into long-term cost savings and potential economic growth that outweighs the front end costs associated with vaccination. In addition, it is important to note there is some risk associated with vaccination. In this regard, the ideal vaccine should be easy to apply, free of side effects, lack residual pathogenicity, have no potential for reversion to virulence and, particularly important for aquaculture, it should pose no threat to the environment (Clark and Cassidy-Hanley, 2005). In addition, if the process involves handling fish, stress may be an adverse effect since stress in fish can translate to periods of anorexia, immunosuppression, and a greater risk of disease by non-target, opportunistic pathogens. Vaccine delivery methods involving injection (mainly by intraperitoneal route) probably induce the most damage in the form of adhesions, granulomas, and pigmentation, especially if oil-based adjuvants are used (Midtlyng, 1997). Other delivery methods, such as immersion or oral vaccination, although less stressful and with minimal side-effects, are still restricted to specific farmed fish species and target a restricted number of diseases, revealing the need for more basic immunology and biotechnology research in pursuit of better and long-lasting vaccination strategies.

A more complete understanding of the fish immune system, in addition to the immune response post-vaccination, will greatly improve our ability to develop new and improved vaccines for global aquaculture. There are estimated to be over 30,000 fish species worldwide with a wide range of susceptibility to different pathogens. As such, we can expect tremendous variability in response to vaccination since the immune function of different culture species may vary. Therefore, a thorough understanding of the pathogenesis of the target pathogens, an exhaustive understanding of the epizootiology of the disease, and a comprehensive understanding of the culture species immune system are required for immunization strategies to be successful.

11.2 Types of mucosal vaccines in aquaculture

11.2.1 Monovalent or polyvalent (multivalent)

At present, the great majority of commercially available mucosal vaccines are monovalent vaccines, meaning they are designed to immunize the host against a single specific antigen or infectious agent. The use of polyvalent vaccines, which consist of vaccines that immunize fish against multiple antigens, saves time and effort. In addition, vaccinated fish are subjected to fewer stressors if multiple agents can be covered within a single vaccine regiment. Additionally, in theory, it should reduce costs of labor and vaccination as ancillary costs from separate vials, labels, packages, cold-chain storage (when necessary), and feed additives. However, a thorough understanding of the fish immune response, particularly the clonal capacities of fish responding to stimulation by multiple antigens as well as the antigenic properties of the vaccines (antigenic cross-reactivity, antigenic competition or interference, affinity maturation, antigen-induced suppression, etc.), is necessary if attempting polyvalent vaccination (Busch, 1997; Nikoskelainen et al., 2007). In addition, the use of multivalent vaccines can have undesirable side-effects associated with a strong local inflammatory response, bringing up animal welfare and production issues that must be explored (Mutoloki et al., 2004).

Cross protection, or indirect immunogenicity, suggests that vaccination of a host against one pathogen confers protection of the host against another agent. This has been demonstrated in laboratory challenges and likely occurs naturally in the environment. The chances of this occurring increase when using strains of the same species or members of the same genus, but have been reported and even commercialized when using nonrelated organisms (Salonius et al., 2005). Hu et al., 2012 reported cross protection given to Japanese flounder (*Paralichthys olivaceus*) against *Vibrio alginolyticus* when vaccinated by immersion with a live attenuated *V. harveyi* mutant. Similarly, a crude bacterin of *Aeromonas salmonicida* administered by immersion to coho salmon (*Onchorhyncus kisutch*) provided significant protection in controlled laboratory challenges against Type 2 *V. anguillarum* and *Yersinia ruckeri* (Busch, 1997). In this particular case, cross-reactivity offers an explanation for the superior protection achieved by polyvalent vaccines against furunculosis and vibriosis compared to vaccination with a monovalent *A. salmonicida* vaccine (Hoel et al., 1997). Salonius et al. (2005) reported protection against *Piscirickettsia salmonis* and *Renibacterium salmoninarum*, the causative agents of Pisciricketsiosis and Bacterial Kidney Disease, respectively, when vaccinating with live *Arthrobacter davidanieli,* a nonpathogenic, gram-negative bacterium. Besides the potential antigenic similarities due to close phylogenetic relationships between those species, the activation of nonspecific innate immune components could be a possible mechanism of action (Wietz et al., 2012). Lastly, Osman et al. (2009) vaccinated tilapia with monovalent, bivalent, and polyvalent formalin killed bacterins of *A. hydrophila*, *A. sobria*, *A. caviae*, and *Pseudomonas fluorescens* via oral and immersion routes. They found polyvalent vaccines administered via immersion provided a high percentage of relative survival upon subsequent rechallenge.

11.2.2 Killed or inactivated vaccines

Historically, vaccination based on killed or inactivated agents via immersion has been a subject of controversy with a wide range of conflicting results. The method used to kill the infectious agent is of great importance because the antigenic determinants of the organism need to be conserved for induction of an efficacious immune response. In veterinary medicine, inactivation of microorganisms is achieved using formaldehyde, acetone, alcohol treatments, or alkylating agents such as ethylene oxide, ethyleneimine, acetylethyleneimine, and β-propiolactone (Tizard, 2009). In aquaculture, formaldehyde and β-propiolactone are the most commonly used (Salgado-Miranda et al., 2013). In general, immersion vaccination using inactivated viral vaccines is not efficacious (Sommerset et al., 2005); however, the use of boosters and the recent adoption of novel delivery methods have brought new insights on the immune stimulation of mucosal vaccines.

Some of the first mucosal vaccines for fish were inactivated bacterins, which, by definition, are suspensions of killed bacteria. In the United States of America, the first commercially available vaccines against enteric redmouth disease, caused by *Y. ruckerii*, and vibriosis, caused by *Vibrio* spp., were based on inactivated bacterial cells applied via immersion (Sommerset et al., 2005). Early studies using both oral and immersion methods for delivery of bacterins provided protection against some pathogens (*Y. ruckerii, V. salmonicida*), but provided less than desirable results for other bacteria (*A. salmonicida*) (Ross and Klontz, 1965; Spence et al., 1965; Egidius and Andersen, 1979; Van Muiswinkel and Nakao, 2014). The use of killed or inactivated vaccines is still one of the most common ways to immunize fish, mainly due to its high stability and ease of storage, minimal risk of reversion to a virulent state, lack of replication in the recipient animal, low environmental risk of spread, and limited costs of development and production (Tizard, 2009).

More recently, Villumsen and Raida (Villumsen and Raida, 2013) successfully immunized rainbow trout against *A. salmonicida* subsp. *salmonicida* using a 5 min bath with formalin-inactivated bacterin, both with and without a booster. Similar results were achieved by Thinh et al. (2009) where a combined immersion and oral vaccination protocol conferred protection of Vietnamese catfish (*Pangasianodon hypophthalmus*) against *Edwardsiella ictaluri*, significantly reducing mortality; however, the need for a booster was necessary to achieve strong protection. Previous reports suggested inefficacy of bacterins to prevent enteric septicemia of catfish (caused by *Edwardsiella ictaluri*) and columnaris disease (caused by *Flavobacterium columnare*) in channel catfish (Sommerset et al., 2005). In other cases, the uptake of antigens following immersion vaccination with bacterins was low, indicating that the delivery of the antigen required injectable methods in order to be successful (Lillehaug, 1989; Tatner and Horne, 1983; Tatner and Manning, 1983). Recently, a different approach was taken by Kai and Chi (Kai and Chi, 2008), who vaccinated grouper larvae against viral nervous necrosis disease (VNN). Bath immunization with nano-encapsulated formalin-inactivated or 0.4 mM binary ethyleneimine inactivated (BEI) betanodavirus vaccine conferred protection after challenge with the wild-type virus. The use of the correct inactivating agent, and new delivery technologies, like nanoparticles, could significantly improve the use of inactivated viruses for mucosal vaccines. This is particularly important due to the high failure rate previously reported using inactivated virus as mucosal vaccines (Bootland et al., 1990; Shao, 2001).

Oral immunization utilizing inactivated microorganisms has also been investigated. Sato and Okamoto (Sato and Okamoto, 2010) orally immunized clonal ginbuna crucian carp (*Carassius auratus langsdorfii*) with inactivated crucian carp hematopoietic necrosis virus (CHNV). After a booster oral dose, significant induction of cytotoxic and antibody response was achieved. The positive induction of antiviral cellular immune response indicates a potential for this type of vaccines in the field. Indian prawn (*Fenneropenaeus indicus*) have also been successfully vaccinated utilizing a formalin-inactivated viral preparation (IVP) derived from WSSV-infected shrimp tissue, at least for short periods of time (Bright Singh et al., 2005). Additionally, oral vaccination has been successfully reported in Atlantic salmon against the gram-negative, intracellular pathogen *Piscirickettsia salmonis* (Tobar et al., 2011). By using inactivated bacterins encapsulated in a proprietary MicroMatrix® technology, oral administration of vaccine during 10 consecutive days was able to induce protection either as prime-vaccination or booster to a primary-IP vaccination in a specific and encapsulating-dependent effect (Tobar et al., 2011). This method has been successfully applied on field as a commercial product available in Chile from Virbac-Centrovet, demonstrating a boost of specific anti-*P. salmonis* IgM antibodies over time; this phenomena has also being observed in viral diseases such as Infectious Salmon Anemia Virus (ISAv) (Tobar et al., personal communication).

11.2.3 Live modified/attenuated vaccines

The use of live modified or attenuated vaccines provides one of the greatest potentials for mucosal vaccines in aquaculture. One of the many advantages of live attenuated vaccines is the strong induction of both arms of immunity (humoral and cell-mediated), which includes the induction of interferon, largely important in fighting viral infections. In general, smaller doses of modified live or attenuated vaccines are required to induce a strong immune response. In addition, minimal adjuvants are required, reducing the chances of hypersensitivity and tissue damage. Moreover, they can be administered through natural routes and generally provide longer lasting protection, often without the need for a boost (Tizard, 2009).

This is particularly true when dealing with intracellular and facultative intracellular pathogens where a strong Th1 response is necessary. Currently there are few live modified or attenuated vaccines commercially available for fish; however, with the advent of molecular methods and the description and characterization of new and safer vectors, more live vaccines are likely to become available in the coming years. Safety concerns related to the potential reversion to a virulent state have been a major drawback in the licensing of many live attenuated vaccines. On some occasions, attenuated microorganisms have been able to revert to virulence (Alexandersen, 1996; Brudeseth et al., 2013); however, a thorough understanding of the pathogenesis of the different infectious agents, the immune response of the host, elucidation of genome sequences of target pathogens, and increased utilization of targeted mutagenesis will aid in the development of stable mutants that will decrease the chances of reversion to virulence. Traditionally, attenuation was achieved by multiple passages of wild-type pathogens through different media or cells, resulting in random, often unknown mutations that lead to attenuation. As such, the increased use of targeted mutagenesis should allow for better control and safety assessment than the random, often ambiguous mutations in a conventionally attenuated vaccine (Frey, 2007; Brudeseth et al., 2013).

As previously stated, the use of live vaccines is particularly important when preventing diseases caused by intracellular or facultative intracellular pathogens. Enteric septicemia of catfish, caused by the facultative intracellular pathogen *Edwardsiella ictaluri*, is one of the most important diseases affecting farm-raised catfish in the southeastern United States. Moreover, emergent strains of *E. ictaluri* were recently described as pathogens in both zebrafish and tilapia (Soto et al., 2012; Hawke et al., 2013). The ability of *E. ictaluri* to replicate both inside and outside of the host leukocytes suggests that an effective immune response towards *E. ictaluri* requires strong stimulation of the cell-mediated arm of the immune system. One of the few commercially available vaccines for the catfish industry is AQUAVAC-ESC, commercially available through Intervet INC., Merck Animal Health. AQUAVAC-ESC is derived from a strain of *E. ictaluri* (RE-33) attenuated by multiple passages (33) in ascending concentrations of rifampin (Klesius and Shoemaker, 1999). Used on immunized fish via immersion in a timed bath treatment, AQUAVAC-ESC has been shown to provide significant protection from disease and mortality when vaccinated catfish are challenged with common virulent or wild-type isolates of *E. ictaluri (online at* http://intervetus.naccvp.com/product/view/1047419).

Choosing the right gene to mutate is also important when developing a live attenuated mutant vaccine. The ideal candidate needs to infect the host cell and persist long enough that an effective immune response is stimulated, yet not result in a lethal septicemia. Elegant target mutagenesis has been reported and experimentally demonstrated for many fish pathogens. Lawrence et al. (1997) constructed an adenine-auxotrophic strain of *E. ictaluri* and provided evidence of its use as a mucosal vaccine via immersion and oral routes. The fact that the mutant persisted for more than 48 h in tissues provided enough time for a strong immune response to develop, but, at the same time, it was significantly attenuated, as demonstrated in lethal and infective dose experiments (Lawrence et al., 1997).

Unfortunately, the commercial availability of live attenuated or modified vaccines against viral pathogens in aquaculture is particularly poor. At this time, the risk that attenuated viral vaccines will revert to a virulent state or that an attenuated virus for one species will maintain its virulence to a different host species has inhibited the development and use of live attenuated or modified viral vaccines in aquaculture (Salgado-Miranda et al., 2013). Currently there are very few commercially available attenuated viral vaccines. Perelberg et al. (2005) created a koi herpesvirus mutant by serial transfer in cell culture followed by irradiation in order to completely attenuate the virus and reduce any chances of reversion back to a virulent state. After a short immersion of fish, the authors explained that the attenuated virus stimulated a strong immune response and protected fish upon subsequent challenges (Perelberg et al., 2005). Recently, a live attenuated vaccine protecting grass carp against spring viremia of carp was launched in China (Brudeseth et al., 2013). Undoubtedly due to the immense need for viral vaccines in aquaculture, further research is needed for the development of safe live vaccines against fish viruses.

11.2.4 Recombinant subunit vaccines

Since the 1970s, large-scale production of recombinant subunit antigens has led to the production of a large number of vaccines in both human and veterinary medicine. Recombinant subunit vaccines are produced using heterologous protein expression systems like bacteria (mainly *Escherichia coli*), yeast (such as *Sacharomyces cerevisiae* or *Pichia pastoris*), insect cells or tissues, protozoa (*Tetrahymena thermophile*), mammalian cell culture, or even plants. One of the biggest advantages over other vaccines is that recombinant subunit vaccines are safer than live attenuated or DNA vaccines since they don't have the ability to invade the host genome or replicate within the environment. Moreover, utilizing some of the newly available expression systems, one can produce high quantities of antigen, and, coupled with novel delivery methods, a strong immune response can be achieved (Clark and Cassidy-Hanley, 2005). One of its main constraints is the generation of misfolded or incorrectly processed membrane antigens that fail to induce a protective immune response and the less than optimal mucosal and cytotoxic T cell response that is key for the clearance of intracellular pathogens. Moreover, the expression of recombinant viral and protozoan membrane antigens has been a challenge. This is of particular importance for the use of recombinant subunit mucosal vaccines against protozoa. Recent advancements have proposed the use of *Tetrahymena thermophile* as an expression system since it possesses the ability to produce protozoa proteins in their correct formation. This strategy has produced promising results in experimental vaccination against *Ichthyophthirius multifiliis* (Clark and Cassidy-Hanley, 2005). Moreover, the availability of multiple novel methods for antigen delivery by immersion or oral mucosal vaccination has resulted in the production of innovative mucosal vaccine strategies. Newly developed vaccination protocols that enhance the uptake of antigens, such as percutaneous administration of immersion vaccines using multiple puncture instruments, have also opened the field to mucosal recombinant subunit antigen vaccination (Nakanishi et al., 2002). Hyper-osmotic infiltration (pretreatment in a hyperosmotic solution, usually NaCl) and mild ultrasound treatments at the time of vaccination also enhance the uptake of soluble antigens via immersion vaccination (Huising et al., 2003; Clark and Cassidy-Hanley, 2005). Lastly, the ability to tag antigens with ligands, which enhances their uptake and increases antigenicity, has also been explored and has the potential to greatly increase the delivery efficiency of mucosal vaccines.

Commercially available recombinant vaccines delivered orally include vaccines against infectious salmon anemia virus (ISAV) via Virbac-Centrovet in Chile, which uses a mix of recombinant hemagglutinin esterase/fusion proteins, and infectious pancreatic necrosis virus (IPNV) via Merck in Canada, which is comprised of a subunit vaccine for the VP2 and VP3 capsid proteins. Experimentally, oral administration of subunit vaccines has proven effective against several other pathogens with potential for large-scale vaccination. Lu et al. (2011) produced a transgenic *E. coli* mutant that expressed a mixture of the VP5 and VP7 outer capsid proteins of grass carp reovirus. Delivered orally to grass carp (*Ctenopharyngon idellus*), this subunit vaccine demonstrated significant protection against wild-type grass carp reovirus. Xue et al. (2013) demonstrated an alternative oral vaccine against grass carp reovirus, this time expressing the VP6 outer membrane protein in silkworm pupae infected with BacFish-vp6, a recombinant baculovirus (Xue et al., 2013). The BacFish-vp6 infected silkworm pupae were used to create a freeze-dried powder that, when mixed with feed and fed to grass carp, resulted in development of the VP6-specific antibody, suggesting that the powder of silkworms infected with BacFish-vp6 has potential as an orally administered vaccine. Similarly, Shivappa et al. (2005) cloned and expressed large genome segments of IPNV in insect cells and larvae using a baculovirus expression system. These structural proteins self-assembled into virus-like particles that were used as an immersion vaccine for rainbow trout (*Oncorhynchus mykiss*) fry and a intraperitoneal immunization of Atlantic salmon (*Salmo salar*) pre-smolts. When challenged with wild-type IPNV, the cumulative mortality of intraperitoneally immunized Atlantic salmon post-smolts was lower than that of the control fish, although there was no indication of protection in the immersion vaccinated rainbow trout fry.

These vaccines have also been successfully used in shrimp. Caipang et al. (2008) used a gram-positive bacterium, *Brevibacillus brevis*, to express the VP28 envelope protein of white spot syndrome virus (WSSV), demonstrating the potential use of this orally delivered vaccine to enhance survival of shrimp. Comparatively, Jha et al. (2007) utilized yeast (*Pichia pastoris*) as an expression vector of the WSSV envelope proteins VP19 and VP28 and provided evidence of protection in post-vaccinated crayfish, *Procambarus clarkia*.

11.2.5 Vectored vaccines

Experimentally, researchers have used molecular tools to clone and express specific antigens of a target agent in a different live attenuated organism, the latter functioning as a vector. The benefit of these methods is an immune response that is generated against both the vector and the antigens expressed from the target organism. Elegant work performed by Noonan et al. (1995) provides evidence of the potential use of these methodologies. This group cloned fragments of the glycoprotein genes of viral hemorrhagic septicemia virus (VHSV) and infectious hematopoietic necrosis virus (IHNV) into a bacterial broad-host-range expression vector, which was mobilized into an attenuated *A. salmonicida* strain. The authors provided evidence of protection in rainbow trout immunized by immersion bath for 30 min, or sprayed for 50 s, against a subsequent challenge with *A. salmonicida*, IHNV, and VHSV. Similar approaches have been utilized in recent years. Min et al. (2012) utilized a plasmid encoding the capsid VP2 gene of IPNV into *Lactobacillus casei* and immunized rainbow trout via oral delivery, stimulating a protective immune response against IPNV demonstrated upon *in vivo* challenges.

Sun et al. (2012) utilized a live attenuated strain of *Edwardsiella tarda* as a carrier host for a *Streptococcus iniae* DNA vaccine. Both oral and immersion routes were utilized by the investigators to immunize and protect Japanese flounder against subsequent challenges with fully virulent bacteria. A key feature of this approach taken by the researchers was to provide cellular stimulation against *E. tarda*, a known facultative intracellular pathogen, and humoral stimulation against *S. iniae*, a classic extracellular pathogen in fish (Sun et al., 2012). A similar approach was taken by Hu et al. (2011), who used a live attenuated *E. tarda* mutant to express a *V. harveyi* antigen. This mutant effectively stimulated immune protection in turbot when vaccinated orally with feed, by immersion, or a combination of both.

Viral vectors have also been utilized to express protective antigens; however, as with attenuated live vaccines, the major concern has been the risk of reversion to a virulent state. Of the fish viruses investigated, IHNV has demonstrated the greatest potential to serve as a vector of important protective antigens from other fish viruses like VHSV, IPNV, ISAV, and sleeping diseases virus (SDV) (Biacchesi, 2011).

11.2.6 DNA vaccines

During the past decade, a vast amount of work has focused on the development of DNA vaccines for aquaculture. In DNA vaccines, DNA encoding a protective antigen is transformed in a plasmid vector under the control of a strong eukaryotic promoter. Once inside a host cell (after vaccination, usually by intramuscular injection), the protective antigen will be expressed intracellularly and presented, inducing an immune response. This technology has great potential for more efficacious vaccines, particularly against intracellular and facultative intracellular bacteria and viruses. The DNA vaccination platform has multiple advantages over other vaccine strategies such as relative simplicity, a high level of safety, activation of both arms of immune response (humoral and cell-mediated), application in small fish and high stability; however, the main concerns to its use are the unknown fate of the plasmid in vaccinated animals or in the environment, the risk of integration of DNA into the host genome and risk of induction of an anti-DNA immune response. These caveats, coupled with the public aversion to genetically modified products in food, have hampered the potential of DNA vaccines in aquaculture (Lorenzen and LaPatra, 2005). However, the tremendous upside of DNA vaccines is that the large body of their research has resulted in commercial availability of DNA vaccines in some countries and markets, although these are limited to injectables. At present, there are no commercially available DNA vaccines for immersion or oral delivery, although research has shown injection of DNA vaccines results in greater stimulation and protection than delivery by other routes.

Romoren et al. (2004) administered a DNA vaccine for luciferase using naked, liposome-formulated or chitosan-formulated DNA by different routes of administration (intramuscular, intraperitoneal, and intravenous injection, immersion, and anal intubation) to rainbow trout (*Oncorhynchus mykiss*). Luciferase expression was only found in internal organs after intravenous, intraperitoneal, and intramuscular injections. No luciferase expression was detected in any of the organs tested following immersion and anal intubation, suggesting these were not effective routes of delivery. However, similar to inactivated and subunit vaccines, the use of newer technology to protect antigens and improve the presentation to the immune system has greatly improved the use of DNA mucosal vaccines.

One of the more novel approaches to delivery of DNA vaccines has been the application of nanoparticles (virus-like particles, liposomes, immune stimulating complexes (ISCOMS), polymeric nanoparticles, etc.) to aid in the protection and delivery of the target molecule. de las Heras et al. (2010) used alginate microspheres to encapsulate a plasmid vector (pDNA) with the capsid VP2 gene of IPNV to vaccinate salmonids. Alginate microspheres were effective in protecting the pDNA encoding the VP2 gene, and the vaccine was effective in immunizing fish, providing protection upon challenge with wild-type IPNV. Similarly, Fernandez-Alonso et al. (2001) vaccinated trout fingerlings by immersion using a plasmid coding for the glycoprotein G gene of viral hemorrhagic septicemia virus (VHSV), which offered protection resulting in both humoral antibody responses and increased survival after VHSV challenge.

In another study, Adomako et al. (2012) used poly (D,L-lactic-*co*-glycolic acid) (PLGA), a polymer approved by the U.S. Food and Drug Administration (FDA) for delivery of DNA vaccines, to vaccinate rainbow trout against IHNV. Fish were fed with a commercial diet coated with PLGA nanoparticles containing the IHNV G gene plasmid. Increased survival was observed in fish challenged 6 weeks post-vaccination, suggesting induction of a protective immune response by oral delivery of a DNA vaccine. However, this protection was short-lived since there was no difference in survival in fish challenged 10 weeks post-vaccination, suggesting that further investigations are required to optimize this vaccination strategy against IHNV. Similarly, Tian et al. (2008a) loaded PLGA microcapsules with plasmid DNA (pDNA) containing the major capsid protein (MCP) of lymphocystis disease virus (LCDV) in order to orally immunize Japanese flounder (*Paralichthys olivaceus*). Their work demonstrated that the PLGA microcapsules protected the pDNA from destruction in the stomach and induced an effective immune response. In a separate study, they observed that chitosan microspheres encapsulate pDNA containing the MCP gene of LCDV for oral vaccination of Japanese flounder (Tian et al., 2008b). Similarly, chitosan was evaluated as a polycationic gene carrier for oral administration of a DNA vaccine against *V. anguillarum*. Fish were fed experimentally prepared fish flakes containing a mixture of chitosan and plasmid DNA encoding the OMP38 gene (pVAOMP38) of *V. anguillarum*. Asian seabass orally immunized with the chitosan-pVAOMP38 complex demonstrated increased survival over nonvaccinated fish when challenged by intramuscular injection with *V. anguillarum* (Rajesh Kumar et al., 2008).

Similar strategies have been used in shrimp. The protective efficacy of an orally administered DNA construct containing the VP28 gene of WSSV encapsulated in chitosan nanoparticles was investigated in black tiger shrimp (*Penaeus monodon*) (Rajesh Kumar et al., 2009). Significant survival was obtained in vaccinated animals upon subsequent rechallenge, providing strong evidence of the utility of mucosal vaccines in shrimp aquaculture.

11.2.7 Synthetic peptides and reverse genetics

The use of reverse genetics in the past 10 years has largely contributed to a better understanding of the biology of many pathogens, especially viruses. This technology has been important in the generation of mutants and gene vectors, providing a potential use as mucosal vaccines (Biacchesi, 2011). Reverse genetics were recently used to create virulent and attenuated viral hemorrhagic septicemia genotype IV virus (VHSV) in efforts to investigate gene function and the potential for this technology to create viral-vectored vaccines (Ammayappan et al., 2011). Similar studies have been conducted with other fish pathogens (Ammayappan et al., 2010), although, at present, there is limited information when using this technology in the delivery of mucosal vaccines in fish.

11.3 Delivery of mucosal vaccines in aquaculture

Multiple delivery methods are utilized to vaccinate fish, each with their own particular advantages and disadvantages. One common method to vaccinate fish is by injection, intraperitoneally or intramuscularly, with the latter being especially important for DNA vaccines. This method is suitable for vaccination with live attenuated, killed, DNA, or subunit vaccines. For the majority of vaccines available, injection induces a strong systemic immune response. However, injection requires fish be handled individually, with the vaccine administered either manually or mechanically (Figure 11.1). In addition, an adjuvant is usually required and injection site lesions are common. The main function of adjuvants is to enhance the immune response and to improve the duration of protection. However, significant growth suppression, internal adhesions, and injection site melanization, resulting in a downgrading of carcass value, have been reported with the use of adjuvants. These are important factors to consider when using adjuvants with fish vaccines (Evensen et al., 2005; Vandenberg, 2004). Although relatively uncomplicated in larger fish, vaccinating small fish by injection can be difficult. In addition, the method is time consuming and, if done manually, labor intensive, and, at the immunological level, injectable vaccines are generally poor inducers of a mucosal response.

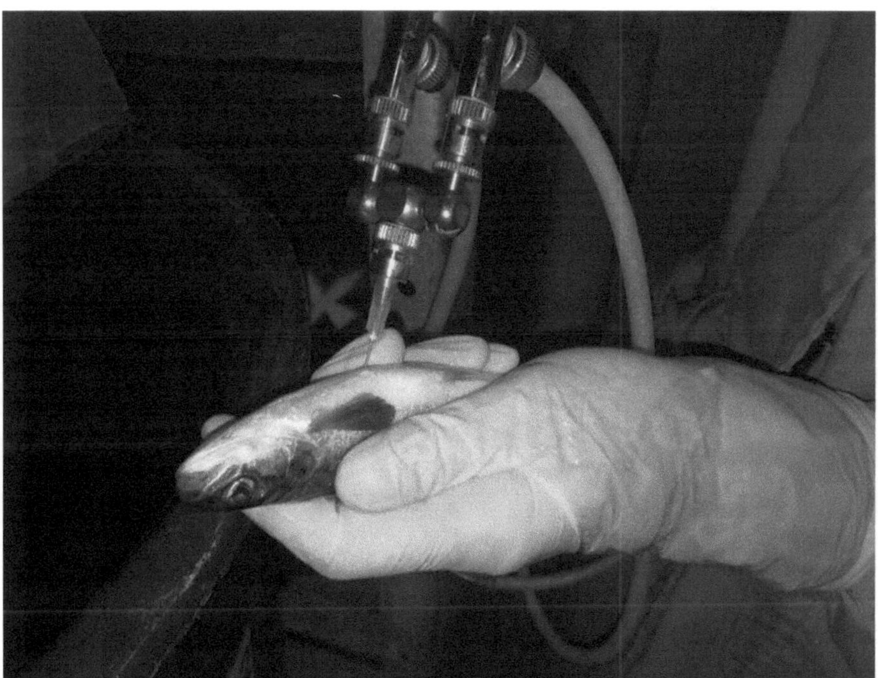

Figure 11.1 Intraperitoneal injection of salmon fingerling.

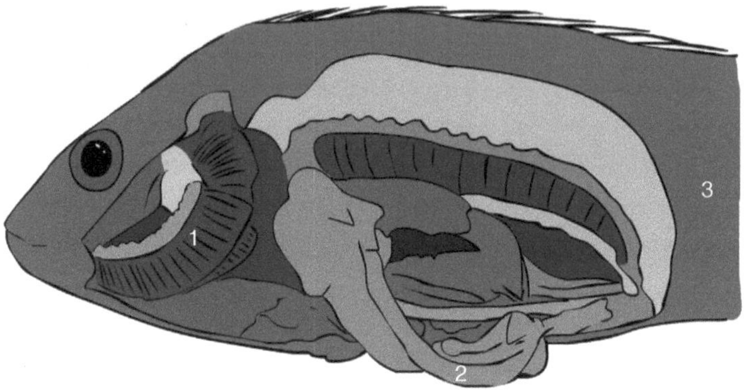

Figure 11.2 Mucosal surfaces in fish include the gill (1), gut (2), and skin (3) epithelia.

Mucosal surfaces represent significant surface areas that are constantly exposed to environmental elements, including commensal and pathogenic microorganisms. In fish, these surfaces include the epithelium of the skin (including lateral line), the gut, and the gills (Figure 11.2). The main goal of mucosal vaccines is to stimulate a strong immune response in these surfaces and, thus, protect the animal from infection when pathogenic organisms are encountered. The growing need for mucosal vaccines is accompanied by a growing need for mucosal adjuvants. This is especially true given the current regulatory climate, as it is unlikely that regulatory agencies will change their view towards live vaccines or genetically modified organisms in the foreseeable future.

In aquaculture, the great majority of vaccines available are either killed or subunit vaccines; thus, the need of effective adjuvants is of the utmost importance. Regrettably, our understanding of the mucosal immune system and the mechanisms governing its activation is limited. Research is only beginning to shed light on the mechanisms involved in mucosal immunity. As we gain a better understanding of the innate and adaptive response associated with mucosal surfaces, it is likely that more efficient adjuvants will emerge. Most recently, a novel microparticle adjuvant containing LPS isolated from meningococcal bacteria was used as an oral adjuvant with a formalin-killed *A. hydrophila* vaccine. Vaccination of African catfish (*Clarias gariepinus*) using this delivery system resulted in significant production of IgM, with increased survival rates upon challenge compared to control groups (Perez et al., 2013).

Many factors must be considered before the decision to vaccinate should be made. Primarily, environmental, chemical, and physiological factors that induce or suppress the immune response of fish directly affect the potential immune stimulation that a vaccine may induce. Temperature, age, species, photoperiod, salinity, heavy-metal contamination, crowding, and handling stress as well as anesthesia (especially true in immersion when gills uptake of antigens is essential) are important factors to consider when implementing vaccination programs (Watts et al., 2001).

Lamentably, our understanding of the mucosal immune response in fish has lagged behind our understanding of the systemic immune response. As such, the majority of vaccines available for aquaculture are based on injectable vaccines. A better understanding of the mucosal immune response, coupled with improved methods to evaluate this response, will greatly enhance our capacity to develop more effective and safer mucosal vaccines. Among the different delivery methods used to stimulate a mucosal immune response, immersion and oral delivery have been the two most common.

11.3.1 Immersion delivery

In immersion vaccines, the main target tissues are the mucosal surfaces of the skin and gills but antigenic uptake can occur in both the anterior and posterior gastrointestinal tract. When utilizing a live attenuated *Francisella noatunensis* mutant, Soto et al. (2013) compared it to the tissue distribution of an iglC live attenuated mutant proposed as a mucosal vaccine delivered by immersion. Over the duration of the 16 day evaluation period, the highest concentration of bacteria, as determined by quantitative PCR and histology, was found in the skin; however, during early stages of infection, the posterior intestine and gills were alternative mucosal sites that presented high levels of bacteria. This would suggest antigenic uptake and presentation was occurring at these sites. After 2 d, bacteria were present in blood-rich visceral organs (spleen and head kidney), indicated by the presence of *F. noatunensis* DNA in these tissues. Utilizing live attenuated *F. noatunensis* mutants, they induced both a mucosal and systemic immune response by immersion (Soto et al., 2011). Immersion vaccines are fairly efficacious and easy to administer. They can serve to vaccinate large numbers of small fish (1–5 g) and usually result in less stress to animals than injectable vaccines and display fewer negligible side effects. However, as previously stated, they usually provide shorter lasting protection with less systemic immune stimulation than injectable vaccines. This is particularly true if immersion baths are performed using inactivated/killed organisms without an additional boost.

There are many variations on the delivery of mucosal immersion vaccines. These variations usually result in improved systemic or/and mucosal immune stimulation. Others allow for less manipulation of the fish, resulting in reduced stress and minimal human/fish contact time. Factors affecting immersion vaccination include antigen concentration, vaccine type, procedure length, fish size, pH, temperature, salt concentration, fish stress, and whether the antigen is a soluble or particulate.

Some different methods to vaccinate fish via immersion include:

11.3.1.1 Direct immersion

In direct immersions, fish are anesthetized and moved to holding tanks where vaccines are added to a predetermined volume of water. Exposure may consist of a short dip (5–60 s) or extended exposures (>30 min), usually with no water circulation and supplemented oxygen (Figure 11.3). After this exposure period, fish are relocated to their original tank. In general, killed or subunit vaccines will require longer "contact" time and higher doses of vaccine than live attenuated mutants. Even at high concentrations, subunit and killed vaccines usually result in variable, although minimal, protection. The inconsistent results achieved from direct immersion methods have driven

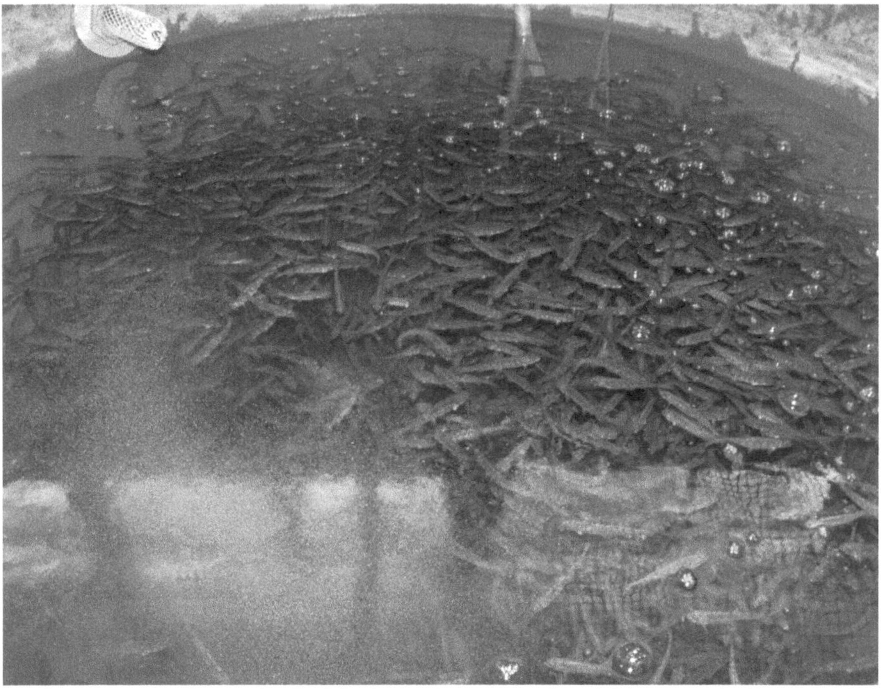

Figure 11.3 Vaccination of salmonids via direct immersion.

the investigation of modifications to this technique. These methods include, but are not limited to, hyperosmotic infiltration, ultrasonic delivery as well as immersion in coordination with puncture or abrasion to facilitate vaccine uptake and stimulate a stronger immune response.

11.3.1.2 Hyperosmotic infiltration

In hyperosmotic infiltration, fish are pre-exposed to a hypertonic solution prior to immersion vaccination. This facilitates the uptake of soluble antigens, although this method has given inconsistent results. Since the fish need to be handled, stress becomes an issue; however, the handling stress is less than injectables and comparable to direct immersion vaccines (Huising et al., 2003). Lio-Po and Wakabayashi (Lio-Po and Wakabayashi, 1986) found no significant immune stimulation or protection when vaccinating tilapia (*Sarotherodon niloticus*) with an *Edwardsiella tarda* bacterin; however, others have reported increased antigen uptake and systemic humoral response when vaccination using an *E. tarda* bacterin was preceded by a hypertonic bath (Nakanishi and Ototake, 1997; Huising et al., 2003; Navot et al., 2004). Huising and co-corkers (Huising et al., 2003) reported significant improvement in mucosal immune stimulation and uptake when pretreating common carp with a NaCl hypertonic solution prior to vaccination with an *A. salmonicida* soluble antigen (LPS), but not with a particulate antigen (*A. salmonicida* bacterin). However, inconclusive and inconsistent results have hindered the adoption of this strategy and it is currently not a common industry practice (Plant and Lapatra, 2011).

11.3.1.3 Low-frequency sonophoresis

Low-frequency (<100 kHz) ultrasound at low intensities have been used to enhance transdermal delivery of macromolecules and hydrophilic molecules in both mammals and fish. The theory operates on the premise that during or preceding immersion vaccination, the use of ultrasonic radiation will increase the uptake of the vaccine, inducing a greater systemic response comparable to injectable vaccines, but with many of the advantages of immersion vaccination (Polat et al., 2010). This technology can be utilized to enhance uptake of nucleic acids in DNA vaccines or antigen molecules, such as killed or subunit vaccines, without the use of adjuvants. However, a careful assessment of this methodology is required since the ultrasounds can damage the skin and gills, and field conditions may expose fish to opportunistic pathogens. Frenkel et al. (1999) reported exposures of $\leq$1.0 W/cm^2, 1 MHz for up to 90 s damaged the external epithelia of fish skin. However, Cobo et al. (2014) reported sonication intensities of 57 mW/cm^2 did not induce erratic swimming or tissue damage in rainbow trout (*Oncorhynchus mykiss*), but resulted in a 3-fold increase in the uptake of an *Aeromonas salmonicida* bacterin into the gill tissue. Navot et al. (2011) effectively immunized goldfish (*Carassius auratus* L.) by applying an *Aeromonas salmonicida* soluble A-layer protein (AP) and formalin-killed bacterin via ultrasound-immersion. Although no antibodies were detected, fish were protected upon challenge. This was particularly interesting since the ultrasound-immersion vaccination without adjuvant provided significantly better cumulative percent survival and less morbidity than subcutaneous injected vaccinated treatments. Similarly, Fernandez-Alonso et al. (2001) successfully vaccinated rainbow trout using short pulses of low-intensity ultrasound to deliver a DNA vaccine (plasmid coding for the glycoprotein G gene of the viral hemorrhagic septicemia virus (VHSV)). Although the proof of this concept is well accepted, application of this technology in commercial aquaculture requires further investigation and an effort composed of interdisciplinary disciplines, such as immunology, veterinary, and engineering, will be needed.

11.3.1.4 Flush

In flush vaccination, a flow-through system is required. In this method, the incoming water is turned off for a short period of time (1–5 min), during which the vaccine is administered into the water. After this brief exposure period, the normal flow of water into the tank is resumed and the vaccine is "flushed" out with the outgoing water. How fast this occurs depends on tank volume and flow rate. This method was used by Anderson et al. (1979) to vaccinate rainbow trout against *Yersinia ruckeri*. Fish were bath-exposed for 2 min with a *Y. ruckeri* O-antigen suspension, after which the flow of water was returned and the antigen was flushed from the system. This procedure was used to investigate the humoral response in vaccinated fish. Both antibody-producing cells and circulating antibodies were detected in animals exposed to the antigen suspension. Similarly, Wise et al. (2000) used a flush vaccination technique to evaluate efficacy of a live attenuated *Edwardsiella ictaluri* isolate (RE-33) in vaccinating mixed and full-sib families of channel catfish (*Ictalurus punctatus*). Fish were held in aquaria and water flow was suspended while fish were exposed to dosages of the attenuated isolate (RE-33) of approximately 1×10^6, 1×10^7, and 2×10^7 CFU/mL of water. After 30 min, water flow was restored. Thirty days later, vaccinated and nonvaccinated fish were exposed similarly to virulent *E. ictaluri* and significantly higher survival rates were observed in vaccinated fish.

11.3.1.5 Shower or spray vaccination

In spray vaccination, fish are usually anesthetized, netted, and rapidly (2–5 s) sprayed with different vaccines to achieve adequate coverage over the exterior body surface. After spraying, they are relocated to a recovery tank to convalesce. One drawback from this method, similar to injection and bath immersion, is that the handling of fish induces stress. However, this method has demonstrated to be efficacious when vaccinating red tilapia hybrids. Fish proved persistent protection following a single spray regimen of formalin-killed *S. agalactiae* bacterin with boosters. Both serum and mucosal IgM antibodies were significantly higher in vaccinated fish, suggesting that the spray regimen conferred protection in vaccinated fish (Noraini et al., 2013).

11.3.1.6 Bath immersion

In bath immersion, the volume on the tank or aquarium is lowered and a determined quantity of vaccine is added to vaccinate fish for a period of time. After vaccination, the volume of water in the tank is restored. A big drawback in this method is the quantity of vaccine in the water needed to effectively immunize the fish. Extending vaccination time improves the immunization, and the use of live attenuated organisms or vectored vaccines significantly reduces the amount of vaccine needed in the water. Moreover, the greatest advantage in this method is the lack of stress induced in the fish.

11.3.1.7 Immersion/puncture

Nakanishi et al. (2002) provided proof for a novel method to vaccinate juvenile rainbow trout against beta-hemolytic *Streptococcus*, utilizing a multiple puncture instrument to create small skin lesions while fish were immersed in a vaccine suspension containing formalin-killed *S. iniae*. Quantitative analysis using fluorescent microspheres revealed that both antigen uptake by skin and delivery to the kidney and spleen were more effective with this method than with immersion alone. The authors reported greater protection conferred by this method than when vaccinating fish via simple immersion and attributed this to greater systemic stimulation and antigen uptake facilitated by this modified immersion technique. However, it should be considered that pinpoint lesions/abrasions/ulcerations created to vaccinate fish could serve as an entry route for other, nontarget opportunistic pathogens. At present, the commercial application of this method has yet to be explored.

11.3.2 Oral mucosal vaccines

In oral vaccines, the target is the digestive system mucosa (particularly the gut-associated lymphoid tissue (GALT)) where macrophages and lymphoid cells are present in relative abundance. Compared to injectables, oral delivery of a vaccine is relatively simple to administer, cost-effective, minimizes procedural stress and side effects, and is suitable for mass immunization of fish of all sizes. However, historically, orally delivered vaccine preparations have required large amounts of antigen, induced weak systemic immune response, and protection failed to persist as long as vaccines delivered by injection (Borgogna et al., 2011). In addition, orally delivered vaccines require protection from digestive hydrolysis, are dependent on uptake in the hind gut, and are contingent on antigens persisting long enough in the GI tract to stimulate mucosal immunity. These problems have been targeted by using novel methods of oral vaccine delivery such as:

11.3.2.1 Subunit vaccines in plants and microalgae

Genetic engineering has made significant contributions to the cultivation of crops for both human and animal consumption and produced enumerable, valuable, and recombinant proteins in the past three decades. This technology has been utilized to create novel oral vaccines in both human and veterinary medicine (Liu Clarke et al., 2013). Companjen et al. (2005) elegantly fused proteins consisting of a gut adhesion molecule and a viral peptide expressed in potato tubers to protect the peptide from degradation in the GI tract, promoting uptake and humoral immune stimulation in carp. Use of microalgae to express antigens of potential pathogens (recombinant subunit vaccine) has been proposed for the development of oral vaccines. Plant cells are of particular interest as an oral delivery platform because their rigid cell walls provide exceptional antigen protection, insuring passage through the stomach into the intestines and facilitating associations with gut-associated lymphoid tissue. Microalgae has advantages over terrestrial plant-based platforms, including scalability and contained growth, rapid transformation, readily available stable cell lines, and consistent transgene expression levels (Siripornadulsil et al., 2007; Surzycki et al., 2009; Specht and Mayfield, 2014). Siripornadulsil et al. 2007 developed a recombinant subunit vaccine expressing *Renibacterium salmoninarum* protein 57 (p57), which was effectively expressed in the microalgae (*Chlamydomonas reinhardtii*). *Chlamydomonas* spp. is a desirable recombinant protein expression system because the organism is easily genetically manipulated (Surzycki et al., 2009). Oral delivery of the p57 recombinant microalgae vaccine to fish induced a systemic antibody response, suggesting that this system has potential as an oral vaccine delivery method in fish (Siripornadulsil et al., 2007; Plant and Lapatra, 2011).

11.3.2.2 Biofilms

Biofilms are aggregates of prokaryotic organisms where surface-associated microbial cells are enclosed in an extracellular polymeric substance matrix, protecting the bacterial community from the environment and enhancing survival (Donlan, 2002). This property has been utilized by researchers to protect live vaccines from digestion and to allow bacteria to persist for longer periods of time in mucosal surfaces, inducing a stronger immune response. Azad et al. (2000) investigated the uptake and processing of biofilm (BF) and free-cell (FC) vaccines of *Aeromonas hydrophila* in catla (*Catla catla*), rohu (*Labeo rohita*), and the common carp (*Cyprinus carpio*). Following a single dose oral vaccination, the pattern of antigen localization was similar in catla, rohu, and common carp; however, in general, there was a distinct difference between BF and FC vaccines in the duration of retention and quantity of uptake in the gut, the kidney, and the spleen (Nayak et al., 2004).

11.3.2.3 Chitosan, alginate and poly (lactide-co-glycolide) (PLGA) polymers

Polymers like chitosan, alginate, and poly (lactide-*co*-glycolide) (PLGA) have been used in aquaculture to encapsulate pathogens or nucleic acids to treat many different fish species. Chitosan derives from the chitin (extracted from crustaceans and insect exoskeleton or from some algae and fungi) and is essentially a polyglucosamine that varies in the degree of acetylation and molecular weight (Borgogna et al., 2011). Vimal et al. (2013) proposed the use of chitosan tripolyphosphate nanoparticles for delivery of a white spot syndrome virus (WSSV) oral DNA vaccine in shrimp. Utilizing serological and molecular methods, expression of the gene was confirmed in fish cell lines. Rajesh Kumar et al. (2009) demonstrated that a DNA vaccine used against WSSV and encapsulated in chitosan nanoparticles significantly protected black tiger shrimp (*Penaeus monodon*) against *in vivo* challenges. Immune stimulation of prophenoloxidase, superoxide dismutase, and superoxide anion in hemolymph probably played a role in the protection of orally vaccinated animals. Several authors have validated the use of chitosan as a polycationic gene carrier for oral vaccination in fish. Rajesh Kumar et al. (2008) constructed a DNA vaccine encoding the porin gene of *Vibrio* (*Listonella*) *anguillarum* and utilized chitosan nanoparticles to deliver the constructed DNA vaccine with feed. The authors reported moderate protection upon *in vivo* challenge. Tian et al. (2008b) utilized a similar approach to orally vaccinate Japanese flounder (*Paralichthys olivaceus*) by utilizing a DNA vaccine containing the major capsid protein (MCP) gene of lymphocystis disease virus (LCDV), encapsulating the vaccine in chitosan microspheres. The authors were able to stimulate a systemic humoral immune response, thus, suggesting conferred protection and demonstrating the potential of this strategy.

Alginate is a polysaccharide of algal or bacterial origin (Borgogna et al., 2011). Similar to chitosan, alginate has been studied as a vaccine delivery method due to its potential to provide protection to the target molecule in the gastro-intestinal tract. Maurice et al. (2004) investigated the immune response and protection conferred by an *Aeromonas salmonicida* A-layer protein (At-R), cloned and modified by the genetic fusion of the protein transduction domain (MTS) and derived from Kaposi fibroblast growth factor (At-MTS). The vaccine was encapsulated in biodegradable alginate gel macrosphere and was then fed to goldfish. Although antibodies were detected, vaccinated fish did not demonstrate resistance to infection with atypical *A. salmonicida* (Maurice et al., 2004). Ballesteros et al. (2012a, 2012b) vaccinated rainbow trout (*Oncorhynchus mykiss*) with an oral DNA-vaccine encoding the VP2 gene of the infectious pancreatic necrosis virus (IPNV) encapsulated in alginates. The authors reported that vaccinated fish qualitatively mimicked both time course and organ transcriptional profiles to naturally infected fish; however, in some cases, the expression of the genes was different. Although further work is necessary, the authors proposed that this vaccination method has the potential to successfully immunize fish.

PLGA is a copolymer that is typically used to improve delivery of antibiotics and vaccines. PLGA was utilized by Harikrishnan et al. (2012) to encapsulate a *Uronema marinum* vaccine and immunize kelp grouper (*Epinephelus bruneus*). The authors reported a significant enhancement of the respiratory burst activity, complement activity, α2-macroglobulin, serum lysozyme activity, antiprotease activity, and antibody levels. Moreover, lower cumulative mortality was found in vaccinated fish than in controls. On the other hand, Adomako et al. (2012) reported mixed results when vaccinating rainbow trout with an oral DNA vaccine utilizing PLGA. PLGA is a promising encapsulating polymer for the delivery of vaccines to fish, although there is still much room for improvement.

11.3.2.4 Liposomes

Liposomes have been utilized as vehicles for administration of vaccines in fish. They are artificially prepared spherical vesicles composed of a lipid bilayer that protects the vaccine molecules from proteases and digestive acids present in the GI tract. Kuruma shrimp (*Marsupenaeus japonicas*) were vaccinated with a liposome-coated recombinant protein VP28 against white spot syndrome virus, demonstrating liposomes improved the efficiency of delivery of the recombinant protein (Mavichak et al., 2010).

11.3.2.5 Bioencapsulation

Different organisms have been used to bioencapsulate vaccines and aid in the delivery of DNA or antigens to the gut mucosa. Members of the genus *Artemia* are aquatic crustaceans, also known as brine shrimp, that have been used as biological antigen carriers. *Artemia* nauplii are indiscriminate filter feeders and are able to incorporate particulate antigens by filter feeding. The nauplii are then fed to the fish, protecting the antigens as they pass through the stomach to the hindgut. Lin et al. (2005) utilized live *Artemia* nauplii to deliver a *Pseudomonas aeuroginosa* recombinant subunit vaccine and immunize zebrafish, protecting them in *in vivo* challenges. However, others have report mixed results when evaluating the uptake of live and inactivated organisms by *Artemia* (Plant and Lapatra, 2011). Similarly, rotifers and water fleas have been investigated for potential delivery of *V. anguillarum* to juvenile ayu (*Plecoglossus altivelis*) (Kawai et al., 1989; Plant and Lapatra, 2011). Although positive results were found when using water fleas, few reports of this technology are available. As such, application of this method in aquaculture remains unknown.

11.3.2.6 Proprietary technologies for fish vaccination

Co-administration of oral vaccines with digestive suppressors (anti-proteases, membrane permeability enhancers, and pH modulators) are the basis of Oralject technology

(PerOs Aquatic, Canada). The use of this technology has been utilized by researchers to vaccinate fish. Shoemaker et al. (2006) successfully immunized Nile tilapia (*Oreochromis niloticus*) by utilizing this technology and provided proof of this concept by protecting the fish upon challenge with virulent bacteria. However, there is a dearth of literature regarding this technology. As such, the application of this method in aquaculture remains unknown.

Another technology that has been successfully applied in aquaculture is Micromatrix technology (Advanced BioNutrition Corp., USA). This technology includes a complex mixture of organic and inorganic components, which together can encapsulate, protect and deliver inactivated antigens into the fish hindgut in order to develop a specific immune response. Using this technology has demonstrated oral protection against *Piscirickettsia salmonis* in Atlantic salmon when fish were fed with Micromatrix-encapsulated bacterins during 10 consecutive days (Tobar et al., 2011).

References

Adomako, M., St-Hilaire, S., Zheng, Y., Eley, J., Marcum, R.D., Sealey, W., Donahower, B.C., Lapatra, S., Sheridan, P.P., 2012. Oral DNA vaccination of rainbow trout, *Oncorhynchus mykiss* (Walbaum), against infectious haematopoietic necrosis virus using PLGA [Poly(D,L-Lactic-*co*-Glycolic Acid)] nanoparticles. J. Fish Dis. 35, 203–214.

Alexandersen, S., 1996. Advantages and disadvantages of using live vaccines risks and control measures. Acta. Vet. Scand. Suppl. 90, 89–100.

Ammayappan, A., Kurath, G., Thompson, T.M., Vakharia, V.N., 2011. A reverse genetics system for the Great Lakes strain of viral hemorrhagic septicemia virus: the NV gene is required for pathogenicity. Mar. Biotechnol. (NY) 13, 672–683.

Ammayappan, A., Lapatra, S.E., Vakharia, V.N., 2010. A vaccinia-virus-free reverse genetics system for infectious hematopoietic necrosis virus. J Virol Methods 167, 132–139.

Anderson, D.P., Dixon, O.W., Roberson, B.S., 1979. Kinetics of the primary immune response in rainbow trout after flush exposure to *Yersinia ruckeri* O-antigen. Dev. Comp. Immunol. 3, 739–744.

Azad, I.S., Shankar, K.M., Mohan, C.V., Kalita, B., 2000. Uptake and processing of biofilm and free-cell vaccines of *Aeromonas hydrophila* in indian major carps and common carp following oral vaccination – antigen localization by a monoclonal antibody. Dis. Aquat. Organ 43, 103–108.

Ballesteros, N.A., Saint-Jean, S.S., Encinas, P.A., Perez-Prieto, S.I., Coll, J.M., 2012a. Oral immunization of rainbow trout to infectious pancreatic necrosis virus (IPNV) induces different immune gene expression profiles in head kidney and pyloric ceca. Fish Shellfish Immunol. 33, 174–185.

Ballesteros, N.A., Saint-Jean, S.S., Perez-Prieto, S.I., Coll, J.M., 2012b. Trout oral VP2 DNA vaccination mimics transcriptional responses occurring after infection with infectious pancreatic necrosis virus (IPNV). Fish Shellfish Immunol. 33, 1249–1257.

Biacchesi, S., 2011. The reverse genetics applied to fish RNA viruses. Vet. Res. 42, 12.

Bootland, L.M., Dobos, P., Stevenson, R.M.W., 1990. Fry age and size effects on immersion immunization of brook trout, *Salvelinus-fontinalis* Mitchell, against infectious pancreatic necrosis virus. J. Fish Dis. 13, 113–125.

Borgogna, M., Bellich, B., Cesaro, A., 2011. Marine polysaccharides in microencapsulation and application to aquaculture: "from sea to sea". Mar. Drugs. 9, 2572–2604.

Bright Singh, I.S., Manjusha, M., Pai, S.S., Philip, R., 2005. *Fenneropenaeus indicus* is protected from white spot disease by oral administration of inactivated white spot syndrome virus. Dis. Aquat. Org. 66, 265–270.

Brudeseth, B.E., Wiulsrod, R., Fredriksen, B.N., Lindmo, K., Lokling, K.E., Bordevik, M., Steine, N., Klevan, A., Gravningen, K., 2013. Status and future perspectives of vaccines for industrialised fin-fish farming. Fish Shellfish Immunol. 35, 1759–1768.

Busch, R.A., 1997. Polyvalent vaccines in fish: the interactive effects of multiple antigens. Dev. Biol. Stand. 90, 245–256.

Caipang, C.M., Verjan, N., Ooi, E.L., Kondo, H., Hirono, I., Aoki, T., Kiyono, H., Yuki, Y., 2008. Enhanced survival of shrimp, *Penaeus* (*Marsupenaeus*) *japonicus* from white spot syndrome disease after oral administration of recombinant VP28 expressed in *Brevibacillus brevis*. Fish Shellfish Immunol. 25, 315–320.

Clark, T.G., Cassidy-Hanley, D., 2005. Recombinant subunit vaccines: potentials and constraints. Dev. Biol. (Basel) 121, 153–163.

Clarke, J.L., Waheed, M.T., Lossl, A.G., Martinussen, I., Daniell, H., 2013. How can plant genetic engineering contribute to cost-effective fish vaccine development for promoting sustainable aquaculture? Plant Mol. Biol. 83, 33–40.

Cobo, C., Makosch, K., Jung, R., Kohlmann, K., Knopf, K., 2014. Enhanced *Aeromonas salmonicida* bacterin uptake and side effects caused by low frequency sonophoresis in rainbow trout (*Oncorhynchus mykiss*). Fish Shellfish Immunol. 36, 444–452.

Companjen, A.R., Florack, D.E., Bastiaans, J.H., Matos, C.I., Bosch, D., Rombout, J.H., 2005. Development of a cost-effective oral vaccination method against viral disease in fish. Dev. Biol. (Basel) 121, 143–150.

de las Heras, A.I., Rodriguez Saint-Jean, S., Perez-Prieto, S.I., 2010. Immunogenic and protective effects of an oral DNA vaccine against infectious pancreatic necrosis virus in fish. Fish Shellfish Immunol. 28, 562–570.

Donlan, R.M., 2002. Biofilms: microbial life on surfaces. Emerg. Infect. Dis. 8, 881–890.

Egidius, E.C., Andersen, K., 1979. Bath-immunization – a practical and non-stressing method of vaccinating sea farmed rainbow trout *Salmo gairdneri* against vibriosis. J. Fish Dis. 2, 405410.

Evensen, O., Brudeseth, B., Mutoloki, S., 2005. The vaccine formulation and its role in inflammatory processes in fish – effects and adverse effects. Dev. Biol. (Basel) 121, 117–125.

FAO, 2010. State of world aquaculture 2010. Online at: http://www.fao.org/fishery/regional-aquaculture-reviews/reviews-2010/en/.

FAO. 2012. State of world aquaculture 2012. Online at: http://www.fao.org/docrep/016/i2727e/i2727e00.htm.

Fernandez-Alonso, M., Rocha, A., Coll, J.M., 2001. DNA vaccination by immersion and ultrasound to trout viral haemorrhagic septicaemia virus. Vaccine 19, 3067–3075.

Frenkel, V., Kimmel, E., Iger, Y., 1999. Ultrasound-induced cavitation damage to external epithelia of fish skin. Ultrasound Med. Biol. 25, 1295–1303.

Frey, J., 2007. Biological safety concepts of genetically modified live bacterial vaccines. Vaccine 25, 5598–5605.

Harikrishnan, R., Balasundaram, C., Heo, M.S., 2012. Poly D,L-lactide-*co*-glycolic acid (PLGA)-encapsulated vaccine on immune system in *Epinephelus bruneus* against *Uronema marinum*. Exp. Parasitol. 131, 325–332.

Hawke, J.P., Kent, M., Rogge, M., Baumgartner, W., Wiles, J., Shelley, J., Savolainen, L.C., Wagner, R., Murray, K., Peterson, T.S., 2013. Edwardsiellosis caused by

Edwardsiella ictaluri in laboratory populations of zebrafish *Danio rerio*. J. Aquat. Anim. Health 25, 171–183.

Hoel, K., Salonius, K., Lillehaug, A., 1997. Vibrio antigens of polyvalent vaccines enhance the humoral immune response to *Aeromonas salmonicida* antigens in Atlantic salmon (*Salmo salar* L.). Fish Shellfish Immunol. 7, 71–80.

Hu, Y.H., Cheng, S., Zhang, M., Sun, L., 2011. Construction and evaluation of a live vaccine against *Edwardsiella tarda* and *Vibrio harveyi*: laboratory vs. mock field trial. Vaccine 29, 4081–4085.

Hu, Y.H., Deng, T., Sun, B.G., Sun, L., 2012. Development and efficacy of an attenuated *Vibrio harveyi* vaccine candidate with cross protectivity against *Vibrio alginolyticus*. Fish Shellfish Immunol. 32, 1155–1161.

Huising, M.O., Guichelaar, T., Hoek, C., Verburg-van Kemenade, B.M., Flik, G., Savelkoul, H.F., Rombout, J.H., 2003. Increased efficacy of immersion vaccination in fish with hyperosmotic pretreatment. Vaccine 21, 4178–4193.

Jha, R.K., Xu, Z.R., Bai, S.J., Sun, J.Y., Li, W.F., Shen, J., 2007. Protection of *Procambarus clarkii* against white spot syndrome virus using recombinant oral vaccine expressed in *Pichia pastoris*. Fish Shellfish Immunol. 22, 295–307.

Kai, Y.H., Chi, S.C., 2008. Efficacies of inactivated vaccines against betanodavirus in grouper larvae (*Epinephelus coioides*) by bath immunization. Vaccine 26, 1450–1457.

Kawai, K., Yamamoto, S., Kusuda, R., 1989. Plankton-mediated oral delivery of *Vibrio anguillarum* vaccine to juvenile Ayu. Nippon Suisan Gakkaishi 55, 35–40.

Kibenge, F.S., Godoy, M.G., Fast, M., Workenhe, S., Kibenge, M.J., 2012. Countermeasures against viral diseases of farmed fish. Antiviral Res. 95, 257–281.

Klesius, P.H., Shoemaker, C.A., 1999. Development and use of modified live *Edwardsiella ictaluri* vaccine against enteric septicemia of catfish. Adv. Vet. Med. 41, 523–537.

Lawrence, M.L., Cooper, R.K., Thune, R.L., 1997. Attenuation, persistence, and vaccine potential of an *Edwardsiella ictaluri purA* mutant. Infect. Immun. 65, 4642–4651.

Lillehaug, A., 1989. A cost-effective study of three different methods of vaccination against vibriosis in salmonids. Aquaculture 83, 227–236.

Lin, J.H., Yu, C.C., Lin, C.C., Yang, H.L., 2005. An oral delivery system for recombinant subunit vaccine to fish. Dev. Biol. (Basel) 121, 175–180.

Lio-Po, G., Wakabayashi, H., 1986. Immuno-response in tilapia *Sarotherodon niloticus* vaccinated with *Edwardsiella tarda* by hyperosmotic infiltration method. Vet. Immunol. Immunopathol. 12, 351–357.

Lorenzen, N., LaPatra, S.E., 2005. DNA vaccines for aquacultured fish. Rev. Sci. Tech. 24, 201–213.

Lu, L., Xu, H., He, Y., Li, J., 2011. Protection of grass carp, *Ctenopharyngon idellus* (*Valenciennes*), through oral administration of a subunit vaccine against reovirus. J. Fish. Dis. 34, 939–942.

Maurice, S., Nussinovitch, A., Jaffe, N., Shoseyov, O., Gertler, A., 2004. Oral immunization of *Carassius auratus* with modified recombinant A-layer proteins entrapped in alginate beads. Vaccine 23, 450–459.

Mavichak, R., Takano, T., Kondo, H., Hirono, I., Wada, S., Hatai, K., Inagawa, H., Takahashi, Y., Yoshimura, T., Kiyono, H., Yuki, Y., Aoki, T., 2010. The effect of liposome-coated recombinant protein VP28 against white spot syndrome virus in kuruma shrimp, *Marsupenaeus japonicus*. J. Fish. Dis. 33, 69–74.

Midtlyng, P.J., 1997. Vaccinated fish welfare: protection versus side-effects. Dev. Biol. Stand. 90, 371–379.

Min, L., Li-Li, Z., Jun-Wei, G., Xin-Yuan, Q., Yi-Jing, L., Di-Qiu, L., 2012. Immunogenicity of *Lactobacillus*-expressing VP2 and VP3 of the infectious pancreatic necrosis virus (IPNV) in rainbow trout. Fish Shellfish Immunol. 32, 196–203.

Mutoloki, S., Alexandersen, S., Evensen, O., 2004. Sequential study of antigen persistence and concomitant inflammatory reactions relative to side-effects and growth of Atlantic salmon (*Salmo salar* L.) following intraperitoneal injection with oil-adjuvanted vaccines. Fish Shellfish Immunol. 16, 633–644.

Nakanishi, T., Kiryu, I., Ototake, M., 2002. Development of a new vaccine delivery method for fish: percutaneous administration by immersion with application of a multiple puncture instrument. Vaccine 20, 3764–3769.

Nakanishi, T., Ototake, M., 1997. Antigen uptake and immune responses after immersion vaccination. Dev. Biol. Stand. 90, 59–68.

Navot, N., Kimmel, E., Avtalion, R.R., 2004. Enhancement of antigen uptake and antibody production in goldfish (*Carassius auratus*) following bath immunization and ultrasound treatment. Vaccine 22, 2660–2666.

Navot, N., Sinyakov, M.S., Avtalion, R.R., 2011. Application of ultrasound in vaccination against goldfish ulcer disease: a pilot study. Vaccine 29, 1382–1389.

Nayak, D.K., Asha, A., Shankar, K.M., Mohan, C.V., 2004. Evaluation of biofilm of *Aeromonas hydrophila* for oral vaccination of *Clarias batrachus* – a carnivore model. Fish Shellfish Immunol. 16, 613–619.

Nikoskelainen, S., Verho, S., Jarvinen, S., Madetoja, J., Wiklund, T., Lilius, E.M., 2007. Multiple whole bacterial antigens in polyvalent vaccine may result in inhibition of specific responses in rainbow trout (*Oncorhynchus mykiss*). Fish Shellfish Immunol. 22, 206–217.

Noonan, B., Enzmann, P.J., Trust, T.J., 1995. Recombinant infectious hematopoietic necrosis virus and viral hemorrhagic septicemia virus glycoprotein epitopes expressed in *Aeromonas salmonicida* induce protective immunity in rainbow trout (*Oncorhynchus mykiss*). Appl. Environ. Microbiol. 61, 3586–3591.

Noraini, O., Sabri, M.Y., Siti-Zahrah, A., 2013. Efficacy of spray administration of formalin-killed *Streptococcus agalactiae* in hybrid red tilapia. J. Aquat. Anim. Health 25, 142–148.

Osman, K.M., Mohamed, L.A., Abdel Rahman, E., Soliman, W., 2009. Trials for vaccination of tilapia fish against *Aeromonas* and *Pseudomonas* infections using monovalent, bivalent and polyvalent vaccines. World J. Fish Mar. Sci. 1, 297–304.

Perelberg, A., Ronen, A., Hutoran, M., Smith, Y., Kotler, M., 2005. Protection of cultured *Cyprinus carpio* against a lethal viral disease by an attenuated virus vaccine. Vaccine 23, 3396–3403.

Perez, O., Romeu, B., Cabrera, O., Gonzalez, E., Batista-Duharte, A., Labrada, A., Perez, R., Reyes, L.M., Ramirez, W., Sifontes, S., Fernandez, N., Lastre, M., 2013. Adjuvants are key factors for the development of future vaccines: lessons from the Finlay adjuvant platform. Front Immunol. 4, 407.

Plant, K.P., Lapatra, S.E., 2011. Advances in fish vaccine delivery. Dev. Comp. Immunol. 35, 1256–1262.

Polat, B.E., Blankschtein, D., Langer, R., 2010. Low-frequency sonophoresis: application to the transdermal delivery of macromolecules and hydrophilic drugs. Expert. Opin. Drug Deliv. 7, 1415–1432.

Rajesh Kumar, S., Venkatesan, C., Sarathi, M., Sarathbabu, V., Thomas, J., Anver Basha, K., Sahul Hameed, A.S., 2009. Oral delivery of DNA construct using chitosan nanoparticles to protect the shrimp from white spot syndrome virus (WSSV). Fish Shellfish Immunol. 26, 429–437.

Rajesh Kumar, S., Ishaq Ahmed, V.P., Parameswaran, V., Sudhakaran, R., Sarath Babu, V., Sahul Hameed, A.S., 2008. Potential use of chitosan nanoparticles for oral delivery of DNA vaccine in Asian sea bass (*Lates calcarifer*) to protect from *Vibrio* (*Listonella*) *anguillarum*. Fish Shellfish Immunol. 25, 47–56.

Rijkers, G.T., Frederix-Wolters, E.M., van Muiswinkel, W.B., 1980. The immune system of cyprinid fish. Kinetics and temperature dependence of antibody-producing cells in carp (*Cyprinus carpio*). Immunology 41, 91–97.

Romoren, K., Thu, B.J., Evensen, O., 2004. Expression of luciferase in selected organs following delivery of naked and formulated DNA to rainbow trout (*Oncorhynchus mykiss*) by different routes of administration. Fish Shellfish Immunol. 16, 251–264.

Ross, A.J., Klontz, G.W., 1965. Oral immunization of rainbow trout against etiological agent of redmouth disease. J. Fish. Res. Board Can. 22, 713–719.

Salgado-Miranda, C., Loza-Rubio, E., Rojas-Anaya, E., Garcia-Espinosa, G., 2013. Viral vaccines for bony fish: past, present and future. Expert Rev. Vaccines 12, 567–578.

Salonius, K., Siderakis, C., MacKinnon, A.M., Griffiths, S.G., 2005. Use of *Arthrobacter davidanieli* as a live vaccine against *Renibacterium salmoninarum* and *Piscirickettsia salmonis* in salmonids. Dev. Biol. (Basel) 121, 189–197.

Sato, A., Okamoto, N., 2010. Induction of virus-specific cell-mediated cytotoxic responses of isogeneic ginbuna crucian carp, after oral immunization with inactivated virus. Fish Shellfish Immunol. 29, 414–421.

Shao, Z.J., 2001. Aquaculture pharmaceuticals and biologicals: current perspectives and future possibilities. Adv. Drug Deliv. Rev. 50, 229–243.

Shivappa, R.B., McAllister, P.E., Edwards, G.H., Santi, N., Evensen, O., Vakharia, V.N., 2005. Development of a subunit vaccine for infectious pancreatic necrosis virus using a baculovirus insect/larvae system. Dev. Biol. (Basel) 121, 165–174.

Shoemaker, C.A., Vandenberg, G.W., Désormeaux, A., Klesius, P.H., Evans, J.J., 2006. Efficacy of a *Streptococcus iniae* modified bacterin delivered using Oralject™ technology in Nile tilapia, *Oreochromis niloticus*. Aquaculture 255, 151–156.

Siripornadulsil, S., Dabrowski, K., Sayre, R., 2007. Microalgal vaccines. Adv. Exp. Med. Biol. 616, 122–128.

Sommerset, I., Krossoy, B., Biering, E., Frost, P., 2005. Vaccines for fish in aquaculture. Expert Rev. Vaccines 4, 89–101.

Soto, E., Griffin, M., Arauz, M., Riofrio, A., Martinez, A., Cabrejos, M.E., 2012. *Edwardsiella ictaluri* as the causative agent of mortality in cultured Nile tilapia. J. Aquat. Anim. Health 24, 81–90.

Soto, E., Kidd, S., Mendez, S., Marancik, D., Revan, F., Hiltchie, D., Camus, A., 2013. *Francisella noatunensis* subsp. *orientalis* pathogenesis analyzed by experimental immersion challenge in Nile tilapia, *Oreochromis niloticus* (L.). Vet. Microbiol. 164, 77–84.

Soto, E., Wiles, J., Elzer, P., Macaluso, K., Hawke, J.P., 2011. Attenuated *Francisella asiatica* iglC mutant induces protective immunity to francisellosis in tilapia. Vaccine 29, 593–598.

Specht, E.A., Mayfield, S.P., 2014. Algae-based oral recombinant vaccines. Front Microbiol. 5, 60.

Spence, K.D., Fryer, J.L., Pilcher, K.S., 1965. Active and passive immunization of certain salmonid fishes against *Aeromonas salmonicida*. Can. J. Microbiol. 11, 397–405.

Sun, Y., Hu, Y.H., Liu, C.S., Sun, L., 2012. A *Streptococcus iniae* DNA vaccine delivered by a live attenuated *Edwardsiella tarda* via natural infection induces cross-genus protection. Lett. Appl. Microbiol.

Surzycki, R., Greenham, K., Kitayama, K., Dibal, F., Wagner, R., Rochaix, J.D., Ajam, T., Surzycki, S., 2009. Factors effecting expression of vaccines in microalgae. Biologicals 37, 133–138.

Tatner, M.F., Horne, M.T., 1983. Susceptibility and immunity to *Vibrio anguillarum* in post-hatching rainbow trout fry, *Salmo gairdneri* Richardson 1836. Dev. Comp. Immunol. 7, 465–472.

Tatner, M.F., Manning, M.J., 1983. The ontogeny of cellular immunity in the rainbow trout, *Salmo gairdneri* Richardson, in relation to the stage of development of the lymphoid organs. Dev. Comp Immunol. 7, 69–75.

Thinh, N.H., Kuo, T.Y., Hung, L.T., Loc, T.H., Chen, S.C., Evensen, O., Schuurman, H.J., 2009. Combined immersion and oral vaccination of Vietnamese catfish (*Pangasianodon hypophthalmus*) confers protection against mortality caused by *Edwardsiella ictaluri*. Fish Shellfish Immunol. 27, 773–776.

Tian, J., Sun, X., Chen, X., Yu, J., Qu, L., Wang, L., 2008a. The formulation and immunisation of oral poly(DL-lactide-*co*-glycolide) microcapsules containing a plasmid vaccine against lymphocystis disease virus in Japanese flounder (*Paralichthys olivaceus*). Int. Immunopharmacol. 8, 900–908.

Tian, J.Y., Sun, X.Q., Chen, X.G., 2008b. Formation and oral administration of alginate microspheres loaded with pDNA coding for lymphocystis disease virus (LCDV) to Japanese flounder. Fish Shellfish Immunol. 24, 592–599.

Tizard, I.R., 2009. Vaccines and Their Production in: Veterinary Immunology. An Introduction, Edition 8 Elsevier, St. Louis Missouri, USA, pp. 255–270.

Tobar, J.A., Jerez, S., Caruffo, M., Bravo, C., Contreras, F., Bucarey, S.A., Harel, M., 2011. Oral vaccination of Atlantic salmon (*Salmo salar*) against salmonid rickettsial septicaemia. Vaccine 29, 2336–2340.

Van Muiswinkel, W.B., Nakao, M., 2014. A short history of research on immunity to infectious diseases in fish. Dev Comp Immunol. 43, 130–150.

Vandenberg, G.W., 2004. Oral vaccines for finfish: academic theory or commercial reality? Anim. Health Res. Rev. 5, 301–304.

Villumsen, K.R., Raida, M.K., 2013. Long-lasting protection induced by bath vaccination against *Aeromonas salmonicida* subsp. *salmonicida* in rainbow trout. Fish Shellfish Immunol. 35, 1649–1653.

Vimal, S., Abdul Majeed, S., Taju, G., Nambi, K.S., Sundar Raj, N., Madan, N., Farook, M.A., Rajkumar, T., Gopinath, D., Sahul Hameed, A.S., 2013. Chitosan tripolyphosphate (CS/TPP) nanoparticles: preparation, characterization and application for gene delivery in shrimp. Acta Trop. 128, 486–493.

Watts, M., Munday, B.L., Burke, C.M., 2001. Immune responses of teleost fish. Aust. Vet. J. 79, 570–574.

Wietz, M., Mansson, M., Bowman, J.S., Blom, N., Ng, Y., Gram, L., 2012. Wide distribution of closely related, antibiotic-producing *Arthrobacter* strains throughout the Arctic Ocean. Appl. Environ. Microbiol. 78, 2039–2042.

Wise, D.J., Klesius, P.H., Shoemaker, C.A., Wolters, W.R., 2000. Vaccination of mixed and full-sib families of channel catfish *Ictalurus punctatus* against septicemia of catfish with a live attenuated *Edwardsiella ictaluri* isolate (RE-33). J. World Aquacult. Soc. 31, 206–212.

World Bank, 2013. Fish to 2030: prospects for fisheries and aquaculture. Online at: http://documents.worldbank.org/curated/en/2013/12/18882045/fish-2030-prospects-fisheries-aquaculture.

Xue, R., Liu, L., Cao, G., Xu, S., Li, J., Zou, Y., Chen, H., Gong, C., 2013. Oral vaccination of BacFish-vp6 against grass carp reovirus evoking antibody response in grass carp. Fish Shellfish Immunol. 34, 348–355.

Mucosal immunity in mollusks

12

Bassem Allam; Emmanuelle Pales Espinosa
School of Marine and Atmospheric Sciences, Stony Brook University, Stony Brook, New York, USA

Chapter Outline

12.1 Introduction

In the extraordinarily diverse world of invertebrates, *Mollusca* (from the Latin word "mollis," meaning soft) is one of the major animal phyla on earth and in the oceans with about 100,000 described species of recent organisms and 35,000 extinct species (Ruppert et al., 2004), making this group the second largest phylum of animals after the arthropods. Another particularity of mollusks is the incredible dissimilarities

Mucosal Health in Aquaculture

(internal and external morphology, size, and habitat) between the species that compose the group. It is difficult to believe that limpet, clam, snail, octopus, and squid are all mollusks (Pechenik, 2000)! However, they share some characteristics that distinguish the members from other phyla. Mollusks feature a soft, unsegmented body that consists of three basic parts: a muscular foot, a visceral mass, and a mantle. Their soft tissue is covered with mucus secretions that provide an efficient physical barrier to help isolate these animals from their environment and provide protection (Simkiss and Wilbur, 1977). They usually harbor a calcium carbonate shell and a radula, or a rasping tongue that is unique to this group (Castro and Huber, 1997). This phylum is divided into 7 or 8 classes (Barnes et al., 1993; Pechenik, 2000), two of which, the gastropods and the bivalves, contain 98% of the known living species (Barnes et al., 1993).

Mollusks represent an important source of food and valuable goods (shell, pearl) around the world. In 2012, 22.1 million tons of mollusks were captured or produced from seas or inland waters worldwide (FAO, 2014), representing a commercial value of about 27 billion US dollars. Clams, cockles, and ark shells represent the most important group produced with 5.6 million tons. By continent, Asia is by far the first producer with 13.9 million tons, followed by Europe with 0.6 million tons. Aquaculture production represented 70% of landings in 2012. A continuous growth over the last few decades has resulted in a doubling of production in the last 15 years (Figure 12.1). Over 86% of the production was made by members of the suspension-feeding bivalves (Lamellibranchia or Pelecypoda) such as clams, oysters, and mussels (Figure 12.1).

The growing economic importance of mollusks has been associated with an increased awareness of and attention to infectious diseases affecting these animals. Currently, there are eight infectious diseases impacting mollusks that are listed by the Office International des Epizooties (OIE, the World Organization for Animal Health),

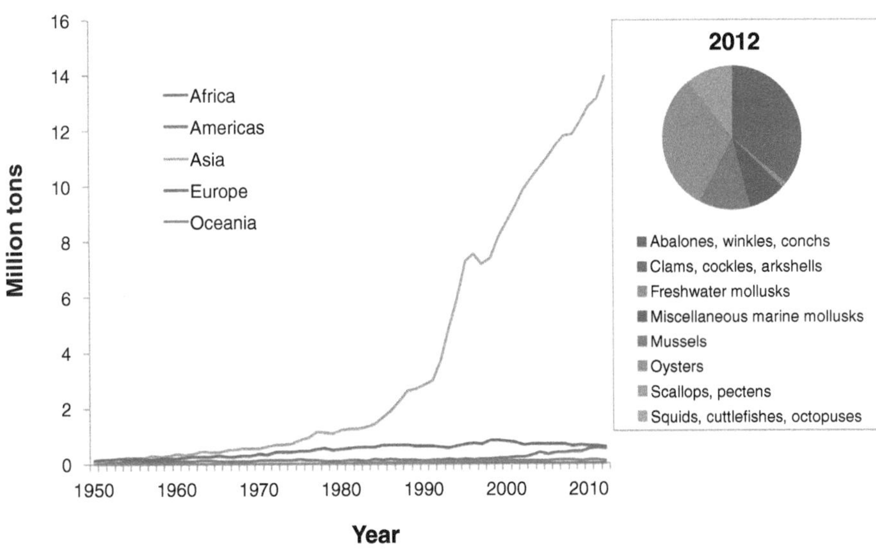

Figure 12.1 Mollusk aquaculture production worldwide between 1950 and 2012 (data from the FAO).

including two viral infections, a prokaryote infection, and five infections caused by protist pathogens. There has also been a growing interest in the study of molluscan immunity and in the exploration of mechanisms used by these organisms to fight and resist infectious agents (Cheng, 1981; Bayne, 1983; Fisher, 1988; Bachère et al., 1995; Loker, 2010; Song et al., 2010). However, most of these investigations targeted internal immune effectors associated with the circulating hemolymph (blood), and very little attention has been given to defense factors associated with molluscan mucosal surfaces. In fact, while a rich body of literature exists on host–pathogen interactions in mollusks once infection is established, the interactions of microbes and their hosts at interfaces during initial encounters remain poorly characterized. The current knowledge on these early host–pathogen interactions in mollusks is exacerbated by the fact that most economically important infections affecting these animals are not vector-transmitted (besides infections caused by *Perkinsus marinus* in the American oyster that was shown to be facultatively transmitted by the blood-feeding snail *Boonea impressa*) (White et al., 1987), implying the primary role of mucosal surfaces in initial interactions with invading microbes. This chapter summarizes some of the information available on the characteristics of mucosal tissues and mucosal secretions in mollusks and their role in host–microbe interactions and overall animal health.

12.2 Molluscan mucosal epithelia

The morphological diversity of mollusks is translated into a large structural and anatomical diversity among different taxa (i.e., presence or absence of various organs such as shell, adductor muscles, foot, etc.). In fact, there is not a single obvious key character present throughout the phylum (Trueman and Clarke, 1988). Some of the general characteristics include the presence of a simple epidermis made of a single layer of cells covered with mucus secretion and supported by a basement membrane. The three main cell types of the molluscan skin are microvillated epidermal cells, ciliated cells, and glandular cells (i.e., mucocytes, Figure 12.2). These three generic cell types are the main constituents of the epithelia of both the external and internal organs. Additional cell types present in some species (i.e., common octopus) include pigmented cells known as chromatophores. The skin (external epithelium of the mantle, for instance) supports the production of the shell that provides the first line of physical defense. Another common morphological feature is the pallial cavity, which is the space outside the body wall delimited by the mantle, or pallium, and that contains respiratory organs, such as ctenidia or gills, or that itself constitutes improvised lungs in some groups (i.e., pulmonates). The spatial extent and role of the pallial cavity are very diverse among the different taxa, ranging from a semi-open, large cavity that encloses the entire soft tissue in bivalves (Figure 12.3) to a partial or complete loss of the cavity in the opisthobranch gastropods (Lindberg and Ponder, 2001). The pallial cavity represents a major interface for exchange between suspension-feeding bivalves and the aquatic environment. The mantle in suspension-feeding bivalves is constituted by two simple epithelial layers separated by a connective tissue: an external layer supporting the shell and a mucus-rich internal layer delimiting the pallial cavity

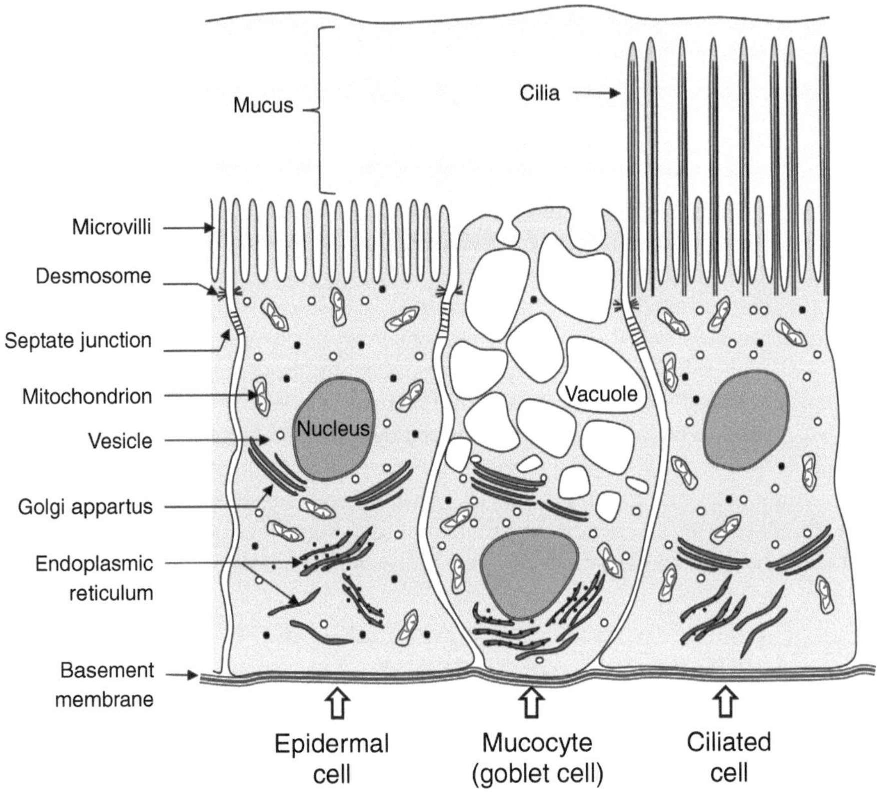

Figure 12.2 Schematic representation of the three main types of epithelial cells in mollusks (redrawn from Simkiss (1988)). Not to scale.

(Figure 12.3). In these animals, the pallial cavity encloses a pair of semi-branchiate gills that allow the capture of oxygen and food particles. The gills, also covered by a simple mucus-rich epithelium, are well irrigated by the blood (hemolymph) and are highly convoluted to increase gas exchange (Figure 12.3). Particles captured during the suspension-feeding process are directed towards the labial palps that contribute to the processing of food particles. The foot, when present, is delimited by a relatively thin epithelium covered by a thick layer of mucus produced, for the most part, by sub-epithelial mucosal glands (Figure 12.3). The opening and closing of the pallial cavity as well as water flow over the pallial organs are tightly controlled by the animal. Respiration and feeding activities expose the soft tissues of the pallial organs (mantle, gills, labial palps, foot, and body wall) to an extremely large amount of waterborne microbes. For example, oysters filter over 10 L h-1 g-1 of dry tissue (Jordan, 1987), equating to over 25,000 microbes/s, considering that a 1 g oyster and a modest 10^4 microbes ml^{-1} of seawater-microbial concentration in estuarine areas is often orders of magnitude higher. The convolution of pallial organs also greatly increases the effective surface of these interfaces and enhances their exposure to waterborne microbes, highlighting the need for an efficient defense system associated with the pallial mucosa.

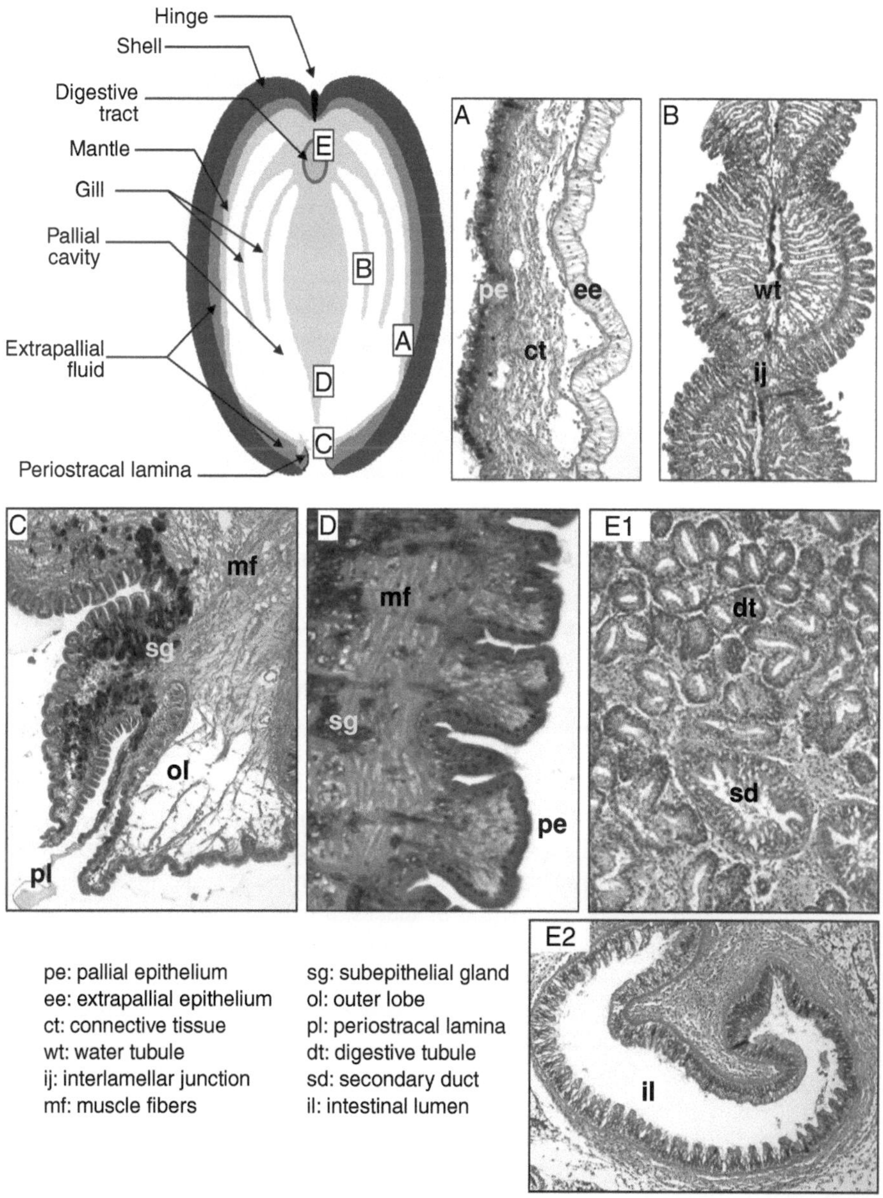

Figure 12.3 A–E Main mucosal epithelia in bivalves.

As in vertebrates, epithelium lining the digestive tract represents another important mucosal interface that can mediate pathogen acquisition. The structure of the digestive tract is diverse between and within each molluscan class with common traits in commercially important bivalves, including the presence of a relatively short esophagus, a stomach equipped with a gastric shield, and a crystalline style that "grinds" food particles by rotating movements, a digestive diverticula (or gland), and a fairly narrow intestine that convolutes into several intestinal loops (Salvini-Plawen, 1988; Langdon and Newell, 1996). Nevertheless, because of its efficient mechanical and chemical processes, the bivalve digestive tract seems to represent a good barrier against infectious agents, and most fatal infections affecting bivalve mollusks are initiated in pallial organs. This is the case of the protist parasites *Haplosporidium nelsoni* (MSX) and Quahog Parasite Unknown (QPX), which affect the oyster *Crassostrea virginica* and the clam *Mercenaria mercenaria*, respectively (Ragone Calvo et al., 1998; Smolowitz et al., 1998; Ford et al., 2002; Burreson and Ford, 2004; Dahl et al., 2010b). The paramyxean *Marteilia sydneyi* has also been shown to initiate infections in the pallial organs of oysters (Kleeman et al., 2002). This route of infection seems to be common to members of the genus *Perkinsus*, which infect clams and oysters worldwide (Azevedo, 1989; Navas et al., 1992; Rodriguez and Navas, 1995; Villalba et al., 2004; Allam et al., 2013a), further stressing the role of pallial mucosa in host–microbe interactions.

12.3 Mucus matrix composition and structure

Mucus is a slimy fluid that, in metazoans, is secreted by submucosal glands or specialized cells (goblet, club, and mucocytes) lining epithelia. It is made of water, mucin-like molecules (protein-polysaccharide complex), electrolytes, epithelial and blood cells, and a wide range of bioactive molecules produced by mucus-secreting cells (Schachter and Williams, 1982). In metazoans, mucus is produced by all epithelia that have living cells on their surfaces such as on the internal organs of vertebrates (i.e., gastrointestinal and tracheobronchial tracts) and the epidermis of amphibians, fish, cnidarians, and mollusks. Simkiss and Wilbur (1977) reported that mucus in mollusks is often the resulting product of various glands/groups of mucocytes, some of which are specialized in the production of mucus with a specific viscosity, mixed with exudates from epithelial cells (i.e., the limpet snail (*Patella vulgata*) (Grenon and Walker, 1978); or the American oyster (*Crassostrea virginica*) (Beninger and Dufour, 1996)). The consistency, viscosity, and elasticity of mucus are generally attributed to polymers within the gel and to the physical entanglement of these polymers with other molecules (Rose et al., 1984; Audie et al., 1993; Smith, 2002). These polymers are mucoproteins associated with carbohydrates, such as high molecular weight mucins and mucin-like glycoproteins 200 kDa–200 MDa (Kesimer and Sheehan, 2012) that are heavily glycosylated (up to 90% of carbohydrates) with short carbohydrate chains (Allen, 1977; Hafez, 1977; Silberberg and Meyer, 1982; Andersch-Björkman et al., 2007), whose charges are slightly negative. These oligosaccharide chains are either O-linked (most common) or N-linked to asparagine residues of the proteins (Gottschalk, 1972; Pearson et al., 1982). Although most mucins share these general features, they differ in complexity with regard to their saccharide chains, polypeptide backbones, and related physical properties (Rose et al., 1984). The viscoelasticity of mucus depends on the polymers concentration (Wolf et al., 1977; Cone, 2009) and cross-linkage between polymeric compounds. Thus, when mucin concentrations reach

2–4%, the molecules entangle and form a gel (Allen, 1977). At low concentrations of mucins, however, the viscosity of mucus can be equal to that of water (Cone, 2009). In addition to large mucin-type glycoproteins, mucus matrices in marine invertebrates, including mollusks, have also been found to contain repetitive, highly sulfated polysaccharides (Smith, 2002; Coddeville et al., 2011) and a wide variety of bioactive molecules (Rollins-Smith et al., 2005; Moraes et al., 2006; Pales Espinosa et al., 2009; Pales Espinosa and Allam, 2013). Based on the biochemical diversity of molecules contained in mucus, it is not surprising that these gels are involved in various functions as speculated by Auld as early as 1920. It should be noted that mucus secretions in metazoans are three-dimensionally structured with the presence of two distinct layers covering epithelial cells (Ross and Corrsin, 1974). The first layer is in direct contact with the cells and is often made of low viscosity mucus that allows for tetherless cilia beating. The external layer is typically made of viscous secretions that entrap environmental and commensal microbes and is directed by cilia movements. The viscoelasticity of mucus secretions is primordial and has to be perfectly regulated in order to ensure normal transport of particles along epithelial surfaces (Wolf et al., 1977). This two-layered model has also been confirmed in bivalves and seems to represent a general model for mucociliary transport in metazoans (Beninger et al., 1997).

12.4 The diverse functions of mollusk mucus

Mucus is produced from virtually all molluscan epithelia (Simkiss and Wilbur, 1977) and plays a role in several biological functions (Davies and Hawkins, 1998) such as locomotion and navigation (Barr, 1926; Prezant and Chalermwat, 1984; Denny, 1989; Smith et al., 1999; Smith, 2002), freeze protection (Hargens and Shabica, 1973), attachment (Smith, 2002), and defense against predators (Gavagnin et al., 1994). One of the major functions of mucus is protection of coated organs against physical, chemical, and biological damages (Schmidt-Nielsen et al., 1971; Hargens and Shabica, 1973). Thus, mucus secretions are known to protect animals against desiccation. When exposed to air, gastropods (such as limpets and snails) produce a thin layer of mucus as a mechanism for minimizing desiccation (Wolcott, 1973; Denny, 1989) or damages caused by freezing temperatures (Hargens and Shabica, 1973). Interestingly, mollusks have also been reported to be able to sequester in their mucus poison from their food and use this toxin to avoid predators (Gustafson and Andersen, 1985; Avila et al., 1991). In addition, mucus gels containing low percentages of polymers reduce friction between moving surfaces and are widely used by animals as lubricants (Simkiss and Wilbur, 1977; Smith et al., 1999). Mucus is also commonly used in mollusks to trap and transport particles on ciliated epithelia for cleansing or feeding through mucociliary transport (Morton, 1977). Most prior work investigating bivalve pallial mucus was performed in the framework of studies of the suspension-feeding process (reviewed in Ward and Shumway, 2004). Mucus is involved in all of these steps (Beninger et al., 1993; Ward et al., 1993; Barille and Cognie, 2000; Urrutia et al., 2001). Particles directed as pseudofeces are embedded in mucus and rejected back into the environment as masses of mucoid substances, entangling live unwanted cells, debris, and abiotic material of low nutritional value. Those directed to the mouth are ingested in a cohesive mucus string. The pallial mucus layer is also the first host factor encountered by microbes that attach to the surface of pallial organs before the establishment of mutualistic (i.e., sulfo-oxidant bacteria in gill bacteriocytes) or parasitic (most lethal parasites of bivalves initiate infection in pallial organs) associations (Burreson and Ford, 2004; Villalba et al., 2004; Dubilier et al., 2008; Dahl et al., 2010a; Allam et al., 2013b). In other words, pallial mucus is involved in the processing of any and all waterborne microbes entering the pallial cavity that are captured by the pallial organs, regardless of whether it leads to predation, mutualism, commensalism, or parasitism. Therefore, an efficient processing of waterborne microbes by pallial mucus is essential for bivalves to maintain their health given the extraordinarily large number of microbes they encounter through their suspension-feeding. Owing it to their role as a barrier against diffusion (Grimm-Jørgensen et al., 1986) and in selective ion transport (Ahn et al., 1988), mucosal secretions also play an important role in animal response to changes in the chemical composition of their surrounding environment (Sze and Lee, 1995). The importance of mucus in the biology of these animals is well reflected in the energy allocated to mucus production, sometimes exceeding 15% of the total energy gained from food (Davies and Hawkins, 1998).

12.5 Host–microbe interactions at mucosal interfaces in metazoans

For both vertebrates and invertebrates, mucosal epithelial tissues represent the major interface for exchange between animals and their environment, and mucus itself is one of the most important lines of defense against microbial invaders. The primary role of mucosal immunity in maintaining animal health is now well recognized in vertebrates. Mucus itself is an excellent physical barrier to cells or microorganisms. The net created by cross-linked glycoproteins (mucoprotein matrices) contained in mucus traps microorganisms before they can reach the soft tissues. In addition to representing an efficient physical barrier, mucus matrices contain various cells and bioactive molecules and have gained prominence in the last few decades as a main component of the innate and acquired immune system.

Understandably, the most recent research on the role of mucus in host–microbe interactions was performed on medically relevant models, and results highlight an intriguing central role of these surfaces in animal health with an elaborate mechanism of feedback controls for the maintenance of mucosal (and overall host) homeostasis. This results in the establishment of a robust, but well-controlled, population of adapted microbes. Any alteration to this balance (i.e., changes in mucus physicochemical characteristics) can lead to a dramatic change in microbial dynamics, resulting in infection and disease.

Due to its carbohydrate- and protein-rich composition, mucus is an excellent environment for microorganism growth (Cognie and Barille, 1999; Davies and Beckwith, 1999;

Koren and Rosenberg, 2006; Ritchie, 2006; Laabir et al., 2007) that can, in turn, produce molecules that enter in the mucus composition (Banin et al., 2001) or that alter host mucus (Brun et al., 2000). In fact, the adhesion of pathogenic microorganisms to mucosal surfaces is considered to be the first step in many infections in vertebrates and invertebrates (Paerregaard et al., 1991; Allam et al., 1996; Finlay and Falkow, 1997; Tuomola et al., 1999). Glycoproteins and peptidoglycans contained in mucus promote sugar–protein interactions that lead to the recognition and adhesion of microorganisms via adhesins that bind specific mucosal ligands. Among microbial adhesins, lectins are proteins that exhibit high structural diversity and specifically and reversibly bind to carbohydrate moieties associated, for example, with extracellular matrices (i.e., mucins) or those covering living host cells (Olafsen, 1986; Fisher and Dinuzzo, 1991). Microbes often have multiple lectins with different carbohydrate specificities, and modulation of surface receptor density or topographical distributions of these receptors on cell membranes regulates adhesion. As an example, *Helicobacter pylori* binds to mucin oligosaccharides via at least four adhesins, which differ substantially with anatomical sites along the digestive tract, infection route, mucin type, pH, and disease status (Teneberg et al., 1997; Mahdavi et al., 2002; Lindén et al., 2004). Thus, for *H. pylori*, binding to mucins (and host colonization) differs along the oral-to-gastric niches and during long-term infection. At the same time, host mucosal lectins can serve as anchor sites for carbohydrates present on microbial surfaces (Cash et al., 2006; Pales Espinosa et al., 2009, 2010b; 2010c).

Previous studies on marine animals have shown that mucus secretions can favor the attachment and growth of adapted (or specialized) microbes and mediate symbiont recognition. For instance, fish mucus contains factors that enhance or inhibit the growth of different bacterial species (Ebran et al., 1999; Nagashima et al., 2003; Vine et al., 2004). In fact, the involvement of mucus in facilitating symbiotic association is not surprising and has been demonstrated in several marine invertebrates. For example, bacterial growth is enhanced, including that of the opportunistic pathogen *Vibrio alginolyticus*, in media supplemented with coral mucus (Ducklow and Mitchell, 1979; Ritchie, 2006). Always in corals, bacterial communities living in the surface mucus layer have been found to be different from those present in the water column, suggesting that mucus recruits and maintains specific microorganisms (Brown and Bythell, 2005; Ritchie, 2006). Similarly, the mucus of the nematode *Laxus oneistus* was shown to contain a C-type lectin that has been suggested to facilitate the aggregation and recruitment of symbionts (Bulgheresi et al., 2006). Even though the examples from mollusks are very limited, accumulated evidence suggests that the colonization of mucus represents the first step in specific interactions between waterborne microbes and their hosts. In their investigations of host/symbiont association in the squid *Euprymna scolopes*, Nyholm and collaborators (Nyholm et al. 2000; Nyholm and McFall-Ngai 2003) demonstrated that the symbiont *Vibrio fischeri* specifically accumulates and remains retained within the mucus, covering the squid's light organ. Davidson (Davidson et al., 2004) further demonstrated that mucus actually regulates the dynamics of microbial communities of the light organ to favor the survival and growth of *V. fischeri*. These studies concluded that the specificity of the squid-*Vibrio* symbiosis begins early in the interaction within the mucus itself. In another squid species, *Illex argentinus*, mucus was suggested to trap and fertilize microorganisms entering

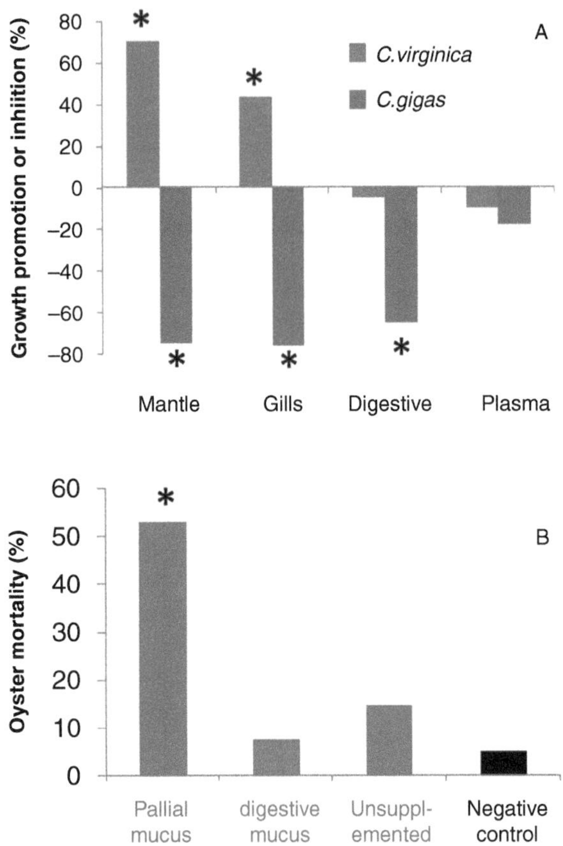

Figure 12.4 Effect of oyster pallial mucus on *Perkinsus marinus* growth (A) and virulence (B). In (B), *P. marinus* cultures were supplemented with *Crassostrea virginica* mucus before injection into the pallial cavity of naive oysters. *indicates significant difference as compared to unsupplemented cultures (data from Pales Espinosa et al. 2013).

in the diet of young individuals (Vidal and Haimovici, 1998). In symbiotic members of *Thyasiridae* (venerid bivalves), pallial mucus is thought to be the main contributor to the recruitment of chemosynthetic bacterial symbionts (Southward, 1986; Dufour, 2005). Recent investigations in the oyster *Crassostrea virginica* showed significant regulation of the proliferation and virulence of the alveolate parasite *Perkinsus marinus* following exposure to host mucus (Allam et al., 2013b; Pales Espinosa et al., 2013, 2014a). While mucus collected from oyster pallial organs enhanced the proliferation of the parasite (the mantle in particular), mucus collected from the digestive gland was inhibitory (Figure 12.4). Interestingly, pallial mucus of the noncompatible host, the Pacific oyster (*Crassostrea gigas*), was strongly inhibitory, suggesting that *P. marinus* host specificity may begin in the mucus (Pales Espinosa et al., 2013). The *in vivo* virulence of *P. marinus* was also significantly enhanced when the parasite was exposed to pallial mucus from *C. virginica*. Mortality was significantly higher (up to 10-fold) in oysters injected with parasite cultures supplemented with pallial mucus as compared to oysters injected with parasite cells supplemented with digestive mucus or unsupplemented cultures (Figure 12.4). RNASeq experiments showed that increased *in vivo* virulence of *P. marinus* following exposure to mucus was associated with a significant up-regulation of potent virulence-related factors (Pales Espinosa et al., 2014a).

It should be noted that specialized microbes are capable of altering the structure and composition of mucus, and this is an important feature of pathogenesis. For example, the protozoan parasite *Entamoeba histolytica* uses its cysteine proteases to cleave the mammalian MUC2 mucin (a major structural component of the mucus of higher vertebrates), causing a local disintegration of mucus. Similarly, most mucosal viruses produce neuraminidases capable of degrading mucin carbohydrates, and these enzymes are a basic requirement for their pathogenicity (Linden et al., 2008).

Overall, mucus offers numerous advantages for microbes. Microbes capable of colonizing mucus can avoid rapid expulsion from the host. Microbial colonization of mucus may, thus, lead to a growth advantage. Both commensal and pathogenic bacteria would derive significant benefits from an ability to chemically regulate mucus synthesis or secretion, and, in fact, many of these microbes do so (Chadee and Meerovitch, 1985; Mack et al., 1999). For example, the cholera toxin of *Vibrio cholerae* triggers a massive secretion and release of mucin via a cAMP-dependent mechanism (Lencer et al., 1990; Epple et al., 1997). Another well-described example of direct microbial effects on mucus secretion is the case of *E. histolytica*, which regulates the synthesis and release of mucus from the intestinal mucosa (Chadee et al., 1991; Keller et al., 1992). Increases in mucus production were also reported in mucus-producing cell lines following exposure to specific Gram-positive (i.e., *Staphylococcus aureus*) and -negative (i.e., *P. aeruginosa* or *E. coli*) bacteria (Dohrman et al., 1998; Li et al., 1998). In contrast, other infectious agents, such as *Clostridium difficile*, were shown to inhibit mucus secretions (Branka et al., 1997). A similar inhibition of mucin synthesis and release with down-regulation of mucin-producing genes MUC1 and MUC5AC was noted in response to *H. pylori* (Micots et al., 1993; Byrd et al., 2000). Bioactive molecules that are present in mucus secretions may also be altered by infectious microbes. For example, Sperandio et al. (2008) has reported that virulent *Shigella flexneri* is able to suppress the transcription of several host genes encoding antimicrobial peptides, including a β-defensin, allowing for progression of the pathogen in the human intestine. Similarly, live enterobacteria *Salmonella enterica* serovar Typhimurium decreases the expression of defensins and lysozyme in the small intestinal crypts of mice (Salzman et al., 2003). Finally, the infection of Atlantic salmon by salmon louse (*Lepeophtheirus salmonis*) causes a significant change in mucus composition and, more specifically, protease activity (Firth et al., 2000).

There is undeniable evidence that host mucus can serve not only as an anchor site, but also as a trigger that allows adapted microbes to initiate the machinery needed for colonization (and invasion, in the case of pathogens). Interestingly, there appears to be a correlation between the type of glycoconjugate to which microbes preferentially bind and the glycoconjugate-cleavage machinery of the respective microorganisms

(Hoyer et al., 1992; Slomiany et al., 1992; Bravo and Correa, 1999; Vimal et al., 2000). Furthermore, it has been suggested that adhesion to mucin can trigger the production of various mucolytic strategies to overcome mucus entrapment. For example, the hemagglutinin protease A of *V. cholerae*, which has both mucinolytic and cytotoxic activity, is induced by mucin. This causes a reduction of the viscosity of mucus, allowing the bacteria to move easily through the matrix and reach the epithelial cells (Silva et al., 2003). Intestinal mucus significantly enhances the production of toxins and the *in vivo* virulence of *E. coli* (Melton-Celsa et al., 1996). Similarly, salmon gastrointestinal mucus induces the production of a metalloprotease in the bacteria *V. anguillarum* (Denkin and Nelson 1999). Fish skin mucus also caused a change in the proteomic profile of *V. salmonicida* with overexpression of the proteins involved in bacterial motility (Uttakleiv Ræder et al., 2007).

The fact that both commensal and pathogenic microbes are capable of attaching and degrading mucus highlights the imbricated ecological issues associated with mucus involvement in pathogen resistance compared to its mediation of colonization by beneficial bacteria (Deplancke and Gaskins, 2001). As stated above, mucus production and composition have a direct impact on microbes, which themselves can alter and regulate mucus secretion both in vertebrates and invertebrates. Therefore, available data indicates that direct cross-talk between microbes and mucus-producing cells is likely. This leads to changes in mucus quantity and quality in response to cues received from commensals, pathogens, or both (Deplancke and Gaskins, 2001). Such changes can induce some commensals to become transient opportunistic pathogens or can cause complete alteration in the microbial flora favoring pathogens. This is particularly true in the marine environment where the limit between commensals and opportunistic pathogens may be extremely small. Indeed, many opportunistic pathogens affecting marine organisms are ubiquitous in the environment and are considered common inhabitants of their hosts, only causing infection and disease under conditions that are unfavorable to this host (environmental stress, reproductive status, etc.) (reviewed in Burge et al., 2013).

12.6 Mucosal immunity in mollusks

In higher vertebrates, it is currently recognized that microbes colonizing mucosal surfaces serve as a primary stimulus for the development of both innate and acquired components of the immune system (Gaskins, 1997). Mucosal surfaces of higher vertebrates contain a wide range of innate and adaptive immune factors, including potent antimicrobial factors such as defensins, cathelicidins, and lysozymes as well as immunoglobulin A (IgA), the main antibody present in mucus (Sansonetti, 2004). Vertebrate mucus secretions were also found to contain protease inhibitors (Fritz, 1988; Kido et al., 1992) as well as several cytokines (i.e., IL-4, IL-6 or anti-inflammatory IL-10). These cytokines are regulated in response to infectious and noninfectious diseases (Scavuzzo et al., 2003). In contrast, mollusks lack the specificity and long-lasting memory of the adaptive immune system to fight pathogens and they only rely on their "generic" innate immune factors even though recent research suggested a certain level of specificity and "memory" in the innate immune system of invertebrates (Kurtz and Franz, 2003; Loker et al., 2004; Rowley and Powell, 2007; Song et al., 2010; Zhang et al., 2014). Because of their location, molluscan mucosal tissues have developed a wide range of defense mechanisms in response to exposure to microbial attacks. The components of mucosal immunity in the mollusks described here include pathogen recognition factors, mechanisms of immune activation, and cell signaling and effectors of innate immunity (antimicrobial proteins, hydrolytic enzymes, and antioxidant molecules) as well as phagocytic activities of the cellular components of the mucosa.

12.7 Immune recognition

The ability of an organism to distinguish between self and non-self is a crucial step in innate immunity. Recognition and/or adhesion is essential to properly recognize and initiate the destruction of invaders or nonhealthy cells. Invertebrates have developed a complex system of designated pattern recognition receptors (PRR) made of dissolved or cell surface-associated proteins that are able to identify microbe-associated molecular patterns (MAMP) present mostly in microorganisms (such as bacterial lipopolysaccharides and peptidoglycans or fungal glycans) as well as damage-associated molecular patterns (DAMP) expressed by damaged host cells. Several groups of PRRs have been identified in mollusks (Ford, 1992; Loker, 2010; Song et al., 2010), but information on PRRs in molluscan mucosa (i.e., epithelial cells or mucus) is extremely scarce. Previous findings highlight the presence of peptidoglycan recognition proteins (PGRP), lectins, and thioester-containing proteins (TEP) in mucosa.

12.7.1 Peptidoglycan recognition proteins

Peptidoglycan recognition proteins have only been identified very recently in mucosal secretions of the eastern oyster (Pales Espinosa et al., 2014b) even though several transcripts coding for PGRPs have been shown to be specifically expressed in mucosal tissues. For example, four cDNA sequences of PGRPs (namely, CgPGRP-S1S, CgPGRP-S1L, CgPGRP -S2, and CgPGRP -S3) were identified by Itoh and Takahashi (2008) in the Pacific oyster (*Crassostrea gigas*) and were suggested to play a role in bacterial recognition. A phylogenetic analysis indicated that the four PGRPs were similar to each other, but, more interestingly, they showed different tissue expression patterns, suggesting specific roles in various host tissues. For instance, CgPGRP-S1S was expressed only in the mantle and the gill (mucus-rich organs exposed to waterborne microbes), -S1L only, but strongly, in the mantle, -S2 weakly in the hemocytes, and -S3 in the digestive diverticula (also an important mucus-rich organ exposed to environmental microbes). The same authors noted that the cDNA sequences of PGRPs expressed in the mantle and the gills (CgPGRP-S1S and -S1L) also contain β-defensin-like (antimicrobial peptide) domains and suggested that these molecules act as antimicrobial proteins. The study did not report a precise location in organs (epithelial, connective, etc.), but, due the presumed defense function, it is assumed that three of these molecules (except CgPGRP-S2, which was expressed in hemocytes) contribute to mucosal immunity in organs that are exposed to bacterial invasions.

Another pattern recognition protein, namely HdPRP, was identified in the abalone *Haliotis discus discus* (Nikapitiya et al., 2008). Phylogenetic analysis grouped HdPRP with the PRPs identified from other mollusk species, including *Biomphalaria glabrata* peptidoglycan recognition proteins (BgGRP) and *Chlamys farreri* lipopolysaccharides and peptidoglycans-binding protein (CfLGBP). HdPRP was mostly expressed in the gill, whereas the expression level is slightly lower in the mantle and the digestive tract and weak in hepatopancreas and hemocytes. Challenge experiments showed that mRNA expression of HdPRP increases significantly following the injection of *Vibrio alginolyticus*, lipopolysaccharides (LPS) and beta-1,3-glucan (cell wall of yeast). The authors concluded that HdPRP plays an important role in the abalone immune defense mechanism. Again, even though this study did not provide a precise location of HdPRP in tissues, the preponderance of its expression in pallial organs suggests that it may be involved in mucosal immunity.

12.7.2 Lectins

The most significant progress in the understanding of immune recognition in molluscan mucosal tissues was made on lectins. The term "lectin" commonly refers to a wide range of carbohydrate-binding proteins and glycoproteins. Most of these molecules are organized as homo-oligomers or hetero-oligomers of noncovalently bound polypeptide subunits displaying one or more carbohydrate-recognition domains (CRD) that bind to their corresponding sugar ligands, usually a nonreducing terminal monosaccharide or oligosaccharide (reviewed in Vasta, 2009). They recognize and bind carbohydrates present on cell surfaces of several unicellular organisms, agglutinating and enhancing the destruction of microbes by specialized immune cells (reviewed in Olafsen, 1986). Lectins, including C-type lectins and galectins, are known to serve multiple purposes in the immune system (Weiss et al., 1998; Zelensky and Gready, 2005; Vasta, 2009). In molluscan mucosa, lectins or lectin-like activities have been described in gastropods (Fountain and Campbell, 1984; Iguchi et al., 1985), in cephalopods (Marthy, 1974) and in bivalves (McDade and Tripp, 1967b; Fisher, 1992; Tripp, 1992; Pales Espinosa et al., 2009, 2010b, 2011; Jing et al., 2011). These molecules were shown to be involved in microbial binding, for the most part, and no bactericidal activity has been demonstrated for mucosal lectins so far.

Fountain and collaborators (Fountain, 1985; Fountain and Campbell, 1984) purified and characterized a lectin-like molecule in the mucus of the snail *Helix aspersa*. This molecule was able to agglutinate rabbit red blood cells, and this agglutination activity was inhibited by *N*-acetyl-galactosamine (GalNAc) and, to a lesser extent, by *N*-acetyl-glucosamine (GlcNAc) and galactose. The authors concluded that this agglutinin represents an important component of the mucosal immunity of the snail. Mitra (Mitra et al., 1988) identified an agglutinin from the mucus of another snail species, *Achatina fulica*. In this case, inhibition tests showed specificity for galactose residues. A C-type lectin (achatinin) was also isolated from the mucus of the giant African snail (*Achatina fulica*). This lectin did not show any bactericidal activity but was able to agglutinate vertebrate red blood cells, and its activity was inhibited by *N*-acetyl-neuraminic acid (Iguchi et al., 1985). More recently, another lectin, AfHML, was also purified from the mucus of *A. fulica* (Itoh et al., 2011). In the presence of calcium, this lectin was able to agglutinate rabbit red blood cells as well as Gram-positive and Gram-negative bacteria, and its activity was inhibited by galactose. AfHML, however, did not inhibit bacterial growth. Tissue immunolocalization of AfHML revealed that the lectin was expressed in the tissues of the mantle collar. Based on these results, these two lectins were suggested to play a role in the agglutination and immobilization of pathogens, but not in their direct destruction.

References are very rare on the presence of mucosal lectins in cephalopods, and only one study reports the presence of a hemagglutinin from the epithelial mucus of the European squid *Loligo vulgaris* (Marthy, 1974). In contrast, several lectins or agglutinins have been found in bivalve mucus. The presence of "agglutinins" in the pallial mucus of the eastern (American) oyster (*Crassostrea virginica*) was initially reported in 1967(b) by McDade and Tripp. In 1992, Fisher reported that *C. virginica* pallial mucus agglutinates a variety of bacteria, including *Aeromonas hydrophila*, *Vibrio cholerae*, and *V. fluvialis*. More recently, studies have shown that mucus covering the gills and labial palps of *C. virginica* (Pales Espinosa et al., 2009) and *Mytilus edulis* (Pales Espinosa et al., 2010a) agglutinates red blood cells and several microalgae species. Agglutination was inhibited to various degrees by different carbohydrates, suggesting the presence of several lectins in mucus. Further, several putative C-type lectins have been identified in the transcriptomes of the oyster *C. virginica* (CvML) (Jing et al., 2011), *C. gigas* (CgCLec-1) (Yamaura et al., 2008), and the mussel *M. edulis* (MeML) (Pales Espinosa et al., 2010b). Gene transcription analysis coupled with *in situ* hybridization revealed that CvML and MeML were specifically localized in mucocytes lining the epithelium of the pallial organs (Figure 12.5), while CgCLec-1 was expressed only in the digestive gland. In addition, CvML and MeML gene transcription levels were significantly up-regulated after bivalve starvation, suggesting that these molecules are involved in food particle capture (Pales Espinosa et al., 2010b, 2013; Jing et al., 2011). More interestingly, CvML mRNA levels increased significantly in oysters exposed to a bacterial challenge, *Vibrio alginolyticus*, but only following bath exposure and not bacterial injection into the circulatory system, which shows that this lectin responds to external cues associated with the presence of pathogens in the pallial cavity, but not in tissues, and highlights its role in mucosal immunity (Jing et al., 2011). In the symbiotic clam *Codakia orbicularis*, which harbors sulfo-oxidant bacteria in its gills, a calcium-dependent C-type lectin (codakine) was identified and purified from gill tissues (Gourdine et al., 2007). These authors hypothesized this lectin to be involved in the recognition of symbiotic and possibly pathogenic bacteria alike. Finally, several lectins (including a galectin and a c-type lectin) were up-regulated in mantle tissues, and hemocytes transmigrated to the extrapallial cavity in clams affected by brown ring disease, a shell disease caused by *Vibrio tapetis* (Allam et al., 2014). Similar trends were also identified for several immunoglobulin-like sialic-acid-binding lectins (c1q domain-containing proteins), which seem to display an elaborate, tailored response to

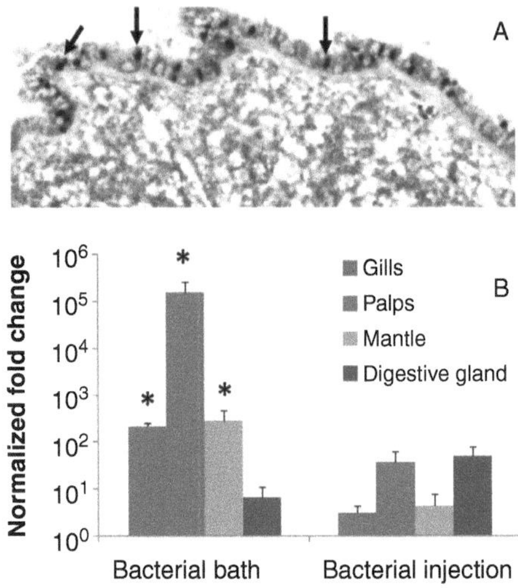

Figure 12.5 A. Detection of *Crassostrea virginica* mucocyte lectin (CvML) in mucocytes (arrows) lining oyster mantle epithelium by *in situ* hybridization using specific cRNA probes. B. Relative expression of CvML (Log scale, normalized to 18S) in different organs determined by qRT-PCR after exposure to *V. alginolyticus*. For each organ, *indicates significantly higher expression (t-test, $p < 0.05$) in challenged oysters compared to controls represented by the x-axis (from Jing et al. 2011).

various microbial challenges affecting mucosal tissues (Allam et al., 2014). Overall, molluscan mucosal tissues and secretions appear to contain a large repertoire of lectins that seem to vary with the reproductive cycle and overall physiological conditions of the animals (Pales Espinosa and Allam, 2013).

12.7.3 Fibrinogen-related proteins

The family of fibrinogen-related proteins (FREP) is a group of highly diversified proteins (different subfamilies as well as alternative splicing of each family member) with fibrinogen-like domains that play important roles as pattern recognition receptors in innate immune responses. For the most part, molluscan FREPs act as calcium-dependent lectins that bind pathogen ligands (Loker, 2010). FREPs have been detected in the tissue of several molluscan species (Adema et al., 1997; Romero et al., 2011; Venier et al., 2011; Zhang et al., 2012), although information on their contribution to mucosal immunity remains very scarce. Li and Graham (Li and Graham, 2007) demonstrated that the major protein found in the epiphragm mucus (membrane covering the opening of the shell) from the snail *Cernuella virgata* contains a fibrinogen-related domain (FReD) that is homologous to the fibrinogen-related proteins (FREP) found in the hemolymph of freshwater snails. These authors suggested that this protein may serve as an adhesive or contributes towards defense against microbial attacks. More recently, Yang et al. (2014) demonstrated the presence in the scallop *Argopecten irradians* of a FREP (designated AiFREP-2) that is orders of magnitude more expressed in gill and mantle tissues as compared to adductor muscle or hemocytes. They further showed that AiFREP-2 binds Gram-negative and -positive bacteria as well as fungal cells and is overexpressed following scallop exposure to microbe-associated molecular patterns (lipopolysaccharide, peptidoglycan, and β-glucan), highlighting its possible role as an important player in scallop immunity. FREPs have not yet been identified in molluscan mucus secretions.

12.7.4 Thioester-containing proteins

The superfamily of thioester-containing proteins (TEP) includes complement components C3, C4, C5, protease inhibitors (alpha 2-macroglobulin), clusters of differentiation 109 (CD109), and several insect TEPs (Song et al., 2010). Among this group, the C3-like molecules and insect TEP were suggested to play a role as PRRs. In mollusks, several TEPs were identified (Zhang et al., 2007; Prado-Álvarez et al., 2009; Mone et al., 2010), including some that display alternative molecular splicing based on the animal sex or the nature of pathogen challenge (Zhang et al., 2009), but very few TEPs were shown to be specifically associated with mucosal tissues. For instance, proteins similar to complement component C3 were identified in the digestive glands of the scallop *Chlamys farreri* (Zhang et al., 2007) and carpet shell clams (*Ruditapes decussatus*) (Prado-Álvarez et al., 2009), but the same molecules were also detected in other tissues, including hemocytes or gonads, suggesting that these molecules may be systemically present (via hemocytes) and not specifically produced in mucosal tissues. A sequence similar to complement component C3 (Es-C3) was also identified in the Hawaiian bobtail squid (*Euprymna scolopes*) by Castillo (Castillo et al., 2009). The gene encoding C3 was expressed in all tissues tested, and immunocytochemistry using an antibody against Es-C3 revealed that the protein is produced principally in the apical surfaces of epithelial cells of all tissues analyzed, including those of the light organ surface, a specialized structure within the squid where the symbiotic *Vibrio fisheri* bacteria reside in close contact with the host epithelia.

12.7.5 Toll-like receptors

Toll-like receptors (TLR) are also among the most important families of pattern recognition receptors (PRR). These are transmembrane receptors characterized by the presence of extracellular leucine-rich repeats and are highly expressed in sentinel immune cells such as dendritic cells and macrophages as well as mucosal epithelia (i.e., TLR4 and TLR5 in the gut) of higher vertebrates (Ortega-Cava et al., 2003; Vijay-Kumar et al., 2010). They are able to selectively recognize and initiate response against a large number of varied and complex MAMPs (Arancibia et al., 2007). Initially discovered to play a major role in *Drosophila* immunity (Lemaitre et al., 1996), the Toll pathway has consequently shown to be highly conserved in metazoans, and TLRs have already been identified in several molluscan species (Tanguy et al., 2004; Goodson et al., 2005; Perrigault et al., 2009). In mollusks, TLRs have been shown to be highly expressed in circulatory hemocytes and were reported to have a wide tissue distribution (possibly as an outcome of the systemic distribution of hemocytes) even though previous studies show TLRs to be also highly expressed in pallial organs (the mantle in particular), which are in direct contact with environmental microbes (Perrigault et al., 2009; Zhang et al., 2011). Significant up-regulation of TLR has also been reported in bivalve mucosal tissues (the mantle and, to a lesser extent, gills) following microbial challenge (Perrigault et al., 2009).

12.8 Immune activation and cell signaling

In mollusks, the innate immune system is controlled by a complex network of signaling pathways that are activated by pathogen invasion and other stimuli. Many pathogen recognition receptors are involved in the activation of corresponding signaling pathways, which, in turn, induces a cascade of reactions and a targeted or systemic immune response to eliminate pathogens (Song et al., 2010). Several regulatory pathways have been identified in mollusks, including the nuclear factor kappa B pathway (NF-kB), the mitogen-activated protein kinase pathway (MAPK), the Janus kinase/signal transducers and activators of transcription pathway (JAK-STAT) and Toll-like receptor pathways that have been described in detail in the reviews by Loker et al. (2004), Loker (2010) and Song et al. (2010). The NF-kB is a key factor that modulates the transcription of a diverse group of genes involved in many biological processes in a multitude of cell types such as development, immunity, apoptosis, homeostatic mechanisms, and cellular differentiation (Li and Stark, 2002). NF-kB is particularly known to be involved in the regulation of many immune molecules, including cytokines, antimicrobial peptides, and apoptosis inhibitors (Silverman and Maniatis, 2001). Similarly, in addition to mediating immune responses, the MAPK and JAK-STAT pathways are also involved in multiple processes, including cell growth, differentiation, and death (Rincón et al., 2000; Arthur and Ley, 2013). Because of their multiple roles, members of these pathways are widely distributed in various types of cells/tissues, and there is little information on their role in regulating specific immune effectors in mollusks and even less so for mucosal immune factors.

12.9 Effector molecules

The mucus matrix, made of glycoproteins and polysaccharides, is an excellent carrier for bioactive molecules since it provides an unstirred surface layer in which the factors can be held to prevent their dispersion in water (Denny, 1989). Mollusks possess a wide range of active molecules that contribute to their immunity, effectively eliminating pathogens or responding to local stimuli or stress, including antimicrobial peptides (AMP) (Yamazaki et al., 1990; Charlet et al., 1996; Mitta et al., 1999a), bactericidal/permeability-increasing proteins (BPI) (Gonzalez et al., 2007b), lysozymes and proteases (Cheng et al., 1975; Xue et al., 2007) as well as antioxidant molecules (Orbea et al., 2000), heat shock proteins and metallothioneins (Moraga et al., 2005). Many of these have been shown to be associated with mucosal tissues and secretions.

12.9.1 Antimicrobial peptides and proteins

Antimicrobial peptides (AMP) are small molecules able to rapidly destroy microorganisms (Tincu and Taylor, 2004). They are classified into 4 groups (β-sheet, α-helical, loop, and extended peptides) (Peters et al., 2010) depending on their molecular structure, but most of them are cationic and display both hydrophilic and hydrophobic areas, which allows these peptides to partition into the membrane lipid bi-layer, disrupting the integrity of or forming pores into the microbial membrane (Yeaman and Yount, 2003). Among the AMPs, defensins represent an important family of small peptides that are abundant and ubiquitous in both vertebrates and invertebrates. They are involved in host defense against a wide range of bacteria and fungi (Lehrer and Ganz, 2002). Several defensins have been reported in mollusks (Charlet et al., 1996; Mitta et al., 1999a): up to 6 in the oyster *C. gigas* (Gueguen et al., 2006; Gonzalez et al., 2007a; Rosa et al., 2011) and 7 in the Manila clam *R. philippinarum* (Allam et al., 2014), some of which are present in epithelial cells. For instance, Gueguen et al. (2006) characterized a defensin mRNA (*Cg*-Def) from the oyster *C. gigas*, specifically expressed and present as a mature protein in the mantle edge. The spectrum of activity of recombinant *Cg*-Def was efficient against Gram-positive bacteria, but was limited against Gram-negative bacteria and fungi. Interestingly, a bacterial challenge did not affect *Cg*-Def expression, which suggests that this protein is constitutively expressed in the mantle and probably plays a role as the first line of defense against pathogen colonization. In contrast, a hemocyte defensin and a big defensin were detected in the mantle and gills of the hard clam (*Mercenaria mercenaria*) and were shown to be significantly regulated following pathogen challenge (Perrigault et al., 2009). Similarly, up-regulation in defensin expression was reported in mantle tissues and extrapallial hemocytes in clams, *R. philippinarum*, infected with the bacterium *Vibrio tapetis* (Allam et al., 2014). Another defensin, dubbed MGD1, was identified in the mussel *Mytilus galloprovincialis* (Mitta et al., 1999b). Immunocytochemical detection of the protein revealed that MGD1 was present not only in hemocytes, but also in granular structures contained in enterocytes lining the epithelium of the intestine, which strongly suggests its involvement in mucosal immunity.

Antimicrobial peptides have also been identified in molluscan mucosal secretions. For instance, an antimicrobial factor (called Dolabellanin B2) was isolated from the skin and mucus of the sea hare *Dolabella auricularia* (Iijima et al., 2003). This factor was described as a small peptide (33 amino acid residues) with cytotoxic activity against a large spectrum of pathogenic microorganisms, including fungi, Gram-positive and Gram-negative bacteria. More recently, a cysteine-rich antimicrobial peptide (mytimacin-AF) was purified and characterized from mucus secretions of the snail of *Achatina fulica* (Zhong et al., 2013). This AMP also displayed wide spectral antimicrobial activity against fungi, Gram-negative, and Gram-positive bacteria.

In addition to AMPs, the antimicrobial arsenal of the innate immune system includes large proteins with potent antibacterial activity. Among these, the bactericidal/permeability-increasing protein (BPI) was initially identified in human neutrophils and was also found in other tissues like mucosa (Canny et al., 2002). BPIs are larger cationic proteins than AMPs (about 50 KDa) (Elsbach, 1998) and are characterized by a high selective cytotoxicity towards Gram-negative bacteria (Boman, 1995). A cDNA sequence similar to the LPS-binding protein and BPI family was identified and characterized in the oyster *Crassostrea gigas* (*Cg*-BPI) (Gonzalez et al., 2007b). The recombinant *Cg*-BPI protein was able to bind LPS, to modify bacterial membrane integrity and to kill the Gram-negative *E. coli. In situ* hybridization showed that *Cg*-BPI is transcribed in various epithelia of the oysters, specifically those in contact with the external environment (mantle, gills, gut, and digestive gland). The authors concluded that this antimicrobial peptide may provide a first line of defense against potential bacterial invasion. Beside bivalves, large antibacterial proteins have also been identified in the mucosal secretions of gastropods. The presence of antibacterial activity was reported in the body surface mucus of the African giant snail (*Achatina fulica*) (Iguchi et al., 1982). Additional studies on the same snail species allowed the isolation of a glycoprotein (Achasin, ~71kDa) with potent activity against Gram-positive and -negative bacteria (Kubota et al., 1985; Obara et al., 1992; Otsuka-Fuchino et al., 1992).

12.9.2 Hydrolytic enzymes

In complement to antimicrobial peptides, enzymes (i.e., lysozyme and proteases) that can degrade specific substrates that make microbial cell walls (i.e., bacterial peptidoglycan) have also been reported in molluscan mucus. McDade and Tripp (1967a) described the presence of lysozyme (N-acetylmuramide glycanhydrolase) in oyster mantle mucus and suggested that this formed an antimicrobial defense. McHenery et al. (1979, 1986) reported the presence of lysozyme activity in mantle, gills, and digestive gland of several bivalve species and hypothesized lysozyme to play a dual role in immunity and digestion. Several lysozymes have also been reported in certain oysters, *Crassostrea gigas* and *C. virginica*, including some that are mainly expressed in the epithelial cells of the digestive gland and other mucosal tissues (Itoh and Takahashi, 2007; Xue et al., 2007, 2010; Itoh et al., 2010). In addition, a goose-type lysozyme (CFLysG) was identified and cloned from the Zhikong scallop (*Chlamys farreri*) (Zhao et al., 2007). The mRNA transcripts of CFLysG were found to be mostly expressed in the digestive gland and gills; there was a weak expression in hemocytes and mantle. Recombinant CFLysG inhibited the growth of both Gram-positive and Gram-negative bacteria. Authors suggested that the high levels of expression of CFLysG mRNA in gills, a water-processing organ covered with mucus, implied that this lysozyme made a significant contribution to the prevention of microbial infections (Zhao et al., 2007). Mantle tissues and secretions were also shown to be particularly rich (in terms of diversity and quantity) in lysozyme activity in various bivalve species including clams (Allam and Paillard, 1998) and oysters (Itoh et al., 2010). Lysozyme activity is widely thought to protect mantle tissues from microbial invasions. In fact, lysozyme activity in mantle secretions (extrapallial fluid) was shown to increase in response to pathogen exposure, supporting this scenario (Allam et al., 2000a, 2000b). These conclusions were also supported by the findings of Perrigault et al. (2009), who reported a significant increase in lysozyme transcription levels in the mantle of hard clams following exposure to the thraustochytrid pathogen QPX. A significant increase in lysozyme transcription levels was also measured in the mantle and hemocytes from the extrapallial fluid of the clams *Ruditapes philippinarum* infected with *Vibrio tapetis* (Allam et al., 2014). Overall, there is strong evidence that the repertoire of lysozymes is diverse in mollusks with most members mainly expressed in mucosal tissues (mantle, gills, and digestive gland), helping with the degradation of microbial food particles and providing a "generic" immune protection from environmental microbes.

Mucus covering the gills of some oysters, *C. virginica*, was also shown to contain several proteases, including a putative acid protease (96 kDa), a zinc metalloprotease (64 kDa), and a serine protease (33 kDa) (Brun et al., 2000). The authors noted a change in the mucosal protease profile in response to infection by the turbellarian worm (*Urastoma cyprinae*). Similarly, significant regulation was reported for a member of the cathepsin L family of proteases in mantle tissues from the clam *R. philippinarum* infected with *V. tapetis* (Allam et al., 2014). In fact, members of this group of cysteine proteases were suggested to play an important role in immunity after they were shown to be upregulated following bacterial exposure in mucosal tissues (mantle, gills, and digestive gland) of several molluscan species, including the pearl oyster (Ma et al., 2010) and the razor clam (Niu et al., 2013). Together with proteases, molluscan mucosal tissues and secretions were also shown to contain an array of protease inhibitors. Habets et al. (1979) showed the presence of an agglutinin that displays potent proteinase-inhibiting properties within the mucus of the snail *Arion empiricorum*, as demonstrated by the inhibition of casein-digestion by trypsin and plasmin. The authors further reported that carbohydrates played a minor role in the inhibition of its agglutination activity and suggested that the primary role of this agglutinin is protease inhibition. The involvement of protease inhibitors in host defense remains largely unexplored in mollusks even though previous studies suggested that they may provide protection against proteases produced by invading microorganisms (Xue et al., 2006; La Peyre et al., 2010; Yu et al., 2011). In that regard, there is strong evidence for the involvement of host protease inhibitors as determinant factors for the resistance of infectious diseases in several animal taxa (Usselman and Cone, 1983; Zintzen et al., 2011), including mollusks (Spungin and Silberberg, 1984; Sleigh, 1989). A recent investigation showed an up-regulation of several transcripts matching serine protease inhibitors in the mantle tissues and secretions of clams infected by a shell disease called brown ring disease (Allam et al., 2014).

12.9.3 Antioxidant enzymes

Host cells activated by exposure to pathogens/MAMPs can produce large amounts of potentially toxic reactive oxygen species (ROS, including the superoxide anion and hydrogen peroxide) that represent important components of the antimicrobial defenses in both vertebrates and invertebrates (Adema et al., 1991). Although ROS play an important role in host defense, they can also damage host cells if produced in high or uncontrolled quantities. Consequently, the host cells initiate a protective mechanism by producing antioxidants, such as various members of the family of superoxide dismutases (SOD), to control the production of ROS. For this reason, antioxidant compounds are commonly found in normal mucosal tissues and secretions of higher vertebrates and are thought to facilitate ROS homeostasis of this microbe-rich environment (Buffinton and Doe, 1995). Information on the presence of anti-oxidant compounds in mucus secretions in mollusks is limited, but antioxidants have been reported in mucosal tissues. For example, a superoxide dismutase (HdCuZnSOD) was detected in mucosal tissues, in particular gills, of the abalone *Haliotis discus discus* (Nikapitiya et al., 2008). The expression of HdCuZnSOD mRNA was significantly regulated after abalone exposure to *Vibrio*, lipopolysaccharides (LPS) and beta- 1,3-glucan, suggesting a protective role against oxidative stress initiated by superoxide production following activation of host cells by exposure to MAMPs. Superoxide dismutases as well as catalases and glutathione peroxidases (i.e., antioxidant enzymes) were also found to be associated with the epithelium of the gut in bivalves. For example, Orbea et al. (2000) used immunohistochemical studies to show that the digestive gland epithelium (including tubule cells and ducts) was strongly immunostained for catalase and Cu, Zn, Mn-SOD in mussels, *Mytilus galloprovincialis*, and oysters, *Crassostrea* sp.

12.9.4 Other protective proteins

Molluscan mucosal tissues were also shown to actively produce two additional groups of proteins known to contribute to host resistance to stress: heat shock proteins (HSP) and metallothioneins (MT). HSP, which are induced by several stimuli, including pathogen exposure and thermal stress, are involved in the re-folding of damaged or misfolded proteins. In vertebrates, HSP production in intestinal epithelia was shown to be enhanced by exposure to probionts, providing increased protection against infectious and noninfectious stress (Tao et al., 2006). In mollusks, Moraga et al. (2005) showed the presence of HSP in epithelial cells lining the digestive gland and gills of the oyster *C. gigas*. The transcription level of HSP was also shown to be up-regulated in mantle tissues from clams infected with brown ring disease (Allam et al., 2014). Since MT are particularly involved in animal resistance to metal exposure, their presence in mucosal tissues is not surprising because these tissues are directly exposed to environmental contaminants. MT are also involved in the scavenging of free radicals and in inflammatory response to injury (Kanekiyo et al., 2002), highlighting their role in mucosal health. In fact, previous studies in bivalves showed significant regulation in MT expression in mucosal tissues in response to challenge with pathogenic bacteria or protists (Canesi et al., 2010; Perrigault and Allam, 2012; Fang et al., 2013).

12.10 Endocytic activity by epithelial cells

Phagocytosis is an important defense mechanism in vertebrates and invertebrates. This mechanism allows the recognition, uptake, and digestion/elimination of non-self-particles and/or dead/damaged self-cells by circulating hemocytes. While phagocytic activity of blood cells is a hallmark of the innate immune system and has been well described in mollusks (reviewed in Cheng et al., 1981; Loker, 2010; Song et al., 2010), the phagocytic activity of epithelial cells also contributes to microbial homeostasis at mucosal interfaces. Virtually all mucosal epithelia of mollusks are capable of endocytosing biotic and abiotic particles and colloids, including epithelial cells lining the external (extrapallial) and internal (pallial) surfaces of the mantle (Bevelander and Nakahara, 1966; Nakahara, 1967; McLean, 1980), the gills (George et al., 1976; Johnson and Le Pennec, 1995), and the foot (Ryder and Bowen, 1977; Grenon and Walker, 1982) or epithelial cells lining different sections of the digestive gland and gut (Yonge, 1926, 1928, 1935). Phagocytic activity performed by these epithelia provides a dual nutritional/defense function by enhancing the uptake and digestion of food particles and by maintaining microbial homeostasis and limiting infections. Particles phagocytosed by epithelial cells are then exposed to toxic/reactive oxygen species produced by the host cells during the respiratory burst associated with phagocytosis and also undergo hydrolytic digestion in phagosomes/phagolysosomes. Microbes that inhibit or that are able to resist intracellular digestion can initiate infection in epithelial cells. This is typically the case for members of the Chlamydiales and Rickettsiales that infect mucosal epithelial cells throughout various taxa, including mollusks (Fryer and Lannan, 1994).

12.11 Hemocytes

Most mollusks have an open circulatory system populated by hemocytes (molluscan blood cells, sometimes referred to as amaebocytes) that circulate in hemolymph vessels and sinuses as well as throughout soft tissues. Hemocytes represent the backbone of the molluscan immune system (Anderson and Good, 1976; Malham et al., 1997; Loker, 2010; Song et al., 2010; Castellanos-Martínez and Gestal, 2013). They are multi-potent and contribute to several biological functions (reviewed in Cheng, 1981, 1996). Of course they play a major role in phagocytosis of invading microbes and encapsulation of larger or refractive invaders, but they are also involved in wound healing, food digestion, and transport of nutrients, reproduction, excretion, shell formation, and production and secretion of humoral factors (Cheng, 1981, 1986; Loker 2010). Little is known about hemocyte formation in mollusks, and the hematopoietic organ (often dubbed the "amebocyte-producing organ") has been identified only in a few classes including cephalopods and gastropods such as the medically important snail *Biomphalaria glabrata* (Lie et al., 1975). In bivalves, incidental evidence suggests that hemocytes may be produced from differentiation of connective tissue cells (Smolowitz et al., 1989; Cheng, 1996). Molluscan hemocytes are generally classified based on morphological appearance and "granularity" of the cytoplasm, which adds to the ambiguity and lack of consistencies between different studies within the same species and across various species within and across taxa. An important feature of hemocytes is their ability to perform chemotaxis towards microbial products (Cheng and Howland, 1979; Howland and Cheng, 1982). Chemotactic movement of hemocytes represents the first step in phagocytosis. This is followed by the attachment of hemocytes to the particles recognized as non-self, preceding endocytosis. After endocytosis, particles are neutralized using a series of microbicidal processes, including the production of a suite of reactive oxygen and nitrogen species as well as a wide range of antimicrobial factors packed in lysosomes (Cheng, 1981; Pipe, 1992; Adema et al., 1993; Malham et al., 1997; Gourdon et al., 2001; Wootton et al., 2003; Buggé and Allam, 2007; Song et al., 2010). When phagocytosis fails or when particles are too large to undergo phagocytosis, hemocytes are recruited in large numbers to surround and encapsulate the invader and release cytotoxic products for extracellular killing (Loker et al., 1982; Meuleman et al., 1986). Encapsulation can lead to granuloma formation when hemocytes accumulate in thin layers surrounding the parasite.

As mentioned above, mucosal tissues are often well irrigated by the blood due to their primary role in exchanges with the surrounding environment for processes such as oxygen or nutrient extraction. In fact, connective tissues of the gills and sub-epithelial tissues along the digestive tract are among the most hemocyte-rich tissues in mollusks. These hemocytes are able to cross the basement membrane and wander on the surface of the epithelial barrier in close association with the mucus layer (Figure 12.6). Transepithelial migration of immune cells is well described in vertebrates where mucus contains representatives of innate and adaptive immune cells, such as neutrophils and dendritic cells, that cross epithelial surfaces to interact with environmental microbes and mount an appropriate host response (Rescigno et al., 2001). In mollusks, the pioneering works by Yonge (1926) and Takatsuki (1934) were the first to report the presence of hemocytes associated with mucosal secretions covering the pallial cavity and in the gut lumen. Both authors showed that these hemocytes were functionally active and were capable of phagocytosing biotic and abiotic particles and transferring phagocytosed materials across the epithelial barrier. In fact, several reports suggested hemocytes trafficking across epithelial barriers to be bidirectional, at least in the gut (Feng et al., 1977). Interestingly, these authors reported the presence, in oyster circulatory hemocytes, of carotenoid pigments known to be synthesized only in plants, suggesting that these pigments are acquired by hemocytes through phagocytosis of algal cells during excursions into the gut lumen before transmigrating back and carrying these products to the circulatory system. More recently, trans-epithelial migration of hemocytes has been reported in the clam *Ruditapes philippinarum* (Allam, 1998; Allam and Paillard, 1998) and the oyster *C. virginica* (Lau et al., 2013b) where hemocytes were found in association with the pallial mucus. Hemocytes identified in bivalve extrapallial fluid and those associated with pallial mucus are functionally active as demonstrated by their ability to phagocytose biotic and abiotic particles and to secrete hydrolytic and antimicrobial compounds (Takatsuki, 1934; Allam, 1998; Allam and Paillard, 1998; Lau et al., 2013b). While hemocytes present in the extrapallial compartment are thought to play a primary role in biomineralization and shell growth, hemocytes lining pallial epithelia (which are in contact with environmental microbes) are thought to play a sentinel role in providing a first alert system and secreting humoral factors that become an integral part of the mucus.

These findings provide a body of evidence that can explain how aquatic mollusks sense and respond to changes in the microbial makeup of their environment. Again, accumulated evidence shows the presence in molluscan mucosal secretions

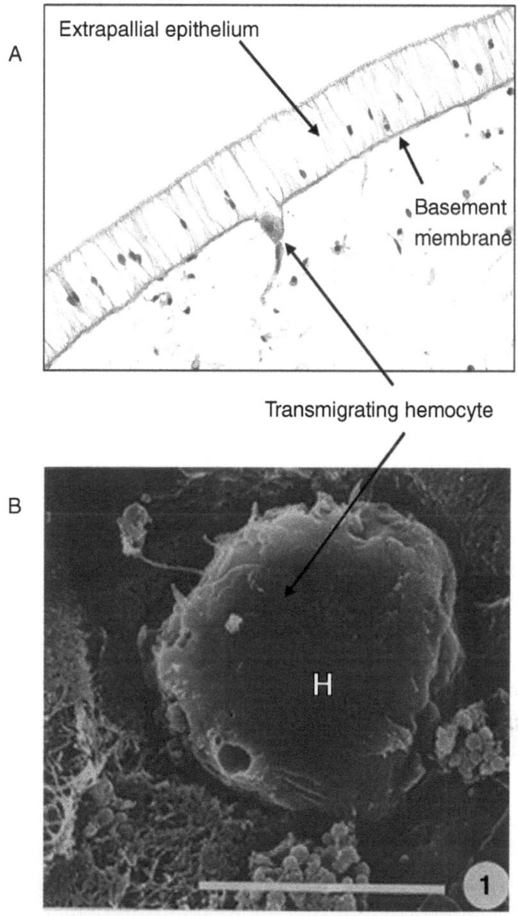

Figure 12.6 A hemocyte transmigrating across the extrapallial epithelium of clams *Mercenaria mercenaria* (A) and *Ruditapes philippinarum* (B). In (A), the hemocyte is seen crossing the basement membrane. In (B), the hemocyte is visible at the apical surface of the epithelial layer.

of functionally active hemocytes that are capable of phagocytosing microbes before migrating back inside tissues (Takatsuki, 1934; Feng et al., 1977; Allam, 1998; Lau et al., 2013b). Through transepithelial migration, oyster hemocytes were shown to translocate from pallial surfaces to underlying tissues and the circulatory system within hours (Lau et al., 2013a). Therefore, these hemocytes seem to play a sentinel role similar to that of dendritic cells in vertebrates, which migrate across epithelial barriers and venture along mucosal surfaces to "sample" environmental microbes (Rescigno et al., 2001). In fact, "pallial hemocytes" in oysters had higher phagocytic activity than circulating hemocytes (Lau et al., 2013b). They also showed epitope signatures (surface carbohydrates and clusters of differentiation) different from those of circulating hemocytes (Lau et al., 2013b), suggesting that they represent a specialized category of hemocytes. Specifically, labeling with the cluster of differentiation 14 (CD14, a receptor of lipopolysaccharides and other MAMPs) was significantly higher in pallial hemocytes compared to that of circulatory cells underlining a higher expression of this pattern recognition receptor and highlighting a sentinel role for these cells. The fact that CD14 is a common constituent of mucosal secretions of vertebrates (Uehara et al., 2003) suggests that this may represent a conserved mechanism of mucosal innate immunity in metazoans.

The occurrence of two-way movements of hemocytes across mucosal epithelia raises the possibility for these cells to serve as vehicles, allowing the acquisition of adapted microbes that are capable of surviving phagocytosis. In fact, previous investigations showed the ability of the obligate oyster parasite *Perkinsus marinus* to take advantage of transepithelial migration of pallial hemocytes in order to gain access to the internal tissues of its oyster host (Allam and Parvez, 2007). Furthermore, exposure of naïve oysters to *P. marinus* was shown to increase transepithelial migration of hemocytes, likely resulting in higher infection rates (Lau et al., 2013a). In contrast, exposure of oysters to the opportunistic bacteria *Vibrio alginolyticus* did not cause any change in transmigration, which suggests that change in transepithelial migration rates is not a generic response to microbial exposure. Overall, a better characterization of mucosal hemocytes (functional characterization, turnover rate, etc.) is needed for a better evaluation of their role in mucosal immunity and interactions with pathogens.

12.12 Melanization and biomineralization

Melanization of pathogens and damaged tissues is a major innate defense process in invertebrates, especially arthropods (Cerenius et al., 2010). In addition to aggregation and encapsulation, specialized hemocytes can promote the formation of melanotic nodules that limit the spread of infecting microorganisms or damaged tissues. Melanin biosynthesis is highly regulated (phenoloxidase cascade) and is mediated by a diverse group of enzymes designated under the generic name of phenoloxidases that encompass several metalloproteins, including tyrosinases, catechol oxidases, and laccases (Walker and Ferrar, 1998). Melanization is a normal process during shell formation in mollusks (Waite and Wilbur, 1976), but is also an important mechanism involved in wound healing and encapsulation of non-self-entities. Hemocytes as well as all pallial epithelia in mollusks were shown to support melanization, particularly the external epithelium of the mantle. In fact, melanization response of the mantle is a major trait of several microbial infections affecting this organ. This is the case for the response of American oysters to *Roseovarius* oyster disease (ROD, previously known as juvenile oyster disease or JOD, caused by *Roseovarius crassostreae*) or that of Manila clams to brown ring disease (BRD, caused by *Vibrio tapetis*). In both cases, mantle tissues and secretions (extrapallial fluid and hemocytes contained within) produce copious amounts of melanin to wall off the pathogens, leading to major rearrangements of shell matrix deposition (Ford and Borrero, 2001; Paillard, 2004). Several tyrosinases have been identified in mollusks and are considered to represent key enzymes in the melanogenic pathway that catalyze the initial rate-determining production of melanin. For instance, a cDNA sequence encoding a putative tyrosinase (OT47) was detected in the pearl oyster (*Pinctada fucata*) and was shown (by PCR and *in situ* hybridization) to be expressed only in the epithelial cells of the mantle edge (Zhang et al., 2006), a strategic area for both defense against pathogens and shell formation even though no functional investigations were performed on this transcript. In parallel, previous studies showed a regulation in the expression of melanogenic enzymes in response to infections. This was the case for a laccase that was shown to be up-regulated in the mantle of clams affected by BRD (Allam et al., 2014).

Melanization of foreign bodies in mollusks is sometimes followed by a biomineralization mechanism that embeds melanized invaders in new calcified shell layers. This is the mechanism of the nacrezation process during pearl formation. There have been many studies focusing on the mechanisms of pearl formation in mollusks (Bevelander and Nakahara, 1969; Addadi and Weiner, 1997), but rarely from an immune perspective. In fact, nacrezation and pearl formation is a common response in mollusks to irritants (including parasites and pathogens as well as abiotic irritants) affecting pallial organs, particularly the mantle. Good examples include infections caused by trematodes in different bivalve species (Jameson and Nicoll, 1913; Stunkard and Uzmann, 1958). Mantle tissues and secretions are heavily involved in this process and previous studies have shown significant changes in the expression of biomineralization-related proteins in response to infection. For example, several genes involved in calcium binding and biomineralization were regulated in mantle tissues and extrapallial hemocytes in clams affected by BRD (Allam et al., 2014). These included several perlucin-like transcripts (which contain C-type lectin-like domains) that were up-regulated in diseased clams. Perlucin nucleates the growth of calcium carbonate crystals in mollusks (Weiss et al., 2000; Blank et al., 2003) and was suggested to play a dual role as organic support for biomineralization and as a potential defense molecule against pathogenic microorganisms (Wang et al., 2008).

12.13 Enhancement of mucosal immunity

It is now well established that beneficial microbial symbionts of mucus can favor host resistance to infections directly or indirectly. In their recent study, Barr et al. (2013) showed an affinity of bacteriophages to mucosal secretions in different taxa (i.e., humans, fish, and corals) and demonstrated that this enhanced viral population protects their metazoan hosts from bacterial infections. This led the authors to designate this virus-mucus association as a "non-host derived immune system." Similarly, probiotic bacteria (*Lactobacillus johnsonii*) reduced the attachment of pathogenic bacteria to human intestinal mucus by competitive exclusion (Tuomola et al., 1999). Probiotic bacteria can also act indirectly. For instance, previous studies have shown that the probiotic strains *L. plantarum* and *L. rhamnosus* increase mucin secretion in host cells, leading to a better resistance toward *E. coli* infection (Mack et al., 1999). The use of probionts has become a common practice in aquaculture, particularly for crustaceans (Verschuere et al., 2000), and several studies have demonstrated the beneficial effects of probionts on mollusk resistance to infection (Douillet and Langdon, 1994; Gibson et al., 1998; Kesarcodi-Watson et al., 2012). This protective effect has often been linked to the production of antibiotic compounds by probionts that inhibit the growth of pathogenic microbes, leading to the establishment of a robust beneficial mucosal microflora. The elegant studies by Dao et al. (2012) and Abd Karim (2012) used probiont mutants to demonstrate the implication of genes involved in biofilm formation in oyster protection from pathogenic bacteria. These authors also concluded that the production of antibiotic compounds is not a requirement for good probionts and that competitive exclusion and immune priming contribute to host protection. Overall, our understanding of the mechanisms of action of probionts on mucosal tissues and secretions in mollusks is in its infancy. How mucosa respond to probionts and how changes in mucus physicochemical characteristics (either caused by disease, by other beneficial/harmful microbes, or by natural cycles) affect microbial homeostasis at mucosal surfaces are among the many questions that still need to be answered.

12.14 The promise of new technologies

Recent progress in "omics" technologies provides the resources and tools needed to make significant progress in our understanding of the role of mucosal immunity in mollusks. There are currently six more or less complete molluscan genomes that are publically available: the pearl oyster Pinctada fucata, the Pacific oyster *C. gigas*, the Mediterranean mussel (*M. galloprovincialis*), the owl limpet *Lottia gigantea*, the California sea hare *Aplysia californica*, and the snail *Biomphalaria glabrata*. As well-assessed by Loker (Loker, 2010), a synthetic comparative interpretation of the molluscan immunome is currently lacking and should be addressed. Nevertheless, combined with new development in transcriptomic and proteomic tools, this resource opens the door to thorough, in-depth investigations of the nature and the dynamics of the effectors of mucosal immunity. Recent quantitative proteomic analysis (using a combination of publically available genomic and transcriptomic resources as a reference) unraveled the extensive diversity of defense-related molecules in oyster and mussel pallial mucus (Pales Espinosa et al., 2014b). In oyster mucus, a total of 1,500 proteins were identified with about 200 matching proteins known to be involved in immunity and defense against pathogens, including antimicrobial peptides, lysozyme, several lectins, and other pathogen recognition receptors as well as several proteases and protease inhibitors. While promising, these findings showing the diversity of antimicrobial molecules in mucus are a clear reminder of the daunting little extent of our current knowledge on mucosal immune effectors and their regulation in mollusks. More interestingly, mucus contained several proteins with no match in current databases, highlighting the potential for the discovery of novel bioactive compounds in these matrices.

12.15 Concluding remarks

Mucosal immunity has gained a prime importance in higher vertebrates over the last two decades. In these animals, it is now well established that microbial homeostasis at mucosal interfaces represents a major factor affecting overall animal health. This is often accomplished through complex interactions and specific cross-talk between mucosa and microbial symbionts. Mucosal immunity is promising in mollusks. Several species in this group have great worldwide importance as aquaculture products, and molluscan aquaculture is growing at unprecedented rates. At the same time, microbial infections are very common in this group and, for the most part, are initiated at mucosal interfaces. The mucosal layer in these animals plays an essential role in functions as diverse as lubrication, feeding, protection from environmental stress (contaminants, desiccation, or freezing), and a physical and biological barrier against infections. Our current understanding underlines the diversity and the dynamic nature of immune effectors at molluscan mucosal interfaces. Evidence showed a certain level of specificity among mucosal immune responses where some immune effectors are regulated in response to specific stimuli (Xing et al., 2011). Of great concern is the fact that most studies on molluscan immunity focus on the circulating hemocytes and the humoral defense factors in the plasma while the most relevant host-microbe interactions occur at mucosal interfaces. In fact, the studies that compared immune effectors in mucosal tissues and secretions with those in molluscan hemolymph showed that the assessment of defense factors in hemolymph is rarely a good proxy for animal resistance or, in many instances, response to infections. In most of these cases, results indicate that focal responses at the initial infection sites (mucosa) are better indicators of immune performance than systemic responses measured in the circulatory system (Allam et al., 2000a, 2001, 2014; Xing et al., 2011). Among the burning questions that still need to be answered are how mollusks keep microbial symbionts in check, how mucosal immune factors are regulated in response to environmental or pathologic stress, and how the behavior and performance of opportunistic pathogens compares to that of obligate parasites. With regard to this last topic, preliminary evidence obtained with the *Perkinsus*-oyster study model suggests that this obligate parasite can divert mucosal factors to its advantage to colonize and invade the host (Pales Espinosa et al., 2013, 2014a). This context raises fascinating questions around host-microbe cross-talk and feedback controls of these interactions and calls for appealing inquisitive research in the years to come.

Acknowledgments

The authors would like to acknowledge financial support provided by the National Science Foundation (projects IOS 1050596 and IOS 1146920) and by the New York Sea Grant program (projects R/XG-19 and R/FBM-34). We thank the many collaborators, colleagues and friends who directly or indirectly contributed to this work via discussions, exchanges and passionate arguments.

References

Abd Karim, M.M., 2012. Mechanisms of Protection of Probiotics Against Bacterial Pathogens in Oyster Aquaculture. Fisheries, Animal and Veterinary Science, Ann Arbor.

Addadi, L., Weiner, S, 1997. Biomineralization: a pavement of pearl. Nature 389, 912–915.

Adema, C., van Deutekom-Mulder, E., van der Knaap, W., Sminia, T., 1993. NADPH-oxidase activity: the probable source of reactive oxygen intermediate generation in hemocytes of the gastropod *Lymnaea stagnalis*. J. Leukoc. Biol. 54, 379–383.

Adema, C., Vanderknaap, W., Sminia, T, 1991. Molluscan hemocyte-mediated cytotoxicity – the role of reactive oxygen intermediates. Rev. Aquat. Sci. 4, 201–223.

Adema, C.M., Hertel, L.A., Miller, R.D., Loker, E.S., 1997. A family of fibrinogen-related proteins that precipitates parasite-derived molecules is produced by an invertebrate after infection. Proc. Natl. Acad. Sci. 94, 8691–8696.

Ahn, H.Y., Sue, L.F., Ma, J.K.H., Pinkstaff, C.A., Pore, R.S., Overman, D.O., Malanga, C.J., 1988. Synthesis and secretion of mucus glycoprotein by the gill of *Mytilus edulis*. 1. histochemical and chromatographic analysis of c-14 glucosamine bioincorporation. Biochim. Biophys. Acta 966, 122–132, doi: 10.1016/0304-4165(88)90136-5.

Allam, B., 1998. Role of extrapallial fluids in bivalve immunity: the case of brown ring disease in the clam, *Ruditapes philippinarum*. Ph.D. Dissertation. University of Western Brittany, Brest, France.

Allam, B., Ashton-Alcox, K.A., Ford, S.E., 2001. Haemocyte parameters associated with resistance to brown ring disease in *Ruditapes* spp. clams. Dev. Comp. Immunol. 25, 365–375, doi: 10.1016/s0145-305x(00)00072-0.

Allam, B., Carden, W., Ward, J.E., Ralph, G.M., Winnicki, S., Parvez, N., Pales Espinosa, E., 2013a. Evidence that *Perkinsus marinus* is acquired by oysters during rejection of water-borne particles as pseudofeces. Integr. Comp. Biol. 53, E3–E13.

Allam, B., Carden, W.E., Ward, J.E., Ralph, G., Winnicki, S., Pales Espinosa, E., 2013b. Early host-pathogen interactions in marine bivalves: evidence that the alveolate parasite *Perkinsus marinus* infects through the oyster mantle during rejection of pseudofeces. J. Invertebr. Pathol. 113, 26–34, doi: 10.1016/j.jip.2012.12.011.

Allam, B., Paillard, C., 1998. Defense factors in clam extrapallial fluids. Dis. Aquat. Org. 33, 123–128, doi: 10.3354/dao033123.

Allam, B., Paillard, C., Auffret, M., 2000a. Alterations in hemolymph and extrapallial fluid parameters in the Manila clam, *Ruditapes philippinarum*, challenged with the pathogen *Vibrio tapetis*. J Invertebr Pathol 76, 63–69.

Allam, B., Paillard, C., Howard, A., Le Pennec, M., 2000. Isolation of the pathogen *Vibrio tapetis* and defense parameters in brown ring diseased Manila clams *Ruditapes philippinarum* cultivated in England. Dis Aquat Org 41, 105–113, doi 10.3354/dao041105.

Allam, B., Paillard, C., Maes, P., 1996. Localization of the pathogen Vibrio P1 in clams affected by Bbrown Rring Ddisease. Dis Aquat Org 27, 149–155, doi 10.3354/dao027149.

Allam, B., Pales Espinosa, E., Tanguy, A., Jeffroy, F., Le Bris, C., Paillard, C., 2014. Transcriptional changes in Manila clam *Ruditapes philippinarum* in response to brown ring disease. Fish Shellfish Immunol.

Allam, B., Parvez, N., 2007. Uptake of *Perkinsus marinus* at pallial interfaces in the oyster, *Crassostrea virginica*. Meeting of the World Aquaculture Society, San Antonio, Texas, USA.

Allen, A., 1977. Structure and function in gastric mucus. In: Elstein, M., Parke, D. (Eds.), Mucus in Health and Disease. Advances in Experimental Medicine and Biology. Plenum Press, New York, pp. 283–299.

Andersch-Björkman, Y., Thomsson, K.A., Larsson, J.M.H., Ekerhovd, E., Hansson, G.C., 2007. Large scale identification of proteins, mucins, and their O-glycosylation in the endocervical mucus during the menstrual cycle. Mol. Cell Proteomics 6, 708–716.

Anderson, R.S., Good, R.A., 1976. Opsonic involvement in phagocytosis by mollusk hemocytes. J. Invertebr. Pathol. 27, 57–64.

Arancibia, S.A., Beltrán, C.J., Aguirre, I.M., Silva, P., Peralta, A.L., Malinarich, F., Hermoso, M.A., 2007. Toll-like receptors are key participants in innate immune responses. Biol. Res. 40, 97–112.

Arthur, J.S.C., Ley, S.C., 2013. Mitogen-activated protein kinases in innate immunity. Nat. Rev. Immunol. 13, 679–692.

Audie, J., Janin, A., Porchet, N., Copin, M., Gosselin, B., Aubert, J., 1993. Expression of human mucin genes in respiratory, digestive, and reproductive tracts ascertained by in situ hybridization. JHC 41, 1479–1485.

Auld, A.G., 1920. The function of mucus. Br. Med. J. 1920, 681–1681.

Avila, C., Cimino, G., Fontana, A., Gavagnin, M., Ortea, J., Trivellone, E, 1991. Defensive strategy of two *Hypselodoris* nudibranchs from Italian and Spanish coasts. J. Chem. Ecol. 17, 625–636.

Azevedo, C., 1989. Fine structure of *Perkinsus atlanticus* n. sp. (Apicomplexa, Perkinsea) parasite of the clam *Ruditapes decussatus* from Portugal. J. Parasitol. 75, 627–635.

Bachere, E., Mialhe, E., Noel, D., Boulo, V., Morvan, A., Rodriguez, J., 1995. Knowledge and research prospects in marine mollusc and crustacean immunology. Aquaculture 132, 17–32.

Banin, E., Israely, T., Fine, M., Loya, Y., Rosenberg, E., 2001. Role of endosymbiotic zooxanthellae and coral mucus in the adhesion of the coral-bleaching pathogen *Vibrio shiloi* to its host. FEMS Microbiol. Lett. 199, 33–37, doi: 10.1111/j.1574-6968.2001.tb10647.x.

Barille, L., Cognie, B, 2000. Revival capacity of diatoms in bivalve pseudofaeces and faeces. Diatom. Res. 15, 11–17.

Barnes, R.S.K., Calow, P., Olive, P.J., 1993. The Invertebrates: A New Synthesis. Blackwell Scientific Publications Ltd.

Barr, J.J., Auro, R., Furlan, M., Whiteson, K.L., Erb, M.L., Pogliano, J., Stotland, A., Wolkowicz, R., Cutting, A.S., Doran, K.S., 2013. Bacteriophage adhering to mucus provide a non-host–derived immunity. Proc. Natl. Acad. Sci. 110, 10771–10776.

Barr, R.A., 1926. Some observations on the pedal gland of Milax. Q. J. Microsc. Sci. 70, 647–667.

Bayne, C, 1983. Molluscan immunobiology. In: Saleuddin, A.S.M., Wilbur, K.M. (Eds.), The Mollusca. Academic Press, San Diego, pp. 408–486.

Beninger, P., Dufour, S, 1996. Mucocyte distribution and relationship to particle transport on the pseudolamellibranch gill of *Crassostrea virginica* (Bivalvia: Ostreidae). Mar. Ecol. Prog. Ser. 137, 133–138, doi: 10.3354/meps137133.

Beninger, P.G., Lynn, J.W., Dietz, T.H., Silverman, H., 1997. Mucociliary transport in living tissue: the two-layer model confirmed in the mussel *Mytilus edulis* L. Biol. Bull. 193, 4–7.

Beninger, P.G., Stjean, S., Poussart, Y., Ward, J.E., 1993. Gill function and mucocyte distribution in *Placopecten magellanicus* and *Mytilus edulis* (Mollusca, Bivalvia) -- the role of mucus in particle-transport. Mar. Ecol. Prog. Ser. 98, 275–282.

Bevelander, G., Nakahara, H, 1966. Correlation of lysosomal activity and igestion by mantle epithelium. Biol. Bull. 131, 76–82, doi: 10.2307/1539648.

Bevelander, G., Nakahara, H., 1969. An electron microscope study of the formation of the nacreous layer in the shell of certain bivalve molluscs. Calcif. Tissue Res. 3, 84–92, doi: 10.1007/bf02058648.

Blank, S., Arnoldi, M., Khoshnavaz, S., Treccani, L., Kuntz, M., Mann, K., Grathwohl, G., Fritz, M., 2003. The nacre protein perlucin nucleates growth of calcium carbonate crystals. J. Microsc. 212, 280–291.

Boman, H.G., 1995. Peptide antibiotics and their role in innate immunity. Annu. Rev. Immunol. 13, 61–92.

Branka, J., Vallette, G., Jarry, A., Bou-Hanna, C., Lemarre, P., Van, P.N., Laboisse, C., 1997. Early functional effects of *Clostridium difficile* toxin A on human colonocytes. Gastroenterology 112, 1887–1894.

Bravo, J.C., Correa, P., 1999. Sulphomucins favour adhesion of *Helicobacter pylori* to metaplastic gastric mucosa. J. Clin. Pathol. 52, 137–140.

Brown, B., Bythell, J., 2005. Perspectives on mucus secretion in reef corals. Mar. Ecol. Prog. Ser. 296, 291–309.

Brun, N.T., Ross, N.W., Boghen, A.D., 2000. Changes in the electrophoretic profiles of gill mucus proteases of the Eastern oyster *Crassostrea virginica* in response to infection by the turbellarian *Urastoma cyprinae*. J. Invertebr. Pathol. 75, 163–170, doi: 10. 1006/jipa. 1999.

Buffinton, G.D., Doe, W.F., 1995. Depleted mucosal antioxidant defences in inflammatory bowel disease. Free Radic. Biol. Med. 19, 911–918.

Buggé, D.M., Allam, B., 2007. Effects of starvation and macroalgae extracts on the survival and growth of quahog parasite unknown (QPX). J. Exp. Mar. Biol. Ecol. 348, 60–69, doi: 10.1016/j.jembe.2007.04.013.

Bulgheresi, S., Schabussova, I., Chen, T., Mullin, N.P., Maizels, R.M., Ott, J.A., 2006. A new C-type lectin similar to the human immunoreceptor DC-SIGN mediates symbiont acquisition by a marine nematode. Appl. Environ. Microbiol. 72, 2950–2956, doi: 10.1128/aem.72.4.2950-2956.2006.

Burge, C.A., Kim, C.J.S., Lyles, J.M., Harvell, C.D., 2013. Oceans and humans health: the ecology of marine opportunists. Microb. Ecol. 65, 869–879, Special issue; doi: 10.1007/s00248-013-0190-7.

Burreson, E.M., Ford, S.E., 2004. A review of recent information on the *Haplosporidia*, with special reference to *Haplosporidium nelsoni* (MSX disease). Aquat. Living Resour. 17, 499–517, doi: 10.1051/alr:2004056.

Byrd, J.C., Yunker, C.K., Xu, Q.S., Sternberg, L.R., Bresalier, R.S., 2000. Inhibition of gastric mucin synthesis by *Helicobacter pylori*. Gastroenterology 118, 1072–1079, doi: 10.1016/s0016-5085(00)70360-x.

Canesi, L., Barmo, C., Fabbri, R., Ciacci, C., Vergani, L., Roch, P., Gallo, G., 2010. Effects of vibrio challenge on digestive gland biomarkers and antioxidant gene expression in *Mytilus galloprovincialis*. Comp. Biochem. Physiol. C Toxicol. Pharmacol. 152, 399–406.

Canny, G., Levy, O., Furuta, G.T., Narravula-Alipati, S., Sisson, R.B., Serhan, C.N., Colgan, S.P., 2002. Lipid mediator-induced expression of bactericidal/ permeability-increasing protein (BPI) in human mucosal epithelia. Proc. Natl. Acad. Sci. 99, 3902–3907, doi: 10.1073/pnas.052533799.

Cash, H.L., Whitham, C.V., Behrendt, C.L., Hooper, L.V., 2006. Symbiotic bacteria direct expression of an intestinal bactericidal lectin. Science 313, 1126–1130.

Castellanos-Martínez, S., Gestal, C., 2013. Pathogens and immune response of cephalopods. J. Exp. Mar. Biol. Ecol. 447, 14–22.

Castillo, M.G., Goodson, M.S., McFall-Ngai, M., 2009. Identification and molecular characterization of a complement C3 molecule in a lophotrochozoan, the Hawaiian bobtail squid *Euprymna scolopes*. Dev. Comp. Immunol. 33, 69–76, doi: http://dx.doi.org/10.1016/j.dci.2008.07.013.

Castro, P., Huber, M.E., 1997. Marine Biology. Wm. C. Brown Publishers.

Cerenius, L., Jiravanichpaisal, P., Liu H-p, Soderhall, I., 2010. Crustacean Immunity Invertebrate Immunity. Springer, pp. 239–259.

Chadee, K., Keller, K., Forstner, J., Innes, D.J., Ravdin, J.I., 1991. Mucin and nonmucin secretagogue activity of *Entamoeba histolytica* and cholera-toxin in rat colon. Gastroenterology 100, 986–997.

Chadee, K., Meerovitch, E., 1985. *Entamoeba histolytica*: early progressive pathology in the cecum of the gerbil (*Meriones unguiculatus*). Am. J. Trop. Med. Hyg. 34, 283–291.

Charlet, M., Chernysh, S., Philippe, H., Hetru, C., Hoffmann, J.A., Bulet, P., 1996. Innate immunity Isolation of several cysteine-rich antimicrobial peptides from the blood of a mollusc, *Mytilus edulis*. J. Biol. Chem. 271, 21808–21813.

Cheng, T.C., 1981. Invertebrate blood cells. In: Ratcliffe, N.A., Rowley, A.F. (Eds.), Bivalves. Academic Press, London, pp. 233–300.

Cheng, T.C., 1996. Hemocytes: forms and functions. In: Kennedy, V., Newell, R., Eble, A. (Eds.), The Eastern Oyster *Crassostrea virginica*. Maryland Sea Grant Book, College Park, MD, USA, pp. 299–333.

Cheng, T.C., Howland, K.H., 1979. Chemotactic attraction between hemocytes of the oyster, *Crassostrea virginica*, and bacteria. J. Invertebr. Pathol. 33, 204–210.

Cheng, T.C., Rodrick, G.E., Foley, D.A., Koehler, S.A., 1975. Release of lysozyme from hemolymph cells of *Mercenaria mercenaria* during phagocytosis. J. Invertebr. Pathol. 25, 261–265.

Coddeville, B., Maes, E., Ferrier-Pages, C., Guerardel, Y., 2011. Glycan profiling of gel forming mucus layer from the scleractinian symbiotic coral *Oculina arbuscula*. Biomacromolecules 12, 2064–2073.

Cognie, B., Barille, L., 1999. Does bivalve mucus favour the growth of their main food source, microalgae? Oceanologica Acta 22, 441–450.

Cone, R.A., 2009. Barrier properties of mucus. Adv. Drug Delivery Rev. 61, 75–85, doi: http://dx.doi.org/10.1016/j.addr.2008.09.008.

Dahl, S., Thiel, J., Allam, B., 2010a. QPX disease progress in cultured and wild type hard clams in New York waters. J. Shellfish Res. 29, 83–90.

Dahl, S.F., Thiel, J., Allam, B., 2010b. Field performance and QPX disease progress in cultured and wild-type strains of *Mercenaria mercenaria* in New York waters. J. Shellfish Res. 29, 83–90, doi: 10.2983/035.029.0131.

Dao, C., Zhao, W., Karim, M., Gómez-Chiarri, M., Nelson, D., Rowley, D., 2012. Investigation of interactions between host, pathogens, and probiotic bacteria. Planta Med. 78, PI84.

Davidson, S.K., Koropatnick, T.A., Kossmehl, R., Sycuro, L., McFall-Ngai, M.J., 2004. NO means 'yes' in the squid-vibrio symbiosis: nitric oxide (NO) during the initial stages of a beneficial association. Cell Microbiol. 6, 1139–1151, doi: 10.1111/j.1462-5822.2004.00429.x.

Davies, M.S., Beckwith, P., 1999. Role of mucus trails and trail-following in the behaviour and nutrition of the periwinkle *Littorina littorea*. Mar. Ecol. Prog. Ser. 179, 247–257, doi: 10.3354/meps179247.

Davies, M.S., Hawkins, S.J., 1998. Mucus from marine molluscs. Blaxter, J.H.S., Southward, A.J., Tyler, P.A. (Eds.), Advances in Marine Biology, 34, Academic Press Ltd-Elsevier Science Ltd, London, pp. 1–71.

Denkin, S.M., Nelson, D.R., 1999. Induction of protease activity in *Vibrio anguillarum* by gastrointestinal mucus. Appl. Environ. Microbiol. 65, 3555–3560.

Denny, M.W., 1989. Invertebrate mucus secretions: functional alternatives to vertebrate paradigms. In: Chantler, E., Ratcliffe, N.A. (Eds.), Symposia of the Society for Experimental Biology, XLIII Mucus and related topics. The Company of Biologists Limited, Cambridge, pp. 337–366.

Deplancke, B., Gaskins, H.R., 2001. Microbial modulation of innate defense: goblet cells and the intestinal mucus layer. Am. J. Clin. Nutr. 73, 1131S–1141S.

Dohrman, A., Miyata, S., Gallup, M., Li, J.-D., Chapelin, C., Coste, A., Escudier, E., Nadel, J., Basbaum, C., 1998. Mucin gene (*MUC 2* and *MUC 5AC*) upregulation by gram-positive

and gram-negative bacteria. Biochimica et Biophysica Acta (BBA)-Molecular Basis of Disease 1406, 251–259.
Douillet, P.A., Langdon, C.J., 1994. Use of a probiotic for the culture of larvae of the pacific oyster (*Crassostrea gigas* Thunberg). Aquaculture 67 (119), 25–40.
Dubilier, N., Bergin, C., Lott, C., 2008. Symbiotic diversity in marine animals: the art of harnessing chemosynthesis. Nat. Rev. Microbiol. 6, 725–740, doi: 10.1038/nrmicro1992.
Ducklow, H.W., Mitchell, R., 1979. Bacterial populations and adaptations in the mucus layers on living corals. Limnol. Oceanogr. 24, 715–725, doi: 10.2307/2835723.
Dufour, S.C., 2005. Gill anatomy and the evolution of symbiosis in the bivalve family Thyasiridae. Biol. Bull. 208, 200–212, doi: 10.2307/3593152.
Ebran, N., Julien, S., Orange, N., Saglio, P., Lemaitre, C., Molle, G., 1999. Pore-forming properties and antibacterial activity of proteins extracted from epidermal mucus of fish. Comp. Biochem. Physiol. A-Mol. Integr. Physiol. 122, 181–189, doi: 10.1016/s1095-6433(98)10165-4.
Elsbach, P., 1998. The bactericidal/permeability-increasing protein (BPI) in antibacterial host defense. J. Leukoc. Biol. 64, 14–18.
Epple, H., Kreusel, K., Hanski, C., Schulzke, J., Riecken, E., Fromm, M., 1997. Differential stimulation of intestinal mucin secretion by cholera toxin and carbachol. Pflügers. Archiv. 433, 638–647.
Fang, Y., Yang, H., Liu, B., Zhang, L., 2013. Transcriptional response of lysozyme, metallothionein, and superoxide dismutase to combined exposure to heavy metals and bacteria in *Mactra veneriformis*. Comp. Biochem. Physiol. C Toxicol. Pharmacol. 157, 54–62.
FAO, 2014. http://www.fao.org/fishery/statistics/global-aquaculture-production/en.
Feng, S., Feng, J., Yamasu, T., 1977. Roles of *Mytilus coruscus* and *Crassostrea gigas* blood cells in defense and nutrition Comp Pathobio. Springer 3, 31–67.
Finlay, B.B., Falkow, S., 1997. Common themes in microbial pathogenicity revisited. Microbiol. Mol. Biol. Rev. 61, 136–169.
Firth, K.J., Johnson, S.C., Ross, N.W., 2000. Characterization of proteases in the skin mucus of Atlantic salmon (*Salmo salar*) infected with the salmon louse (*Lepeophtheirus salmonis*) and in whole-body louse homogenate. J. Parasitol., 1199–1205.
Fisher, W.S., 1988. Disease Processes in Marine Bivalve Molluscs. American Fisheries Society, USA, special publication, p. 315.
Fisher, W.S., 1992. Occurrence of agglutinins in the pallial cavity mucus of oysters. J. Exp. Mar. Biol. Ecol. 162, 1–13.
Fisher, W.S., Dinuzzo, A.R., 1991. Agglutination of bacteria and erythrocytes by serum from 6 species of marine mollusks. J. Invertebr. Pathol. 57, 380–394.
Ford, L.A., 1992. Host defense mechanisms of cephalopods. Ann. Rev. Fish Dis. 2, 25–41, doi: 10.1016/0959-8030(92)90054-2.
Ford, S.E., Borrero, F.J., 2001. Epizootiology and pathology of juvenile oyster disease in the Eastern oyster, *Crassostrea virginica*. J. Invertebr. Pathol. 78, 141–154.
Ford, S.E., Chintala, M.M., Bushek, D., 2002. Comparison of in vitro-cultured and wild-type *Perkinsus marinus*. I. Pathogen virulence. Dis. Aquat. Org. 51, 187–201, doi: 10.3354/dao051187.
Fountain, D.W., 1985. The lectin-like activity of Helix aspersa mucus. Comp. Biochem. Physiol. B-Comp. Biochem. 80 (4), 795–800.
Fountain, D.W., Campbell, B.A., 1984. A lectin isolate from mucus of *Helix asJ360persa*. Comp. Biochem. Physiol. B-Biochem. Mol. Biol. 77, 419–425.
Fritz, H., 1988. Human mucus proteinase inhibitor (human MPI). Human seminal inhibitor I (HUSI-I), antileukoprotease (ALP), secretory leukocyte protease inhibitor (SLPI). Biol. Chem. Hoppe Seyler. 369 (Suppl), 79–82.

Fryer, J.L., Lannan, C.N., 1994. Rickettsial and chlamydial infections of freshwater and marine fishes, bivalves, and crustaceans. Zool. Stud. 33, 95–107.

Gaskins, H, 1997. Immunological aspects of host/microbiota interactions at the intestinal epithelium. In: Mackie, R., White, B., Isaacson, R. (Eds.), Gastrointestinal Microbiology. Chapman & Hall, New York, pp. 537–587.

Gavagnin, M., Spinella, A., Castelluccio, F., Cimino, G., Marin, A., 1994. Polypropionates from the Mediterranean mollusk *Elysia timida*. J. Nat. Prod. 57, 298–304.

George, S., Pirie, B., Coombs, T., 1976. The kinetics of accumulation and excretion of ferric hydroxide in *Mytilus edulis* (I.) and its distribution in the tissues. J. Exp. Mar. Biol. Ecol. 23, 71–84.

Gibson, L.F., Woodworth, J., George, A.M., 1998. Probiotic activity of *Aeromonas* media on the Pacific oyster, *Crassostrea gigas*, when challenged with *Vibrio tubiashii*. Aquaculture 169, 111–120, doi: 10. 1016/s0044-8486(98)00369-x.

Gonzalez, M., Gueguen, Y., Desserre, G., de Lorgeril, J., Romestand, B., Bachère, E., 2007a. Molecular characterization of two isoforms of defensin from hemocytes of the oyster *Crassostrea gigas*. Dev. Comp. Immunol. 31, 332–339, doi: http://dx.doi.org/10.1016/j.dci.2006.07.006.

Gonzalez, M., Gueguen, Y., Destoumieux-Garzón, D., Romestand, B., Fievet, J., Pugnière, M., Roquet, F., Escoubas, J.-M., Vandenbulcke, F., Levy, O., 2007b. Evidence of a bactericidal permeability increasing protein in an invertebrate, the *Crassostrea gigas* Cg-BPI. Proc. Nat.l. Acad. Sci. 104, 17759–17764.

Goodson, M.S., Kojadinovic, M., Troll, J.V., Scheetz, T.E., Casavant, T.L., Soares, M.B., McFall-Ngai, M.J., 2005. Identifying components of the NF-κB pathway in the beneficial *Euprymna scolopes–Vibrio fischeri* light organ symbiosis. Appl. Environ. Microbiol. 71, 6934–6946.

Gottschalk, A., 1972. Glycoproteins: their composition, structure and function. In: Gottschalk, A. (Ed.), Glycoproteins. Elsevier, New York, pp. 470–476.

Gourdine, J.P., Markiv, A., Smith-Ravin, J., 2007. The three-dimensional structure of codakine and related marine C-type lectins. Fish and Shellfish Immunol. 23, 831–839, doi: 10.1016/j.fsi.2007.03.009.

Gourdon, I., Guerin, M.-C., Torreilles, J., Roch, P., 2001. Nitric oxide generation by hemocytes of the mussel *Mytilus galloprovincialis*. Nitric Oxide 5, 1–6.

Grenon, J.-F., Walker, G., 1978. The histology and histochemistry of the pedal glandular system of two limpets, *Patella vulgata* and *Acmaea tessulata* (Gastropoda: Prosobranchia). J. Mar. Biol. Assoc. UK 58, 803–816.

Grenon, J.-F., Walker, G., 1982. Further fine structure studies of the "space" layer which underlies the foot sole epithelium of the limpet, Patella vulgata L. J. Molluscan. Stud. 48, 55–63.

Grimm-Jørgensen, Y., Ducor, M.E., Piscatelli, J., 1986. Surface mucus production in gastropods is dependent on environmental salinity and humidity. Comp. Biochem. Physiol. A: Physiol. 83, 415–419, doi: 10.1016/0300-9629(86)90125-8.

Gueguen, Y., Herpin, A., Aumelas, A., Garnier, J., Fievet, J., Escoubas, J.-M., Bulet, P., Gonzalez, M., Lelong, C., Favrel, P, 2006. Characterization of a defensin from the oyster *Crassostrea gigas*: recombinant production, folding, solution structure, antimicrobial activities, and gene expression. J. Biol. Chem. 281, 313–323.

Gustafson, K., Andersen, R.J., 1985. Chemical studies of British Columbia nudibranchs. Tetrahedron 41, 1101–1108, doi: 10.1016/s0040-4020(01)96478-6.

Habets, L., Vieth, U.C., Hermann, G., 1979. Isolation and new biological properties of *Arion empiricorum* lectin. Biochim. Biophys. Acta 582, 154–163, doi: http://dx.doi.org/10.1016/0304-4165(79)90298-8.

Hafez, E., 1977. Functional anatomy of mucus-secreting cells. Mucus in Health and Disease. Springer, pp 19–38.

Hargens, A.R., Shabica, S.V., 1973. Protection against lethal freezing temperatures by mucus in an Antarctic limpet. Cryobiology 10, 331–337.

Howland, K.H., Cheng, T.C., 1982. Identification of bacterial chemoattractants for oyster (*Crassostrea virginica*) hemocytes. J. Invertebr. Pathol. 39, 123–132, doi: 10.1016/0022-2011(82)90001-5.

Hoyer, L.L., Hamilton, A.C., Steenbergen, S.M., Vimr, E.R., 1992. Cloning, sequencing and distribution of the Salmonella typhimurium lt2 sialidase gene, NANH, provides evidence for interspecies gene-transfer. Mol. Microbiol. 6, 873–884, doi: 10.1111/j.1365-2958.1992.tb01538.x.

Iguchi, S.M.M., Aikawa, T., Matsumoto F. J.J., 1982. Antibacterial activity of snail mucus mucin. Comp. Biochem. Physiol. A: Physiol. 72, 571–574, doi: http://dx.doi.org/10.1016/0300-9629(82)90123-2.

Iguchi, S.M.M., Momoi, T., Egawa, K., Matsumoto, J.J., 1985. An N-acetylneuraminic acid-specific lectin from the body-surface mucus of African giant snail. Comp. Biochem. Physiol. B-Biochem. Mol. Biol. 81, 897–900, doi: 10.1016/0305-0491(85)90085-9.

Iijima, R., Kisugi, J., Yamazaki, M., 2003. A novel antimicrobial peptide from the sea hare *Dolabella auricularia*. Dev. Comp. Immunol. 27, 305–311, doi: http://dx.doi.org/10.1016/S0145-305X(02)00105-2.

Itoh, N., Okada, Y., Takahashi, K.G., Osada, M., 2010. Presence and characterization of multiple mantle lysozymes in the Pacific oyster *Crassostrea gigas*. Fish Shellfish Immunol. 29, 126–135.

Itoh, N., Takahashi, K.G., 2007. cDNA cloning and *in situ* hybridization of a novel lysozyme in the Pacific oyster, *Crassostrea gigas*. Comp. Biochem. Physiol. B-Biochem. Mol. Biol. 148, 160–166.

Itoh, N., Takahashi, K.G., 2008. Distribution of multiple peptidoglycan recognition proteins in the tissues of Pacific oyster, *Crassostrea gigas*. Comp. Biochem. Physiol. B-Biochem. Mol. Biol. 150, 409–417, doi: http://dx.doi.org/10.1016/j.cbpb.2008.04.011.

Itoh, N., Xue, Q.-G., Schey, K.L., Li, Y., Cooper, R.K., La Peyre, J., 2011. Characterization of the major plasma protein of the eastern oyster, *Crassostrea virginica*, and a proposed role in host defense. Comp. Biochem. Physiol. B-Biochem. Mol. Biol. 158, 9–22, doi: 10.1016/j.cbpb.2010.06.006.

Jameson, H.L., Nicoll, W., 1913. On some parasites of the scoter duck (*Oedemia nigra*), and their relation to the pearl-inducing trematode in the edible mussel (*Mytilus edulis*). Proc. Zool. Soc. Lond. 1913, 53–63.

Johnson, M.A., Le Pennec, M., 1995. Association between the mollusk bivalve *Loripes lucinalis* and a *Chlamydia*-like organism, with comments on its pathogenic impact, life-cycle and possible mode of transmission. Mar. Biol. 123, 523–530, doi: 10.1007/bf00349231.

Jordan, S.J., 1987. Sedimentation and remineralization associated with biodeposition by the American oyster *Crassostrea virginica* (Gmelin). Ph.D. dissertation. University of Maryland, College Park, Maryland, USA.

Kanekiyo, M., Itoh, N., Kawasaki, A., Matsuyama, A., Matsuda, K., Nakanishi, T., Tanaka, K., 2002. Metallothionein modulates lipopolysaccharide-stimulated tumour necrosis factor expression in mouse peritioneal macrophages. Biochem. J. 361, 363–369, doi: 10.1042/0264-6021:3610363.

Keller, K., Olivier, M., Chadee, K., 1992. The fast release of mucin secretion from human colonic cells induced by *Entamoeba histolytica* is dependent on contact and protein kinase C activation. Arch. Med. Res. 23, 217.

Kesarcodi-Watson, A., Miner, P., Nicolas, J.L., Robert, R., 2012. Protective effect of four potential probiotics against pathogen-challenge of the larvae of three bivalves: Pacific oyster (*Crassostrea gigas*), flat oyster (*Ostrea edulis*) and scallop (*Pecten maximus*). Aquaculture 344, 29–34, doi: 10.1016/j.aquaculture.2012.02.029.

Kesimer, M., Sheehan, J., 2012. Mass spectrometric analysis of mucin core proteins. Methods Mol. Biol. 842, 67–79.

Kido, H., Yokogoshi, Y., Sakai, K., Tashiro, M., Kishino, Y., Fukutomi, A., Katunuma, N., 1992. Isolation and characterization of a novel trypsin-like protease found in rat bronchiolar epithelial Clara cells. A possible activator of the viral fusion glycoprotein. J. Biol. Chem. 267, 13573–13579.

Kleeman, S., Adlard, R., Lester, R., 2002. Detection of the initial infective stages of the protozoan parasite *Marteilia sydneyi* in *Saccostrea glomerata* and their development through to sporogenesis. Int. J. Parasitol. 32, 767–784.

Koren, O., Rosenberg, E., 2006. Bacteria associated with mucus and tissues of the coral *Oculina patagonica* in summer and winter. Appl. Environ. Microbiol. 72, 5254–5259, doi: 10.1128/aem.00554-06.

Kubota, Y., Watanabe, Y., Otsuka, H., Tamiya, T., Tsuchiya, T., Matsumoto, J.J., 1985. Purification and characterization of an antibacterial factor from snail mucus. Comp. Biochem. Physiol. C. 82, 345–348.

Kurtz, J., Franz, K., 2003. Innate defence: evidence for memory in invertebrate immunity. Nature 425, 37–38.

La Peyre, J.F., Xue, Q.-G., Itoh, N., Li, Y., Cooper, R.K., 2010. Serine protease inhibitor cvSI-1 potential role in the eastern oyster host defense against the protozoan parasite *Perkinsus marinus*. Dev. Comp. Immunol. 34, 84–92, doi: 10.1016/j.dci.2009.08.007.

Laabir, M., Amzil, Z., Lassus, P., Masseret, E., Tapilatu, Y., De Vargas, R., Grzebyk, D., 2007. Viability, growth and toxicity of *Alexandrium catenella* and *Alexandrium minutum* (Dinophyceae) following ingestion and gut passage in the oyster *Crassostrea gigas*. Aquat. Living. Resour. 20, doi: 10.1051/alr:2007015.

Langdon, C., Newell, R., 1996. Digestion and nutrition in larvae and adults. The Eastern Oyster Crassostrea virginica Maryland Sea Grant College. University of Maryland, College Park, Maryland, pp. 231–269.

Lau, J., Gambino, L., Pales Espinosa, E., Allam, B., 2013a. What are the source and function of hemocytes associated with oyster pallial mucus?, https://www.was.org/meetings/ShowAbstract.aspx?Id=28539

Lau, J., Sussman, L., Katalai, S., Pales Espinosa, E., Allam, B., 2013b. Characterization of hemocytes from different body fluids of the eastern oyster *Crassostrea virginica*, https://www.was.org/meetings/ShowAbstract.aspx?Id=29070.

Lehrer, R.I., Ganz, T., 2002. Defensins of vertebrate animals. Curr. Opin. Immunol. 14, 96–102.

Lemaitre, B., Nicolas, E., Michaut, L., Reichhart, J.M., Hoffmann, J.A., 1996. The dorsoventral regulatory gene cassette spatzle/Toll/cactus controls the potent antifungal response in *Drosophila* adults. Cell 86, 973–983, doi: 10.1016/s0092-8674(00)80172-5.

Lencer, W., Reinhart, F., Neutra, M., 1990. Interaction of cholera toxin with cloned human goblet cells in monolayer culture. Am. J. Physiol.-Gastr. L. 258, G96–G102.

Li, D., Graham, L.D., 2007. Epiphragmin, the major protein of epiphragm mucus from the vineyard snail *Cernuella virgata*. Comp. Biochem. Physiol. B Biochem. Mol. Biol. 148, 192–200.

Li, J.D., Feng, W.J., Gallup, M., Kim, J.H., Gum, J., Kim, Y., Basbaum, C., 1998. Activation of NF-kappa B via a Src-dependent Ras-MAPK-pp90rsk pathway is required for *Pseudomonas aeruginosa*-induced mucin overproduction in epithelial cells. Proc. Natl. Acad. Sci. USA 95, 5718–5723, doi: 10.1073/pnas.95.10.5718.

Li, X.X., Stark, G.R., 2002. NF kappa B-dependent signaling pathways. Exp. Hematol. 30, 285–296, doi: 10.1016/s0301-472x(02)00777-4.

Lie, K., Heyneman, D., Lim, H., 1975. Studies on resistance in snails: specific resistance induced by irradiated miracidia of *Echinostoma lindoense* in *Biomphalaria glabrata* snails. Int. J. Parasitol. 5, 627–631.

Lindberg, D.R., Ponder, W.F., 2001. The influence of classification on the evolutionary interpretation of structure a re-evaluation of the evolution of the pallial cavity of gastropod molluscs. Org. Divers. Evol. 1, 273–299.

Lindén, S., Boren, T., Mahdavi, J., Hedenbro, J., Carlstedt, I., 2004. Effects of pH on *Helicobacter pylori* binding to human gastric mucins: identification of binding to non-MUC5AC mucins. Biochem. J. 384, 263–270.

Linden, S., Sutton, P., Karlsson, N., Korolik, V., McGuckin, M., 2008. Mucins in the mucosal barrier to infection. Mucosal immunol. 1, 183–197.

Loker, E.S., 2010. Gastropod immunobiology Invertebrate immunity. Springer 708, 17–43.

Loker, E.S., Adema, C.M., Zhang, S.M., Kepler, T.B., 2004. Invertebrate immune systems – not homogeneous, not simple, not well-understood. Immunol. Rev. 198, 10–24.

Loker, E.S., Bayne, C.J., Buckley, P.M., Kruse, K.T., 1982. Ultrastructure of encapsulation of *Schistosoma mansoni* mother sporocysts by hemocytes of juveniles of the 10-r2 strain of *Biomphalaria glabrata*. J. Parasitol. 68, 84–94, doi: 10.2307/3281328.

Ma, J., Zhang, D., Jiang, J., Cui, S., Pu, H., Jiang, S., 2010. Molecular characterization and expression analysis of cathepsin L1 cysteine protease from pearl oyster *Pinctada fucata*. Fish Shellfish Immunol. 29, 501–507.

Mack, D.R., Michail, S., Wei, S., McDougall, L., Hollingsworth, M.A., 1999. Probiotics inhibit enteropathogenic *E. coliadherence* in vitro by inducing intestinal mucin gene expression. Am. J. Physiol.-Gastr. L. 276, G941–G950.

Mahdavi, J., Sondén, B., Hurtig, M., Olfat, F.O., Forsberg, L., Roche, N., Ångström, J., Larsson, T., Teneberg, S., Karlsson K-A, 2002. *Helicobacter pylori* SabA adhesin in persistent infection and chronic inflammation. Science 297, 573–578.

Malham, S.K., Runham, N., Secombes, C., 1997. Phagocytosis by haemocytes from the lesser octopus *Eledone cirrhosa*. Iberus 15, 1–11.

Marthy, H.J., 1974. Evidence and significance of a hemagglutinin from skin of cephalopods. Zeitschrift Fur Immunitats-Forschung Experimentelle Und Klinische Immunologie 148, 225–234.

McDade, J.E., Tripp, M.R., 1967a. Lysozyme in oyster mantle mucus. J. Invertebr. Pathol. 9, 581–582, doi: 10.1016/0022-2011(67)90146-2.

McDade, J.E., Tripp, M.R., 1967b. Mechanism of agglutination of red blood cells by oyster hemolymph. J. Invertebr. Pathol. 9, 523–530, doi: 10.1016/0022-2011(67)90133-4.

McHenery, J., Allen, J., Birkbeck, T., 1986. Distribution of lysozyme-like activity in 30 bivalve species. Comp. Biochem. Physiol. B 85, 581–584.

McHenery, J.G., Birkbeck, T.H., Allen, J.A., 1979. The occurrence of lysozyme in marine bivalves. Comp. Biochem. Physiol. B 63, 25–28.

McLean, N., 1980. Phagocytosis by epidermal-cells of the mantle in *Mytilus edulis*-1 (mollusca, bivalvia). Comp. Biochem. Physiol. A-Physiol. 66, 367–369, doi: 10.1016/0300-9629(80)90180-2.

Melton-Celsa, A.R., Darnell, S.C., O'Brien, A.D., 1996. Activation of Shiga-like toxins by mouse and human intestinal mucus correlates with virulence of enterohemorrhagic *Escherichia coli* O91: H21 isolates in orally infected, streptomycin-treated mice. Infect. Immun. 64, 1569–1576.

Meuleman, E.A., van der Knaap, W.P.W., Mulder, E.C., 1986. Encapsulation of schistosome parasites by the haemocytes of the snail *Lyminea stagnilis*. Dev. Comp. Immunol. 10, 635–636, doi: http://dx.doi.org/10.1016/0145-305X(86)90214-4.

Micots, I., Augeron, C., Laboisse, C., Muzeau, F., Megraud, F., 1993. Mucin exocytosis: a major target for *Helicobacter pylori*. J. Clin. Pathol. 46, 241–245.
Mitra, D., Sarkar, M., Allen, A.K., 1988. Purification and characterization of an agglutinin from mucus of the snail *Achatina fulica*. Biochimie 70, 1821–1829, doi: 10.1016/0300-9084(88)90044-2.
Mitta, G., Hubert, F., Noël, T., Roch, P., 1999a. Myticin, a novel cysteine-rich antimicrobial peptide isolated from haemocytes and plasma of the mussel *Mytilus galloprovincialis*. Eur. J. Biochem. 265, 71–78.
Mitta, G., Vandenbulcke, F., Hubert, F., Roch, P., 1999b. Mussel defensins are synthesised and processed in granulocytes then released into the plasma after bacterial challenge. J. Cell. Sci. 112, 4233–4242.
Mone, Y., Gourbal, B., Duval, D., Du Pasquier, L., Kieffer-Jaquinod, S., Mitta, G., 2010. A large repertoire of parasite epitopes matched by a large repertoire of host immune receptors in an invertebrate host/parasite model. PLoS Negl. Trop. Dis. 4, 18, doi: 10.1371/journal.pntd.0000813.
Moraes, T.B., Ribas Ferreira, J.L., da Rosa, C.E., Sandrini, J.Z., Votto, A.P., Trindade, G.S., Geracitano, L.A., Abreu, P.C., Monserrat, J.M., 2006. Antioxidant properties of the mucus secreted by *Laeonereis acuta* (Polychaeta, Nereididae): A defense against environmental pro-oxidants? Comp. Biochem. Physiol. C-Toxicol. Pharmacol. 142, 293–300, doi: http://dx.doi.org/10.1016/j.cbpc.2005.10.017.
Moraga, D., Meistertzheim, A.L., Tanguy-Royer, S., Boutet, I., Tanguy, A., Donval, A., 2005. Stress response in Cu2+ and Cd2+ exposed oysters (*Crassostrea gigas*): An immunohistochemical approach. Comp. Biochem. Physiol. C-Toxicol. Pharmacol. 141, 151–156, doi: 10.1016/j.cca.2005.05.014.
Morton, B., 1977. The hypobranchial gland in the Bivalvia. Can. J. Zool. 55, 1225–1234, doi: 10.1139/z77-161.
Nagashima, Y., Kikuchi, N., Shimakura, K., Shiomi, K., 2003. Purification and characterization of an antibacterial protein in the skin secretion of rockfish *Sebastes schlegeli*. Comp. Biochem. Physiol. C-Toxicol. Pharmacol. 136, 63–71, doi: 10.1016/s1532-0456(03)00174-1.
Nakahara, H., Bevelander, G., 1967. Ingestion of particulate matter by outer surface cells of mollusc mantle. J. Morphol. 122, 139–145, doi: 10.1002/jmor.1051220206.
Navas, J., Castillo, M., Vera, P., Ruiz-Rico, M., 1992. Principal parasites observed in clams, *Ruditapes decussatus* (L.), *Ruditapes philippinarum* (Adams et Reeve), *Venerupis pullastra* (Montagu) and *Venerupis aureus* (Gmelin), from the Huelva coast (SW Spain). Aquaculture 107, 193–199.
Nikapitiya, C., De Zoysa, M., Lee, J., 2008. Molecular characterization and gene expression analysis of a pattern recognition protein from disk abalone, *Haliotis discus discus*. Fish Shellfish Immunol. 25, 638–647, doi: 10.1016/j.fsi.2008.08.002.
Niu, D., Jin, K., Wang, L., Feng, B., Li, J., 2013. Molecular characterization and expression analysis of four cathepsin L genes in the razor clam, *Sinonovacula constricta*. Fish Shellfish Immunol. 35 (2), 581–588.
Nyholm, S.V., McFall-Ngai, M.J., 2003. Dominance of *Vibrio fischeri* in secreted mucus outside the light organ of *Euprymna scolopes*: The first site of symbiont specificity. Appl. Environ. Microbiol. 69, 3932–3937, doi: 10.1128/aem.69.7.3932-3937.2003.
Nyholm, S.V., Stabb, E.V., Ruby, E.G., McFall-Ngai, M.J., 2000. Establishment of an animal-bacterial association: recruiting symbiotic vibrios from the environment. Proc. Natl. Acad. Sci. USA 97, 10231–10235, doi: 10.1073/pnas.97.18.10231.
Obara, K., Otsuka-Fuchino, H., Sattayasai, N., Nomomura, Y., Tsuchiya, T., Tamiya, T., 1992. Molecular cloning of the antibacterial protein of the giant African snail, *Achatina fulica Ferussac*. Eur. J. Biochem. 209, 1–6.

Olafsen, J.A., 1986. Invertebrate lectins: biochemical heterogeneity as a possible key to their biological function. In: Brehelin, M. (Ed.), Immunity in Invertebrates. Springer-Verlag, Berlin, pp. 94–111.

Orbea, A., Fahimi, H.D., Cajaraville, M.P., 2000. Immunolocalization of four antioxidant enzymes in digestive glands of mollusks and crustaceans and fish liver. Histochem. Cell. Biol. 114, 393–404.

Ortega-Cava, C.F., Ishihara, S., Rumi, M.A., Kawashima, K., Ishimura, N., Kazumori, H., Udagawa, J., Kadowaki, Y., Kinoshita, Y., 2003. Strategic compartmentalization of Toll-like receptor 4 in the mouse gut. J. Immunol. 170, 3977–3985.

Otsuka-Fuchino, H., Watanabe, Y., Hirakawa, C., Tamiya, T., Juichiro, M., Tsuchiya, T., 1992. Bactericidal action of a glycoprotein from the body surface mucus of giant African snail. Comp. Biochem. Physiol. C 101, 607–613, doi: http://dx.doi.org/10.1016/0742-8413(92)90094-N.

Paerregaard, A., Espersen, F., Jensen, O.M., Skurnik, M., 1991. Interactions between *Yersinia enterocolitica* and rabbit ileal mucus: growth, adhesion, penetration, and subsequent changes in surface hydrophobicity and ability to adhere to ileal brush border membrane vesicles. Infect. Immun. 59, 253–260.

Paillard, C., 2004. A short-review of brown ring disease, a vibriosis affecting clams, *Ruditapes philippinarum* and *Ruditapes decussatus*. Aquat. Living Resour. 17, 467–475.

Pales Espinosa, E., Allam, B., 2013. Food quality and season affect gene expression of the mucosal lectin MeML and particle sorting in the blue mussel *Mytilus edulis*. Mar. Biol. 160, 1441–1450, doi: 10.1007/s00227-013-2196-6.

Pales Espinosa, E., Corre, E., Allam, B., 2014a. Pallial mucus of the oyster *Crassostrea virginica* regulates the expression of putative virulence genes of its pathogen *Perkinsus marinus*. Int. J. Parasitol. 44, 305–317.

Pales Espinosa, E., Hassan, D., Ward, J.E., Shumway, S.E., Allam, B., 2010a. Role of epicellular molecules in the selection of particles by the blue mussel, *Mytilus edulis*. Biol. Bull. 219, 50–60.

Pales Espinosa, E., Jing, X., Perrigault, M., Allam, B., 2011. Mucosal c-type lectins in *Crassostrea virginia* and *Mytilus edulis*: potential involvement in particle capture and mucosal immunity. J. Shellfish Res. 30, 503–1503.

Pales Espinosa, E., Koller, A., Allam, B., 2014b. Shotgun proteomic characterization of the pallial mucus of the oyster *Crassostrea virginica* National shellfish Association meeting, Jacksonville. Fl.

Pales Espinosa, E., Perrigault, M., Allam, B., 2010b. Identification and molecular characterization of a mucosal lectin (MeML) from the blue mussel *Mytilus edulis* and its potential role in particle capture. Comp. Biochem. Physiol. A-Mol. Integr. Physiol. 156, 495–501, doi: 10.1016/j.cbpa.2010.04.004.

Pales Espinosa, E., Perrigault, M., Ward, J.E., Shumway, S.E., Allam, B., 2009. Lectins associated with the feeding organs of the oyster, *Crassostrea virginica*, can mediate particle selection. Biol. Bull. 217, 130–141.

Pales Espinosa, E., Perrigault, M., Ward, J.E., Shumway, S.E., Allam, B., 2010c. Microalgal cell surface carbohydrates as recognition sites for particle sorting in suspension-feeding bivalves. Biol. Bull. 218, 75–86.

Pales Espinosa, E., Winnicki, S.M., Allam, B., 2013. Early host-pathogen interactions in marine bivalves: Pallial mucus of *Crassostrea virginica* modulates the growth and virulence of its pathogen *Perkinsus marinus*. Dis. Aquat. Org. 104, 237–247, doi: 10.3354/dao02599.

Pearson, J.P., Kaura, R., Taylor, W., Allen, A., 1982. The composition and polymeric structure of mucus glycoprotein from human gallbladder bile. Biochimica et Biophysica Acta (BBA) – Protein Structure and Molecular Enzymology 706, 221–228, doi: http://dx.doi.org/10.1016/0167-4838(82)90490-3.

Pechenik, J., 2000. Biology of the Invertebrates. McGraw-Hill, Boston, MA.

Perrigault, M., Allam, B., 2012. Differential immune response in the hard clam (*Mercenaria mercenaria*) against bacteria and the protistan pathogen QPX (quahog parasite unknown). Fish Shellfish Immunol. 32, 1124–1134, doi: 10.1016/j.fsi.2012.03.018.

Perrigault, M., Tanguy, A., Allam, B., 2009. Identification and expression of differentially expressed genes in the hard clam, *Mercenaria mercenaria,* in response to quahog parasite unknown (QPX). BMC Genomics 10, 17, doi: 37710.1186/1471-2164-10-377.

Peters, B.M., Shirtliff, M.E., Jabra-Rizk, M.A., 2010. Antimicrobial peptides: primeval molecules or future drugs? PLoS Pathog. 6, e1001067.

Pipe, R.K., 1992. Generation of reactive oxygen metabolites by the hemocytes of the mussel *Mytilus edulis*. Dev. Comp. Immunol. 16, 111–122, doi: 10.1016/0145-305x(92)90012-2.

Prado-Álvarez, M., Rotllant, J., Gestal, C., Novoa, B., Figueras, A., 2009. Characterization of a C3 and a factor B-like in the carpet-shell clam, *Ruditapes decussatus*. Fish Shellfish Immunol. 26, 305–315.

Prezant, R.S., Chalermwat, K., 1984. Flotation of the bivalve *Corbicula fluminea* as a means of dispersal. Science 225, 1491–1493, doi: 10.1126/science.225.4669.1491.

Ragone Calvo, L.M., Walker, J.G., Burreson, E.M., 1998. Prevalence and distribution of QPX, Quahog Parasite Unknown, in hard clams, *Mercenaria mercenaria* in Virginia. USA. Dis. Aquat. Org. 33, 209–219.

Rescigno, M., Urbano, M., Valzasina, B., Francolini, M., Rotta, G., Bonasio, R., Granucci, F., Kraehenbuhl, J.-P., Ricciardi-Castagnoli, P., 2001. Dendritic cells express tight junction proteins and penetrate gut epithelial monolayers to sample bacteria. Nat. Immunol. 2, 361–367.

Rincón, M., Conze, D., Weiss, L., Diehl, N.L., Fortner, K.A., Yang, D., Flavell, R.A., Enslen, H., Whitmarsh, A., Davis, R.J., 2000. Do T cells care about the mitogen-activated protein kinase signalling pathways? Immunol. Cell Biol. 78, 166–175.

Ritchie, K.B., 2006. Regulation of microbial populations by coral surface mucus and mucus-associated bacteria. Mar. Ecol. Prog. Ser. 322, 1–14, doi: 10.3354/meps322001.

Rodriguez, F., Navas, J., 1995. A comparison of gill and hemolymph assays for the thioglycollate diagnosis of *Perkinsus atlanticus* (Apicomplexa, Perkinsea) in clams, *Ruditapes decussatus* (L.) and *Ruditapes philippinarum* (Adams et Reeve). Aquaculture 132, 145–152.

Rollins-Smith, L.A., King, J.D., Nielsen, P.F., Sonnevend, A., Conlon, J.M., 2005. An antimicrobial peptide from the skin secretions of the mountain chicken frog *Leptodactylus fallax* (Anura:Leptodactylidae). Regul. Pept. 124, 173–178, doi: http://dx.doi.org/10.1016/j.regpep.2004.07.013.

Romero, A., Dios, S., Poisa-Beiro, L., Costa, M.M., Posada, D., Figueras, A., Novoa, B, 2011. Individual sequence variability and functional activities of fibrinogen-related proteins (FREPs) in the Mediterranean mussel (*Mytilus galloprovincialis*) suggest ancient and complex immune recognition models in invertebrates. Dev. Comp. Immunol. 35, 334–344.

Rosa, R.D., Santini, A., Fievet, J., Bulet, P., Destoumieux-Garzón, D., Bachère, E., 2011. Big defensins, a diverse family of antimicrobial peptides that follows different patterns of expression in hemocytes of the oyster *Crassostrea gigas*. PLoS ONE 6, e25594.

Rose, M.C., Voter, W.A., Brown, C.F., Kaufman, B., 1984. Structural features of human tracheobronchial mucus glycoprotein. Biochem. J. 222, 371–377.

Ross, S., Corrsin, S., 1974. Results of an analytical model of mucociliary pumping. J. Appl. Physiol. 37, 333–340.

Rowley, A.F., Powell, A., 2007. Invertebrate immune systems – specific, quasi-specific, or nonspecific? J. Immunol. 179, 7209–7214.

Ruppert, E.E., Fox, R.S., Barnes, R.D., 2004. Invertebrate Zoology. Brooks/Cole, Belmont, CA, 963.

Ryder, T., Bowen, I., 1977. Endocytosis and aspects of autophagy in the foot epithelium of the slug *Agriolimax reticulatus* (Müller). Cell Tissue Res. 181, 129–141.

Salvini-Plawen, L.v., 1988. The structure and function of molluscan digestive systems. The Mollusca 11, 301–379.

Salzman, N.H., Chou, M.M., de Jong, H., Liu, L., Porter, E.M., Paterson, Y., 2003. Enteric Salmonella Infection Inhibits Paneth Cell Antimicrobial Peptide Expression. Infect. Immun. 71, 1109–1115, doi: 10.1128/iai.71.3.1109-1115.2003.

Sansonetti, P.J., 2004. War and peace at mucosal surfaces. Nat. Rev. Immunol. 4, 953–964.

Scavuzzo, M.C., Rocchi, V., Fattori, B., Ambrogi, F., Carpi, A., Ruffoli, R., Manganelli, S., Giannessi, F., 2003. Cytokine secretion in nasal mucus of normal subjects and patients with allergic rhinitis. Biomed. Pharmacother. 57, 366–371, doi: http://dx.doi.org/10.1016/S0753-3322(03)00097-0.

Schachter, H., Williams, D., 1982. Biosynthesis of mucus glycoproteins. In: Chantler, E., Elder, J., Elstein, M. (Eds.), Mucus in Health and Disease – II. Plenum Press, New York, USA, pp. 3–28.

Schmidt-Nielsen, K., Taylor, C., Shkolnik, A., 1971. Desert snails: problems of heat, water and food. J. Exp. Biol. 55, 385–398.

Silberberg, A., Meyer, F., 1982. Structure and function of mucus. In: Chantler, E., Elder, J., Elstein, M. (Eds.), Mucus in Health and Disease – II. Plenum Press, New York, USA, pp. 53–74.

Silva, A.J., Pham, K., Benitez, J.A., 2003. Haemagglutinin/protease expression and mucin gel penetration in El Tor biotype *Vibrio cholerae*. Microbiology 149, 1883–1891.

Silverman, N., Maniatis, T., 2001. NF-kappa B signaling pathways in mammalian and insect innate immunity. Genes. Dev. 15, 2321–2342, doi: 10.1101/gad.909001.

Simkiss, k., Wilbur, K.M., 1977. The molluscan epidermis and its secretions. Symp. Zool. Soc. Lond. 39, 35–76.

Simkiss, K., 1988. Molluscan skin (excluding cephalopods). Trueman, E.R., Wilbur, Karl M., Clarke, M.R. (Eds.), The Mollusca: Form and Function, vol. 11, Academic Press, London, UK, pp. 11–34.

Sleigh, M.A., 1989. Adaptations of ciliary systems for the propulsion of water and mucus. Comp. Biochem. Physiol. A Physiol. 94, 359–364.

Slomiany, B.L., Murty, V.L.N., Piotrowski, J., Liau, Y.H., Sundaram, P., Slomiany, A., 1992. Glycosulfatase activity of *Helicobacter pylori* toward gastric mucin. Biochem. Biophys. Res. Commun. 183, 506–513, doi: 10.1016/0006-291x(92)90511-i.

Smith, A.M., 2002. The structure and function of adhesive gels from invertebrates. Integr. Comp. Biol. 42, 1164–1171.

Smith, A.M., Quick, T.J., Peter, R.S., 1999. Differences in the composition of adhesive and non-adhesive mucus from the limpet Lottia limatula. Biol. Bull. 196, 34–44.

Smolowitz, R., Leavitt, D., Perkins, F., 1998. Observations of a protistan disease similar to QPX in *Mercenaria mercenaria* (hard clams) from the coast of Massachusetts. J. Invertebr. Pathol. 71, 9–25, doi: S0022201197947066 [pii].

Smolowitz, R., Miosky, D., Reinisch, C., 1989. Ontogeny of leukemic cells of the soft shell clam. J. Invertebr. Pathol. 53, 41–51.

Song, L., Wang, L., Qiu, L., Zhang, H., 2010. Bivalve immunity Invertebrate Immunity. Springer, 44–65.

Southward, E.C., 1986. Gill symbionts in Thyasirids and other bivalve molluscs. J. Mar. Biol. Assoc. UK 66, 889–914, doi: 10.1017/S0025315400048517.

Sperandio, B., Regnault, B., Guo, J., Zhang, Z., Stanley, S.L., Sansonetti, P.J., Pédron, T., 2008. Virulent *Shigella flexneri* subverts the host innate immune response through manipulation of antimicrobial peptide gene expression. JEM 205, 1121–1132.

Spungin, B., Silberberg, A., 1984. Stimulation of mucus secretion, ciliary activity, and transport in frog palate epithelium. Am. J. Physiol. Cell Physiol. 247, C299–C308.

Stunkard, H.W., Uzmann, J.R., 1958. Studies on digenetic trematodes of the genera *Gymnophallus* and *Parvatrema*. Biol. Bull. 115, 276–302.

Sze, P.W.C., Lee, S.Y., 1995. The potential role of mucus in the depuration of copper from the mussels *Perna viridis* (L.) and *Septifer virgatus* (Wiegmann). Mar. Pollut. Bull. 31, 390–393, doi: http://dx.doi.org/10.1016/0025-326X(95)00140-I.

Takatsuki, S.I., 1934. On the nature and functions of the amoebocytes of *Ostrea edulis*. Q. J. Microsc. Sci. 76, 379–431.

Tanguy, A., Guo, X., Ford, S.E., 2004. Discovery of genes expressed in response to *Perkinsus marinus* challenge in Eastern (*Crassostrea virginica*) and Pacific (*C. gigas*) oysters. Gene 338, 121–131.

Tao, Y., Drabik, K.A., Waypa, T.S., Musch, M.W., Alverdy, J.C., Schneewind, O., Chang, E.B., Petrof, E.O., 2006. Soluble factors from *Lactobacillus* GG activate MAPKs and induce cytoprotective heat shock proteins in intestinal epithelial cells. Am. J. Physiol.-Cell Physiol. 290, C1018–C1030.

Teneberg, S., Miller-Podraza, H., Lampert, H.C., Evans, D.J., Evans, D.G., Danielsson, D., Karlsson K-A, 1997. Carbohydrate binding specificity of the neutrophil-activating protein of *Helicobacter pylori*. J. Biol. Chem. 272, 19067–19071.

Tincu, J.A., Taylor, S.W., 2004. Antimicrobial peptides from marine invertebrates. Antimicrob. Agents Chemother. 48, 3645–3654.

Tripp, M.R., 1992. Agglutinins in the hemolymph of the hard clam, *Mercenaria mercenaria*. J. Invertebr. Pathol. 59, 228–234.

Trueman, E., Clarke, M., 1988. Introduction. Trueman, E., Clarke, M. (Eds.), The mollusca form and function, 11, Academic Press, New York.

Tuomola, E.M., Ouwehand, A.C., Salminen, S.J., 1999. The effect of probiotic bacteria on the adhesion of pathogens to human intestinal mucus. FEMS Immunol. Med. Microbiol. 26, 137–142, doi: 10.1111/j.1574-695X.1999.tb01381.x.

Uehara, A., Sugawara, S., Watanabe, K., Echigo, S., Sato, M., Yamaguchi, T., Takada, H., 2003. Constitutive expression of a bacterial pattern recognition receptor, CD14, in human salivary glands and secretion as a soluble form in saliva. Clin. Diagn. Lab Immunol. 10, 286–292.

Urrutia, M.B., Navarro, E., Ibarrola, I., Iglesias JIP, 2001. Preingestive selection processes in the cockle *Cerastoderma edule*: mucus production related to rejection of pseudofaeces. Mar. Ecol. Prog. Ser. 209, 177–187, doi: 10.3354/meps209177.

Usselman, M.C., Cone, R.A., 1983. Rat sperm are mechanically immobilized in the caudal epididymis by "immobilin," a high molecular weight glycoprotein. Biol. Reprod. 29, 1241–1253, doi: 10.1095/biolreprod29.5.1241.

Uttakleiv Ræder, I., Paulsen, S., Smalås, A., Willassen, N., 2007. Effect of fish skin mucus on the soluble proteome of *Vibrio salmonicida* analysed by 2-D gel electrophoresis and tandem mass spectrometry. Microb. Pathog. 42, 36–45.

Vasta, G., 2009. Roles of galectins in infection. Nat Rev. Microbiol. 7, 424–438.

Venier, P., Varotto, L., Rosani, U., Millino, C., Celegato, B., Bernante, F., Lanfranchi, G., Novoa, B., Roch, P., Figueras, A., 2011. Insights into the innate immunity of the Mediterranean mussel *Mytilus galloprovincialis*. BMC Genomics 12, 69.

Verschuere, L., Rombaut, G., Sorgeloos, P., Verstraete, W., 2000. Probiotic bacteria as biological control agents in aquaculture. Microbiol. Mol. Biol. Rev. 64, 655–671.

Vidal, E.A., Haimovici, M., 1998. Feeding and the possible role of the proboscis and mucus cover in the ingestion of microorganisms by rhynchoteuthion paralarvae (Cephalopoda: Ommastrephidae). Bull. Mar. Sci. 63, 305–316.

Vijay-Kumar, M., Aitken, J.D., Carvalho, F.A., Cullender, T.C., Mwangi, S., Srinivasan, S., Sitaraman, S.V., Knight, R., Ley, R.E., Gewirtz, A.T., 2010. Metabolic syndrome and altered gut microbiota in mice lacking Toll-like receptor 5. Science 328, 228–231.

Villalba, A., Reece, K.S., Ordas, M.C., Casas, S.M., Figueras, A., 2004. Perkinsosis in molluscs: a review. Aquat. Living. Resour. 17, 411–432, doi: 10.1051/alr:2004050.

Vimal, D., Khullar, M., Gupta, S., Ganguly, N., 2000. Intestinal mucins: the binding sites for *Salmonella typhimurium*. Mol. Cell Biochem. 204, 107–117.

Vine, N.G., Leukes, W.D., Kaiser, H., 2004. In vitro growth characteristics of five candidate aquaculture probiotics and two fish pathogens grown in fish intestinal mucus. FEMS Microbiol. Lett. 231, 145–152, doi: 10.1016/s0378-1097(03)00954-6.

Waite, J.H., Wilbur, K.M., 1976. Phenoloxidase in periostracum of marine bivalve *Modiolus demissus* dillwyn. J. Exp. Zool. 195, 359–367, doi: 10.1002/jez.1401950304.

Walker, J.R., Ferrar, P.H., 1998. Diphenol oxidases, enzyme-catalysed browning and plant disease resistance. Biotechnol Genet. Eng. Rev. 15, 457–498.

Wang, N., Lee, Y.H., Lee, J.H., 2008. Recombinant perlucin nucleates the growth of calcium carbonate crystals: molecular cloning and characterization of perlucin from disk abalone, *Haliotis discus discus*. Comp. Biochem. Physiol. B-Biochem. Mol. Biol. 149, 354–361, doi: 10.1016/j.cbpb.2007.10.007.

Ward, J.E., Macdonald, B.A., Thompson, R.J., Beninger, P.G., 1993. Mechanisms of suspension-feeding in bivalves – resolution of current controversies by means of endoscopy. Limnol. Oceanogr. 38, 265–272.

Ward, J.E., Shumway, S.E., 2004. Separating the grain from the chaff: particle selection in suspension- and deposit-feeding bivalves. J. Exp. Mar. Biol. Ecol. 300, 83–130, doi: 10.1016/j.jembe.2004.03.002.

Weiss, I.M., Kaufmann, S., Mann, K., Fritz, M., 2000. Purification and characterization of perlucin and perlustrin, two new proteins from the shell of the mollusc *Haliotis laevigata*. Biochem. Biophys. Res. Commun. 267, 17–21.

Weiss, L., Ma, Y., Takvorian, P., Tanowitz, H., Wittner, M., 1998. Bradyzoite development in *Toxoplasma gondii* and the hsp70 stress response. Infect. Immun. 66, 3295–3302.

White, M.E., Powell, E., Ray, S., Wilson, E., 1987. Host-to-host transmission of Perkinsus marinus in oyster (*Crassostrea virginica*) populations by the ectoparasitic snail *Boonea impressa* (Pyramidellidae). J. Shellfish Res. 6, 1–5.

Wolcott, T.G., 1973. Physiological ecology and intertidal zonation in limpets (Acmaea): a critical look at "limiting factors". Biol. Bull. 145, 389–422.

Wolf, D.P., Blasco, L., Khan, M.A., Litt, M., 1977. Human cervical-mucus .1. Rheologic characteristics. Fertil. Steril. 28, 41–46.

Wootton, E., Dyrynda, E., Ratcliffe N, 2003. Bivalve immunity: comparisons between the marine mussel (*Mytilus edulis*), the edible cockle (*Cerastoderma edule*) and the razor-shell (*Ensis siliqua*). Fish Shellfish Immunol. 15, 195–210.

Xing, J., Pales Espinosa, E., Perrigault, M., Allam, B., 2011. Identification, molecular characterization and expression analysis of a mucosal C-type lectin in the eastern oyster, *Crassostrea virginica*. Fish Shellfish Immunol. 30, 851–858, doi: 10.1016/j.fsi.2011.01.007.

Xue, Q.-G., Itoh, N., Schey, K., Li, Y.-L., Cooper, R., La Peyre, J., 2007. A new lysozyme from the eastern oyster (*Crassostrea virginica*) indicates adaptive evolution of i-type lysozymes. Cell Mol. Life. Sci. 64, 82–95.

Xue, Q., Hellberg, M.E., Schey, K.L., Itoh, N., Eytan, R.I., Cooper, R.K., La Peyre, J.F., 2010. A new lysozyme from the eastern oyster, *Crassostrea virginica*, and a possible evolutionary pathway for i-type lysozymes in bivalves from host defense to digestion. BMC Evol Biol 10, 213.

Xue, Q.-G., Waldrop, G.L., Schey, K.L., Itoh, N., Ogawa, M., Cooper, R.K., Losso, J.N., La Peyre, J.F., 2006. A novel slow-tight binding serine protease inhibitor from eastern oyster *Crassostrea virginica* plasma inhibits perkinsin, the major extracellular protease of the oyster protozoan parasite *Perkinsus marinus*. Comp. Biochem. Physiol. B Biochem. Mol. Biol. 145, 16–26.

Yamaura, K., Takahashi, K.G., Suzuki, T., 2008. Identification and tissue expression analysis of C-type lectin and galectin in the Pacific oyster, *Crassostrea gigas*. Comp. Biochem. Physiol. B-Biochem. Mol. Biol. 149, 168–175, doi: 10.1016/j.cbpb.2007.09.004.

Yamazaki, M., Ohye, H., Kisugi, J., Kamiya, H., 1990. Bacteriostatic and cytolytic activity of purple fluid from the sea hare. Dev. Comp. Immunol. 14, 379–383.

Yang, C., Wang, L., Zhang, H., Wang, L., Huang, M., Sun, Z., Sun, Y., Song, L., 2014. A new fibrinogen-related protein from *Argopecten irradians* (AiFREP-2) with broad recognition spectrum and bacteria agglutination activity. Fish Shellfish Immunol. 38, 221–229.

Yeaman, M.R., Yount, N.Y., 2003. Mechanisms of antimicrobial peptide action and resistance. Pharmacol. Rev. 55, 27–55, doi: 10.1124/pr.55.1.2.

Yonge, C.M., 1926. Structure and physiology of the organs of feeding and digestion in *Ostrea edulis*. J. Mar. Biol. Assoc. UK 14, 295–386, doi: 10.1017/S002531540000789X.

Yonge, C.M., 1928. Feeding mechanisms in the invertebrates. Biol. Rev. 3, 21–76, doi: 10.1111/j.1469-185X.1928.tb00882.x.

Yonge, C.M., 1935. On some aspects of digestion in ciliary feeding animals. J. Mar. Biol. Assoc. UK 20, 341–346, doi: 10.1017/S0025315400045252.

Yu, H., He, Y., Wang, X., Zhang, Q., Bao, Z., Guo, X., 2011. Polymorphism in a serine protease inhibitor gene and its association with disease resistance in the eastern oyster (*Crassostrea virginica* Gmelin). Fish Shellfish Immunol. 30, 757–762, doi: 10.1016/j.fsi.2010.12.015.

Zelensky, A.N., Gready, J.E., 2005. The C-type lectin-like domain superfamily. FEBS J. 272, 6179–6217, doi: 10.1111/j.1742-4658.2005.05031.x.

Zhang, L., Li, L., Zhang, G., 2011. A *Crassostrea gigas* Toll-like receptor and comparative analysis of TLR pathway in invertebrates. Fish Shellfish Immunol. 30, 653–660.

Zhang, L., Li, L., Zhang, G., 2012. Sequence variability of fibrinogen-related proteins (FREPs) in *Crassostrea gigas*. Chin. Sci. Bull. 57, 3312–3319.

Zhang, T., Qiu, L., Sun, Z., Wang, L., Zhou, Z., Liu, R., Yue, F., Sun, R., Song, L., 2014. The specifically enhanced cellular immune responses in Pacific oyster (*Crassostrea gigas*) against secondary challenge with *Vibrio splendidus*. Dev. Comp. Immunol. 45, 141–150, doi: http://dx.doi.org/10.1016/j.dci.2014.02.015.

Zhang, H., Song, L., Li, C., Zhao, J., Wang, H., Gao, Q., Xu, W., 2007. Molecular cloning and characterization of a thioester-containing protein from Zhikong scallop *Chlamys farreri*. Mol. Immunol. 44, 3492–3500, doi: http://dx.doi.org/10.1016/j.molimm.2007.03.008.

Zhang, H., Wang, L., Song, L., Zhao, J., Qiu, L., Gao, Y., Song, X., Li, L., Zhang, Y., Zhang, L., 2009. The genomic structure, alternative splicing and immune response of *Chlamys farreri* thioester-containing protein. Dev. Comp. Immunol. 33, 1070–1076.

Zhang, C., Xie, L.P., Huang, J., Chen, L., Zhang, R.Q., 2006. A novel putative tyrosinase involved in periostracum formation from the pearl oyster (*Pinctada fucata*). Biochem. Biophys. Res. Commun. 342, 632–639, doi: 10.1016/j.bbrc.2006.01.182.

Zhao, J., Song, L., Li, C., Zou, H., Ni, D., Wang, W., Xu, W., 2007. Molecular cloning of an invertebrate goose-type lysozyme gene from *Chlamys farreri*, and lytic activity of the recombinant protein. Mol Immunol. 44, 1198–1208.

Zhong, J., Wang, W., Yang, X., Yan, X., Liu R, 2013. A novel cysteine-rich antimicrobial peptide from the mucus of the snail of *Achatina fulica*. Peptides 39, 1–5, doi: http://dx.doi.org/10.1016/j.peptides.2012.09.001.

Zintzen, V., Roberts, C.D., Anderson, M.J., Stewart, A.L., Struthers, C.D., Harvey ES, 2011. Hagfish predatory behaviour and slime defence mechanism. Sci. Rep. 1, doi: http://www.nature.com/srep/2011/111027/srep00131/abs/srep00131.html#supplementary-information.

New frontiers in mucosal health in aquaculture

13

Benjamin H. Beck; Eric Peatman***
*Stuttgart National Aquaculture Research Center, Stuttgart, Arkansas, USA
**School of Fisheries, Aquaculture, and Aquatic Sciences, Auburn University, Alabama, USA

Chapter Outline

As this book came together, one continuous theme that emerged was, despite the recent burst of research in the areas documented in previous chapters, how little we currently know about the mucosal health of cultured aquatic organisms. Many of the gaps in our knowledge seem to lie at the intersection of previously distinct disciplines – between nutrition and immunity, between water quality and microbiology, between host genetics and the resident microbiome. Researchers and producers interested in the health of cultured species must seek to understand and manage the fundamentally interconnected nature of all aspects of aquaculture. For example, a hatchery owner needs to understand how the soil chemistry of the land he chose for his fingerling ponds will change his water chemistry parameters, impact algal populations, shift water and fish-based microbial communities, alter pathogen growth and adhesion dynamics, and, ultimately, control feeding rates and survival. This continuum of co-regulated environmental and host parameters can be regarded as the mucosal interactome (Figure 13.1). A variety of new approaches, tools, and models are allowing us to understand these connections that, heretofore, were often only anecdotal observations based on the behavior and performance of captive organisms. These approaches have the potential to bring mechanistic understanding to fundamental questions such as: (1) Why does withholding feed change pathogen susceptibility?; (2) How do biofloc approaches change pathogen prevalence and host susceptibility?; (3) How do genetic strains with differing disease susceptibilities differ in associated microbial flora?; (4) What is the mechanism by which dietary additive X promotes "gut health" and faster growth? Below, we highlight some promising technologies and avenues for research that should broadly advance our knowledge of aquatic animal health while facilitating the continued, sustainable growth of aquaculture.

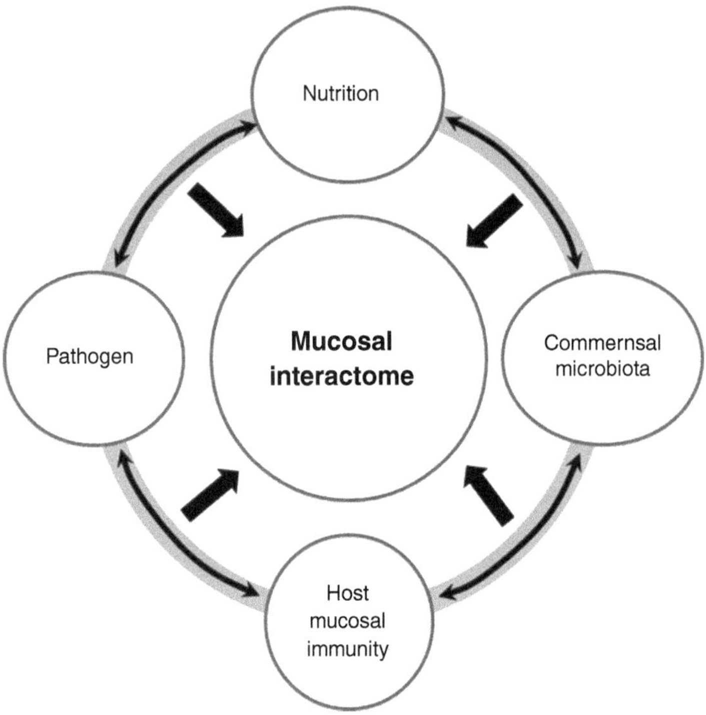

Figure 13.1 Mucosal interactome.

13.1 Next-generation sequencing-based approaches

The dramatic decline in sequencing costs brought about by a shift in the last 5–10 years to massively parallel sequencing platforms has far-reaching consequences for the study of mucosal health in aquaculture. The genomes of cultured organisms can be affordably sequenced (DNA-seq), with Atlantic salmon, cod, tilapia, Pacific oyster, rainbow trout, catfish, sole, carp (among others) now among the list of completed genomes. A genome sequence is of considerable benefit in examining genetic differences underlying phenotypic trait performance in strains/lines of fish and shellfish. Actors in pathogen recognition, goblet cell differentiation, mucous secretion, etc. may be identified and further functionally characterized. QTL or association studies can be carried out with mined microsatellite or SNP markers, identifying markers linked to pathogen resistance.

Transcriptome sequencing and gene expression profiling (RNA-seq) offer a rapid approach to characterizing actors in mucosal tissues and cell types and their changes following disease challenge, environmental perturbation, nutritional change, or a combination thereof. Our labs (Peatman and Beck) have focused on basal and treatment-induced expression in mucosal tissues (skin, gill, gut) in catfish, for example, revealing early mechanisms of pathogen adhesion and invasion unanticipated by classical examinations of mammalian immune factors in fish (Sun et al., 2012; Beck et al., 2012; Liu et al., 2013; Peatman et al., 2013; Li et al., 2014a). Our group has recently utilized channel catfish (*Ictalurus punctatus*) and *F. columnare* as a host-pathogen model to understand teleost mucosal dynamics. Global transcriptome profiling of the channel catfish gill revealed a rhamnose-binding lectin (RBL) whose expression was induced greater than 100-fold soon after *F. columnare* experimental infection (Sun et al., 2012). Saturation of the RBL with its ligands, L-rhamnose, or D-galactose, lowered its expression and decreased *F. columnare* mortality in a dosage-dependent manner in a subsequent challenge infection (Beck et al., 2012). Additionally, RBL expression was found to be inversely correlated with host resistance to *F. columnare* infection. Taken together, these results suggested that the host lectin is mediating *F. columnare* binding to the surface mucosa. We next asked if changes in feeding, previously tied to *F. columnare* susceptibility (Klesius et al., 1999), may impact RBL expression. Indeed, a period of 7 d fasting up-regulated RBL expression in the catfish gill greater than 120-fold (Beck et al., 2012; Figure 13.2).

This striking co-regulation of a surface lectin by both infection and nutritional status led us to a broader examination by RNA-seq of shared host gene signatures in fasted vs. fed and *F. columnare* resistant vs. susceptible catfish. Our results indicated, that beyond RBL, critical components of the innate immune response governing host susceptibility to *F. columnare* were perturbed by short-term feed deprivation (Peatman et al., 2013; Liu et al., 2013; Li et al., 2014a). Both *F. columnare* susceptible and fasted (7 d) channel catfish were characterized by altered arginine metabolism pathways, critical for production of inducible nitric oxide synthase (iNOS) and its effector nitric oxide (NO). iNOS expression, which we found to be extremely abundant in the fed catfish gill, was down-regulated greater than 17-fold following fasting. We also found evidence of immuno-nutritional co-regulation of lysozyme levels, MHC class I/II profiles, mucin secretion, and the chemokine repertoire (Liu et al., 2013; Li et al., 2014a).

We highlight these studies as an illustration of how sequencing approaches can reveal key mucosal players and pathways missed by leaning too heavily on our knowledge of mammalian immunity. To bring these RNA-seq studies from the level of interesting observation to application, we are currently studying the impact of rhamnose on both host susceptibility and pathogen virulence, formulating diets to experimentally modulate goblet cell formation and mucin secretion, and pursuing RBL knockout fish lines.

One common, deserved critique of many RNA-seq studies in fish to-date, is that they have focused on heterogeneous tissue level changes in expression rather than looking at component cell types, e.g., goblet cells, mast cells, epithelia. Approaches utilizing laser capture micro-dissection of specific cells coupled with RNA-seq, both basally and after pathogen invasion, are becoming more common in some species (Vannucci et al., 2013), but are needed in aquaculture research in the near future. Efforts to understand the effector functions of these cell types should dovetail with considerable, ongoing efforts in mucosal cell mapping (Pittman et al., 2013). Norwegian researchers are reporting significant progress with diets that enhance mucous cell density in Atlantic salmon and result in the repulsion of sea lice, with mucosal measures being a far more reliable indicator of sea lice resistance than genetic family

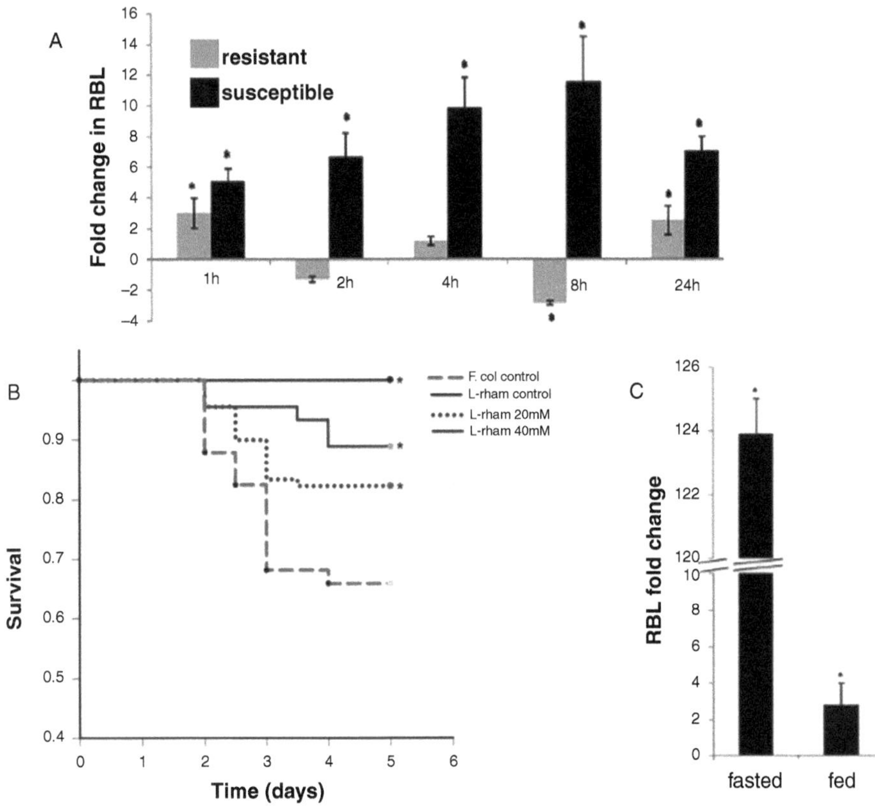

Figure 13.2 Foe and famine: striking co-regulation of rhamnose-binding lectin expression by infection and nutritional status. (A) Fish from a columnaris disease susceptible family strongly up-regulate RBL expression after pathogen encounter. (B) Saturation of RBL receptors with ligand (L-rhamnose) protects fish from columnaris disease in a dose-dependent manner. (C) RBL expression in the gill is markedly up-regulated after short-term feed deprivation in channel catfish.

(http://www.quantidoc.net/en/methodology/mucosal-mapping/). These techniques are also being applied to understanding soy diet-based enteritis and responses to a range of therapeutants.

Beyond host genome and transcriptome profiling is the wide open frontier of microbial profiling using next-generation sequencing. As highlighted in Chapter 9, the microbiome is widely regarded as the largest missing link in our understanding of the mucosal interactome. While microbiome studies to date in aquaculture have largely been confined to establishing baselines for natural microbiomes, studies underway or recently published have begun to examine how host genetics, diet, and environmental factors can shift these baselines for good or ill (Semova et al., 2102; Boutin et al., 2014; Bolnick et al., 2014). Recently developed Illumina-based microbial amplicon sequencing techniques offer greater depth of coverage and lower per sample costs than existing 454 sequencing-driven approaches, making it more likely that microbiome profiling will become a common aspect of disease, nutrition, and water quality studies in the near future (Llewellyn et al., 2014). Gained knowledge as to how diet and environmental factors can be used to shift the microbial community in a manner that excludes pathobionts from replicating and/or adhering to culture organisms will be critical in sustaining the rapid growth of aquaculture. One key tool, in this regard, are gnotobiotic models that start with germ-free larvae. Following pioneering work in zebrafish (Rawls et al., 2004), similar lines are under study in sea bass (Rekecki et al., 2013), cod (Forberg et al., 2012), and tilapia (Situmorang et al., 2014). Using these models, researchers can determine the system parameters most likely to foster the early, stable development of beneficial microbial communities in larvae (often the most sensitive culture stage). Additionally, they can study the impact of the microbiota on pathogen invasion and transplant various artificial microbiota to recolonize the gnotobiotic fish.

A final area of application of next-generation sequencing-based approaches to mucosal health is in the area of pathogen genomics. Sequencing of the pathogen genome and studies of pathogen gene expression, as with the host, provides understanding of mechanism of virulence, attachment, and host immune system evasion. These functional elements may be targeted as the basis of attenuated vaccines or provide clues to the enemy's plan of attack so that tailored countermeasures in the form of chemical prophylactic treatments or specialized diets can be deployed.

13.2 Gene-editing

Our understanding of host and pathogen gene function at the mucosal surface is on the cusp of a significant expansion, thanks to advances in gene editing within the last 2 years. Coding or noncoding sequences in host or pathogen determined to be important for mucosal health can be accurately, rapidly, and affordably targeted with CRISPR/Cas9 systems (Jiang et al., 2013; Li et al., 2014b), inducing single nucleotide mutants or knocking-in other short sequence segments. An advancement beyond earlier zinc finger nuclease and TALEN systems that required extensive protein engineering, CRISPR technology has already been deployed to generate loss-of-function mutant lines in tilapia (Li et al., 2014b) and zebrafish (Hruscha et al., 2013) with high heritability and efficiencies as high as 95%. While no published studies yet report targeting of pathways of mucosal immunity in fish, several studies are known to be currently underway. Low-hanging fruit for gene modification include genes governing goblet cell differentiation, mucin secretion, and reactive oxygen species release as well as genes hijacked as receptors for pathogen binding. More detailed targeting of gene regulatory elements could fine-tune host gene expression to create a mucosal environment conducive to commensal growth and unfavorable to pathobionts. The resulting lines from these studies may be used to further our understanding of mucosal health in unedited aquaculture species (like lab mice), or, depending on regulatory changes, may be the basis of breeding nuclei for robust, disease-resistant, cultured organisms.

13.3 Conclusions

The integration of the still-evolving technologies of next-generation sequencing and gene-editing with tools such as gnotobiotic fish lines and techniques such as mucosal mapping and laser-capture microdissection should lead to a dramatic expansion of our knowledge of the mucosal barriers of aquaculture organisms in the near future (and a 2nd edition of this text reaching into the thousands of pages!). As we determine the critical control points modulating beneficial microbial communities and optimal host health at each surface, we can focus our attention on crafting diets, rearing systems, vaccines, and therapeutants that foster and maintain these conditions predictably and efficiently. Ultimately, our goal should be to harness our understanding of mucosal health in aquaculture species to minimize disease-based losses and to ensure that aquaculture continues to be a sustainable source of protein for growing world populations.

References

Beck, B.H., Farmer, B.D., Straus, D.L., Li, C., Peatman, E., 2012. Putative roles for a rhamnose binding lectin in *Flavobacterium columnare* pathogenesis in channel catfish *Ictalurus punctatus*. Fish Shellfish Immunol. 33, 1008–1015.

Bolnick, D.I., Snowberg, L.K., Gregory Caporaso, J., Lauber, C., Knight, R., Stutz, W.E., 2014. Major histocompatibility complex class IIβ polymorphism influences gut microbiota composition and diversity. Mol. Ecol. 23 (19), 4831–4845, doi: 10.1111/mec.12846.

Boutin, S., Sauvage, C., Bernatchez, L., Audet, C., Derome, N., 2014. Inter individual variations of the fish skin microbiota: host genetics basis of mutualism? PLoS One 97, e102649.

Forberg, T., Vestrum, R.I., Arukwe, A., Vadstein, O., 2012. Bacterial composition and activity determines host gene-expression responses in gnotobiotic Atlantic cod (*Gadus morhua*) larvae. Vet. Microbiol. 157, 420–427.

Hruscha, A., Krawitz, P., Rechenberg, A., Heinrich, V., Hecht, J., Haass, C., Schmid, B., 2013. Efficient CRISPR/Cas9 genome editing with low off-target effects in zebrafish. Development 140, 4982–4987.

Jiang, W., Bikard, D., Cox, D., Zhang, F., Marraffini, L.A., 2013. RNA-guided editing of bacterial genomes using CRISPR-Cas systems. Nat. Biotechnol. 31, 233–239.

Klesius, P., Lim, C., Shoemaker, C., 1999. Effect of feed deprivation on innate resistance and antibody response to *Flavobacterium columnare* in channel catfish, *Ictalurus punctatus*. Bull. Eur. Assoc. Fish Pat. 19, 156–158.

Klesius, P.H., Shoemaker, C.A., Evans, J.J., 2008. *Flavobacterium columnare* chemotaxis to channel catfish mucus. FEMS Microbiol. Lett. 288, 216–220.

Li, C., Beck, B.H., Peatman, E., 2014a. Nutritional impacts on gene expression in the surface mucosa of blue catfish (Ictalurus furcatus). Dev. Comp. Immunol. 44 (1), 226–234.

Li, M., Yang, H., Zhao, J., Fang, L., Shi, H., Li, M., Sun, Y., Zhang, X., Jiang, D., Zhou, L., Wang, D., 2014b. Efficient and heritable gene targeting in tilapia by CRISPR/Cas9. Genetics 197, 591–599.

Liu, L., Li, C., Su, B., Beck, B.H., Peatman, E., 2013. Short-term feed deprivation alters immune status of surface mucosa in channel catfish (*Ictalurus punctatus*). PLoS One 8, e74581.

Llewellyn, M.S., Boutin, S., Hoseinifar, S.H., Derome, N., 2014. Teleost microbiomes: the state of the art in their characterization, manipulation and importance in aquaculture and fisheries. Front Microbiol. 5, 207.

Peatman, E., Li, C., Peterson, B.C., Straus, D.L., Farmer, B.D., Beck, B.H., 2013. Basal polarization of the mucosal compartment in *Flavobacterium columnare* susceptible and resistant channel catfish (*Ictalurus punctatus*). Mol. Immunol. 56, 317–327.

Pittman, K., Pittman, A., Karlson, S., Cieplinska, T., Sourd, P., Redmond, K., Ravnøy, B., Sweetman, E., 2013. Body site matters: an evaluation and application of a novel histological methodology on the quantification of mucous cells in the skin of Atlantic salmon *Salmo salar* L. J Fish Dis. 36, 115–127.

Rawls, J.F., Samuel, B.S., Gordon, J.I., 2004. Gnotobiotic zebrafish reveal evolutionarily conserved responses to the gut microbiota. Proc. Natl. Acad. Sci. USA 101, 4596–4601.

Rekecki, A., Ringø, E., Olsen, R., Myklebust, R., Dierckens, K., Bergh, O., Laureau, S., Cornelissen, M., Ducatelle, R., Decostere, A., Bossier, P., Van den Broeck, W., 2013. Luminal uptake of Vibrio (*Listonella*) *anguillarum* by shed enterocytes – a novel early defence strategy in larval fish. J. Fish Dis. 36, 419–426.

Semova, I., Carten, J.D., Stombaugh, J., Mackey, L.C., Knight, R., Farber, S.A., Rawls, J.F., 2102. Microbiota regulate intestinal absorption and metabolism of fatty acids in the zebrafish. Cell Host Microbe. 123, 277–288.

Situmorang, M.L., Dierckens, K., Mlingi, F.T., Van Delsen, B., Bossier, P., 2014. Development of a bacterial challenge test for gnotobiotic Nile tilapia *Oreochromis niloticus* larvae. Dis. Aquat. Organ. 109, 23–33.

Sun, F., Peatman, E., Li, C., Liu, S., Jiang, Y., Zhou, Z., Liu, Z., 2012. Transcriptomic signatures of attachment, NF-κB suppression and IFN stimulation in the catfish gill following columnaris bacterial infection. Dev. Comp. Immunol. 38, 169–180.

Vannucci, F.A., Foster, D.N., Gebhart, C.J., 2013. Laser microdissection coupled with RNA-seq analysis of porcine enterocytes infected with an obligate intracellular pathogen (*Lawsonia intracellularis*). BMC Genomics 14, 421.

Subject Index

N